Skills Performance Checklists

for

Clinical Nursing Skills & Techniques

Skills Performance Checklists
for

Clinical Nursing Skills & Techniques

Perry, Potter, Ostendorf, Laplante

*11*th
edition

ELSEVIER
MOSBY

Elsevier
3251 Riverport Lane
St. Louis, Missouri 63043

SKILLS PERFORMANCE CHECKLISTS FOR CLINICAL NURSING
SKILLS & TECHNIQUES, ELEVENTH EDITION

ISBN: 978-0-443-11330-7

Notices

Knowledge and best practice in this field are constantly changing. As new research and experience broaden our understanding, changes in research methods, professional practices, or medical treatment may become necessary. Practitioners and researchers must always rely on their own experience and knowledge in evaluating and using any information, methods, compounds or experiments described herein. Because of rapid advances in the medical sciences, in particular, independent verification of diagnoses and drug dosages should be made. To the fullest extent of the law, no responsibility is assumed by Elsevier, authors, editors or contributors for any injury and/or damage to persons or property as a matter of products liability, negligence or otherwise, or from any use or operation of any methods, products, instructions, or ideas contained in the material herein.

Previous editions copyrighted 2022, 2018, 2014, 2010, 2006, 2002, 1998, 1994, 1990, 1986.

Senior Content Strategist: Brandi Graham
Senior Content Development Manager: Lisa Newton
Content Development Specialist: Andrew Schubert
Publishing Services Manager: Deepthi Unni
Project Manager: Sindhuraj Thulasingam
Design Direction: Gopalakrishnan Venkatraman

Printed in India

Last digit is the print number: 9 8 7 6 5 4 3 2 1

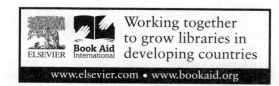

Contents

Student _____ Date _____

Instructor _____ Date _____

PERFORMANCE CHECKLIST SKILL 2.1 **ESTABLISHING THE NURSE-PATIENT RELATIONSHIP**

	S	U	NP	Comments
ASSESSMENT				
1. Prepared for orientation phase of therapeutic communication.	——	——	——	_____
2. Identified patient using two identifiers.	——	——	——	_____
3. Assessed patient and family caregiver health literacy.	——	——	——	_____
4. Assessed the patient's ability to hear. Ensured hearing aid was functional if worn. Ensured patient could hear and understand words.	——	——	——	_____
5. Determined how the patient would like to be addressed. Addressed patient by name and introduced self and role on the health care team.	——	——	——	_____
6. Assessed the following during initial interaction: patient's needs, coping strategies, defenses, and adaptation styles.	——	——	——	_____
7. Determined patient's need to communicate.	——	——	——	_____
8. Observed patient's pattern of communication and verbal or nonverbal behavior.	——	——	——	_____
a. Observed for signs that patient had barriers in being allowed to communicate that might have indicated abuse or human trafficking.	——	——	——	_____
9. Assessed reason patient needed health care.	——	——	——	_____
10. Assessed and reflected upon variables that influence communication.	——	——	——	_____
11. Assessed personal barriers to communicating with patient.	——	——	——	_____
12. Assessed patient's use of language and ability to speak.	——	——	——	_____
13. Assessed resources available in selecting communication methods.	——	——	——	_____
a. Reviewed information in electronic health record (EHR) and reflected on past patient communication experiences.	——	——	——	_____
b. Consulted with family, health care provider, and other health care team members concerning patient's condition, problems, and impressions.	——	——	——	_____

	S	U	NP	Comments

14. Before initiating the working phase of nurse-patient relationship, assessed patient's readiness to work toward goal attainment.

15. Considered when patient was due to be discharged or transferred from health care agency. Shared that information with patient and family caregiver.

PLANNING

1. Determined expected outcomes following completion of procedure.

2. Prepared patient physically and provided an appropriate environment.

3. Prepared communication aids and initial communication approach.

   a. Used appropriate communication tools.

   b. Prepared open-ended questions to identify strategies for developing a plan to meet patient health goals.

IMPLEMENTATION

1. Working phase:

   a. Observed patient's nonverbal behaviors.

   b. When verbal behaviors did not match nonverbal behaviors, sought clarification from patient.

2. Explained purpose of interaction when information was to be shared.

3. Continued to use therapeutic communication skills.

4. Used questions carefully and appropriately.

5. Explored ways the health care team could meet patient's expectations in seeking health care.

6. Encouraged patient to ask for clarification at any time.

7. Set mutual goals.

   a. Used therapeutic communication skills to identify and clarify strategies for attainment of mutually agreed-on goals.

   b. Discussed and prioritized problem areas.

   c. Provided information to patients and helped them to express needs and feelings.

   d. Avoided communication barriers.

2

	S	U	NP	Comments

8. Termination phase: Communicated with the patient.   S ___ U ___ NP ___ _____

  a. Prepared by identifying methods of summarizing and synthesizing information pertinent for patient's aftercare.   ___ ___ ___ _____

  b. Used therapeutic communication skills to discuss discharge or termination issues and guided discussion related to specific patient changes in thoughts and behaviors.   ___ ___ ___ _____

  c. Summarized with patient what was discussed during interaction, including goal setting and achievement.   ___ ___ ___ _____

9. For hospitalized patients, ensured nurse call system was within patient's reach, side rails were raised appropriately, bed was in lowest position and locked into position.   ___ ___ ___ _____

EVALUATION

1. Observed patient's verbal and nonverbal responses to communication; noted his or her willingness to share information and concerns during orientation phase.   ___ ___ ___ _____

2. Noted own response to patient and patient's response. Reflected on effectiveness of therapeutic techniques used in establishing rapport with patient.   ___ ___ ___ _____

3. During working phase, evaluated patient's ability to work toward identified goals. Elicited feedback (verbal and nonverbal) to determine success of goal attainment. Evaluated patient's health status in relation to identified goals. Reevaluated and identified barriers when patient goals were not met.   ___ ___ ___ _____

4. During termination phase, summarized and restated. Reinforced patient's strengths, outlined issues still requiring work, and developed an action plan.   ___ ___ ___ _____

5. Used Teach-Back. Revised instruction if patient or family caregiver was not able to teach back correctly.   ___ ___ ___ _____

DOCUMENTATION

1. Documented communication pertinent to patient's health, response to illness or therapies, and responses that demonstrated understanding or lack of understanding.   ___ ___ ___ _____

2. Documented teach-back and any changes to teaching plan.   ___ ___ ___ _____

HAND-OFF REPORTING

1. Reported any relevant information obtained through patient's verbal and nonverbal behaviors to members of health care team.

____ ____ ____ _____

Student _____ Date _____

Instructor _____ Date _____

PERFORMANCE CHECKLIST SKILL 2.2 **COMMUNICATING WITH PATIENTS WHO HAVE DIFFICULTY COPING**

	S	U	NP	Comments

ASSESSMENT

1. Identified the patient using at least two identifiers, then provided a brief, simple introduction. ____ ____ ____ _____

2. Assessed patient's/family caregiver's health literacy. ____ ____ ____ _____

3. Assessed factors influencing communication with patient. ____ ____ ____ _____

4. Observed for physical, behavioral, and verbal cues that indicated patient was anxious. ____ ____ ____ _____

5. Assessed for possible factors causing patient anxiety. ____ ____ ____ _____

6. Discussed possible causes of patient's anxiety, anger or depression with family members, including past history of the illness, if necessary. ____ ____ ____ _____

7. Assessed for physical, behavioral, and verbal cues that indicated patient was depressed. ____ ____ ____ _____

8. Assessed for possible factors causing patient's depression. ____ ____ ____ _____

9. Observed for behaviors that indicated that the patient was angry and/or expressions that indicated anger. ____ ____ ____ _____

10. Assessed factors that influenced the angry patient's communication. ____ ____ ____ _____

11. Assessed for resources available to help in communicating with potentially violent patient. ____ ____ ____ _____

12. Assessed for underlying medical conditions that might have potentially led to violent behavior. ____ ____ ____ _____

PLANNING

1. Determined expected outcomes following completion of procedure. ____ ____ ____ _____

2. Prepared for therapeutic intervention by considering patient goals, time allocation, and resources. ____ ____ ____ _____

	S	U	NP	Comments

3. Recognized personal level of anxiety and consciously tried to remain calm when communicating with an anxious, angry, or depressed patient. Remained nonjudgmental.

    ____ ____ ____ _____

4. Prepared a quiet, calm area, allowing ample personal space.

    ____ ____ ____ _____

5. Prepared for de-escalation for an angry patient.

    ____ ____ ____ _____

    a. Paused to collect own thoughts, feelings, and reactions.

    ____ ____ ____ _____

    b. Determined what patient was saying.

    ____ ____ ____ _____

    c. Prepared the environment to de-escalate a potentially violent patient:

    ____ ____ ____ _____

      (1) Encouraged other people to leave room or area.

    ____ ____ ____ _____

      (2) Maintained an adequate distance and opened exit. Positioned self appropriately.

    ____ ____ ____ _____

      (3) When anger began to disturb others, closed door.

    ____ ____ ____ _____

      (4) Reduced disturbing factors in room.

    ____ ____ ____ _____

IMPLEMENTATION

1. Used appropriate nonverbal behaviors and active listening skills.

    ____ ____ ____ _____

2. Used appropriate verbal techniques that were clear and concise to respond to anxious patient.

    ____ ____ ____ _____

3. Helped patient acquire alternative coping strategies.

    ____ ____ ____ _____

4. Provided necessary comfort measures.

    ____ ____ ____ _____

5. Used open-ended questions.

    ____ ____ ____ _____

6. Encouraged and rewarded small decisions and independent actions. Made decisions as needed. Presented situations that required no decision making.

    ____ ____ ____ _____

7. Accepted patient as he or she was and focused on his or her positive aspects; provided positive feedback.

    ____ ____ ____ _____

8. Was honest and empathic.

    ____ ____ ____ _____

9. De-escalated an angry patient appropriately:

    ____ ____ ____ _____

    a. Maintained personal space.

    ____ ____ ____ _____

    b. Maintained nonthreatening verbal and nonverbal approach.

    ____ ____ ____ _____

    c. Used therapeutic silence and allowed patient to vent feelings. Used active listening. Did not argue with patient.

    ____ ____ ____ _____

6

	S	U	NP	Comments

d. Responded to anger therapeutically. ___ ___ ___ _____

e. Answered questions calmly and honestly as appropriate. ___ ___ ___ _____

f. When patient made verbal threats to harm others, remained calm yet professional and continued to set limits on inappropriate behavior. ___ ___ ___ _____

g. When patient appeared to be calm and anger was defused, explored alternatives to situation or feelings of anger. ___ ___ ___ _____

EVALUATION

1. Observed for continuing presence of physical signs and symptoms or behaviors reflecting anxiety, anger, or depression. ___ ___ ___ _____

2. Asked patient to describe ways to cope with anxiety, depression, or anger in the future and make decisions about own care. ___ ___ ___ _____

3. Evaluated patient's ability to discuss factors causing anxiety, depression, or anger. ___ ___ ___ _____

4. Noted patient's ability to answer questions and problem solve. ___ ___ ___ _____

5. Used Teach-Back. Revised instruction if patient or family caregiver was not able to teach back correctly. ___ ___ ___ _____

DOCUMENTATION

1. Documented cause of patient's anxiety/anger/depression, any exhibited signs and symptoms of behaviors, and any methods used to enhance coping. Included direct quotes from patient demonstrating patient viewpoint. ___ ___ ___ _____

2. Documented de-escalation technique used and patient's response to de-escalation efforts. ___ ___ ___ _____

3. Documented evaluation of patient and family caregiver learning. ___ ___ ___ _____

HAND-OFF REPORTING

1. Reported methods used to relieve anxiety/anger/depression and patient's response to ensure continuity of care between nurses. ___ ___ ___ _____

2. Reported technique used to de-escalate and patient's response to nurse in charge. ___ ___ ___ _____

Student _____ Date _____

Instructor _____ Date _____

PERFORMANCE CHECKLIST SKILL 2.3 **COMMUNICATING WITH A COGNITIVELY IMPAIRED PATIENT**

	S	U	NP	Comments

ASSESSMENT

1. Identified patient using two identifiers.   ___ ___ ___ _____

2. Initially approached patient from the front. Assessed for physical, behavioral, and verbal cues that indicated that a patient was cognitively impaired. Assessed orientation status of patient and performed a mini-mental examination.   ___ ___ ___ _____

3. Assessed patient's or family caregiver's health literacy with simplest literacy screening tool.   ___ ___ ___ _____

4. Reviewed EHR and assessed for possible factors causing patient's cognitive impairment.   ___ ___ ___ _____

5. Assessed factors influencing communication with patient.   ___ ___ ___ _____

6. Discussed possible causes of patient's cognitive impairment with family caregivers.   ___ ___ ___ _____

7. Discussed with family how patient typically communicates.   ___ ___ ___ _____

8. Ascertained the most effective means of communication.   ___ ___ ___ _____

PLANNING

1. Determined expected outcomes following completion of procedure.   ___ ___ ___ _____

2. Prepared for communication by considering type of cognitive impairment, communication impairments, time allocation, and resources.   ___ ___ ___ _____

3. Was aware of own nonverbal cues that could affect communication with the cognitively impaired patient; remained nonjudgmental.   ___ ___ ___ _____

4. Prepared environment physically by providing a quiet, calm area.   ___ ___ ___ _____

IMPLEMENTATION

1. Approached patient from the front and faced him or her when speaking.   ___ ___ ___ _____

8

	S	U	NP	Comments

2. Provided brief, simple introduction.

3. Used appropriate nonverbal behaviors and active listening skills.

4. Used clear and concise verbal techniques to respond to patient.

5. Asked one question at a time and allowed time for response; did not interrupt patient.

6. Repeated sentences using a steady voice and avoided raising own voice or being too quick to guess what patient was trying to express.

7. Used augmentative and assistive communication devices.

8. Ensured patient was wearing eyeglasses or hearing aids.

9. Did not argue with patient or correct him or her if mistakes were made.

10. Maintained meaningful interactions with patients and used creative modes of communication based on patient's comfort level and abilities.

11. Used individualized coping strategies.

EVALUATION

1. Observed patient's response for clarity and understanding of messages sent and received.

2. Observed verbal and nonverbal behaviors.

3. Used Teach-Back. Revised instruction if patient or family caregiver was not able to teach back correctly.

DOCUMENTATION

1. Documented objective and subjective behaviors the patient displayed, and objective behaviors observed.

2. Documented methods used to communicate with the patient and patient's response.

3. Documented evaluation of patient and family caregiver learning.

HAND-OFF REPORTING

1. Reported the methods used to communicate and the patient's response.

Student _____ Date _____

Instructor _____ Date _____

PERFORMANCE CHECKLIST SKILL 2.4 **COMMUNICATING WITH COLLEAGUES**

	S	U	NP	Comments

ASSESSMENT

1. Identified purpose of interaction with colleague.

2. Assessed factors influencing communication with others.

3. Assessed own level of stress in the situation.

PLANNING

1. Prepared for communication with members of the health care team who may have differing needs or concerns.

2. Was aware of own nonverbal cues affecting communication with others; remained nonjudgmental.

3. Prepared environment physically.

4. Was aware of hierarchical differences among members of the health care team as a common barrier to effective communication and collaboration.

IMPLEMENTATION

1. Approached colleague from the front and faced him or her when speaking; maintained appropriate eye contact.

2. Provided brief, simple introduction.

3. Was aware of own body language and tone.

4. Acknowledged and responded to a range of views.

5. Used oral communication skills appropriately.

6. Used a range of workplace written communication methods.

7. Encouraged discussion of both positive and negative feelings.

8. Summarized key themes in the discussion and helped develop alternative solutions to the issue.

	S	U	NP	Comments
EVALUATION				
1. Confirmed clarity and understanding of messages sent and received.	___	___	___	_____
2. Observed verbal and nonverbal behaviors.	___	___	___	_____

Student _____ Date _____

Instructor _____ Date _____

PERFORMANCE CHECKLIST SKILL 2.5   **WORKPLACE VIOLENCE AND SAFETY**

	S	U	NP	Comments
ASSESSMENT				
1. Assessed baseline knowledge of agency staff regarding workplace violence	___	___	___	_____
2. Identified organizational risk factors for workplace violence.	___	___	___	_____
3. Identified patient- and setting-related risk factors for workplace violence.	___	___	___	_____
4. Assessed patient for signs and symptoms of potentially violent behavior.	___	___	___	_____
PLANNING				
1. Determined expected outcomes following completion of procedure.	___	___	___	_____
IMPLEMENTATION				
1. Used notification system for identifying high-risk patients.	___	___	___	_____
2. Removed opportunity for any type of weapon to be used by patients or visitors.	___	___	___	_____
3. Did not work alone when feeling uncomfortable with a patient; used measures to prevent or control workplace hazards.	___	___	___	_____
4. Ensured all staff were trained to cope with physical and verbal abuse using appropriate de-escalation techniques.	___	___	___	_____
5. Notified security staff to intervene when patient began unruly behavior or when additional information was needed to determine potential for violence.	___	___	___	_____
6. When an incident occurred, initiated first aid and emergency care for the injured workers and prevented further injury.	___	___	___	_____
7. Debriefed using standard postincident procedures and services.	___	___	___	_____
8. Referred colleague to agency program for medical and psychological counseling and debriefing for staff who had experienced and witnessed assaults or violent incidents.	___	___	___	_____

	S	U	NP	Comments

EVALUATION

1. Evaluated staff comprehension of workplace violence program and deescalation strategies. ___ ___ ___ _____

2. Monitored prevention impact. ___ ___ ___ _____

3. When there was a violent incident, evaluated safety of all persons involved; provided prompt medical treatment for victims of workplace violence. ___ ___ ___ _____

4. When there was an incident, immediately evaluated the effectiveness of the de-escalation techniques implemented. ___ ___ ___ _____

DOCUMENTATION

1. Documented hazard assessment and strategies used to promote a safe environment. ___ ___ ___ _____

2. Documented escalating behaviors exhibited by patient, any injuries, de-escalation techniques used by staff, any treatment, and outcome of incident. ___ ___ ___ _____

HAND-OFF REPORTING

1. Provided detailed assessment of potentially hazardous situation. ___ ___ ___ _____

2. Reported patients who were flagged as high risk for potentially violent behaviors. ___ ___ ___ _____

3. Reported strategies implemented to prevent escalating behaviors. ___ ___ ___ _____

4. Reported any violent incidents and outcomes associated with the incidents. ___ ___ ___ _____

Student _____ Date _____

Instructor _____ Date _____

PERFORMANCE CHECKLIST PROCEDURAL GUIDELINE 4.1   **GIVING A HAND-OFF REPORT**

	S	U	NP	Comments

PROCEDURAL STEPS

1. Planned to use an organized format for delivering report that provided a description of patient needs and problems.

2. Identified the patient using at least two identifiers.

3. Gathered information from documentation sources, AP report, or other relevant documents.

4. Prioritized information on the basis of patient's problems and nursing diagnoses.

5. For each patient included:

   • Situation

   • Background information

   • Assessment data

   • Recommendations

6. Asked staff from oncoming shift about any questions regarding information provided and clarified any confusion or misinformation.

7. When report given at bedside, encouraged patient to ask questions and asked if there were any decisions he or she wished to add to treatment plan.

Student _____ Date _____

Instructor _____ Date _____

PERFORMANCE CHECKLIST PROCEDURAL GUIDELINE 4.2   **ADVERSE EVENT REPORTING**

	S	U	NP	Comments

PROCEDURAL STEPS

1. When adverse event was witnessed, assessed extent of any injury to patient or others. ____ ____ ____ _____

2. When the adverse event involved an injury, took steps to restore individual's safety and assessed for further injuries. ____ ____ ____ _____

3. When patient sustained an injury, called the health care provider immediately. ____ ____ ____ _____

4. Used clinical judgment skills to assess what was involved in the event. Either reported the event as witnessed or determined from AP specifically what occurred. ____ ____ ____ _____

5. Notified risk management department per agency protocol. ____ ____ ____ _____

6. Provided any treatment ordered or prepared patient for any diagnostic tests. ____ ____ ____ _____

7. When visitor or staff member sustained an injury, referred to emergency department or appropriate treatment setting. ____ ____ ____ _____

8. Completed adverse occurrence event report form appropriately: ____ ____ ____ _____

   a. Documented time of event and described in chronological order exactly what occurred or was observed, using objective findings and observations. Documented nurse involved, condition of patient when discovered or observed, and observation of factors that possibly contributed to incident. Used language that did not allow for subjective interpretation. Did not include personal opinions or feelings. ____ ____ ____ _____

   b. Described measures taken by any caregivers at time of event. ____ ____ ____ _____

   c. Documented victim's interpretation of event by using quotes. When there were witnesses, used quotation marks to frame their statements. ____ ____ ____ _____

	S	U	NP	Comments

9. Submitted completed report and notified management team per agency policy. ___ ___ ___ _____

10. When patient was involved, documented events of incident in patient's chart. ___ ___ ___ _____

   a. Entered only objective description of what happened. ___ ___ ___ _____

   b. Documented any assessment and intervention activities initiated as a result of event. ___ ___ ___ _____

   c. Did not duplicate all information from report. ___ ___ ___ _____

   d. Did not document in record that an occurrence report was completed. ___ ___ ___ _____

11. Submitted the report promptly with the risk-management department or designated people. ___ ___ ___ _____

12. Conducted an adverse event huddle. ___ ___ ___ _____

Student _____ Date _____

Instructor _____ Date _____

PERFORMANCE CHECKLIST SKILL 5.1   **MEASURING BODY TEMPERATURE**

	S	U	NP	Comments

ASSESSMENT

1. Identified patient using at least two identifiers according to agency policy.

2. Reviewed patient's EHR to determine need to measure patient's body temperature.

    a. Noted patient's risks for temperature alterations.

    b. Determined previous baseline temperature and measurement site when available.

3. Assessed patient's or family caregiver's health literacy.

4. Performed hand hygiene.

5. Assessed for factors that influence temperature.

6. Determined appropriate measurement site and device for patient; used disposable thermometer for patient on isolation precautions.

7. Assessed patient's knowledge of and prior experience with temperature measurement and feelings about the procedure.

PLANNING

1. Determined expected outcomes following completion of procedure.

2. Provided privacy and explained procedure and importance of maintaining proper position until temperature reading was complete.

3. Organized and set up any equipment needed to perform procedure.

4. When measuring oral temperature verified that patient had not had anything to eat or drink and had not chewed gum or smoked within the past 20 minutes.

IMPLEMENTATION

1. Performed hand hygiene again. Helped patient to comfortable position that provided easy access to temperature measurement site.

	S	U	NP	Comments

2. Obtained temperature reading correctly.

   a. Obtained oral temperature (electronic) correctly:

     (1) Optional: Applied clean gloves when appropriate.

     (2) Removed thermometer pack from charging unit. Attached oral thermometer probe stem (blue tip) to thermometer unit. Grasped top of probe stem without applying pressure on ejection button.

     (3) Slid disposable plastic probe cover over thermometer probe stem until cover locked in place.

     (4) Asked patient to open mouth; observed for any inflammatory process. When present, considered an alternate route. Placed thermometer probe under tongue in posterior sublingual pocket lateral to center of lower jaw.

     (5) Asked patient to hold thermometer probe with lips closed and to refrain from talking.

     (6) Left thermometer probe in place until audible signal indicated completion and patient's temperature appeared on digital display; removed thermometer probe; noted temperature reading.

     (7) Pushed ejection button on thermometer probe stem to discard plastic probe cover into appropriate receptacle. Returned thermometer probe stem to storage position of thermometer unit.

     (8) When wearing gloves, removed, disposed of in appropriate receptacle, and performed hand hygiene.

   b. Obtained rectal temperature (electronic) correctly:

     (1) With patient in side-lying or left lateral recumbent position with upper leg flexed, exposed only anal area. Kept patient's upper body and lower extremities covered with sheet or blanket.

     (2) Applied clean gloves. Cleansed anal region when feces and/or secretions were present. Removed soiled gloves, performed hand hygiene and reapplied clean gloves.

	S	U	NP	Comments

(3) Removed thermometer pack from charging unit. Attached rectal thermometer probe stem (red tip) to thermometer unit. Grasped top of probe stem; did not apply pressure on ejection button. ___ ___ ___ _____

(4) Slid disposable plastic probe cover over thermometer probe stem until cover locked in place. ___ ___ ___ _____

(5) Using a single-use package, squeezed a liberal amount of lubricant on tissue. Dipped probe cover of thermometer, blunt end, into lubricant, covering 2.5 to 3.5 cm (1 to 1½ inches) for adult. ___ ___ ___ _____

(6) With nondominant hand, separated patient's buttocks to expose anus; asked patient to breathe slowly and relax. ___ ___ ___ _____

(7) Inserted thermometer into anus in direction of umbilicus 3.5 cm (1½ inches) for adult; did not force thermometer. ___ ___ ___ _____

(8) Held thermometer probe in place until audible signal indicated completion and patient's temperature appeared on digital display; removed thermometer probe and noted temperature reading. ___ ___ ___ _____

(9) Pushed ejection button on thermometer stem to discard plastic probe cover into appropriate receptacle, wiped probe stem with antiseptic swab, allowed probe stem to dry, and returned probe stem to recording unit. ___ ___ ___ _____

(10) Cleaned patient's anal area and discarded tissue. Performed perineal hygiene as needed. Replaced gown and linen. ___ ___ ___ _____

(11) Removed and disposed of gloves in appropriate receptacle. Performed hand hygiene. ___ ___ ___ _____

c. Obtained axillary temperature (electronic) correctly: ___ ___ ___ _____

(1) Provided patient privacy, helped patient to supine or sitting position, removed clothing from shoulder and arm. ___ ___ ___ _____

(2) Removed thermometer pack from charging unit. Attached oral thermometer probe stem (blue tip) to thermometer unit. Grasped top of thermometer probe stem, did not apply pressure on ejection button. ___ ___ ___ _____

(3) Slid disposable plastic probe cover over thermometer stem until cover locked in place.

___ ___ ___ _____

(4) Raised patient's arm away from torso. Inspected for skin lesions and excessive perspiration; dried axilla or selected alternative site as needed. Inserted thermometer probe into center of axilla, lowered arm over probe and placed arm across patient's chest.

___ ___ ___ _____

(5) Held probe in place until audible signal indicated completion and patient's temperature appeared on digital display; removed thermometer probe from axilla. Noted temperature reading.

___ ___ ___ _____

(6) Pushed ejection button on thermometer stem to discard plastic probe cover into appropriate receptacle. Returned thermometer stem to storage position of recording unit.

___ ___ ___ _____

(7) Replaced linen or gown. Performed hand hygiene.

___ ___ ___ _____

d. Obtained tympanic membrane temperature correctly:

___ ___ ___ _____

(1) Helped patient to assume comfortable position with head turned away toward side. When patient had been lying on one side, used upper ear. Noted if there was cerumen in patient's ear canal. Obtained temperature from patient's right ear if right-handed; or from patient's left ear if left-handed.

___ ___ ___ _____

(2) Removed thermometer handheld unit from charging base, did not apply pressure to ejection button.

___ ___ ___ _____

(3) Slid disposable speculum cover over otoscope-like lens tip until it locked in place. Did not touch lens cover.

___ ___ ___ _____

(4) Inserted speculum into ear canal per manufacturer instructions.

___ ___ ___ _____

(a) Adults: pulled ear pinna backward, up, and out. Children younger than 3 years of age: pulled pinna down and back; pointed covered probe toward midpoint between eyebrow and sideburns. Children older than 3 years: pulled pinna up and back.

___ ___ ___ _____

	S	U	NP	Comments

(b) Fit speculum tip snugly in canal, pointed toward nose. Optional: Moved thermometer in figure-eight pattern.

    — — — _____

(5) Pressed scan button on handheld unit. Left speculum in place until audible signal indicated completion and temperature appeared on digital display.

    — — — _____

(6) Removed speculum, noted temperature reading. Pushed ejection button on handheld unit to discard speculum cover into appropriate receptacle.

    — — — _____

(7) When temperature was abnormal or second reading was necessary, replaced probe cover and waited 2 minutes before repeating in same ear or repeated measurement in other ear. Considered an alternative temperature site or instrument.

    — — — _____

(8) Returned handheld unit to thermometer base.

    — — — _____

(9) Performed hand hygiene.

    — — — _____

e. Obtained temporal artery temperature correctly:

    — — — _____

(1) Ensured forehead was dry; dried as needed.

    — — — _____

(2) Placed sensor firmly on patient's forehead.

    — — — _____

(3) Pressed red scan button with thumb, slowly slid thermometer across forehead, kept scan button depressed, lifted sensor, and touched sensor on neck behind earlobe, read temperature when clicking sound stopped, released scan button.

    — — — _____

(4) Cleaned sensor with alcohol swab, returned to charging storage unit, and performed hand hygiene.

    — — — _____

3. Informed patient of temperature reading and documented per agency policy.

    — — — _____

4. Helped patient into comfortable position.

    — — — _____

5. Raised side rails (as appropriate) and lowered bed to lowest position, locking into position.

    — — — _____

6. Placed nurse call system in an accessible location within patient's reach.

    — — — _____

7. Performed hand hygiene.

    — — — _____

	S	U	NP	Comments

EVALUATION

1. When assessing temperature for the first time, established it as baseline if within acceptable range.

2. Compared temperature reading with patient's previous baseline and acceptable temperature range for patient's age-group.

3. When patient had a fever, took temperature 30 minutes after administering antipyretics and every 4 hours until temperature stabilized.

4. Used Teach-Back. Revised instruction if patient/family caregiver was not able to teach back correctly.

DOCUMENTATION

1. Documented temperature and route appropriately.

2. Documented temperature after administration of specific therapies, as applicable.

3. Documented evaluation of patient and family caregiver learning.

HAND-OFF REPORTING

1. Reported abnormal findings appropriately.

2. Reported measures taken to reduce or increase temperature and need for reassessment.

Student _____ Date _____

Instructor _____ Date _____

PERFORMANCE CHECKLIST SKILL 5.2 **ASSESSING RADIAL PULSE**

	S	U	NP	Comments

ASSESSMENT

1. Identified patient using at least two identifiers according to agency policy. ___ ___ ___ _____

2. Reviewed patient's EHR for need to assess radial pulse. ___ ___ ___ _____

3. Determined previous pulse rate and measurement site (when available) from patient's record. ___ ___ ___ _____

4. Assessed patient's and family caregiver's health literacy. ___ ___ ___ _____

5. Assessed for factors that influence radial pulse rate and rhythm. ___ ___ ___ _____

6. Performed hand hygiene. ___ ___ ___ _____

7. Assessed for signs and symptoms of altered cardiac function. ___ ___ ___ _____

8. Assessed for signs and symptoms of peripheral vascular disease. ___ ___ ___ _____

9. Assessed patient's knowledge of and prior experience with pulse measurement and feelings about procedure. ___ ___ ___ _____

PLANNING

1. Determined expected outcomes following completion of procedure. ___ ___ ___ _____

2. Provided privacy for patient, explained procedure, and encouraged patient to relax. ___ ___ ___ _____

3. Obtained and organized equipment needed. ___ ___ ___ _____

IMPLEMENTATION

1. Performed hand hygiene and positioned patient in supine or sitting position. ___ ___ ___ _____

2. When patient was supine, placed patient's forearm straight alongside or across lower chest or upper abdomen. When sitting, bent patient's elbow 90 degrees and supported lower arm. Placed tips of first two or middle three fingers of hand over groove along radial or thumb side of patient's inner wrist. Slightly extended or flexed wrist with palm down until strongest pulse was noted. ___ ___ ___ _____

	S	U	NP	Comments

3. Lightly compressed pulse against radius, losing pulse initially; relaxed pressure so pulse became easily palpable.

4. Determined strength of pulse. Noted whether thrust of vessel against fingertips was bounding (4+); full increased, strong (3+); expected (2+); barely palpable, diminished (1+); or absent, not palpable (0).

5. After palpating a regular pulse, looked at watch second hand and began to count rate. Counted the first beat after the second hand hit the number on the dial; counted as one, then two, and so on.

6. When pulse was regular, counted rate for 30 seconds and multiplied total by 2.

7. Helped patient to comfortable position.

8. Discussed findings with patient and documented according to agency policy.

9. Disposed of all contaminated supplies in appropriate receptacle; removed and disposed of gloves if worn. Performed hand hygiene.

10. Raised side rails (as appropriate), placed bed in lowest position, and locked into position.

11. Placed nurse call system in an accessible location within patient's reach.

EVALUATION

1. When assessing pulse for first time, established radial pulse as baseline when within acceptable range.

2. Compared pulse rate and character with patient's previous baseline and acceptable range for patient's age.

3. Used teach-back. Revised instruction if patient/family caregiver was not able to teach back correctly.

DOCUMENTATION

1. Documented pulse rate and site appropriately.

2. Documented pulse after administration of specific therapies, as applicable.

3. Documented evaluation of patient and family caregiver learning.

HAND-OFF REPORTING

1. Reported abnormal findings appropriately.

Student _____ Date _____

Instructor _____ Date _____

PERFORMANCE CHECKLIST SKILL 5.3 **ASSESSING APICAL PULSE**

	S	U	NP	Comments

ASSESSMENT

1. Identified patient using at least two identifiers according to agency policy.   ___ ___ ___ _____

2. Reviewed patient's EHR to determine need to assess apical pulse.   ___ ___ ___ _____

3. Determined previous pulse rate and measurement site (when available) from patient's record.   ___ ___ ___ _____

4. Assessed for factors that influence apical pulse rate and rhythm.   ___ ___ ___ _____

5. Assessed patient and family caregiver health literacy.   ___ ___ ___ _____

6. Assess for presence of latex allergy. If patient had latex allergy, ensured that stethoscope was latex free.   ___ ___ ___ _____

7. Performed hand hygiene.   ___ ___ ___ _____

8. Assessed for signs and symptoms of altered cardiac function.   ___ ___ ___ _____

9. Determined if patient measured apical heart rate at home. Assessed patient's knowledge and skill level.   ___ ___ ___ _____

10. Assessed patient's knowledge and experience with apical pulse measurement and feelings about procedure.   ___ ___ ___ _____

PLANNING

1. Determined expected outcomes following completion of procedure.   ___ ___ ___ _____

2. Provided privacy and explained procedure.   ___ ___ ___ _____

3. Helped patient to supine or sitting position. Moved aside bed linen and gown to expose sternum and left side of chest.   ___ ___ ___ _____

4. Organized and set up equipment needed and performed stethoscope hygiene according to agency policy prior to procedure.   ___ ___ ___ _____

5. Encouraged patient to relax and not speak.   ___ ___ ___ _____

	S	U	NP	Comments

IMPLEMENTATION

1. Performed hand hygiene. Located anatomic landmarks to identify point of maximal impulse (PMI). ___ ___ ___ _____

2. Placed diaphragm of stethoscope in palm of hand for 5 to 10 seconds. ___ ___ ___ _____

3. Placed diaphragm of stethoscope over PMI at fifth ICS, at left MCL, and auscultated for normal S1 and S2 heart sounds. ___ ___ ___ _____

4. After hearing S1 and S2 with regularity, used second hand of watch and began to count rate: when sweep hand hit number on dial, started counting with zero, then one, two, and so on. ___ ___ ___ _____

5. When apical rate was regular, counted for 30 seconds and multiplied by 2. ___ ___ ___ _____

6. Noted regularity of any dysrhythmia. ___ ___ ___ _____

7. Replaced patient's gown and bed linen and helped patient to a comfortable position. ___ ___ ___ _____

8. Discussed findings with patient and documented according to agency policy. ___ ___ ___ _____

9. Disposed of all contaminated supplies in appropriate receptacle; removed and disposed of gloves if worn. Performed hand hygiene. ___ ___ ___ _____

10. Raised side rails (as appropriate) and lowered bed to lowest position, locking into position. ___ ___ ___ _____

11. Placed nurse call system in an accessible location within patient's reach. ___ ___ ___ _____

12. Cleaned earpieces and diaphragm of stethoscope with alcohol swab routinely after each use. Performed hand hygiene. ___ ___ ___ _____

EVALUATION

1. When assessing pulse for first time, established apical rate as baseline when it was within an acceptable range. ___ ___ ___ _____

2. Compared apical rate and character with patient's previous baseline and acceptable range of HR for patient's age. ___ ___ ___ _____

3. Used Teach-Back. Revised instructions if patient/family caregiver was not able to teach back correctly. ___ ___ ___ _____

	S	U	NP	Comments

DOCUMENTATION

1. Documented apical pulse rate and rhythm appropriately. When apical pulse not found at fifth ICS and left MCL, documented location of PMI.   ⎯   ⎯   ⎯   ⎯⎯⎯⎯⎯⎯⎯⎯⎯⎯

2. Documented measurement of apical pulse rate after administration of specific therapies per agency policy.   ⎯   ⎯   ⎯   ⎯⎯⎯⎯⎯⎯⎯⎯⎯⎯

3. Documented evaluation of patient and family caregiver learning.   ⎯   ⎯   ⎯   ⎯⎯⎯⎯⎯⎯⎯⎯⎯⎯

HAND-OFF REPORTING

1. Reported abnormal findings to nurse in charge or health care provider.   ⎯   ⎯   ⎯   ⎯⎯⎯⎯⎯⎯⎯⎯⎯⎯

Student _____ Date _____

Instructor _____ Date _____

PERFORMANCE CHECKLIST SKILL 5.4   **ASSESSING RESPIRATIONS**

	S	U	NP	Comments

ASSESSMENT

1. Identified patient using at least two identifiers according to agency policy.

2. Reviewed patient's EHR to assess for factors that influence the patient's respirations.

3. Determined previous baseline respiratory rate (when available) from patient's EHR.

4. Assessed patient's or family caregiver's health literacy.

5. Performed hand hygiene.

6. Assessed for signs and symptoms that influence the patient's respirations.

7. Assessed for signs and symptoms of respiratory alterations.

8. Assessed patient's knowledge of and prior experience with respiratory measurement and feelings about procedure.

PLANNING

1. Determined expected outcomes following completion of procedure.

2. If patient had been active, waited 5 to 10 minutes before assessing respirations.

3. Ensured that patient was in comfortable position, preferably sitting or lying with head of bed elevated 45 to 60 degrees.

4. Provided privacy and explained procedure to patient.

5. Organized and set up any equipment needed to perform procedure.

6. Ensured that patient's chest was visible. When necessary, moved bed linen or gown.

7. Assessed respirations after pulse measurement in an adult.

	S	U	NP	Comments

IMPLEMENTATION

1. Performed hand hygiene and placed patient's arm in relaxed position across abdomen or lower chest leaving fingertips on the wrist or placed own hand directly over patient's upper abdomen. ___ ___ ___ _____

2. Observed complete respiratory cycle. ___ ___ ___ _____

3. After observing a cycle, looked at second hand of watch and began to count rate: when sweep hand hit number on dial, began time frame, counting one with first full respiratory cycle. ___ ___ ___ _____

4. When rhythm was regular, counted number of respirations in 30 seconds and multiplied by 2. When rhythm was irregular, less than 12, or greater than 20, counted for 1 full minute. ___ ___ ___ _____

5. Noted depth of respirations by observing degree of chest wall movement while counting rate. Assessed depth by palpating chest wall excursion or auscultating posterior thorax after rate counted. Described depth as shallow, normal, or deep. ___ ___ ___ _____

6. Noted rhythm of ventilatory cycle. Did not confuse sighing with abnormal rhythm. ___ ___ ___ _____

7. Replaced bed linen and patient's gown. Helped patient to a comfortable position. ___ ___ ___ _____

8. Informed patient of respiratory rate and documented per agency policy ___ ___ ___ _____

9. Disposed of all contaminated supplies in appropriate receptacle; removed and disposed of gloves if worn. Performed hand hygiene. ___ ___ ___ _____

10. Raised side rails (as appropriate) and lowered bed to lowest position, locking into position. ___ ___ ___ _____

11. Placed nurse call system in an accessible location within patient's reach. ___ ___ ___ _____

EVALUATION

1. When assessing respirations for first time, established rate, rhythm, and depth as baseline when within acceptable range. ___ ___ ___ _____

2. Compared respirations with patient's previous baseline and usual rate, rhythm, and depth. ___ ___ ___ _____

	S	U	NP	Comments

3. Correlated respiratory rate, depth, and rhythm with data obtained from pulse oximetry and ABG measurements when available.

   ____   ____   ____   _____

4. Used Teach-Back. Revised instruction if patient/family caregiver was not able to teach back correctly.

   ____   ____   ____   _____

DOCUMENTATION

1. Documented respiratory rate, depth, and rhythm according to agency policy.

   ____   ____   ____   _____

2. Documented measurement of respiratory rate after administration of specific therapies per agency policy.

   ____   ____   ____   _____

3. Documented evaluation of patient and family caregiver learning.

   ____   ____   ____   _____

4. Documented type and amount of oxygen therapy, when used, per agency policy.

   ____   ____   ____   _____

HAND-OFF REPORTING

1. Reported abnormal findings appropriately.

   ____   ____   ____   _____

2. Reported need for oxygen therapy.

   ____   ____   ____   _____

Student _____ Date _____

Instructor _____ Date _____

PERFORMANCE CHECKLIST SKILL 5.5 **ASSESSING ARTERIAL BLOOD PRESSURE**

	S	U	NP	Comments

ASSESSMENT

1. Identified patient using at least two identifiers according to agency policy.

2. Reviewed patient's EHR to assess for risk factors for BP alterations.

3. Assessed patient's or family caregiver's health literacy.

4. Assessed for factors that influence BP.

5. Determined previous baseline BP and site (when available) from patient's record. Determined any report of latex allergy.

6. Performed hand hygiene.

7. Assessed for factors that influence BP measurement.

8. Assessed for signs and symptoms of BP alterations.

9. Assessed patient's knowledge of and prior experience with BP measurement and feelings about procedure.

PLANNING

1. Determined expected outcomes following completion of procedure.

2. Provided privacy and explained procedure. Ensured that room was warm, quiet, and relaxing.

3. Determined best site for BP assessment.

4. Selected appropriate cuff size. Ensured that sphygmomanometer or electronic BP machine was in patient's room.

5. Organized and set up any equipment needed to perform procedure.

6. Ensured that patient had not exercised, ingested caffeine, or smoked for 30 minutes before assessing BP. Had patient rest at least 5 minutes before measuring lying or sitting BP and 1 minute before measuring standing BP.

	S	U	NP	Comments

7. Explained procedure to patient. Had patient assume sitting or lying position. Allowed the patient to rest 3 to 5 minutes before obtaining a BP. Asked patient not to speak during BP measurement.

IMPLEMENTATION

1. Performed hand hygiene. Performed stethoscope hygiene according to agency policy.

2. Prepared to obtain BP by auscultation.

   a. Upper extremity: With patient sitting or lying, positioned forearm at heart level with palm turned up. Supported arm on table or under own arm. When sitting, supported back and instructed patient to keep feet flat on floor without legs crossed. When supine, instructed patient not to cross legs.

   b. Lower extremity: When upper extremities were inaccessible, lower extremity BP measures were obtained.

      (1) Calf BP measurements: positioned the patient supine.

      (2) Thigh BP measurements: Placed the patient prone. When the patient could not be placed prone, positioned the patient supine with knee slightly bent.

   c. Exposed extremity (arm or leg) fully by removing constricting clothing.

3. Palpated brachial artery (arm) or popliteal artery (thigh) or dorsalis pedis artery or posterior tibial artery (calf). With cuff fully deflated, positioned bladder of cuff appropriately and wrapped evenly and snugly around upper arm or lower extremity.

4. Positioned manometer gauge vertically at eye level no more than 1 meter (1 yard) away.

5. Auscultated BP.

   a. Two-step method:

      (1) Relocated brachial or popliteal pulse. Palpated artery distal to cuff with fingertips of nondominant hand while inflating cuff rapidly to pressure 30 mm Hg above point at which pulse disappears. Slowly deflated cuff and noted point when pulse reappeared. Deflated cuff fully and waited 30 seconds.

      (2) Placed stethoscope earpieces in ears and ensured that sounds were clear, not muffled.

32

	S	U	NP	Comments

(3) Relocated artery and placed bell or diaphragm chest piece of stethoscope over it. Did not allow chest piece to touch cuff or clothing.   ___ ___ ___ _____

(4) Closed valve of pressure bulb clockwise until tight. Quickly inflated cuff to 30 mm Hg above patient's estimated systolic pressure.   ___ ___ ___ _____

(5) Slowly released pressure bulb valve and allowed manometer needle to fall at rate of 2 to 3 mm Hg/second.   ___ ___ ___ _____

(6) Noted point on manometer when first clear sound was heard.   ___ ___ ___ _____

(7) Continued to deflate cuff gradually, noting point at which sound disappeared in adults. Noted pressure to nearest 2 mm Hg. Listened for 20 to 30 mm Hg after last sound and allowed remaining air to escape quickly.   ___ ___ ___ _____

b. One-step method: ___ ___ ___ _____

(1) Placed stethoscope earpieces in ears and ensured that sounds were clear, not muffled.   ___ ___ ___ _____

(2) Relocated brachial or popliteal artery and placed bell or diaphragm chest piece of stethoscope over it. Did not allow chest piece to touch cuff or clothing.   ___ ___ ___ _____

(3) Closed valve of pressure bulb clockwise until tight. Quickly inflated cuff to 30 mm Hg above patient's usual systolic pressure.   ___ ___ ___ _____

(4) Slowly released pressure bulb valve and allowed manometer needle to fall at rate of 2 to 3 mm Hg/s. Noted point on manometer when first clear sound was heard.   ___ ___ ___ _____

(5) Continued to deflate cuff gradually, noting point at which sound disappeared in adults. Noted pressure to nearest 2 mm Hg. Listened for 10 to 20 mm Hg after last sound and allowed remaining air to escape quickly.   ___ ___ ___ _____

6. Assessed SBP by palpation: ___ ___ ___ _____

a. Located and then continually palpated brachial, radial, or popliteal artery with fingertips of one hand. Inflated cuff to pressure 30 mm Hg above point at which pulse could no longer be palpated.   ___ ___ ___ _____

	S	U	NP	Comments

b. Slowly released valve and deflated cuff, allowing manometer needle to fall at rate of 2 mm Hg/s. Noted point on manometer when pulse was again palpable. ___ ___ ___ _____

c. Deflated cuff rapidly and completely. Removed cuff from patient's extremity unless patient condition required repeated measurements. ___ ___ ___ _____

7. Used average of two sets of BP measurements, 2 minutes apart. Used second set of BP measurements as baseline. When readings were different by more than 5 mm Hg, performed additional readings. ___ ___ ___ _____

8. Removed cuff from patient's arm or leg unless repeat measurements needed. ___ ___ ___ _____

9. When this was first assessment of patient, repeated procedure on other arm or leg. ___ ___ ___ _____

10. Disposed of all contaminated supplies in appropriate receptacle; removed and disposed of gloves. Performed hand hygiene. ___ ___ ___ _____

11. Helped patient return to comfortable position and covered upper arm or leg if previously clothed. ___ ___ ___ _____

12. Discussed findings with patient and documented results per agency policy. ___ ___ ___ _____

13. Raised side rails (as appropriate) and placed bed in lowest position, locking into position. ___ ___ ___ _____

14. Placed nurse call system in an accessible location within patient's reach. ___ ___ ___ _____

15. Cleaned earpieces and diaphragm of stethoscope with alcohol swab as needed. Wiped cuff with agency-approved disinfectant when used between patients. ___ ___ ___ _____

16. Performed hand hygiene. ___ ___ ___ _____

EVALUATION

1. When assessing BP for first time, established baseline BP when it was within acceptable range. ___ ___ ___ _____

2. Compared BP reading with patient's previous baseline and usual BP for patient's age. ___ ___ ___ _____

3. Used Teach-Back. Revised instruction if patient/family caregiver was not able to teach back correctly. ___ ___ ___ _____

	S	U	NP	Comments

DOCUMENTATION

1. Documented BP and site(s) assessed. ____ ____ ____ _____

2. Documented measurement of BP and any signs or symptoms of BP alterations after administration of specific therapies. ____ ____ ____ _____

3. Documented evaluation of patient and family caregiver learning. ____ ____ ____ _____

HAND-OFF REPORTING

1. Reported abnormal findings appropriately. ____ ____ ____ _____

2. Reported method of BP measurement. ____ ____ ____ _____

Student _____ Date _____

Instructor _____ Date _____

PERFORMANCE CHECKLIST PROCEDURAL GUIDELINE 5.1 **NONINVASIVE ELECTRONIC BLOOD PRESSURE MEASUREMENT**

	S	U	NP	Comments

PROCEDURAL STEPS

1. Identified patient using at least two identifiers according to agency policy.

2. Assessed risk factors for blood pressure alterations and determined patient's baseline blood pressure.

3. Determined appropriateness of using electronic blood pressure measurement.

4. Assessed patient's/family caregiver's health literacy.

5. Performed hand hygiene and explained procedure to patient. Determined best site for cuff placement; inspected condition of extremities.

6. Collected and brought appropriate equipment to patient's bedside. Selected appropriate cuff size for patient extremity and appropriate cuff for machine.

7. Assisted patient to comfortable lying or sitting position. Plugged device into electric outlet and placed it near patient, ensured that connector hose between cuff and machine reached.

8. Located on/off switch and turned on machine to enable device to self-test computer systems.

9. Removed constricting clothing to ensure proper cuff application.

10. Prepared blood pressure cuff by manually squeezing all the air out of the cuff and connecting it to connector hose.

11. Performed hand hygiene. Wrapped flattened cuff snugly around extremity, verifying that only one finger could fit between cuff and patient's skin. Made sure that "artery" arrow marked on outside of cuff was placed correctly.

12. Verified that connector hose between cuff and machine was not kinked.

	S	U	NP	Comments

13. Followed manufacturer directions, set frequency control for automatic or manual, and pressed the start button.
    ____ ____ ____ _____

14. When deflation was complete, noted that digital display provided most recent values and flash time in minutes that had elapsed since the measurement occurred.
    ____ ____ ____ _____

15. Set frequency of measurements and upper and lower alarm limits for systolic, diastolic, and mean blood pressure readings.
    ____ ____ ____ _____

16. Obtained additional readings by pressing the start button.
    ____ ____ ____ _____

17. When frequent measurements were required, may have left cuff in place. Removed it at least every 2 hours to assess underlying skin integrity and, if possible, alternated measurement sites.
    ____ ____ ____ _____

18. When patient no longer required frequent blood pressure monitoring:
    ____ ____ ____ _____

    a. Helped patient return to comfortable position and covered upper arm or leg if previously clothed.
    ____ ____ ____ _____

    b. Raised side rails (as appropriate) and lowered bed to lowest position, locking into position.
    ____ ____ ____ _____

    c. Placed nurse call system in accessible location within patient's reach; instructed patient in use.
    ____ ____ ____ _____

    d. Wiped cuff with agency-approved disinfectant. Cleaned and stored electronic blood pressure machine.
    ____ ____ ____ _____

19. Performed hand hygiene.
    ____ ____ ____ _____

20. Compared electronic blood pressure readings with auscultatory measurements.
    ____ ____ ____ _____

21. Informed patient of blood pressure.
    ____ ____ ____ _____

22. Used Teach-Back. Revised instruction if patient/family caregiver was not able to teach back correctly.
    ____ ____ ____ _____

23. Documented blood pressure and site assessed in EHR per agency policy; documented any signs or symptoms of blood pressure alterations.
    ____ ____ ____ _____

24. Reported reason for electronic blood pressure and abnormal findings to nurse in charge or health care provider.
    ____ ____ ____ _____

Student _____ Date _____

Instructor _____ Date _____

PERFORMANCE CHECKLIST PROCEDURAL GUIDELINE 5.2   **MEASURING OXYGEN SATURATION (PULSE OXIMETRY)**

	S	U	NP	Comments

PROCEDURAL STEPS

1. Identified patient using at least two identifiers according to agency policy.

2. Determined need to measure patient's oxygen saturation.

3. Assessed patient's/family caregiver's health literacy.

4. Performed hand hygiene. Assessed for signs and symptoms of alterations in oxygen saturation.

5. Determined if patient had a latex allergy.

6. Assessed for factors that influenced measurement of SpO_2.

7. Reviewed patient's EHR for health care provider's order or consulted agency procedure manual for standard of care for measurement of SpO_2.

8. Determined previous baseline SpO_2 (when available) from patient's record.

9. Performed hand hygiene.

10. Determined most appropriate patient-specific site for sensor probe placement by measuring capillary refill. When capillary refill was greater than 2 seconds, selected alternative site.

11. Explained procedure to patient.

12. Arranged equipment at the bedside.

13. Positioned patient comfortably.

14. Attached sensor to monitoring site. If using finger, removed regular fingernail polish from digit with acetone or polish remover. If gel polish was in place, had it removed by patient or nail technician before monitoring, or chose alternate site. Instructed patient that clip-on probe would feel like a clothespin on the finger but would not hurt.

38

15. With sensor in place, turned on oximeter by activating power. Observed pulse waveform/intensity display and audible beep. Correlated oximeter pulse rate with patient's radial pulse. ___ ___ ___ _____

16. Left sensor in place 10 to 30 seconds or until oximeter readout reached constant value and pulse display reached full strength during each cardiac cycle. Informed patient that oximeter alarm would sound if sensor falls off or patient moves it. Read SpO_2 on digital display. ___ ___ ___ _____

17. When planning to monitor SpO_2 continuously, verified SpO_2 alarm limits preset by manufacturer at a low of 85% and a high of 100%. Determined limits for SpO_2 and pulse rate as indicated by patient's condition. Verified that alarms were on. Assessed skin integrity under sensor probe every 2 hours; relocated sensor at least every 4 hours and more frequently when skin integrity was altered, or tissue perfusion compromised. ___ ___ ___ _____

18. When planning intermittent or spot-checking of SpO_2, removed probe, and turned oximeter power off. ___ ___ ___ _____

19. Used Teach-Back. Revised instruction if patient/family caregiver was unable to teach back correctly. ___ ___ ___ _____

20. Discussed findings with patient. ___ ___ ___ _____

21. Cleaned sensor and device per agency policy and stored sensor in appropriate location. Performed hand hygiene. ___ ___ ___ _____

22. Compared SpO_2 with patient's previous baseline, acceptable SpO_2. Correlated reading with data obtained from respiratory rate, depth, and rhythm assessment. ___ ___ ___ _____

23. Documented SpO_2 on vital sign flow sheet in EHR; indicated type and amount of oxygen therapy used by patient during assessment; documented any signs or symptoms of alterations in oxygen saturation in narrative nurses' notes. ___ ___ ___ _____

24. Reported abnormal findings to nurse in charge or health care provider. ___ ___ ___ _____

Student _____ Date _____

Instructor _____ Date _____

PERFORMANCE CHECKLIST SKILL 6.1 **GENERAL SURVEY**

	S	U	NP	Comments

ASSESSMENT

1. Identified patient using at least two identifiers. ___ ___ ___ _____

2. Checked the EHR for important information related to the assessment about to be performed. ___ ___ ___ _____

3. Noted if patient had any acute distress and, if present, deferred general survey until later and focused immediately on affected body system. ___ ___ ___ _____

4. Assessed patient's level of consciousness (LOC) and orientation by observing and talking to him or her. ___ ___ ___ _____

5. Identified self. Used gender-affirming approach. Welcomed others accompanying patient and asked about connections to patient. ___ ___ ___ _____

6. Assessed patient's/family caregiver's health literacy. Obtained an appropriate interpreter if needed and available. ___ ___ ___ _____

7. After reviewing history, confirmed with patient the primary reason he or she sought health care. ___ ___ ___ _____

8. Identified patient's normal height, weight, and body mass index (BMI). If sudden gain or loss in weight had occurred, determined amount of weight change and period of time in which it occurred. Assessed if patient was on a special diet or had recently been dieting or following an exercise program. Used growth chart for children younger than 18 years of age. ___ ___ ___ _____

9. Asked if patient had noticed any changes in condition of skin. ___ ___ ___ _____

10. Reviewed patient's past fluid intake and output (I&O) records. ___ ___ ___ _____

11. Identified patient's general perceptions about personal health. ___ ___ ___ _____

12. Determined history of any allergies or allergic reactions to latex, food, medications, or liquid preparations for skin. Assessed patient for risk factors for developing latex allergies. ___ ___ ___ _____

	S	U	NP	Comments

13. Assessed patient's knowledge, experience, and feelings about physical assessment and personal goals.   ____ ____ ____ _____

PLANNING

1. Determined expected outcomes following completion of procedure.   ____ ____ ____ _____

2. Prepared patient: explained procedure. Asked patient to identify any area that hurt when touched.   ____ ____ ____ _____

3. Anticipated topics for patient teaching.   ____ ____ ____ _____

4. Performed hand hygiene. Assembled necessary equipment and supplies.   ____ ____ ____ _____

5. Closed room doors and/or bedside curtain.   ____ ____ ____ _____

6. Positioned patient initially, either sitting or lying supine with head of bed elevated.   ____ ____ ____ _____

7. Assured patient that assessment was routine and confidential.   ____ ____ ____ _____

IMPLEMENTATION

1. Performed hand hygiene. Throughout assessment noted patient's verbal and nonverbal behaviors.   ____ ____ ____ _____

2. Obtained temperature, pulse, respirations, and blood pressure unless taken within past 3 hours or if serious potential change was noted. Informed patient of vital signs.   ____ ____ ____ _____

3. Asked patient to identify age.   ____ ____ ____ _____

4. When uncertain whether patient understood a question, rephrased or asked a similar question.   ____ ____ ____ _____

5. When patient's responses were inappropriate, asked short, to-the-point questions regarding information patient should know.   ____ ____ ____ _____

6. When patient was unable to respond to questions of orientation, offered simple commands.   ____ ____ ____ _____

7. Assessed affect and mood. Noted if verbal expressions matched nonverbal behavior and if appropriate to situation.   ____ ____ ____ _____

8. Watched patient interact with spouse or partner, older-adult, child, or family caregiver when possible. Was alert for indications of fear, hesitancy to report health status, or willingness to let someone else control assessment interview. Noted if patient had any obvious physical injuries.   ____ ____ ____ _____

9. Observed for signs of abuse.   ____ ____ ____ _____

	S	U	NP	Comments

10. Assessed posture and position, noted alignment of shoulders and hips while patient stood and/or sat. Observed whether patient was slumped, erect, or had bent posture. ____ ____ ____ _____

11. Assessed body movements. ____ ____ ____ _____

12. Assessed pattern of speech. ____ ____ ____ _____

13. Observed hygiene and grooming for presence or absence of makeup, type of clothes, and cleanliness. ____ ____ ____ _____

14. Inspected exposed areas of skin and asked if patient had noted any changes. ____ ____ ____ _____

15. Inspected skin surfaces. Compared color of symmetrical body parts, including areas unexposed to sun. Looked for any patches or areas of skin color variation. ____ ____ ____ _____

16. Carefully inspected color of face, oral mucosa, lips, conjunctiva, sclera, palms of hands, and nail beds. ____ ____ ____ _____

17. Used ungloved fingertips to palpate skin surfaces to feel texture and moisture of intact skin. Made sure hands were warm. ____ ____ ____ _____

   a. Stroked skin surfaces lightly with fingertips to detect texture of surface of skin. Noted whether skin was smooth or rough, thick or thin, or tight or supple and if localized areas of hardness or lesions were present. ____ ____ ____ _____

   b. Palpated any areas that appear irregular in texture. ____ ____ ____ _____

   c. Using dorsum (back) of hand, palpated for temperature of skin surfaces. Compared symmetrical body parts. Compared upper and lower body parts. Noted distinct temperature difference and localized areas of warmth. ____ ____ ____ _____

18. Applied clean gloves. Inspected character of any body secretions; noted color, odor, amount, and consistency. Removed gloves. Performed hand hygiene. ____ ____ ____ _____

19. Assessed skin turgor. ____ ____ ____ _____

20. Assessed condition of skin for pressure areas. If areas of redness were seen, placed fingertip over area, applied gentle pressure, and released. Looked at skin color. ____ ____ ____ _____

	S	U	NP	Comments

21. When a lesion was detected, used adequate lighting to inspect color, location, texture, size, shape, and type. Also noted grouping and distribution. ____ ____ ____ _____

   a. Applied clean gloves if lesion was moist or draining. Gently palpated any lesion to determine mobility, contour, and consistency. ____ ____ ____ _____

   b. Noted if patient reported tenderness with or without palpation. ____ ____ ____ _____

   c. Measured size of lesion with centimeter ruler. ____ ____ ____ _____

22. When patient had medical device using adhesive, assessed for patient's age, inspected skin around where adhesive was applied. ____ ____ ____ _____

23. Removed gloves. Discarded used supplies and gloves in proper receptacle. Proceeded to next examination or helped patient to comfortable position. Performed hand hygiene. ____ ____ ____ _____

24. Placed nurse call system in an accessible location within patient's reach. ____ ____ ____ _____

25. Raised side rails (as appropriate) and lowered bed to lowest position, locking into position. ____ ____ ____ _____

EVALUATION

1. Observed throughout assessment for evidence of physical or emotional distress. ____ ____ ____ _____

2. Compared assessment findings with normal characteristics. ____ ____ ____ _____

3. Asked patient if there was information about physical condition that was not discussed. ____ ____ ____ _____

4. Used Teach-Back. Revised instruction if patient or family caregiver was not able to teach back correctly. ____ ____ ____ _____

DOCUMENTATION

1. Documented assessment findings and patient's VS. ____ ____ ____ _____

2. Described alterations in patient's general appearance and patient's behaviors using objective terminology. Included patient's self-report of signs and symptoms. ____ ____ ____ _____

3. Documented evaluation of patient and family caregiver learning. ____ ____ ____ _____

HAND-OFF REPORTING

1. Reported abnormalities and acute symptoms to nurse in charge or health care provider. ____ ____ ____ _____

Student _____ Date _____

Instructor _____ Date _____

PERFORMANCE CHECKLIST SKILL 6.2 **HEAD AND NECK ASSESSMENT**

	S	U	NP	Comments
ASSESSMENT				
1. Identified patient using two identifiers. Determined patient's level of consciousness, primary language, and literacy level.	___	___	___	_____
2. Checked the EHR for history of any conditions that had implications for the assessment to be performed.	___	___	___	_____
3. Reviewed EHR for history of sexually transmitted disease, especially HPV.	___	___	___	_____
4. Asked patient about history of headache, dizziness, neck pain, or stiffness in head or neck. Asked patient if there was history of difficulty moving neck.	___	___	___	_____
5. Determined if patient had history of eye disease, diabetes mellitus, or hypertension.	___	___	___	_____
6. Asked if patient had experienced blurred vision, flashing lights, halos around lights, or reduced visual field.	___	___	___	_____
7. Asked if patient had experienced ear pain, itching, discharge, vertigo, tinnitus (ringing in the ears), or change in hearing. Determined if the patient used a personal audio device or system.	___	___	___	_____
8. Reviewed patient's occupational history.	___	___		_____
9. Asked if patient had history of seasonal allergies, nasal discharge, epistaxis (nosebleeds), or postnasal drip.	___	___	___	_____
10. Assessed if patient smoked or chewed tobacco.	___	___		_____
11. Assessed patient's knowledge, prior experience with head and neck assessment, and feelings about procedure.	___	___	___	_____
PLANNING				
1. Determined expected outcomes following completion of procedure.	___	___	___	_____
2. Prepared patient by explaining procedure.	___	___	___	_____

		S	U	NP	Comments

3. Anticipated topics for patient teaching.
    S ___ U ___ NP ___ Comments _____

4. Performed hand hygiene. Assembled necessary supplies and equipment at bedside.
    ___ ___ ___ _____

5. Closed room doors or bed curtains.
    ___ ___ ___ _____

6. Positioned patient sitting upright when possible.
    ___ ___ ___ _____

IMPLEMENTATION

1. Inspected head's position and facial features. Looked for symmetry.
    ___ ___ ___ _____

2. Assessed eyes. During examination, included patient teaching.

   a. Inspected position of eyes, color, condition of conjunctiva, and movement.
    ___ ___ ___ _____

   b. Assessed patient's near vision and far vision.
    ___ ___ ___ _____

   c. Inspected pupils for size, shape, and equality.
    ___ ___ ___ _____

   d. Tested pupillary reflexes and accommodation. Observed pupillary response of both eyes, noting briskness and equality.
    ___ ___ ___ _____

3. Assessed ears. During examination, included patient teaching.
    ___ ___ ___ _____

   a. Inspected outer ear and external auditory canal. Gently pressed against tragus and asked if patient noted discomfort.
    ___ ___ ___ _____

   b. Noted patient's response to questions and presence/use of hearing aid. Noted if patient cupped a hand behind ear or tilted ear while listening. When hearing loss was suspected, checked patient's response to whispered voice one ear at a time. Standing behind and to side of patient, exhaled and whispered into ear using a random combination of six letters and numbers. Repeated, gradually increasing voice intensity until patient correctly repeated the words.
    ___ ___ ___ _____

4. Inspected nose.
    ___ ___ ___ _____

   a. Inspected externally for shape, skin color, alignment, drainage, and presence of deformity or inflammation. Noted color of mucosa and any lesions, discharge, swelling, or presence of bleeding. If drainage appeared infectious, consulted with health care provider about obtaining a specimen.
    ___ ___ ___ _____

b. In patients with enteral tubes or nasotracheal (NT) tubes, inspected nares for pressure injury, excoriation, inflammation, or discharge. Using penlight, looked up into each naris. Stabilized tube as needed. Inspected skin around any adhesive stabilization device. ___ ___ ___ _____

c. Inspected sinuses by palpating gently over frontal and maxillary areas. Used thumbs to apply pressure up and under eyebrows to assess frontal sinuses. Used thumbs to apply pressure over maxillary sinuses, approximately 0.4 cm below eyes. ___ ___ ___ _____

5. Assessed mouth. During examination, included patient teaching. ___ ___ ___ _____

a. Applied clean gloves. Inspected lips for color, texture, hydration, and lesions. Had patient remove lipstick, if worn. ___ ___ ___ _____

b. Asked patient to open mouth wide. Inspected teeth and noted position and alignment. Noted color of teeth and presence of dental caries, tartar, and extraction sites. ___ ___ ___ _____

c. Inspected mucosa and gums. Determined if patient wore dentures or retainers and if they were comfortable. Removed dentures to visualize and palpate gums. Used tongue blade to lightly depress tongue and inspect oral cavity with penlight. Inspected oral mucosa, tongue, teeth, and gums for color, hydration, texture, and obvious lesions. ___ ___ ___ _____

d. If oral lesions were present, palpated gently with gloved hand for tenderness, size, and consistency. Removed and dispose of gloves. Performed hand hygiene. ___ ___ ___ _____

6. Inspected and palpated the neck: ___ ___ ___ _____

a. Neck muscles: Inspected neck for bilateral symmetry of muscles. Asked patient to slowly flex and hyperextend neck and turn head side to side. ___ ___ ___ _____

b. Lymph nodes: With patient's chin raised and head tilted slightly, inspected area where lymph nodes were distributed and compared both sides. ___ ___ ___ _____

(1) To examine lymph nodes more closely, had patient relax with neck flexed slightly forward. To palpate, faced or stood to side of patient and used pads of middle three fingers of hand. Palpated gently in rotary motion for superficial lymph nodes. ___ ___ ___ _____

46

	S	U	NP	Comments
(2) Noted if lymph nodes were large, fixed, inflamed, or tender.	___	___	___	_____
7. Discarded used supplies and gloves in proper receptacle. Proceeded to next examination or helped patient to comfortable position. Performed hand hygiene.	___	___	___	_____
8. Placed nurse call system in an accessible location within patient's reach.	___	___	___	_____
9. Raised side rails (as appropriate) and lowered bed to lowest position, locking into position.	___	___	___	_____

EVALUATION

	S	U	NP	Comments
1. Compared assessment findings with normal assessment characteristics or previous assessments.	___	___	___	_____
2. Asked patient to describe common symptoms of eye, ear, sinus, or mouth disease.	___	___	___	_____
3. Asked patient to list occupational safety precautions.	___	___	___	_____
4. Used Teach-Back. Revised instruction if patient or family caregiver was not able to teach back correctly.	___	___	___	_____

DOCUMENTATION

	S	U	NP	Comments
1. Documented all findings.	___	___	___	_____
2. Documented evaluation of patient and family caregiver learning.	___	___	___	_____

HAND-OFF REPORTING

	S	U	NP	Comments
1. Reported unexpected findings or changes to charge nurse or health care provider.	___	___	___	_____

Student _____   Date _____

Instructor _____   Date _____

PERFORMANCE CHECKLIST SKILL 6.3   **THORAX AND LUNG ASSESSMENT**

	S	U	NP	Comments

ASSESSMENT

1. Identified patient, determined patient's level of consciousness, primary language, and health literacy.

2. Checked the EHR for history of lung disease, chest trauma, and VS.

3. Assessed history of tobacco or marijuana use. If patient had quit, determined length of time since smoking stopped. If patient vaped, determined device type, flavor preference and identified the mix of tobacco products used.

4. Asked if patient experienced persistent cough, sputum production, chest pain, worsening shortness of breath, a hoarse voice, orthopnea, dyspnea during exertion, activity intolerance, or recurrent bouts of pneumonia or bronchitis.

5. Determined if patient lived or worked in environment containing pollutants or requiring exposure to radiation.

6. Reviewed history for known or suspected human immunodeficiency virus (HIV) infection; determined risk factors for TB.

7. Asked when patient last had a TB test.

8. Asked if patient had a history of persistent cough, hemoptysis, unexplained weight loss, fatigue, night sweats, and/or fever.

9. Determined if patient had a history of chronic hoarseness.

10. Assessed for history of allergies to pollen, dust, or other airborne irritants and to any foods, drugs, or chemical substances. Determined if patient had history of severe allergic reaction.

11. Reviewed family history for cancer, TB, allergies, asthma, bronchitis, or emphysema.

12. Assessed patient's knowledge, prior experience with chest examination and risk factors for lung problems, and feelings about procedure.

48

	S	U	NP	Comments

PLANNING

1. Determined expected outcomes following completion of procedure. ___ ___ ___ _____

2. Explained procedure to patient. ___ ___ ___ _____

3. Anticipated topics to teach patient during examination. ___ ___ ___ _____

4. Performed hand hygiene. Prepared necessary supplies at bedside. ___ ___ ___ _____

5. Closed room doors or bed curtains. ___ ___ ___ _____

6. Positioned patient sitting upright. For bedridden patient, elevated head of bed 45 to 90 degrees. When unable to tolerate sitting, used supine and side-lying positions. ___ ___ ___ _____

IMPLEMENTATION

1. Removed patient's gown or drape from the posterior chest. Kept front of chest and legs covered. As examination progressed, removed gown from area being examined. ___ ___ ___ _____

2. Explained all steps of procedure, encouraging patient to relax and breathe normally through mouth. ___ ___ ___ _____

3. Posterior thorax:

   a. If possible, stood behind patient. Inspected thorax for shape and symmetry and anteroposterior diameter. ___ ___ ___ _____

   b. Determined rate and rhythm of breathing. Examined thorax as a whole. Had patient relax. ___ ___ ___ _____

   c. Systematically palpated posterior chest wall, costal spaces, and ICS. When patient voiced pain or tenderness, avoided deep palpation. When there was a suspicious mass, palpated lightly for shape, size, and qualities of lesion. ___ ___ ___ _____

   d. Assessed chest expansion, noting movement and symmetry. ___ ___ ___ _____

   e. Auscultated breath sounds, listening to entire inspiration and expiration at each stethoscope position. When sounds were faint, asked patient to breathe harder and faster. Compared breath sounds over right and left sides, listening for normal and adventitious sounds. ___ ___ ___ _____

   f. When auscultating adventitious sounds, had patient cough. Listened again with stethoscope to determine if sound cleared with coughing. ___ ___ ___ _____

	S	U	NP	Comments

4. Lateral thorax:

   a. Instructed patient to raise arms and inspected chest wall for same characteristics as reviewed for posterior chest.

   b. Extended palpation and auscultation of posterior thorax to lateral sides of chest, except for excursion measurement.

5. Anterior thorax:

   a. Inspected accessory muscles while patient was breathing; noted effort to breathe.

   b. Inspected width or spread of costal angle made by costal margins and tip of sternum.

   c. Observed patient's breathing pattern, observing symmetry and degree of chest wall and abdominal movement.

   d. Palpated anterior thoracic muscles and ribs for lumps, masses, tenderness, or unusual movement, following a systematic pattern across and down.

   e. Palpated anterior chest excursion, noting symmetry.

   f. With patient sitting, auscultated anterior thorax; compared right and left sides.

6. Cleaned and stored stethoscope. Proceeded to next examination or helped patient to comfortable position. Performed hand hygiene.

7. Placed nurse call system in an accessible location within patient's reach.

8. Raised side rails (as appropriate) and lowered bed to lowest position, locking into position.

EVALUATION

1. Compared respiratory findings with normal assessment characteristics or previous assessments for thorax and lungs.

2. Had patient identify own risk factors and those factors leading to lung disease.

3. Used Teach-Back. Revised instruction if patient or family caregiver was not able to teach back correctly.

	S	U	NP	Comments

DOCUMENTATION

1. Documented patient's respiratory rate and character; breath sounds, changes noted after coughing, chest excursion, and other physical assessment findings. ___ ___ ___ _____

2. Documented evaluation of patient and family caregiver learning. ___ ___ ___ _____

HAND-OFF REPORTING

1. Reported abnormalities immediately to the health care provider. ___ ___ ___ _____

Student _____   Date _____

Instructor _____   Date _____

PERFORMANCE CHECKLIST SKILL 6.4 **CARDIOVASCULAR ASSESSMENT**

	S	U	NP	Comments

ASSESSMENT

1. Identified patient; determined patient's level of consciousness, primary language, and health literacy.

2. Reviewed EHR and confirmed with patient any medications being taken for cardiovascular function, and patient knowledge about medications.

3. Asked if patient had experienced dyspnea, chest pain or discomfort, palpitations, excess fatigue, reduced ability to exercise, cough, leg pain or cramps, edema of the feet, rapid weight gain from fluid retention, cyanosis, fainting, and orthopnea. Asked if symptoms occurred at rest or during exercise.

4. If patient reported chest pain, determined onset, precipitating factors, quality, region, and severity and whether the pain radiated.

5. Assessed family history for heart disease, diabetes mellitus, high cholesterol and/or lipid levels, hypertension, stroke, or rheumatic heart disease.

6. Asked patient about a history of any preexisting heart conditions, heart surgery, or vascular disease.

7. Determined if patient experienced leg cramps; numbness or tingling in extremities; sensation of cold hands or feet; pain in legs; or swelling or cyanosis of feet, ankles, or hand. Asked about precipitating factors.

8. If patient experienced leg pain or cramping in lower extremities, asked if it was relieved by walking or standing for long periods or if it occurred during sleep.

9. Asked patients about wearing tight-fitting underwear, hosiery, tight-fitting trouser socks, and sitting or lying in bed with legs crossed.

10. Assessed patient's knowledge, prior experience with cardiovascular examination and risks for heart problems, and feelings about procedure.

	S	U	NP	Comments

PLANNING

1. Determined expected outcomes following completion of procedure. ___ ___ ___ _____

2. Explained procedure to patient. ___ ___ ___ _____

3. Anticipated topics to teach patient during examination. ___ ___ ___ _____

4. Performed hand hygiene. Prepared necessary supplies at bedside. Closed room curtains or door. ___ ___ ___ _____

5. Helped patient be as relaxed and comfortable as possible, using a calm tone of voice and purposeful actions. ___ ___ ___ _____

6. Had patient assume semi-Fowler or supine position. ___ ___ ___ _____

IMPLEMENTATION

1. Explained procedure. Avoided facial gestures reflecting concern. ___ ___ ___ _____

2. Ensured that room was quiet. ___ ___ ___ _____

3. Assessed the heart: ___ ___ ___ _____

   a. Visualized location of the heart. ___ ___ ___ _____

   b. Located angle of Louis. Slipped fingers down each side of angle to feel adjacent ribs. ___ ___ ___ _____

   c. Identified the following anatomical landmarks: ___ ___ ___ _____

      (1) Aortic area ___ ___ ___ _____

      (2) Pulmonic area ___ ___ ___ _____

      (3) Second pulmonic area ___ ___ ___ _____

      (4) Tricuspid area ___ ___ ___ _____

      (5) Mitral area ___ ___ ___ _____

      (6) Epigastric area ___ ___ ___ _____

   d. Stood to patient's right to inspect precordium with patient supine. Noted any visible pulsations or exaggerated lifts. Closely inspected area of apex. ___ ___ ___ _____

   e. Stayed in same position. Palpated for pulsations at all anatomic landmarks. ___ ___ ___ _____

   f. Located PMI. ___ ___ ___ _____

   g. Turned patient onto left side if palpating PMI was difficult. ___ ___ ___ _____

   h. Inspected epigastric area and palpated abdominal aorta. ___ ___ ___ _____

	S	U	NP	Comments

i. Auscultated heart sounds: _____ _____ _____ _____

   (1) Had patient sit up and lean slightly forward; then had patient lie supine; and ended examination with patient in left lateral recumbent position. Lifted left breast if necessary. _____ _____ _____ _____

   (2) While auscultating sounds at each anatomic landmark, asked patient not to speak but to breathe comfortably. Began with diaphragm of stethoscope; alternated with bell. Used light pressure for bell. Inched stethoscope along; avoided jumping from one area to another. Did not try to hear all heart sounds at once. _____ _____ _____ _____

   (3) Began at apex or PMI; moved systematically to aortic area, pulmonic area, Erb's point, tricuspid area, and mitral area. _____ _____ _____ _____

   (4) Listened for S2 at each site. _____ _____ _____ _____

   (5) After both sounds were heard clearly as "lub-dub," counted each combination of S1 and S2 as one heartbeat. Counted number of beats for 1 minute. _____ _____ _____ _____

   (6) Assessed heart rhythm by noting time between S1 and S2 (systole) and then time between S2 and the next S1 (diastole). Listened to full cycle at each auscultation area. Noted regular intervals between each sequence of beats. Noted a distinct pause between S1 and S2. _____ _____ _____ _____

   (7) Assessed for pulse deficit. When heart rate was irregular, compared apical and radial pulses. _____ _____ _____ _____

j. Auscultated for extra heart sounds at each site. _____ _____ _____ _____

   (1) Used stethoscope bell and listened for low-pitched extra heart sounds. _____ _____ _____ _____

4. Assessed neck vessels: _____ _____ _____ _____

a. Had patient remain in sitting position to assess carotid arteries. Visualized position of artery. _____ _____ _____ _____

b. Inspected neck on both sides for obvious arterial pulsations. _____ _____ _____ _____

	S	U	NP	Comments

c. Palpated each carotid artery separately with index and middle fingers around medial edge of sternocleidomastoid muscle. Asked patient to raise chin slightly, keeping head straight or slightly away from artery. Noted rate and rhythm, strength, and elasticity of artery. Also noted if pulse changed as patient inhaled and exhaled.

d. Placed bell of stethoscope over each carotid artery, auscultating for blowing sound (bruit). Asked patient to exhale and hold breath for a few heartbeats so respiratory sounds did not interfere with auscultation.

5. Peripheral vascular assessment:

a. Inspected lower extremities for changes in color and condition of skin. Noted skin and nail texture, hair distribution, venous patterns, edema, and scars or impaired skin integrity. Compared skin color with patient lying and standing.

b. Palpated edematous areas, noting mobility, consistency, and tenderness.

c. Assessed for pitting edema.

d. Used tape measure to measure circumference of leg.

e. Checked capillary refill.

f. Asked if patient experienced pain or tenderness and gently palpated for heat, firmness, or localized swelling of calf muscle.

g. Palpated peripheral arteries.

(1) Started at most distal part of each extremity. Palpated each peripheral artery for equality, comparing side to side; elasticity of vessel wall; and strength of pulse.

(2) Palpated radial pulse.

(3) Palpated ulnar pulse.

(4) Palpated brachial pulse.

(5) Palpated dorsalis pedis pulse.

(6) Palpated posterior tibial pulse.

(7) Palpated popliteal pulse.

(8) Applied clean gloves. Palpated femoral pulse.

h. If pulses were difficult to palpate or were not palpable, used a Doppler instrument over pulse site.

   (1) Applied conducting gel to patient's skin over pulse site or onto transducer tip of probe. Turned Doppler on.

   (2) Applied ultrasound probe to skin, changing Doppler angle until pulsation was audible. Adjusted volume as needed. Wiped off gel from patient and Doppler.

6. Removed and discarded gloves and used supplies in proper receptacle. Performed hand hygiene.

7. Proceeded to next examination or helped patient to comfortable position.

8. Placed nurse call system in an accessible location within patient's reach.

9. Raised side rails (as appropriate) and lowered bed to lowest position, locking into position.

EVALUATION

1. Compared findings with normal assessment characteristics or previous assessments of heart and vascular system.

2. If heart sounds were not audible or pulses were not palpable, asked another nurse to confirm assessment.

3. Asked patient to describe own behaviors that increase risk for heart and vascular disease and how to adopt changes for better health.

4. Asked patient to describe schedule, dosage, purpose, and benefits of medications being taken for cardiovascular health

5. Used Teach-Back. Revised instruction if patient or family caregiver was not able to teach back correctly.

DOCUMENTATION

1. Documented quality, intensity, rate, and rhythm of heart sounds and quality and strength of peripheral pulses.

2. Documented additional cardiac findings, jugular vein distention, and condition of extremities.

3. Documented activity level and subjective data related to fatigue, shortness of breath, and chest pain.

4. Documented evaluation of patient and family caregiver learning.

	S	U	NP	Comments

HAND-OFF REPORTING

1. Reported immediately to health care provider any irregularities in heart function and indications of impaired arterial blood flow.   ___ ___ ___ _____

2. Reported to health care provider changes in peripheral circulation.   ___ ___ ___ _____

Student _____ Date _____

Instructor _____ Date _____

PERFORMANCE CHECKLIST SKILL 6.5 **ABDOMINAL ASSESSMENT**

	S	U	NP	Comments

ASSESSMENT

1. Identified patient; determined patient's level of consciousness, health literacy, and primary language. ___ ___ ___ _____

2. Reviewed EHR for family history of cancer, kidney disease, alcoholism, liver disease, hypertension, or heart disease. ___ ___ ___ _____

3. Reviewed patient's history for risk factors. ___ ___ ___ _____

4. If patient had abdominal or low back pain, assessed the character of pain in detail. ___ ___ ___ _____

5. Observed patient's movement and position. ___ ___ ___ _____

6. Assessed patient's normal bowel habits: frequency of stools; character of stools; recent changes in character of stools; measures used to promote elimination such as laxatives (including frequency), enemas, and dietary intake and eating and drinking habits. ___ ___ ___ _____

7. Assessed if patient had recent weight changes or intolerance to diet. ___ ___ ___ _____

8. Assessed for difficulty in swallowing, belching, flatulence, bloody emesis, black or tarry stools, heartburn, diarrhea, or constipation. ___ ___ ___ _____

9. Determined if patient took antiinflammatory medications, iron supplements, or antibiotics. ___ ___ ___ _____

10. Assessed patient's knowledge, prior experience with abdominal examination, and feelings about procedure. ___ ___ ___ _____

PLANNING

1. Determined expected outcomes following completion of procedure. ___ ___ ___ _____

2. Prepared patient; explained procedure. ___ ___ ___ _____

3. Anticipated topics to teach patient during examination. ___ ___ ___ _____

4. Asked if patient needed to empty bladder or defecate. ___ ___ ___ _____

5. Performed hand hygiene. Prepared necessary supplies at bedside. ___ ___ ___ _____

6. Closed room curtains or door. ___ ___ ___ _____

58

	S	U	NP	Comments

7. Helped patient be as relaxed and comfortable as possible, using a calm tone of voice and purposeful actions. Ensured room was warm. ____ ____ ____ _____

8. Positioned patient supine or in dorsal recumbent position with arms down at sides and knees slightly bent. Option: placed small pillow under patient's knees. Kept upper chest and legs draped. ____ ____ ____ _____

IMPLEMENTATION

1. Moved sheet or blanket to expose area from just above xiphoid process down to symphysis pubis. ____ ____ ____ _____

2. Maintained conversation during assessment except during auscultation. Explained steps calmly and slowly. ____ ____ ____ _____

3. Asked patient to point to any tender abdominal areas. ____ ____ ____ _____

4. Identified landmarks that divide abdominal region into quadrants. ____ ____ ____ _____

5. Inspected skin of surface of abdomen for color, scars, venous patterns, rashes, lesions, silvery white striae, and artificial openings. ____ ____ ____ _____

6. If bruising was noted, asked if patient self-administered injections. ____ ____ ____ _____

7. Inspected contour, symmetry, and surface motion of abdomen. Noted any masses, bulging, or distention. ____ ____ ____ _____

8. If abdomen appeared distended, noted if distention was generalized. Looked at flanks on each side. ____ ____ ____ _____

9. If distention was suspected, measured size of abdominal girth by placing tape measure under patient and around abdomen at level of umbilicus. Used marking pen to indicate where tape measure was applied. ____ ____ ____ _____

10. If patient had an enteral tube connected to suction, turned off momentarily to check bowel sounds. ____ ____ ____ _____

11. To auscultate bowel sounds, placed diaphragm of stethoscope lightly over surface of abdomen. Asked patient not to talk. Listened until repeated gurgling or bubbling sounds were heard. Described sounds as normal, hyperactive, hypoactive, or absent. ____ ____ ____ _____

12. Placed bell of stethoscope over epigastric region of abdomen and each quadrant. Auscultated for vascular sounds. ____ ____ ____ _____

	S	U	NP	Comments

13. Performed routine percussion.

14. Lightly palpated over each abdominal quadrant. Palpated painful areas last. When obvious mass was sensed, applied deep palpation.

    a. Noted muscular resistance, distention, tenderness, and superficial masses or organs while observing patient's face for signs of discomfort.

    b. Noted if abdomen was firm or soft to touch.

15. Just below umbilicus and above symphysis pubis, palpated for smooth, rounded mass. While applying light pressure, asked if patient had sensation of needing to void.

16. If masses were palpated, noted size, location, shape, consistency, tenderness, mobility, and texture.

17. Discarded used supplies in proper receptacle. Performed hand hygiene.

18. Proceeded to next examination or helped patient into comfortable position.

19. Placed nurse call system in an accessible location within patient's reach.

20. Raised side rails (as appropriate) and lowered bed to lowest position, locking into position.

EVALUATION

1. Compared assessment findings with previous assessment characteristics or normal findings to identify changes.

2. Asked patient to describe own risks and signs and symptoms of colorectal cancer.

3. Used Teach-Back. Revised instruction if patient or family caregiver was not able to teach back correctly.

DOCUMENTATION

1. Documented appearance of abdomen, quality and location of bowel sounds, presence of distention, abdominal circumference, and presence and location of tenderness.

2. Documented patient's ability to void and defecate, including description of output.

3. Documented evaluation of patient and family caregiver learning.

HAND-OFF REPORTING

1. Reported serious abnormalities to nurse in charge and health care provider.

Student _____ Date _____

Instructor _____ Date _____

PERFORMANCE CHECKLIST SKILL 6.6 **GENITALIA AND RECTUM ASSESSMENT**

	S	U	NP	Comments

ASSESSMENT

1. Identified patient; determined patient's level of consciousness, primary language, and health literacy. _____ _____ _____ _____

2. Assessment of female patients:

   a. Reviewed EHR or asked if patient had signs and symptoms of vaginal discharge, painful or swollen perianal tissues, or genital lesions. _____ _____ _____ _____

   b. Reviewed electronic health record (EHR) for symptoms or history of GU problems. _____ _____ _____ _____

   c. Asked if the patient had signs of bleeding outside of normal menstrual cycle or after menopause or unusual vaginal discharge. _____ _____ _____ _____

   d. Determined if patient had history of HPV. _____ _____ _____ _____

   e. Reviewed electronic health record (EHR) to determine risk factors for ovarian cancer. _____ _____ _____ _____

   f. Determined if patient had risk factors for endometrial cancer. _____ _____ _____ _____

   g. Assessed patient's knowledge, prior experience with risk factors and signs of cervical and other gynecological cancers, and feelings about procedure. _____ _____ _____ _____

3. Assessment of male patients:

   a. Reviewed normal elimination pattern; history of nocturia; character and volume of urine; daily fluid intake; symptoms of burning, urgency, and frequency; difficulty starting stream; and hematuria. _____ _____ _____ _____

   b. Asked if patient noted penile pain or swelling, genital lesions, or urethral discharge. _____ _____ _____ _____

   c. Asked if patient noted heaviness, painless enlargement, or irregular lumps of testis, and whether testicular self-examination is performed regularly. _____ _____ _____ _____

   d. Asked if patient noted any enlargement in the inguinal area and assessed for potential inguinal hernia. _____ _____ _____ _____

	S	U	NP	Comments

e. Reviewed electronic record (EHR) to assess patient for warning signs of prostatic cancer.

f. Asked if patient had experienced warning signs of advanced prostatic cancer and benign prostatic hypertrophy. Assessed if patient had continuing pain in lower back, pelvis, or upper thighs.

g. Assessed patient's knowledge of examination, risk factors, signs of BPH, and prostate and testicular cancer, as well as feelings about procedure.

4. Assessment of all patients:

   a. Determined whether patient had received HPV vaccine.

   b. Determined whether patient had history of risk factors for colorectal cancer.

   c. Determined whether patient had strong family history of colorectal cancer, polyps, or chronic inflammatory bowel disease.

   d. Inquired about dietary habits, including high fat intake, diet high in processed meats, or deficient fiber content.

   e. Assessed medication history for use of laxatives or cathartic medications.

   f. Assessed for use of codeine or iron preparations.

   g. Assessed patient's knowledge of risks and signs of colorectal cancer.

5. Assessed patient's knowledge, prior experience with genital/rectal examination, and feelings about procedure.

PLANNING

1. Determined expected outcomes following completion of procedure.

2. Anticipated topics to teach patient during examination.

3. Asked if patient needed to empty bladder or defecate.

4. Performed hand hygiene. Prepared necessary supplies at bedside.

5. Closed room curtains or door.

6. Kept upper chest and legs draped and kept room warm.

	S	U	NP	Comments

7. Positioned patient appropriately.

   a. Positioned female in dorsal recumbent position with arms by sides and knees bent with small pillow under knees.

   b. Positioned male in supine position with chest, abdomen, and lower legs draped; or had male patient stand during examination.

IMPLEMENTATION

1. Performed hand hygiene. Applied clean gloves.

2. Performed female genitalia examination; taught about STIs and signs and symptoms of cancers.

   a. Exposed perineal area; repositioned sheet as needed.

   b. Inspected surface characteristics of perineum and retracted labia majora; observed for inflammation, edema, lesions, or lacerations. Noted if there was any vaginal discharge.

3. Performed male genitalia examination; taught about STIs and signs and symptoms of cancer.

   a. Exposed perineal area. Observed genitalia for rashes, excoriations, or lesions.

   b. Inspected and palpated penile surfaces.

      (1) Inspected corona, prepuce, glans, urethral meatus, and shaft. Retracted foreskin in uncircumcised males. Observed for discharge, lesions, edema, and inflammation. Returned foreskin to normal position.

   c. Inspected and palpated testicular surfaces.

      (1) Inspected size, color, shape, and symmetry; noted any lesions or swellling.

   d. Palpated testes.

      (1) Noted size, shape, and consistency of tissue.

      (2) Asked if patient experienced tenderness with palpation.

4. Assessed rectum.

   a. Kept female patient in dorsal recumbent position or had her assume side-lying position.

b. Had male patient stand and bend forward with hips flexed and upper body resting across examination table; examined non-ambulatory patient lying in bed in left lateral position with hips and knees flexed.   ___ ___ ___ _____

c. Viewed perianal and sacrococcygeal areas by gently retracting buttocks with non-dominant hand.   ___ ___ ___ _____

d. Inspected anal tissue for skin characteristics, lesions, external hemorrhoids, inflammation, rashes, and excoriation.   ___ ___ ___ _____

5. Removed and discarded gloves and used supplies in proper receptacle. Performed hand hygiene.   ___ ___ ___ _____

6. Proceeded to next examination or helped patient to comfortable position.   ___ ___ ___ _____

7. Placed nurse call system in an accessible location within patient's reach.   ___ ___ ___ _____

8. Raised side rails (as appropriate) and lowered bed to lowest position, locking in position.   ___ ___ ___ _____

EVALUATION

1. Compared assessment findings with previous assessment characteristics or normal findings to identify changes.   ___ ___ ___ _____

2. Asked patient to list warning signs of colorectal cancer: female patient: cervical, endometrial, and ovarian cancer; male patient: testicular and prostate cancer.   ___ ___ ___ _____

3. Asked male patient to explain how to perform self-exam of genitalia.   ___ ___ ___ _____

4. Asked patient to identify guidelines for HPV vaccination.   ___ ___ ___ _____

5. Used Teach-Back. Revised instruction if patient or family caregiver was not able to teach back correctly.   ___ ___ ___ _____

DOCUMENTATION

1. Documented appearance of genitalia, presence and description of any discharge, and any abnormal findings.   ___ ___ ___ _____

2. Documented patient's ability to void, including description of output.   ___ ___ ___ _____

3. Documented evaluation of patient learning.   ___ ___ ___ _____

HAND-OFF REPORTING

1. Reported any abnormalities to nurse in charge and health care provider.   ___ ___ ___ _____

Student _____ Date _____

Instructor _____ Date _____

PERFORMANCE CHECKLIST SKILL 6.7 **MUSCULOSKELETAL AND NEUROLOGICAL ASSESSMENT**

	S	U	NP	Comments

ASSESSMENT

1. Identified patient; determined patient's level of consciousness, health literacy, and primary language.

2. Assessed EHR for history of risk factors for osteoporosis.

3. Determined if patient had been screened for osteoporosis.

4. Asked patient to describe location and history of changes or problems related to bone, muscle, or joint function.

5. Assessed height and weight. Noted if there was a height decrease in women older than 50 by subtracting current height from recall of maximum adult height.

6. Asked patient to describe nature and extent of musculoskeletal pain. If patient reported pain or cramping in lower extremities, asked if walking or stretching relieved or aggravated it. Assessed distance walked and characteristics of pain before, during, and after activity.

7. Determined if patient used analgesics, antipsychotics, antidepressants, nervous system stimulants, or recreational drugs.

8. Determined if patient had recent history of seizures or convulsions. Clarified sequence of events; character of any symptoms; and relationship to time of day, fatigue, or emotional stress.

9. Screened patient for symptoms of CNS dysfunction.

10. Discussed with spouse, family member, or friends (as appropriate) any recent changes in patient's behavior.

11. Determined if patient had noticed change in vision, hearing, smell, taste, or touch.

	S	U	NP	Comments

12. If patient displayed sudden acute confusion, reviewed history for drug toxicity, serious infections, metabolic disturbances, heart failure, and severe anemia. ___ ___ ___ _____

13. Reviewed history for head or spinal cord injury, meningitis, congenital anomalies, neurological disease, or psychiatric counseling. ___ ___ ___ _____

14. Assessed patient's knowledge, prior experience with neuromuscular assessment and knowledge of osteoporosis, and feelings about procedure. ___ ___ ___ _____

PLANNING

1. Determined expected outcomes following completion of procedure. ___ ___ ___ _____

2. Performed hand hygiene. Prepared necessary supplies at bedside. ___ ___ ___ _____

3. Closed room curtains or doors. ___ ___ ___ _____

4. Prepared patient: ___ ___ ___ _____

   a. Integrated musculoskeletal and neurologic assessments during other parts of physical assessment or during nursing care. ___ ___ ___ _____

   b. Planned time for short rest periods during a comprehensive assessment. ___ ___ ___ _____

IMPLEMENTATION

1. Assessed musculoskeletal system; discussed risks. ___ ___ ___ _____

   a. Made a general observation of extremities. ___ ___ ___ _____

   b. Observed ability to use arms and hands for grasping objects and dressing self. ___ ___ ___ _____

   c. To assess hand grasp strength, crossed own hands and had patient grasp index and middle fingers and squeeze them as hard as possible. ___ ___ ___ _____

   d. To assess strength of lower arms or legs, asked patient to extend or flex the joint being tested. Then had patient resist as force was applied against that muscle contraction. Had patient maintain pressure until told to stop. Compared symmetrical muscle groups. Noted weakness and compared right with left. ___ ___ ___ _____

   e. Observed body alignment for sitting, supine, prone, or standing positions. ___ ___ ___ _____

   f. Inspected gait as patient walked. Had patient use assistive device if appropriate. ___ ___ ___ _____

	S	U	NP	Comments

g. Performed the Banner Mobility Assessment Tool (BMAT) or the "timed up and go (TUG)" test if patient was able to ambulate. ____ ____ ____ _____

h. Stood behind patient and observed postural alignment. Looked sideways at cervical, thoracic, and lumbar curves. ____ ____ ____ _____

i. Gently palpated bones, joints, and surrounding tissue in involved areas. Noted any heat, tenderness, edema, stiffness, or resistance to pressure. Did not attempt to move joint when fracture was suspected, or joint was apparently "frozen" by lack of movement over a long period of time. ____ ____ ____ _____

j. Asked patient to put major joint through its full ROM. Used passive ROM instead for patients with deformities, reduced mobility, joint fixation, or weakness. Observed equality of motion in same body parts. ____ ____ ____ _____

   (1) Active motion: Taught patient to move each joint through its normal range. ____ ____ ____ _____

   (2) Active assisted or Passive motion: Had patient relax and moved same joints passively until end of range was felt. Supported extremity at joint. Did not force joint if there was pain or muscle spasm. ____ ____ ____ _____

k. Assessed muscle tone in major muscle groups. ____ ____ ____ _____

2. Neurological Assessment. ____ ____ ____ _____

a. Assessed LOC and orientation by asking patient to identify name, location, day of week, and year; noted behavior and appearance. ____ ____ ____ _____

b. Assessed CNs: ____ ____ ____ _____

   (1) Assessed CNs III, IV, and VI by assessing extraocular muscles (EOMs). ____ ____ ____ _____

   (2) Assessed CN V by applying light sensation with a cotton ball to symmetrical areas of face; had patient tightly clench teeth and palpated muscles over jaw for tone. ____ ____ ____ _____

   (3) Assessed CN VII by noting facial symmetry while the patient frowned, smiled, puffed out cheeks, and raised eyebrows. ____ ____ ____ _____

	S	U	NP	Comments

(4) Assessed CNs IX and X by having patient speak and swallow. Asked patient to say "ah" while using tongue blade and penlight. Checked for midline uvula and symmetrical rise of uvula and soft palate. Used tongue blade and placed on posterior tongue to elicit gag reflex. Assessed CN XII by inspecting tongue for symmetry, tremors, and movement toward nose and chin. ___ ___ ___ _____

(5) Assessed CN XI by having patient shrug shoulders against resistance, then turn head toward each side against resistance. ___ ___ ___ _____

c. Assessed extremities for sensation. Performed all sensory testing with patient's eyes closed. Used minimal stimulation initially and increased gradually until patient was aware of it. ___ ___ ___ _____

(1) Pain: Asked patient to indicate when sharp or dull sensation was felt on skin. Applied in symmetrical areas of extremities. ___ ___ ___ _____

(2) Light touch: Applied light wisp of cotton to different points along surface of skin in symmetrical areas of extremities. ___ ___ ___ _____

(3) Position: Grasped finger or toe and moved it up and down. Asked patient to state when finger was up or down. Repeated with toes. ___ ___ ___ _____

d. Assessed motor and cerebellar function: ___ ___ ___ _____

(1) Gait: Had patient walk across room, turn, and come back. Similarly noted use of assistive devices. ___ ___ ___ _____

(2) Romberg test: Had patient stand with feet together, arms at sides, both with eyes open, and eyes closed. Protected patient's safety by standing at side; observed for swaying. ___ ___ ___ _____

e. Assessed deep tendon reflexes (DTRs) if appropriate. ___ ___ ___ _____

3. Removed and discarded gloves and used supplies in proper receptacle. Performed hand hygiene. ___ ___ ___ _____

4. Asked patient if he or she had any questions about exam findings. ___ ___ ___ _____

5. Helped patient to a comfortable position. ___ ___ ___ _____

	S	U	NP	Comments

6. Placed nurse call system in an accessible location within patient's reach.

7. Raised side rails (as appropriate) and lowered bed to lowest position, locking into position.

EVALUATION

1. Compared muscle strength, posture, and alignment and ROM with previous physical assessment.

2. Compared neurological status with previous physical assessment.

3. Asked patient to explain personal risks for osteoporosis and falls.

4. Used Teach-Back. Revised instruction if patient or family caregiver was not able to teach back correctly.

DOCUMENTATION

1. Documented posture, gait, muscle strength, ROM, LOC, cognition and orientation, pupillary and other CN responses, and sensation.

2. Documented evaluation of patient and family caregiver learning.

HAND-OFF REPORTING

1. Reported to nurse in charge or health care provider acute pain or sudden muscle weakness, change in LOC, or change in size or pupillary reaction.

Student _____ Date _____

Instructor _____ Date _____

PERFORMANCE CHECKLIST PROCEDURAL GUIDELINE 6.1 **MONITORING INTAKE AND OUTPUT**

	S	U	NP	Comments
PROCEDURAL STEPS				
1. Identified patients with conditions that increase fluid loss.	___	___	___	_____
2. Identified patients with impaired swallowing, unconscious patients, and patients with impaired mobility.	___	___	___	_____
3. Identified patients on medications that influence fluid balance.	___	___	___	_____
4. Assessed signs and symptoms of dehydration and fluid overload.	___	___	___	_____
5. Weighed patients daily using the same scale, the same time of day, and with comparable clothing.	___	___	___	_____
6. Monitored laboratory reports.	___	___	___	_____
7. Assessed patient's and family caregiver's literacy level and knowledge of purpose and process of I&O measurement.	___	___	___	_____
8. Explained to patient and family caregiver importance of I&O measurement.	___	___	___	_____
9. Performed hand hygiene.	___	___	___	_____
10. Measured and documented all fluid intake:	___	___	___	_____
a. Liquids with meals, gelatin, custards, ice cream, popsicles, sherbets, ice chips appropriately using the metric system.	___	___	___	_____
b. Counted liquid medicines such as antacids and fluids with medications as fluid intake.	___	___	___	_____
c. Calculated fluid intake from tube feedings.	___	___	___	_____
d. Calculated fluid intake from parenteral fluids, blood components, and total parenteral nutrition solutions.	___	___	___	_____

70

	S	U	NP	Comments

11. Instructed patient and family caregiver to call you or the AP to empty contents of urinal, urine hat, or commode each time patient used it. Had patient and family monitor incontinence, vomiting, and excessive perspiration and report it to the nurse. ___ ___ ___ _____

12. Informed patient and family caregiver that Foley catheter drainage bag and wound, gastric, or chest tube drainage are closely monitored, measured, and documented and explained who was responsible for this. ___ ___ ___ _____

13. Applied clean gloves. Measured drainage at the end of the shift or as indicated, using appropriate containers and noting color and characteristics. If splashing was anticipated, wore mask, eye protection, and/or gown. ___ ___ ___ _____

   a. Measured urine drainage using a "hat" into which patient voided and a graduated container. ___ ___ ___ _____

   b. Observed color and characteristics of urine in Foley tubing and drainage bag. Measure using bag drainage device or with a graduated container. ___ ___ ___ _____

   c. Measured chest tube drainage by marking and documenting the time on the collection chamber at specified intervals. ___ ___ ___ _____

   d. Measured Jackson-Pratt/Hemovac drainage with a medicine cup. ___ ___ ___ _____

   e. Measured gastric drainage or larger drainage pouches by opening clamp and pouring into graduated cup with a 240-mL capacity. ___ ___ ___ _____

14. Removed gloves and disposed of them in appropriate receptacle. Performed hand hygiene. ___ ___ ___ _____

15. Noted I&O balance or imbalance and reported to health care provider any urine output less than 30 mL/h or significant changes in daily weight. ___ ___ ___ _____

16. Documented intake and output. ___ ___ ___ _____

Student _____   Date _____

Instructor _____   Date _____

PERFORMANCE CHECKLIST SKILL 7.1   **URINE SPECIMEN COLLECTION: MIDSTREAM (CLEAN-VOIDED) URINE; STERILE URINARY CATHETER**

	S	U	NP	Comments

ASSESSMENT

1. Identified patient using at least two identifiers according to agency policy.

2. Reviewed patient's electronic health record (EHR), including health care provider's order and nurses' notes.

3. Reviewed EHR for any pathological conditions that might impair collection of urine specimen or impact results.

4. Referred to agency procedures for specimen collection methods.

5. Assessed patient's/family caregiver's health literacy.

6. Asked patient and checked EHR for history of allergies. Checked allergy bracelet.

7. Performed hand hygiene. Assessed patient's weight, level of consciousness, developmental level, ability to cooperate, and mobility.

8. Assessed for signs and symptoms of urinary tract infection (UTI).

9. Assessed patient's knowledge, prior experience with urine specimen collection, and feelings about procedure.

PLANNING

1. Determined expected outcomes following completion of procedure.

2. Provided privacy. Allowed mobile patients to collect specimen in bathroom.

3. Explained the procedure and what was required of the patient.

4. Obtained and organized equipment, labels, and requisition for urine specimen collection at bedside.

5. Arranged for extra personnel to help if necessary.

72

	S	U	NP	Comments

IMPLEMENTATION

1. Collected clean-voided urine specimen.

   a. Performed hand hygiene and applied clean gloves. Gave patient cleaning towelette or towel, washcloth, and soap to clean perineum or helped with cleaning perineum. Helped bedridden patient onto bedpan to facilitate access to perineum. Removed and disposed of gloves. Performed hand hygiene.

   b. Using aseptic technique, opened outer package of commercial specimen kit.

   c. Applied clean gloves.

   d. Poured antiseptic solution over cotton balls as applicable.

   e. Opened specimen container, maintaining sterility of inside specimen container, and placed cap with sterile inside up. Did not touch inside of cap or container.

   f. Used aseptic technique to help patient or allowed patient to independently clean perineum and collect specimen. Informed patient that antiseptic solution would feel cold.

     (1) Male:

       (a) Held penis with one hand; used circular motion and antiseptic towelette, cleaned meatus, moving from center to outside 3 times with different towelettes. Had uncircumcised male patient retract foreskin for effective cleaning of urinary meatus and keep retracted during voiding. Returned foreskin when done.

       (b) If agency procedure indicated, rinsed area with sterile water and dried with cotton balls or gauze pad.

       (c) After patient had initiated urine stream into toilet or bedpan, had him pass urine specimen container into stream and collect 90–120 mL of urine.

     (2) Female:

       (a) Spread labia minora with fingers of nondominant hand.

    (b) With dominant hand, cleaned urethral area with antiseptic swab. Moved from front to back. Used fresh swab each time; cleaned 3 times; began with farthest labial fold, then closest labial fold, and then down center. ___ ___ ___ _____

    (c) If agency procedure indicated, rinsed area with sterile water and dried with cotton ball. ___ ___ ___ _____

    (d) While continuing to hold labia apart, had patient initiate urine stream into toilet or bedpan; after stream was achieved, passed specimen container into stream and collected 90–120 mL of urine. ___ ___ ___ _____

g. Removed specimen container before flow of urine stopped and before releasing labia or penis. Patient finished voiding into bedpan or toilet. Offered to help with personal hygiene as appropriate. ___ ___ ___ _____

h. Replaced cap securely on specimen container, touching only outside. ___ ___ ___ _____

i. Cleaned urine from exterior surface of container. ___ ___ ___ _____

2. Collected urine from indwelling urinary catheter. ___ ___ ___ _____

a. Explained that syringe would be used without need to remove urine through catheter port and that patient would not experience any discomfort. ___ ___ ___ _____

b. Explained need to clamp catheter for 10–15 min before obtaining urine specimen and that urine could not be obtained from the drainage bag. ___ ___ ___ _____

c. Performed hand hygiene and applied clean gloves. Clamped drainage tubing with clamp or rubber band for as long as 15 min below site chosen for withdrawal. ___ ___ ___ _____

d. After 15 min, positioned patient so catheter sampling port was easily accessible. Cleaned port for 15 s with disinfectant swab and allowed to dry. ___ ___ ___ _____

e. Attached needleless Luer-Lok syringe to built-in catheter sampling port. ___ ___ ___ _____

f. Withdrew 3 mL for culture or 20 mL for routine urinalysis. ___ ___ ___ _____

	S	U	NP	Comments

g. Transferred urine from syringe into clean urine container for routine urinalysis or into sterile urine container for culture. ____ ____ ____ _____

h. Placed lid tightly on container. ____ ____ ____ _____

i. Unclamped catheter and allowed urine to flow into drainage bag. Ensured that urine flowed freely. ____ ____ ____ _____

3. Checked label, then securely attached label to container (not lid). In patient's presence, confirmed label identifiers. If patient was female, indicated if she was menstruating. ____ ____ ____ _____

4. Disposed of soiled supplies. Removed and disposed of gloves and performed hand hygiene. ____ ____ ____ _____

5. Offered patient hand hygiene or provided time to wash hands. ____ ____ ____ _____

6. Helped patient to comfortable position. ____ ____ ____ _____

7. Raised side rails (as appropriate) and lowered bed to lowest position, locking into position. ____ ____ ____ _____

8. Placed nurse call system in an accessible location within patient's reach. ____ ____ ____ _____

9. Sent specimen and completed requisition to laboratory within 20 min. Refrigerated specimen if delay could not be avoided. ____ ____ ____ _____

EVALUATION

1. Inspected clean-voided specimen for contamination with toilet paper or stool. ____ ____ ____ _____

2. Evaluated patient's urine C&S report for bacterial growth. ____ ____ ____ _____

3. Observed urinary drainage system in catheterized patient to ensure that it was intact and patent. ____ ____ ____ _____

4. Used Teach-Back. Revised instruction if patient or family caregiver was not able to teach back correctly. ____ ____ ____ _____

DOCUMENTATION

1. Documented method used to obtain specimen, date and time collected, type of test ordered, laboratory receiving specimen, characteristics of specimen, patient's tolerance to procedure of specimen collection, and time specimen sent to the lab. ____ ____ ____ _____

2. Documented evaluation of patient and family caregiver learning. ____ ____ ____ _____

	S	U	NP	Comments

HAND-OFF REPORTING

1. Reported the type of urinalysis, date and time specimen was sent to laboratory.

___ ___ ___ _____

2. Reported any abnormal findings to health care provider.

___ ___ ___ _____

Student _____ Date _____

Instructor _____ Date _____

PERFORMANCE CHECKLIST PROCEDURAL GUIDELINE 7.1 **COLLECTING A TIMED URINE SPECIMEN**

	S	U	NP	Comments

PROCEDURAL STEPS

1. Identified patient using two identifiers according to agency policy. ___ ___ ___ _____

2. Reviewed health provider's order to determine specific test. ___ ___ ___ _____

3. Assessed patient's/family caregiver's health literacy. ___ ___ ___ _____

4. Explained the reason for specimen collection, how patient could help, and that urine must be free of feces and toilet tissue. ___ ___ ___ _____

5. Assessed patient's knowledge, prior experience with time urine collection, and feelings about procedure. ___ ___ ___ _____

6. Placed specimen collection container in the bathroom and, if indicated, in a pan of ice. ___ ___ ___ _____

   a. Posted signs to remind staff, family and visitors, and patient of timed urine collection on patient's door and toileting area. ___ ___ ___ _____

   b. If patient left unit, ensured that personnel in receiving area collected and saved all urine. ___ ___ ___ _____

7. If possible, had patient drink 2–4 glasses of water about 30 min before times of collection to facilitate ability to void at the appropriate time for test to begin. ___ ___ ___ _____

8. Performed hand hygiene and applied clean gloves. Discarded the first voided specimen as the test began. Indicated time test began on laboratory requisition. Began collecting all urine for designated time. Removed and disposed of gloves and performed hand hygiene. ___ ___ ___ _____

9. Measured volume of each voiding if I&O was to be documented. Placed all voided urine in labeled specimen bottle with appropriate additives. ___ ___ ___ _____

10. Unless instructed otherwise, kept specimen bottle in specimen refrigerator or container of ice in bathroom to prevent decomposition of urine. ___ ___ ___ _____

	S	U	NP	Comments

11. Encouraged patient to drink two glasses of water 1 h before timed urine collection ended. Encouraged patient to empty bladder during last 15 min of urine collection period. ___ ___ ___ _____

12. Performed hand hygiene and applied clean gloves. Collected final specimen at end of collection period. Labeled specimen in patient's presence, attached appropriate requisition, and sent to laboratory. Removed and disposed of gloves and performed hand hygiene. Disposed of all contaminated supplies in appropriate receptacle. ___ ___ ___ _____

13. Removed signs. Told patient that specimen collection period was completed. ___ ___ ___ _____

14. Raised side rails (as appropriate) and lowered bed to lowest position, locking into position. ___ ___ ___ _____

15. Placed nurse call system in an accessible location within patient's reach. ___ ___ ___ _____

16. Used Teach-Back. Revised instruction if patient or family caregiver was not able to teach back correctly. ___ ___ ___ _____

17. Placed specimen in biohazard bag or container per agency policy and delivered to appropriate laboratory. ___ ___ ___ _____

18. Documented time 24-hour specimen collection was completed and time sent to lab. ___ ___ ___ _____

19. Provided hand-off report to health care provider of any changes or abnormal findings. ___ ___ ___ _____

Student _____ Date _____

Instructor _____ Date _____

PERFORMANCE CHECKLIST SKILL 7.2 **MEASURING OCCULT BLOOD IN STOOL**

	S	U	NP	Comments

ASSESSMENT

1. Identified patient using at least two identifiers according to agency policy.. ___ ___ ___ _____

2. Reviewed patient's EHR, including health care provider's order and nurses' notes. Noted any health care provider's orders for medication or dietary modifications or restrictions before test. ___ ___ ___ _____

3. Reviewed patient's EHR for GI disorders. ___ ___ ___ _____

4. Reviewed patient's EHR for any patient medications that contribute to bleeding. ___ ___ ___ _____

5. Assessed patient's/family caregiver's health literacy. ___ ___ ___ _____

6. Performed hand hygiene. Assessed patient's weight, level of consciousness, developmental level, ability to cooperate, and mobility. ___ ___ ___ _____

7. Assessed patient's knowledge, prior experience with stool specimen collection, and feelings about procedure. ___ ___ ___ _____

PLANNING

1. Determined expected outcomes following completion of procedure. ___ ___ ___ _____

2. Arranged for any needed dietary or medication restrictions. ___ ___ ___ _____

3. Provided privacy and explained procedure to patient and/or family caregiver. Discussed reason for specimen collection and how patient could help. Explained that feces must be free of urine and toilet tissue. ___ ___ ___ _____

4. Organized and set up any equipment needed to perform procedure. ___ ___ ___ _____

5. Arranged for extra personnel to help as necessary. Organized supplies at bedside. ___ ___ ___ _____

IMPLEMENTATION

1. Performed hand hygiene and applied clean gloves. Obtained uncontaminated stool specimen and placed in clean, dry container not contaminated with urine, water, or toilet tissue. ___ ___ ___ _____

	S	U	NP	Comments

2. Obtained two pieces of stool from two different areas of the specimen using a new wooden applicator for each of the two pieces.   ___ ___ ___ _____

3. Measured for occult blood.   ___ ___ ___ _____

   a. Performed Hemoccult slide test: ___ ___ ___ _____

      (1) Opened flap of Hemoccult slide. Applied thin smear of stool on paper in first box.   ___ ___ ___ _____

      (2) Obtained second fecal specimen from different part of stool with a new applicator and applied thinly to second box of slide.   ___ ___ ___ _____

      (3) Closed slide cover and turned slide over to reverse side. Opened cardboard flap and applied 2 drops of Hemoccult developing solution on each box of guaiac paper.   ___ ___ ___ _____

      (4) Read results of test after 30–60 seconds. Noted color changes.   ___ ___ ___ _____

      (5) Disposed of test slide in proper receptacle.   ___ ___ ___ _____

   b. Performed test using Hematest tablets: ___ ___ ___ _____

      (1) Placed stool on guaiac paper. Then placed Hematest tablet on top of stool specimen. Applied 2 to 3 drops of tap water to tablet, allowing water to flow onto guaiac paper.   ___ ___ ___ _____

      (2) Observed color of guaiac paper within 2 minutes.   ___ ___ ___ _____

      (3) Disposed of tablet and paper in proper receptacle.   ___ ___ ___ _____

4. Wrapped wooden applicator in paper towel, grasped in nondominant hand, removed gloves over wrapped applicator and discarded soiled supplies, and performed hand hygiene.   ___ ___ ___ _____

5. Raised side rails (as appropriate) and lowered bed to lowest position, locking into position.   ___ ___ ___ _____

6. Placed nurse call system in an accessible location within patient's reach.   ___ ___ ___ _____

EVALUATION

1. Noted color changes in guaiac paper.   ___ ___ ___ _____

2. Used Teach-Back. Revised instruction if patient or family caregiver was not able to teach back correctly.   ___ ___ ___ _____

3. Noted character of stool specimen.   ___ ___ ___ _____

DOCUMENTATION

1. Documented results of test and stool characteristics.   ___ ___ ___ _____

	S	U	NP	Comments
2. Documented evaluation of patient and family caregiver learning.	___	___	___	_____

HAND-OFF REPORTING

	S	U	NP	Comments
1. Reported positive test results to health care provider.	___	___	___	_____

Student _____ Date _____

Instructor _____ Date _____

PERFORMANCE CHECKLIST SKILL 7.3　**MEASURING OCCULT BLOOD IN GASTRIC SECRETIONS (GASTROCCULT)**

	S	U	NP	Comments

ASSESSMENT

1. Identified patient using at least two identifiers according to agency policy. ___ ___ ___ _____

2. Reviewed patient's EHR, including health care provider's order and nurses' notes. Noted if occult blood was found previously in gastric secretions. ___ ___ ___ _____

3. Reviewed patient's EHR for patient's medical history for bleeding or GI disorders and drugs that predispose the patient to increased risk of bleeding. ___ ___ ___ _____

4. Assessed patient's/family caregiver's health literacy. ___ ___ ___ _____

5. Assessed patient's knowledge, prior experience with screening for occult blood in gastric secretions, and feelings about procedure. ___ ___ ___ _____

PLANNING

1. Determined expected outcomes following completion of procedure. ___ ___ ___ _____

2. Explained procedure to patient and/or family caregiver. Discussed why specimen collection was necessary. ___ ___ ___ _____

3. Provided privacy and explained procedure. ___ ___ ___ _____

4. Organized and set up any equipment needed to perform procedure. ___ ___ ___ _____

IMPLEMENTATION

1. Performed hand hygiene. Applied clean gloves. ___ ___ ___ _____

2. Verified NG tube placement. ___ ___ ___ _____

3. Obtained specimen. ___ ___ ___ _____

   a. Disconnect suction or gravity drainage tube from NG or NE tube. Using a bulb or catheter tip syringe, aspirate 5 to 10 mL of fluid from NG or NE tube. ___ ___ ___ _____

   b. To obtain sample of emesis, use 3-mL syringe or wooden applicator to obtain sample from emesis basin. ___ ___ ___ _____

4. Performed Gastroccult test: ___ ___ ___ _____

	S	U	NP	Comments

a. Using wooden applicator or syringe, applied 1 drop of gastric sample to Gastroccult blood test slide. ___ ___ ___ _____

b. Applied 2 drops of commercial developer solution over sample and 1 drop between positive and negative performance monitors. ___ ___ ___ _____

c. Verified that performance monitor turned blue in 30 seconds. ___ ___ ___ _____

d. After 60 seconds, compared color of gastric sample with that of performance monitor. ___ ___ ___ _____

5. Disposed of test slide, wooden applicator, and syringe in proper receptacle. If needed, reconnected enteral tube to drainage system or suction. Removed and disposed of gloves. Performed hand hygiene. ___ ___ ___ _____

6. Raised side rails (as appropriate) and lowered bed to lowest position, locking into position. ___ ___ ___ _____

7. Placed nurse call system in an accessible location within patient's reach. ___ ___ ___ _____

EVALUATION

1. Noted character of gastric secretions. ___ ___ ___ _____

2. Noted color changes in guaiac paper. ___ ___ ___ _____

3. Used Teach-Back. Revised instruction if patient or family caregiver was not able to teach back correctly. ___ ___ ___ _____

DOCUMENTATION

1. Documented results of test and presence of any unusual characteristics of gastric contents. ___ ___ ___ _____

2. Documented evaluation of patient and family caregiver learning. ___ ___ ___ _____

HAND-OFF REPORTING

1. Reported positive test results to health care provider. ___ ___ ___ _____

Student _____ Date _____

Instructor _____ Date _____

PERFORMANCE CHECKLIST SKILL 7.4 **COLLECTING NOSE AND THROAT SPECIMENS FOR CULTURE**

	S	U	NP	Comments

ASSESSMENT

1. Identified patient using at least two identifiers.

2. Reviewed patient's electronic health record (EHR), including health care provider's order and nurses' notes. Noted if nose, throat, or both cultures were needed.

3. Reviewed patient's EHR to determine if patient had a fever, chills, or other signs of infection.

4. Assessed patient's/family caregiver's health literacy.

5. Asked whether patient was experiencing post-nasal drip, sinus headache or tenderness, nasal congestion, sore throat, or had exposure to others with similar symptoms.

6. Performed hand hygiene and applied clean gloves. Assessed condition of posterior pharynx.

7. Inspected condition of nares and drainage from nasal mucosa and sinuses.

8. Assessed patient's knowledge, prior experience with nose or throat cultures, and feelings about procedure.

PLANNING

1. Determined expected outcomes following completion of procedure.

2. Planned to do culture before mealtime or at least 1 hour after eating.

3. Provided privacy and explained procedure to patient and/or family caregiver. Discussed reason for specimen collection and how patient could help.

4. Explained sensations to expect during procedure.

5. Organized and set up any equipment needed to perform procedure.

6. Arranged for extra personnel to help, as necessary.

84

	S	U	NP	Comments

IMPLEMENTATION

1. Had swab in tube ready for use. Loosened top so swab could be removed easily. ____ ____ ____ _____

2. Asked patient to sit erect in bed or chair. Positioned acutely ill patient or young child in bed with head of bed raised to 45-degree angle in semi-Fowler position. ____ ____ ____ _____

3. Collected throat culture. ____ ____ ____ _____

   a. Performed hand hygiene and applied clean gloves. ____ ____ ____ _____

   b. Instructed patient to tilt head backward. For patients in bed, placed pillow behind shoulders. ____ ____ ____ _____

   c. Asked patient to open mouth and say "ah." To visualize pharynx, depressed tongue with tongue blade and noted inflamed areas of pharynx or tonsils. Depressed anterior third of tongue only and illuminated with penlight as needed. ____ ____ ____ _____

   d. Inserted swab without touching lips, teeth, tongue, cheeks, or uvula. ____ ____ ____ _____

   e. Gently but quickly swabbed tonsillar area side to side, contacting inflamed or purulent sites. ____ ____ ____ _____

   f. Carefully withdrew swab without touching oral structures. ____ ____ ____ _____

4. Collected nasal culture ____ ____ ____ _____

   a. Performed hand hygiene and applied clean gloves. ____ ____ ____ _____

   b. Encouraged patient to blow nose and then checked nostrils for patency with penlight. Selected nostril with greatest patency. ____ ____ ____ _____

   c. In sitting position, had patient tilt head backward. Provided patients in bed with a small pillow behind shoulders. ____ ____ ____ _____

   d. Gently inserted nasal speculum in one nostril. ____ ____ ____ _____

   e. Carefully passed swab into nostril until it reached that part of mucosa that was inflamed or containing exudate. Rotated swab quickly. ____ ____ ____ _____

   f. Removed swab without touching sides of speculum or nasal canal. ____ ____ ____ _____

	S	U	NP	Comments

g. Carefully removed nasal speculum (if used) and placed in basin. Offered patient facial tissue.

5. Inserted swab into culture tube. Used gauze to protect fingers while crushing ampule at bottom of tube to release culture medium.

6. Placed tip of swab into liquid medium and placed top securely on top of tube.

7. Securely attached completed identification label and laboratory requisition to culture tube and confirmed identifiers, specimen source, and collection date and time in front of patient, according to agency policy. Noted on laboratory requisition if patient was taking antibiotic or if specific organism was suspected.

8. Enclosed specimen in plastic biohazard bag (according to agency policy) and sent immediately to laboratory.

9. Returned patient to position of comfort. Removed and disposed of gloves and performed hand hygiene.

10. Raised side rails (as appropriate) and lowered bed to lowest position, locking into position.

11. Placed nurse call system in an accessible location within patient's reach.

EVALUATION

1. Checked laboratory record for results of culture test.

2. Used Teach-Back. Revised instruction if patient or family caregiver was not able to teach back correctly.

DOCUMENTATION

1. Documented appearance of nasal and oral mucosal structure; documented specimen; and time sent to laboratory.

2. Documented evaluation of patient and family caregiver learning.

HAND-OFF REPORTING

1. Reported unusual test results to health care provider.

Student _____   Date _____

Instructor _____   Date _____

PERFORMANCE CHECKLIST SKILL 7.5   **OBTAINING VAGINAL OR URETHRAL DISCHARGE SPECIMENS**

	S	U	NP	Comments
ASSESSMENT				
1. Identified patient using at least two identifiers.	—	—	—	_____
2. Reviewed patient's electronic health record (EHR), including health care provider's order to determine if culture was to be vaginal or urethral.	—	—	—	_____
3. Reviewed patient's EHR to determine if patient had a fever, chills, or other signs of infection.	—	—	—	_____
4. Assessed patient's/family caregiver's health literacy.	—	—	—	_____
5. Asked patient about dysuria, localized pruritus of genitalia, or lower abdominal pain.	—	—	—	_____
6. If symptoms suggested STI, gathered and documented patient's sexual history.	—	—	—	_____
7. Performed hand hygiene and applied clean gloves. Positioned patient and assessed condition of external genitalia and urethra, meatus, and vaginal orifice. Observed for redness; swelling; complaint of tenderness; and discharge that was whitish, mucoid, or purulent or resembled cottage cheese. Removed and disposed of gloves and performed hand hygiene. Alternately performed this step during collection.	—	—	—	_____
8. Assessed patient's knowledge, prior experience with vaginal or urethral swab, and feelings about procedure.	—	—	—	_____
PLANNING				
1. Determined expected outcomes following completion of procedure.	—	—	—	_____
2. Provided privacy and explained procedure to patient and/or family caregiver. Discussed reason for specimen collection and how patient could help. Instructed female patient not to douche 24 hours before culture was to be obtained. Instructed male patients not to urinate 1 hour before urethral culture was to be obtained.	—	—	—	_____
3. Organized and set up equipment needed to perform procedure.	—	—	—	_____

	S	U	NP	Comments

4. Arranged for extra personnel, usually of the same gender as the patient, to assist specimen collection. Organized supplies at bedside.

IMPLEMENTATION

1. Drew bedside curtains or closed room door. Placed "Do Not Enter" sign on door (if available).

2. Performed hand hygiene and applied clean gloves.

3. Helped patient to proper position, raised gown, and draped body parts to be exposed:

   a. Female: Positioned in dorsal recumbent position with sheet draped over each leg and genitalia.

   b. Male: Positioned sitting on chair or bed or lying supine with sheet draped across lower trunk and genitalia.

4. Directed light source onto perineum as needed.

5. Opened culture tube and held swab in dominant hand.

6. Instructed patient to deep breathe slowly.

7. Obtained specimens.

   a. Female:

   (1) With nondominant hand, fully separated labia to expose vaginal orifice.

   (2) Touched tip of swab into discharge pool, being careful not to touch skin or mucosa along perineum or vaginal canal. If no discharge was visible, gently inserted swab 1–2.5 cm (1/3–1 inch) into vaginal orifice and rotated before removal.

   (3) To expose urethral meatus, used nondominant hand to pull gently on labia minora upward and back to separate.

   (4) Used clean swab; gently applied to tip of meatus where discharge was visible. Avoided touching labia.

   b. Male:

   (1) Grasped patient's penis proximal to glans with nondominant hand; if male was uncircumcised, gently retracted foreskin.

   (2) Used dominant hand to hold swab. Applied gently to area of discharge at urinary meatus.

	S	U	NP	Comments

(3) If no discharge was apparent, health care provider may have ordered swab to be introduced into urinary meatus. Held male genitalia firmly but gently. ___ ___ ___ _____

(4) Returned foreskin to natural position. ___ ___ ___ _____

8. Returned each swab to culture tube and secured top. ___ ___ ___ _____

9. If using commercial culture tube, wrapped ampule with gauze to prevent injury to fingers while crushing. Immediately squeezed end of tube to crush ampule. Pushed tip of swab into fluid medium. ___ ___ ___ _____

10. Removed and disposed of gloves. Performed hand hygiene. ___ ___ ___ _____

11. Labeled each culture tube with identification label, affixed completed requisition, and confirmed identifiers in front of patient. ___ ___ ___ _____

12. Sent specimen to laboratory immediately or refrigerated. ___ ___ ___ _____

13. Helped patient to comfortable position, helped with personal hygiene, and removed and discarded drape. Performed hand hygiene. ___ ___ ___ _____

14. Raised side rails (as appropriate) and lowered bed to lowest position, locking into position. ___ ___ ___ _____

15. Placed nurse call system in an accessible location within patient's reach. ___ ___ ___ _____

EVALUATION

1. Reviewed laboratory results for evidence of pathogens. ___ ___ ___ _____

2. Continued to monitor whether discharge was present; if so, observed color and amount. ___ ___ ___ _____

3. Used Teach-Back. Revised instruction if patient or family caregiver was not able to teach back correctly. ___ ___ ___ _____

DOCUMENTATION

1. Documented types of cultures obtained and date and time sent to laboratory. ___ ___ ___ _____

2. Documented evaluation of patient and family caregiver learning. ___ ___ ___ _____

HAND-OFF REPORTING

1. Reported laboratory results to health care provider. ___ ___ ___ _____

2. Reported abnormal findings. ___ ___ ___ _____

Student _____ Date _____

Instructor _____ Date _____

PERFORMANCE CHECKLIST PROCEDURAL GUIDELINE 7.2 **COLLECTING A SPUTUM SPECIMEN BY EXPECTORATION**

	S	U	NP	Comments

PROCEDURAL STEPS

1. Identified the patient using at least two identifiers. ___ ___ ___ _____

2. Provided opportunity to clean or rinse mouth with water. Did not use mouthwash or toothpaste. ___ ___ ___ _____

3. Assessed patient's/family caregiver's health literacy. ___ ___ ___ _____

4. Assessed patient's knowledge, prior experience with sputum collection, and feelings about procedure. ___ ___ ___ _____

5. Provided privacy and explained procedure to patient. ___ ___ ___ _____

6. Performed hand hygiene and applied clean gloves. Provided sputum cup and instructed patient not to touch the inside of the container. ___ ___ ___ _____

7. Had the patient take three to four deep, slow breaths with full exhalation. Then had patient take a full inhalation followed immediately by a forceful cough, expectorating sputum directly into specimen container. ___ ___ ___ _____

8. Repeated until 5–10 mL of sputum (not saliva) had been collected. ___ ___ ___ _____

9. Secured lid on container tightly. If any sputum was present on outside of container, wiped it off with disinfectant. ___ ___ ___ _____

10. Offered patient tissues after patient expectorated, disposed of tissues, and offered mouth care. ___ ___ ___ _____

11. Securely attached properly completed identification label and laboratory requisition to side of specimen container (not lid). Confirmed identifiers in patient's presence. ___ ___ ___ _____

12. Enclosed specimen in a biohazard bag. ___ ___ ___ _____

13. Removed and disposed of gloves. Performed hand hygiene. ___ ___ ___ _____

14. Helped patient to a comfortable position. ___ ___ ___ _____

	S	U	NP	Comments

15. Raised side rails (as appropriate) and lowered bed to lowest position, locking into position. ____ ____ ____ _____

16. Placed nurse call system in an accessible location within patient's reach. ____ ____ ____ _____

17. Sent specimen to laboratory immediately. ____ ____ ____ _____

18. Used Teach-Back. Revised instruction if patient or family caregiver was not able to teach back correctly. ____ ____ ____ _____

19. Documented time sputum specimen collection was completed and sent to lab. ____ ____ ____ _____

20. Provided handoff report to health care provider including any changes, abnormal findings, or respiratory distress. ____ ____ ____ _____

Student _____ Date _____

Instructor _____ Date _____

PERFORMANCE CHECKLIST SKILL 7.6   **COLLECTING A SPUTUM SPECIMEN BY SUCTION**

	S	U	NP	Comments

ASSESSMENT

1. Identified patient using at least two identifiers.   ___ ___ ___ _____

2. Reviewed electronic health record (EHR) for health care provider's orders for type of sputum analysis and specifications.   ___ ___ ___ _____

3. Assessed patient's/family caregiver's health literacy.   ___ ___ ___ _____

4. Assessed EHR for contraindication to airway suctioning.   ___ ___ ___ _____

5. Assessed when patient last ate meal or had tube feeding.   ___ ___ ___ _____

6. Determined type of help needed by patient to obtain specimen.   ___ ___ ___ _____

7. Performed hand hygiene and performed a respiratory assessment, including respiratory rate, depth, and pattern and color of mucous membranes. Measured BP and attached pulse oximeter and measured oxygen saturation.   ___ ___ ___ _____

8. Assessed patient's knowledge, prior experience with collecting a sputum specimen by suctioning, and feelings about procedure.   ___ ___ ___ _____

PLANNING

1. Determined expected outcomes following completion of procedure.   ___ ___ ___ _____

2. Provided privacy and explained steps of procedure and purpose. Instructed patient to breathe normally during suctioning to prevent hyperventilation.   ___ ___ ___ _____

3. Gathered and organized supplies at bedside.   ___ ___ ___ _____

4. Prepared suction machine or device and determined whether it functioned properly.   ___ ___ ___ _____

5. Positioned patient in high- or semi-Fowler position.   ___ ___ ___ _____

IMPLEMENTATION

1. Performed hand hygiene and applied clean glove to nondominant hand. Prepared suction machine or device and determined if it functioned properly.   ___ ___ ___ _____

2. Connected suction tube to adapter on sputum trap. Opened sterile water.   ___ ___ ___ _____

92

	S	U	NP	Comments

3. Using sterile technique, applied sterile glove to dominant hand or used a clean glove if suction catheter had plastic sleeve. ___ ___ ___ _____

4. With gloved hand connected sterile suction catheter to rubber tubing on sputum trap. ___ ___ ___ _____

5. Lubricated suction catheter tip with sterile water (with suction off). ___ ___ ___ _____

6. Gently inserted tip of suction catheter through nasopharynx, endotracheal tube, or tracheostomy tube without applying suction. ___ ___ ___ _____

7. Gently and quickly advanced catheter into trachea. Warned patient to expect to cough. ___ ___ ___ _____

8. As patient coughed, applied suction for 5–10 seconds, collecting 2–10 mL of sputum. ___ ___ ___ _____

9. Released suction and removed catheter; turned off suction. ___ ___ ___ _____

10. Detached catheter from specimen trap and disposed of catheter in appropriate receptacle. ___ ___ ___ _____

11. Secured top on specimen container tightly. For sputum trap, detached suction tubing and connected rubber tubing on sputum trap to plastic adapter. ___ ___ ___ _____

12. If any sputum was present on outside of container, wiped it off with disinfectant. ___ ___ ___ _____

13. Offered patient tissues after suctioning. Disposed of tissues in emesis basin or appropriate container. ___ ___ ___ _____

14. Labeled specimen with identification label on side of specimen container (not lid). Confirmed identifiers in front of patient. Placed specimen in biohazard bag (or container specified by agency) and attached requisition. ___ ___ ___ _____

15. Removed and disposed of gloves. Performed hand hygiene. ___ ___ ___ _____

16. Offered patient mouth care if desired. Helped patient to comfortable position. ___ ___ ___ _____

17. Raised side rails (as appropriate) and lowered bed to lowest position, locking into position. ___ ___ ___ _____

18. Placed nurse call system in an accessible location within patient's reach. ___ ___ ___ _____

19. Sent specimen immediately to laboratory or refrigerated. ___ ___ ___ _____

	S	U	NP	Comments

EVALUATION

1. Observed patient's respiratory status throughout procedure, especially during suctioning. If in distress, measured oxygen saturation with pulse oximeter. ___ ___ ___ _____

2. Noted anxiety or discomfort in patient. ___ ___ ___ _____

3. Observed character of sputum. ___ ___ ___ _____

4. Referred to laboratory reports for test results. ___ ___ ___ _____

5. Used Teach-Back. Revised instruction if patient or family caregiver was not able to teach back correctly. ___ ___ ___ _____

DOCUMENTATION

1. Documented the method used to obtain specimen, type of test ordered, date and time collected, and transported to laboratory. Described characteristics of sputum specimen. Described patient's tolerance of procedure. ___ ___ ___ _____

2. Documented evaluation of patient and family caregiver learning. ___ ___ ___ _____

3. Documented on specimen requisition if patient was receiving antibiotics and name of antibiotic. ___ ___ ___ _____

HAND-OFF REPORTING

1. Reported any change in respiratory status and/or unusual sputum characteristics to nurse in charge or health care provider. ___ ___ ___ _____

2. Reported abnormal findings to health care provider. If acid-fast bacillus sputum culture was positive, initiated appropriate isolation techniques. ___ ___ ___ _____

Student _____ Date _____

Instructor _____ Date _____

PERFORMANCE CHECKLIST SKILL 7.7 **OBTAINING WOUND DRAINAGE SPECIMENS**

	S	U	NP	Comments

ASSESSMENT

1. Identified patient using at least two identifiers according to agency policy.

2. Reviewed patient's electronic health record (EHR), including health care provider's order. Noted if specimen was for aerobic or anaerobic culture.

3. Reviewed patient's EHR for fever, and if laboratory results reported whether white blood cell (WBC) count was elevated.

4. Assessed patient's/family caregiver's health literacy.

5. Asked patient about extent and type of pain at wound site and use a scale of 0 to 10 to assess severity. If patient required analgesic before dressing changes, gave medication 30 minutes before beginning procedure to reach peak effect.

6. Determined when dressing change was scheduled. Performed wound assessment as part of actual procedure.

7. Performed hand hygiene and applied clean gloves. Removed old dressings covering wound. Folded soiled sides of dressing together and disposed of properly. Removed and disposed of gloves and performed hand hygiene. Applied sterile gloves to palpate wound. Observed for swelling, separation of wound edges, inflammation, and drainage. Palpated gently along wound edges and noted tenderness or drainage. Removed and disposed of gloves and performed hand hygiene.

8. Assessed patient's knowledge, prior experience with wound specimen collection, and feelings about procedure.

PLANNING

1. Determined expected outcomes following completion of procedure.

2. Determined if analgesia was necessary. Administered analgesic 30 minutes before dressing change and/or specimen collection.

	S	U	NP	Comments

3. Provided privacy and explained reason for wound culture and how it would be collected.   ____ ____ ____ _____

4. Explained that patient might feel tickling sensation when wound was swabbed.   ____ ____ ____ _____

5. Organized and set up equipment needed to perform procedure.   ____ ____ ____ _____

6. Arranged for extra personnel to help as necessary. Organized supplies at bedside.   ____ ____ ____ _____

IMPLEMENTATION

1. Performed hand hygiene and applied clean gloves.   ____ ____ ____ _____

2. Cleaned area around wound edges with antiseptic swab or sterile saline as ordered. Wiped from edges outward. Removed old exudate.   ____ ____ ____ _____

3. Discarded swab and removed and disposed of soiled gloves in appropriate receptacle. Performed hand hygiene.   ____ ____ ____ _____

4. Opened packages containing sterile culture tube and dressing supplies. Applied sterile gloves.   ____ ____ ____ _____

5. Obtained cultures.   ____ ____ ____ _____

   a. Aerobic culture

     (1) Took swab from culture tube, inserted tip into wound in area of drainage, and rotated swab gently. Removed swab and returned to culture tube (wrapped outside of ampule with gauze to prevent injury). Crushed ampule of medium and pushed swab into fluid.   ____ ____ ____ _____

   b. Anaerobic culture

     (1) Took swab from special anaerobic culture tube, swabbed deeply into draining body cavity of viable tissue, and rotated gently. Removed swab and returned to culture tube.   ____ ____ ____ _____

   Or

     (2) Inserted tip of syringe (without needle) into wound and aspirated 5–10 mL of exudate. Attached 19-gauge needle, expelled all air, and injected drainage into special culture tube.   ____ ____ ____ _____

6. Removed and disposed of gloves. Performed hand hygiene.   ____ ____ ____ _____

7. Placed correct specimen label on each culture tube. Verified identifiers in front of patient. NOTE: Indicated on specimen if patient was receiving antibiotics.   ____ ____ ____ _____

	S	U	NP	Comments

8. Sent specimens to laboratory within 30 minutes.

9. Cleaned wound per health care provider's order. Applied new sterile dressing using aseptic technique. Secured dressing with tape or ties.

10. Removed and disposed of gloves and soiled supplies in appropriate receptacle according to agency policy. Performed hand hygiene.

11. Helped patient to comfortable position.

12. Raised side rails (as appropriate) and lowered bed to lowest position, locking into position.

13. Placed nurse call system in an accessible location within patient's reach.

EVALUATION

1. Obtained laboratory report for results of cultures.

2. Observed character of wound drainage.

3. Observed edges of wound for redness and bleeding.

4. Used Teach-Back. Revised instruction if patient or family caregiver was not able to teach back correctly.

DOCUMENTATION

1. Documented types of specimens obtained, source, and time and date sent to laboratory and described appearance of wound and characteristics of any drainage.

2. Documented evaluation of patient and family caregiver learning.

3. Documented patient's tolerance of procedure, dressing change, and response to analgesics.

HAND-OFF REPORTING

1. Reported any evidence of infection to the health care provider.

Student _____ Date _____

Instructor _____ Date _____

PERFORMANCE CHECKLIST SKILL 7.8   **COLLECTING BLOOD SPECIMENS AND CULTURE BY VENIPUNCTURE (SYRINGE AND VACUTAINER METHOD)**

	S	U	NP	Comments

ASSESSMENT

1. Identified patient using at least two identifiers.

2. Reviewed patient's electronic health record (EHR) for health care provider's orders for type of tests.

3. Reviewed patient's EHR for possible risks associated with venipuncture.

4. Assessed patient's or family caregiver's health literacy.

5. Determined if special conditions needed to be met before specimen collection.

6. Performed hand hygiene and assessed patient for contraindicated sites for venipuncture.

7. Identified patient's risk for medical adhesive sensitivities.

8. Identified if patient allergic to latex or povidone-iodine (Betadine) or other antiseptic.

9. Before drawing blood cultures, assessed for systemic signs and symptoms of bacteremia, including fever and chills.

10. Assessed patient's knowledge, prior experience with blood collection, and feelings about procedure.

PLANNING

1. Determined expected outcomes following completion of procedure.

2. Provided privacy and explained procedure to patient.

3. Gathered and organized equipment at bedside.

IMPLEMENTATION

1. Raised or lowered bed to comfortable working height.

98

	S	U	NP	Comments

2. Performed hand hygiene and applied gloves. Helped patient to supine or semi-Fowler position with arms extended to form straight line from shoulders to wrists. Placed small pillow or towel under upper arm. (Option: Lowered arm briefly so it filled veins in hand and arm with blood.) ____ ____ ____ _____

3. Applied tourniquet so it could be removed by pulling one end with a single motion. ____ ____ ____ _____

   a. Positioned tourniquet 5–10 cm (2–4 inches) above venipuncture site selected. ____ ____ ____ _____

   b. Crossed tourniquet over patient's arm. ____ ____ ____ _____

   c. Held tourniquet between fingers close to arm. Tucked loop between patient's arm and tourniquet. ____ ____ ____ _____

4. Did not keep tourniquet on patient longer than 1 minute. ____ ____ ____ _____

5. Quickly inspected extremity for best venipuncture site, looking for straight, prominent vein without swelling or hematoma. ____ ____ ____ _____

6. Palpated selected vein with finger. Noted if vein was firm and rebounded when palpated or if it felt rigid or cordlike and rolled when palpated. Avoided vigorously slapping vein, which can cause vasospasm. ____ ____ ____ _____

7. Obtained blood specimen. ____ ____ ____ _____

   a. Syringe method

     (1) Had syringe with appropriate needle securely attached. ____ ____ ____ _____

     (2) Cleaned venipuncture site with antiseptic swab, allowed to dry. ____ ____ ____ _____

       (a) If drawing sample for blood alcohol level or blood cultures, used only antiseptic swab rather than alcohol swab. ____ ____ ____ _____

     (3) Removed needle cover and checked needle for burrs. ____ ____ ____ _____

     (4) Placed thumb or forefinger of nondominant hand 2.5 cm (1 inch) below site and gently pulled skin taut. Stretched skin steadily until vein was stabilized. ____ ____ ____ _____

     (5) Held syringe and needle at 15- to 30-degree angle from patient's arm with bevel up. ____ ____ ____ _____

     (6) Slowly inserted needle into vein, stopping when "pop" was felt as needle entered vein. ____ ____ ____ _____

	S	U	NP	Comments

(7) Held syringe securely and pulled back gently on plunger.

(8) Observed for blood return.

(9) Obtained desired amount of blood, kept needle stabilized.

(10) After obtaining specimen, released tourniquet.

(11) Applied 2 × 2–inch gauze pad without applying pressure. Quickly withdrew needle from vein.

(12) Immediately applied pressure over venipuncture site with gauze or antiseptic pad for 2 to 3 minutes or until bleeding stopped. Observed for hematoma. Taped gauze dressing securely.

(13) Activated safety cover and immediately discarded needle in appropriate container.

(14) Attached blood-filled syringe to needle-free blood transfer device. Attached tube and allowed vacuum to fill tube to specified level. Removed and filled other tubes as appropriate. Gently rotated each tube back and forth 8–10 times.

b. Vacutainer system method

(1) Attached double-ended needle to Vacutainer tube holder.

(2) Had proper blood specimen tube resting inside Vacutainer holder but did not puncture rubber stopper.

(3) Cleaned venipuncture site. Allowed to dry.

(4) Removed needle cover and informed patient that "stick" would occur, lasting only a few seconds.

(5) Placed thumb or forefinger of nondominant hand 2.5 cm (1 inch) below site and gently pulled skin taut. Stretched skin down until vein stabilized.

(6) Held Vacutainer needle at 15- to 30-degree angle from arm with bevel up.

(7) Slowly inserted needle into vein.

(8) Grasped Vacutainer securely and advanced specimen tube into needle of holder (did not advance needle in vein).

(9) Noted flow of blood into tube.

	S	U	NP	Comments

(10) After filling specimen tube, grasped Vacutainer firmly and removed tube. Inserted additional specimen tubes as needed. Gently rotated each tube back and forth 8–10 times. ____ ____ ____ _____

(11) After last tube was filled and removed from Vacutainer, released tourniquet. ____ ____ ____ _____

(12) Applied 2 × 2–inch gauze pad over puncture site without applying pressure and withdrew needle with Vacutainer from vein. ____ ____ ____ _____

(13) Immediately applied pressure over venipuncture site with gauze or antiseptic pad for 2–3 min or until bleeding stopped. Observed for hematoma. Taped gauze dressing securely. ____ ____ ____ _____

(14) Disposed of syringe, needle, gauze, and other supplies in appropriate containers. ____ ____ ____ _____

c. Blood culture

(1) Loosened tourniquet to prepare site and culture bottles. Cleaned venipuncture site with chlorhexidine antiseptic swab for 30 seconds or followed agency policy. Allowed to dry. ____ ____ ____ _____

(2) Removed protective flip-top overcap and prepped the rubber septum of the blood culture bottles with alcohol swab; allowed to dry for 1 minute. ____ ____ ____ _____

(3) Reapplied tourniquet and located vein. ____ ____ ____ _____

(4) Connected the Vacutainer holder to the Luer connector of the blood culture collection set. ____ ____ ____ _____

(5) Removed and disposed of gloves. Applied clean pair of gloves. Applied tourniquet. ____ ____ ____ _____

(6) Performed venipuncture. When the needle was in the vein, secured it with tape or held in place. ____ ____ ____ _____

(7) Inserted the aerobic bottle first into the Vacutainer holder and pressed down to penetrate the septum. Allowed bottle to fill (approximately 10 mL). Repeated with anaerobic bottle. ____ ____ ____ _____

(8) Gently rotated (did not shake) the bottles to mix the blood and broth. ____ ____ ____ _____

(9) Placed gauze pad over needle and removed gently. Applied pressure. ____ ____ ____ _____

(10) Repeated venipuncture at another site (usually other arm). ____ ____ ____ _____

d. Central venous catheter (CVC) collection

(1) Applied a barrier gown or prepared a sterile drape work surface (per agency policy). Selected appropriate port on IV catheter. Turned off all IV pumps and clamped lumens. ____ ____ ____ _____

(2) Wiped all Luer-Lok caps with alcohol-wipe antiseptic solution or removed Luer-Lok alcohol-impregnated cap (Dual Cap System). Attached 10-mL saline prefilled syringe to selected port. Released clamp. Aspirated gently for blood return. Flushed with 5–10 mL normal saline (NS) (check agency policy). Did not use syringe smaller than 10 mL. Removed syringe.

____ ____ ____ _____

(3) Wiped port with alcohol wipe. For syringe method, attached syringe to selected port, aspirated 5 mL of blood, and discarded. Reclamped catheter. Wiped port, attached 10- to 20-mL Luer-Lok syringe, unclamped catheter, and aspirated desired amount of blood. Reclamped catheter and removed syringe. Cleaned catheter port with alcohol. To transfer blood from syringe to specimen tube, used Vacutainer holder with Luer-Lok attachment. Inserted appropriate specimen tube into Vacutainer holder. Attached syringe to Luer-Lok attachment and filled desired tubes.

____ ____ ____ _____

(4) For Vacutainer method, clamped catheter and attached needleless connector to Vacutainer holder. Placed blood tube into Vacutainer holder. Disinfected injection or access cap with alcohol. Inserted Vacutainer needleless connector into injection or access cap, unclamped catheter, and advanced blood tube into holder to activate blood flow. Allowed blood to fill tube, clamped catheter, and discarded first tube in appropriate biohazard container. Attached specimen tubes to Vacutainer with Luer-Lok adapter, unclamped catheter, and obtained blood specimens.

____ ____ ____ _____

(5) After all specimens were collected, clamped catheter. Removed Vacutainer holder and needleless connector from injection or access cap and disinfected cap with alcohol.

____ ____ ____ _____

(6) Attached 10-mL prefilled NS syringe and flushed with 5–10 mL NS using push-pause method. Ensured positive pressure for lumen. If cap with spring automatically had positive pressure, syringe could be removed and lumen locked. For caps without positive pressure, held syringe plunger steady at completion of flush, locked off lumen with slide clamp, and removed syringe. Reattached alcohol-impregnated cap.

____ ____ ____ _____

	S	U	NP	Comments

(7) Gently rotated blood tubes back and forth 8 to 10 times. Removed gown or drape and disposed in receptacle.   ___ ___ ___ _____

8. Checked tubes for any sign of external contamination with blood. Decontaminated with 70% alcohol if necessary.   ___ ___ ___ _____

9. Securely attached properly completed identification label to each tube and affixed proper requisition. Verified identifiers in front of patient.   ___ ___ ___ _____

10. Placed specimens in plastic biohazard bag and sent to laboratory within 30 minutes.   ___ ___ ___ _____

11. Disposed of syringe, needle, gauze, and other supplies in appropriate containers.   ___ ___ ___ _____

12. Removed and disposed of gloves and performed hand hygiene after specimen was obtained and any spillage cleaned.   ___ ___ ___ _____

13. Helped patient to a comfortable position.   ___ ___ ___ _____

14. Raised side rails (as appropriate) and lowered bed to lowest position, locking into position.   ___ ___ ___ _____

15. Placed nurse call system in an accessible location within patient's reach.   ___ ___ ___ _____

EVALUATION

1. Inspected venipuncture site for hemostasis.   ___ ___ ___ _____

2. Determined if patient remained anxious or fearful.   ___ ___ ___ _____

3. Checked laboratory report for test results.   ___ ___ ___ _____

4. Used Teach-Back. Revised instruction if patient or family caregiver was not able to teach back correctly.   ___ ___ ___ _____

DOCUMENTATION

1. Documented method used to obtain blood specimen, date and time collected, type of test ordered, time specimen was sent to the laboratory, and description of venipuncture site   ___ ___ ___ _____

2. Documented evaluation of patient and family caregiver learning.   ___ ___ ___ _____

HAND-OFF REPORTING

1. Reported any STAT or abnormal test results to health care provider.   ___ ___ ___ _____

Student _____ Date _____

Instructor _____ Date _____

PERFORMANCE CHECKLIST SKILL 7.9 **BLOOD GLUCOSE MONITORING**

	S	U	NP	Comments

ASSESSMENT

1. Identified patient using at least two identifiers. ___ ___ ___ _____

2. Reviewed patient's electronic health record (EHR) for health care provider's order for time or frequency of measurement. ___ ___ ___ _____

3. Reviewed patient's EHR to determine if risks existed for performing skin puncture. ___ ___ ___ _____

4. Determined if specific conditions needed to be met before or after sample collection. ___ ___ ___ _____

5. Assessed patient's/family caregiver's health literacy. ___ ___ ___ _____

6. Assessed area of skin to be used as puncture site. Inspected for edema, inflammation, cuts, or sores. Avoided areas of bruising and open lesions. ___ ___ ___ _____

7. For patient with diabetes who performed test at home, assessed ability to handle skin-puncturing device. Allowed patient to choose to continue self-testing while in hospital. ___ ___ ___ _____

8. Assessed patient's knowledge, prior experience with blood glucose monitoring, and feelings about procedure. ___ ___ ___ _____

PLANNING

1. Determined expected outcomes following completion of procedure. ___ ___ ___ _____

2. Provided privacy and explained procedure and purpose to patient and/or family caregiver. Offered patient and family caregiver opportunity to practice testing procedures. Provided resources/teaching aids for patient and family caregiver. ___ ___ ___ _____

3. Organized and set up any equipment needed to perform procedure. ___ ___ ___ _____

IMPLEMENTATION

1. Performed hand hygiene. Instructed adult to perform hand hygiene, including forearm (if applicable) with soap and water. Rinsed and dried. ___ ___ ___ _____

2. Positioned patient comfortably in chair or in semi-Fowler position in bed. ___ ___ ___ _____

104

	S	U	NP	Comments

3. Applied clean gloves. Removed reagent strip from vial and tightly sealed cap. Checked code on test strip vial. Used only test strips recommended for glucose meter. ___ ___ ___ _____

4. Inserted strip into meter. Did not bend strip or touch the sensor where the specimen of blood was to be obtained. ___ ___ ___ _____

5. Removed unused reagent strip from meter and placed on paper towel or clean, dry surface with test pad facing up ___ ___ ___ _____

6. Meter displayed code on screen that matched code from test strip vial. Pressed button on meter to confirm matching codes. ___ ___ ___ _____

7. Prepared single-use lancet or multiple-use lancet device. Removed cap from lancet device; inserted new lancet. ___ ___ ___ _____

   a. Twisted off protective cover on tip of lancet. Replaced cap of lancet device. ___ ___ ___ _____

   b. Cocked lancet device, adjusting for proper puncture depth. ___ ___ ___ _____

8. Obtained blood sample. ___ ___ ___ _____

   a. Wiped patient's finger or forearm lightly with antiseptic swab and allowed to dry. Chose vascular area for puncture site. Avoided central tip of finger. ___ ___ ___ _____

   b. Held area to be punctured in dependent position. Did not milk or massage finger site. ___ ___ ___ _____

   c. Held tip of lancet device against area of skin chosen for test site. Pressed release button on device. Removed device. ___ ___ ___ _____

   d. Watched for blood sample to appear. Otherwise, gently squeezed or massaged fingertip until round drop of blood formed. ___ ___ ___ _____

9. Obtained test results. ___ ___ ___ _____

   a. Ensured meter was still on. Brought test strip in meter to drop of blood until blood was wicked onto test strip. Followed specific meter instructions to obtain an adequate sample. ___ ___ ___ _____

   b. Blood glucose test result appeared on screen. ___ ___ ___ _____

10. Turned meter off, if necessary. Disposed of test strip, lancet, and gloves in proper receptacles. ___ ___ ___ _____

11. Performed hand hygiene. ___ ___ ___ _____

12. Discussed test results with patient and encouraged questions and eventual participation in care if this was a new diabetes mellitus diagnosis. ___ ___ ___ _____

	S	U	NP	Comments
13. Helped patient to a comfortable position.	___	___	___	_____
14. Raised side rails (as appropriate) and lowered bed to lowest position, locking into position.	___	___	___	_____
15. Placed nurse call system in an accessible location within patient's reach.	___	___	___	_____

EVALUATION

	S	U	NP	Comments
1. Inspected puncture site for bleeding or tissue injury.	___	___	___	_____
2. Compared glucose meter reading with normal blood glucose levels and previous test results.	___	___	___	_____
3. Used Teach-Back. Revised instruction if patient or family caregiver was not able to teach back correctly.	___	___	___	_____

DOCUMENTATION

	S	U	NP	Comments
1. Documented procedure and glucose level according to agency policy.	___	___	___	_____
2. Documented action taken for abnormal range.	___	___	___	_____
3. Described patient response, including appearance of puncture site.	___	___	___	_____
4. Described any patient education provided.	___	___	___	_____
5. Documented evaluation of patient and family caregiver learning.	___	___	___	_____

HAND-OFF REPORTING

	S	U	NP	Comments
1. Reported abnormal blood glucose levels.	___	___	___	_____
2. Reported interventions implemented to correct high or low blood glucose levels.	___	___	___	_____

Student _____ Date _____

Instructor _____ Date _____

PERFORMANCE CHECKLIST SKILL 7.10   **OBTAINING AN ARTERIAL SPECIMEN FOR BLOOD GAS MEASUREMENT**

	S	U	NP	Comments

ASSESSMENT

1. Identified patient using at least two identifiers according to agency policy.

2. Reviewed patient's electronic health record (EHR) for health care provider's order for time or frequency of measurement.

3. Reviewed patient's EHR to identify medications that influenced ABG measurement.

4. Assessed patient's/family caregiver's health literacy.

5. Assessed for factors that influenced ABG measurements.

   a. Assessed respiratory status.

   b. Assessed body temperature.

6. Reviewed criteria for choosing site for ABG sample.

   a. Assessed collateral blood flow. Performed Allen test.

      (1) Performed hand hygiene and applied gloves. Had patient make tight fist and raise hand above heart.

      (2) Applied direct pressure to radial and ulnar arteries.

      (3) Had patient lower and open hand.

      (4) Released pressure over ulnar artery; observed color of fingers, thumbs, and hand.

   b. Assessed accessibility of vessel.

   c. Assessed tissue surrounding artery.

   d. Assessed that arteries were not directly adjacent to veins.

7. Assessed arterial sites for use in obtaining specimen.

8. Removed and disposed of gloves. Performed hand hygiene.

9. Reviewed the EHR for baseline ABG values for patient.

10. Assessed patient's knowledge, prior experience with obtaining an ABGs, and feelings about procedure.

	S	U	NP	Comments

PLANNING

1. Determined expected outcomes following completion of procedure. ___ ___ ___ _____

2. Prepared heparinized syringe (if not in commercial kit). ___ ___ ___ _____

   a. Aspirated 0.5 mL sodium heparin (1000 units/mL) into syringe from vial or ampule. ___ ___ ___ _____

   b. Withdrew plunger entire length of syringe. Maintained asepsis. ___ ___ ___ _____

   c. Ejected all heparin in barrel out of syringe. ___ ___ ___ _____

3. Provided privacy and explained procedure. ___ ___ ___ _____

4. Organized and set up any additional equipment needed to perform procedure at bedside. ___ ___ ___ _____

5. Arranged for extra personnel to help if necessary. ___ ___ ___ _____

IMPLEMENTATION

1. Performed hand hygiene. ___ ___ ___ _____

2. Palpated selected radial, femoral, or brachial site with fingertips. ___ ___ ___ _____

3. Using radial artery, elevated patient's wrist with small pillow and asked patient to extend fingers downward. Stabilized artery by slight hyperextension of wrist. ___ ___ ___ _____

4. Applied clean gloves. Cleaned area of maximal impulse with alcohol swab or antiseptic swab. Wiped in circular motion away from site or used back-and-forth strokes. Allowed to dry. ___ ___ ___ _____

5. Held 2 × 2 inch–gauze pad with same fingers used to palpate artery. ___ ___ ___ _____

6. Used corner of sterile gauze pad or alcohol wipe to point to chosen site. ___ ___ ___ _____

7. Held needle bevel up and inserted at 45-degree angle into artery. Prepared patient for needlestick. ___ ___ ___ _____

8. Stopped advancing needle when blood was noted returning into hub of needle or syringe. ___ ___ ___ _____

9. Allowed arterial pulsations to pump 2–3 mL of blood into heparinized syringe slowly. ___ ___ ___ _____

10. When sampling was complete, held 2×2–inch gauze pad over puncture site, withdrew syringe and needle, and activated safety guard over needle. ___ ___ ___ _____

11. Applied pressure over and just proximal to puncture site with pad. ___ ___ ___ _____

	S	U	NP	Comments

12. Maintained continuous pressure on and proximal to site for 3–5 min (approximately 15 min if patient was undergoing anticoagulant therapy or had bleeding disorder). Had another nurse remove safety needle and attach filter cap to syringe if prolonged pressure was needed.   ___ ___ ___ _____

13. Visually inspected site for signs of bleeding or hematoma formation.   ___ ___ ___ _____

14. Palpated artery below or distal to puncture site.   ___ ___ ___ _____

15. Took syringe, if not done by another nurse, removed safety needle, and discarded needle in appropriate biohazard container. Attached filter cap to syringe to expel air or covered tip of syringe with 2×2–inch sterile gauze to expel air (per agency procedure).   ___ ___ ___ _____

16. Prepared syringe for laboratory analysis per agency policy.   ___ ___ ___ _____

    a. Placed patient identification label on syringe in front of patient; confirmed identifiers.   ___ ___ ___ _____

    b. Placed syringe in cup of crushed ice.   ___ ___ ___ _____

    c. Attached properly labeled laboratory requisition to blood gas sample. Added appropriate patient data.   ___ ___ ___ _____

17. Placed sample in biohazard bag. Sent sample to laboratory immediately.   ___ ___ ___ _____

18. Removed and disposed of gloves and performed hand hygiene.   ___ ___ ___ _____

19. Assisted patient to a comfortable position.   ___ ___ ___ _____

20. Raised side rails (as appropriate) and lowered bed to lowest position, locking into position.   ___ ___ ___ _____

21. Placed nurse call system in an accessible location within patient's reach.   ___ ___ ___ _____

EVALUATION

1. Inspected puncture site and area distal to puncture site for complications.   ___ ___ ___ _____

2. Reviewed results of sample as soon as possible.   ___ ___ ___ _____

3. Used Teach-Back. Revised instruction if patient or family caregiver was not able to teach back correctly.   ___ ___ ___ _____

DOCUMENTATION

1. Documented results of Allen test, location and condition of puncture site, patient's tolerance of procedure, use of supplemental oxygen, and time specimen was sent to the laboratory.   ___ ___ ___ _____

	S	U	NP	Comments

2. Documented evaluation of patient and family caregiver learning. ___ ___ ___ _____

3. Documented results of ABG. ___ ___ ___ _____

HAND-OFF REPORTING

1. Reported ABG results to health care provider as soon as available. ___ ___ ___ _____

2. Reported patient's fraction of inspired oxygen concentration (FiO_2) and any ventilator settings. ___ ___ ___ _____

Student _____ Date _____

Instructor _____ Date _____

PERFORMANCE CHECKLIST SKILL 8.1   **INTRAVENOUS MODERATE SEDATION**

	S	U	NP	Comments

ASSESSMENT

1. Identified patient using at least two identifiers. ___ ___ ___ _____

2. Assessed patient's/family caregiver's health literacy. ___ ___ ___ _____

3. Referred to health care provider order and verified type of procedure scheduled and procedure site with patient. ___ ___ ___ _____

4. Verified that a preprocedure medication reconciliation and history and physical (H&P) examination were completed. ___ ___ ___ _____

5. Verified that informed consent was obtained before administering any sedatives. ___ ___ ___ _____

6. Assessed patient's history of adverse reaction to IV sedation. ___ ___ ___ _____

7. Verified patient's ASA physical status classification. ___ ___ ___ _____

8. Reviewed EHR for history of airway abnormalities, liver failure, lung disease, heart failure, hypotonia, sleep apnea, and history of adverse reaction to sedatives. ___ ___ ___ _____

9. Assessed patient's current or history for substance abuse or liver/kidney disease. ___ ___ ___ _____

10. Verified that patient had not ingested food or fluids, except for oral medications, for at least 4 h. ___ ___ ___ _____

11. Determined if patient was allergic to latex, antiseptic, tape, medications used for induction, or anesthetic solutions. ___ ___ ___ _____

12. Performed hand hygiene. Assessed baseline heart rate, breath sounds, respiratory rate, blood pressure, level of consciousness, pain level, and oxygen saturation (SpO_2). ___ ___ ___ _____

13. Determined patient's height and weight. ___ ___ ___ _____

14. Assessed patient's baseline status via designated scoring system of agency. ___ ___ ___ _____

15. Assessed patient's knowledge, prior experience with IV sedation, and feelings about procedure. ___ ___ ___ _____

111

	S	U	NP	Comments

PLANNING

1. Determined expected outcomes following completion of procedure. ___ ___ ___ _____

2. Provided privacy and explained to patient that IV sedation would cause relaxation and amnesia but maintain wakefulness during procedure. If patient would not be able to verbalize because of nature of procedure, taught him or her agreed-on nonverbal signals such as "yes," "no," and "pain." ___ ___ ___ _____

3. Explained that close monitoring of vital signs (VS) and frequent checks to determine that patient was awake were normal and did not mean that there were problems. ___ ___ ___ _____

4. Explained to patient major steps of procedure. ___ ___ ___ _____

5. Organized and set up any equipment needed to perform procedure. ___ ___ ___ _____

6. Positioned patient as needed for procedure. ___ ___ ___ _____

IMPLEMENTATION

1. Performed hand hygiene. Applied clean gloves, mask, and other PPE as needed. Established peripheral IV access ___ ___ ___ _____

2. Implemented Universal Protocol for second time in presence of appropriate health care team members (as applicable) and in accordance with agency policy. ___ ___ ___ _____

3. During diagnostic procedure, monitored heart rate and SpO_2 continuously. Monitored patient's airway patency, respiratory rate and depth, blood pressure, and level of consciousness and responsiveness every 5 min. Kept oxygen and suction equipment nearby. ___ ___ ___ _____

4. Observed for verbal or nonverbal evidence of pain, facial grimacing, and eye opening. ___ ___ ___ _____

5. Assessed level of sedation using Modified Ramsay Sedation Scale or other criteria adopted by agency. ___ ___ ___ _____

6. Repositioned patient as needed without interrupting diagnostic procedure. ___ ___ ___ _____

7. Disposed of all contaminated supplies in appropriate receptacle, removed and disposed of gloves, mask, and other PPE. ___ ___ ___ _____

8. Helped patient to a comfortable position. ___ ___ ___ _____

9. Raised side rails (as appropriate) and lowered bed to lowest position, locking into position. ___ ___ ___ _____

	S	U	NP	Comments

10. Placed nurse call system in an accessible location within patient's reach.
— — — _____

11. Performed hand hygiene.
— — — _____

EVALUATION

1. Monitored patient throughout procedure using the Modified Ramsay Sedation Scale (or other criteria adopted by the agency).
— — — _____

2. After procedure: Used PADSS and monitored level of consciousness, respiratory rate, SpO_2, blood pressure, heart rate and rhythm, and pain score according to agency policy.
— — — _____

3. Had patient's "designated driver" explain any postprocedure education and sign appropriate documents if patient was unable to sign.
— — — _____

4. Used Teach-Back. Revised instruction if patient or family caregiver was not able to teach back correctly.
— — — _____

DOCUMENTATION

1. Documented VS, SpO_2, end-tidal CO_2, and sedation level at baseline, then every 5 minutes during the procedure, and every 15 minutes for at least 30 minutes after the procedure according to agency policy.
— — — _____

2. Documented dosage, route, and time of administration for drugs given during and after the procedure, including reversal agents.
— — — _____

3. Documented significant patient reactions during the procedure. Included IV fluids and blood products if administered.
— — — _____

4. Documented discharge teaching, medication reconciliation, discontinuation of IV access, final/discharge assessment, and whom/how discharged.
— — — _____

5. Documented evaluation of patient and family caregiver learning.
— — — _____

HAND-OFF REPORTING

1. Immediately reported to patient's health care provider any respiratory distress, cardiac compromise, or unexpected altered mental status.
— — — _____

Student _____ Date _____

Instructor _____ Date _____

PERFORMANCE CHECKLIST SKILL 8.2 **ARTERIOGRAM (ANGIOGRAM)**

	S	U	NP	Comments

ASSESSMENT

1. Identified patient using at least two identifiers. ___ ___ ___ _____

2. Assessed patient's/family caregiver's health literacy. ___ ___ ___ _____

3. Referred to health care provider order and verified type of procedure scheduled and procedure site with patient. ___ ___ ___ _____

4. Verified that informed consent was obtained before administering any sedatives. ___ ___ ___ _____

5. Determined if patient was taking anticoagulants, aspirin, or any nonsteroidal medication. ___ ___ ___ _____

6. Assessed patient for history of any allergies to iodine dye or shellfish and whether patient had previous reaction to contrast agent. If so, notified cardiologist or radiologist. ___ ___ ___ _____

7. Reviewed EHR for contraindications to procedure. Determined whether patient took metformin hydrochloride within previous 48 hours. If so, notified health care provider immediately. ___ ___ ___ _____

8. Assessed patient's bleeding and coagulation status and renal function before procedure. Assessed electrolytes. ___ ___ ___ _____

9. Performed hand hygiene. Obtained VS and peripheral pulses. For arterial procedures, marked patient's peripheral pulses before procedure. For cardiac catheterization, also auscultated heart and lungs and obtained weight. ___ ___ ___ _____

10. Assessed patient's hydration status, including condition of mucous membranes, skin turgor, and recent 24-hour intake. ___ ___ ___ _____

11. Determined type of arteriogram scheduled. If cardiac catheterization, verified if test was for right or left side of heart or both. For IVP asked if study was for one or both kidneys. ___ ___ ___ _____

12. Determined and documented last time of ingested food, drink, or medications. ___ ___ ___ _____

13. Reviewed health care provider's orders for preprocedure medications, hydration, antihistamines, and IV sedation. ___ ___ ___ _____

114

	S	U	NP	Comments

14. Assessed patient's knowledge, prior experience with contrast media studies, and feelings about procedure.   ___ ___ ___ _____

PLANNING

1. Determined expected outcomes following completion of procedure.   ___ ___ ___ _____

2. Provided privacy and explained to patient purpose of and what will happen during procedure.   ___ ___ ___ _____

3. Had patient empty bladder before procedure.   ___ ___ ___ _____

4. Removed all of patient's jewelry, metal objects, and body piercings.   ___ ___ ___ _____

5. Performed preprocedure preparation: ___ ___ ___ _____

   a. For IVP: Verified that patient had completed necessary bowel preparation of orally administered evacuation preparation 24 hours before test and evacuation enema 8 hours before test per agency policy.   ___ ___ ___ _____

   b. For cardiac catheterization: Determined whether hair at site of catheter insertion needed clipping or preparation with antiseptic just before procedure. Allowed antiseptic to dry. Did not shave site.   ___ ___ ___ _____

6. For cardiac catheterization, verified availability of emergent cardiac surgery. Verified patient's ASA classification before procedure.   ___ ___ ___ _____

7. Organized and set up any equipment needed to perform procedure.   ___ ___ ___ _____

IMPLEMENTATION

1. Opened and prepared supplies in procedure room using sterile technique.   ___ ___ ___ _____

2. Prepared cardiac monitor, pulse oximeter, and/or end-tidal CO_2 monitor.   ___ ___ ___ _____

3. Performed hand hygiene and applied clean gloves and appropriate protective equipment.   ___ ___ ___ _____

4. Provided IV access using large-bore cannula. Removed and disposed of gloves and performed hand hygiene.   ___ ___ ___ _____

5. Helped patient assume a comfortable supine position on x-ray table, or slight Trendelenburg position if appropriate. Immobilized extremity to be injected. Padded any bony prominences.   ___ ___ ___ _____

6. Took time-out to verify patient's name, type of procedure to be performed, and procedure site with patient.   ___ ___ ___ _____

	S	U	NP	Comments

7. Began monitoring VS, pulse oximetry (SpO$_2$), end-tidal CO$_2$; and, for arterial procedures, palpated peripheral pulses.

8. Informed patient that during injection of dye it was common to experience some chest pain and a severe hot flash.

9. All health care team members applied appropriate PPE.

10. Physician cleansed arterial puncture site for catheter with antiseptic.

11. Draped patient with sterile drapes, leaving puncture site exposed. Physician anesthetized skin overlying arterial puncture site.

12. For arterial procedures physician:

   a. Punctured artery, inserted introducer into artery, inserted guidewire through introducer and advanced, and inserted flexible catheter over guidewire and advanced into heart.

   b. Advanced catheter to desired artery or cardiac chamber, removed guidewire, and injected contrast medium through catheter.

13. During dye injection specialized machinery took rapid sequence of x-ray films.

14. If iodinated dye was used, observed patient for signs of anaphylaxis.

15. During cardiac catheterization, assisted with measuring cardiac volumes and pressure.

16. Nurse administering IV sedation monitored levels of sedation, level of consciousness, and VS.

17. Physician withdrew catheter and applied manual pressure to puncture site until homeostasis occurred. Used vascular closure device if appropriate.

18. If a percutaneous coronary intervention (PCI) such as a percutaneous transluminal coronary angioplasty (PTCA) or directional coronary atherectomy (DCA) was performed during cardiac catheterization, a femoral introducer/sheath may have been left in place and removed in several hours.

19. Disposed of all contaminated supplies in appropriate receptacle; removed and disposed of gloves and other PPE.

20. Raised side rails (as appropriate) and lowered bed or stretcher to lowest position, locking into position.

116

	S	U	NP	Comments

21. Placed nurse call system in an accessible location within patient's reach.
    — — — _____

22. Performed hand hygiene.
    — — — _____

23. Postprocedure:

  a. For arterial procedures:

    (1) Kept affected extremity extended and immobilized after removal of sheath per agency policy. Used orthopedic bedpan for female patient as needed for bowel or bladder evacuation while on bed rest.
    — — — _____

    (2) Emphasized need to lie flat for 4 to 8 hours, or overnight if sheath was left in groin.
    — — — _____

    (3) Encouraged patient to drink fluids after procedure.
    — — — _____

EVALUATION

1. Evaluated patient's body position and comfort during procedure.
    — — — _____

2. Monitored VS and SpO_2 and assessed for signs of cardiac complications every 15 minutes for 1 hour, every 30 minutes for 2 hours, or until patient was stable.
    — — — _____

3. Monitored for complications:
    — — — _____

  a. Performed neurovascular checks by palpating peripheral pulses on affected extremity and comparing right and left extremities for skin color, temperature, and sensation. Used Doppler ultrasonic stethoscope to locate pulses that were not palpable.
    — — — _____

  b. Assessed vascular access site for bleeding and hematoma.
    — — — _____

  c. Auscultated heart and lungs and compared with preprocedure findings.
    — — — _____

  d. Observe patient for possible delayed reaction to iodine dye (if used).
    — — — _____

4. Evaluated level of sedation, level of consciousness, and SpO_2. Used PADSS scale.
    — — — _____

5. Assessed postprocedure laboratory values.
    — — — _____

6. Had patient rate pain acuity on pain scale of 0 to 10.
    — — — _____

7. Used Teach-Back. Revised instruction if patient or family caregiver was not able to teach back correctly.
    — — — _____

	S	U	NP	Comments

DOCUMENTATION

1. Documented patient's status: VS, SpO_2/end-tidal CO_2, status of peripheral pulses for equality and symmetry, BP for hypotension, temperature and color of catheterized extremity, condition of IV site, and level of patient responsiveness.

2. Documented any drainage from puncture site, appearance of dressing, and condition of puncture site.

3. Documented evaluation of patient and family caregiver learning.

HAND-OFF REPORTING

1. Reported to health care provider any VS change, excessive bleeding or increasing hematoma at puncture site, decreased or absent peripheral pulses, persistent pain, altered neurological status, dysrhythmias, decreased SpO_2 or increased end-tidal CO_2, or decreased responsiveness after sedation.

Student _____ Date _____

Instructor _____ Date _____

PERFORMANCE CHECKLIST SKILL 8.3 **CARE OF PATIENTS UNDERGOING ASPIRATIONS: BONE MARROW ASPIRATION/BIOPSY, LUMBAR PUNCTURE, PARACENTESIS, AND THORACENTESIS**

	S	U	NP	Comments
ASSESSMENT				
1. Identified patient using at least two identifiers.	___	___	___	_____
2. Verified type of procedure scheduled, purpose, and procedure site with patient and EHR.	___	___	___	_____
3. Verified that informed consent was obtained before administering any analgesia or antianxiety agents.	___	___	___	_____
4. Reviewed EHR for contraindications.	___	___	___	_____
5. Determined patient's ability to assume position for procedure. Discussed with health care provider need for premedication for anxious patients.	___	___	___	_____
6. Assessed patient's/family caregiver's health literacy.	___	___	___	_____
7. Performed hand hygiene. Obtained VS, oxygen saturation (SpO_2)/end-tidal carbon dioxide (CO_2) value, and weight. For paracentesis, obtained abdominal girth measurement. (Used ink pen to mark measurement location for abdominal girth measurement.) For LP assessed lower extremity movement, sensation, and muscle strength.	___	___	___	_____
8. Instructed patient to empty bladder.	___	___	___	_____
9. Assessed patient's coagulation status.	___	___	___	_____
10. Determined whether patient was allergic to antiseptic, latex, or anesthetic solutions.	___	___	___	_____
11. Assessed patient's character of pain and rated acuity on pain scale of 0 to 10.	___	___	___	_____
12. Assessed patient's knowledge, prior experience with aspiration, and feelings about procedure.	___	___	___	_____

	S	U	NP	Comments

PLANNING

1. Determined expected outcomes following completion of procedure.

2. Provided privacy and explained procedure.

3. Organized and set up any equipment needed to perform procedure at bedside.

4. If ordered, premedicated for pain or anxiety 30 min before procedure.

5. Before thoracentesis verified recent chest x-ray film examination.

IMPLEMENTATION

1. Performed hand hygiene. Applied clean gloves. Donned additional PPE if appropriate.

2. Set up sterile tray or opened supplies to make accessible for health care provider.

3. Took time-out to verify patient's name, type of procedure scheduled, and procedure site with patient and health care team.

4. Helped patient maintain correct position. Reassured patient while explaining procedure.

5. Explained to patient that pain could occur when lidocaine was injected into tissues and that pressure could also occur when tissue or fluid was aspirated.

6. Physician and members of health care team in procedure applied sterile gloves, mask, gown, and goggles; physician cleaned patient's skin with antiseptic solution; and draped site with sterile drape.

7. Physician injected local anesthetic and allowed time for anesthesia to occur.

8. Physician inserted needle or trocar into spinal space or body cavity involved. To aspirate tissue or body fluids for specimen analysis, syringe was attached to trocar or needle, and aspirate was placed into specimen container.

9. Nurse assessed patient's condition during procedure, including respiratory status, VS if indicated, and any complaints of pain or feelings of anxiety. Maintained conversation to provide distraction.

10. Noted characteristics of aspirate.

	S	U	NP	Comments

11. Properly labeled specimens in presence of patient and transported to laboratory in proper containers. Labeled specimens in order of collection. ____ ____ ____ _____

12. Physician removed needle/trocar and applied pressure over insertion site until drainage ceased. If necessary, helped with direct pressure and application of a small gauze dressing. ____ ____ ____ _____

13. All health care team members in procedure removed and disposed of protective equipment and discarded in appropriate receptacle. ____ ____ ____ _____

14. Helped patient to comfortable postprocedure position. ____ ____ ____ _____

15. Raised side rails (as appropriate) and lowered bed to lowest position, locking into position. ____ ____ ____ _____

16. Placed nurse call system in an accessible location within patient's reach. ____ ____ ____ _____

17. Performed hand hygiene. ____ ____ ____ _____

EVALUATION

1. Monitored level of consciousness, VS, lung sounds, and SpO_2/end-tidal CO_2. Followed agency policy. ____ ____ ____ _____

2. Inspected dressing over puncture site for bleeding, swelling, tenderness, and erythema. Inspected area under patient for bleeding. Avoided disrupting healing clot at site if pressure dressing was present. ____ ____ ____ _____

3. Evaluated character of patient's pain and whether pain acuity was a score of 4 or less on pain scale of 0 to 10. ____ ____ ____ _____

4. Following paracentesis, measured abdominal girth and respirations and compared to preprocedure measurements. ____ ____ ____ _____

5. Used Teach-Back. Revised instruction if patient or family caregiver was not able to teach back correctly. ____ ____ ____ _____

DOCUMENTATION

1. Documented name of procedure; preprocedure preparation; location of puncture site; amount, consistency, and color of fluid drained or specimen obtained; duration of procedure; patient's tolerance and comfort level; laboratory tests ordered and specimen sent; type of dressing; postprocedure activities; and other procedure-specific assessments. ____ ____ ____ _____

	S	U	NP	Comments

2. Documented evaluation of patient and family caregiver learning.

HAND-OFF REPORTING

1. Immediately reported to health care provider any change in vital signs and SpO$_2$, unexpected pain/discomfort, and any excessive drainage from dressing over puncture site.

Student _____ Date _____

Instructor _____ Date _____

PERFORMANCE CHECKLIST SKILL 8.4 **CARE OF A PATIENT UNDERGOING BRONCHOSCOPY**

	S	U	NP	Comments

ASSESSMENT

1. Identified patient using at least two identifiers.

2. Verified type of procedure scheduled and procedure site with patient and EHR.

3. Verified that informed consent was obtained before administration of any sedatives.

4. Determined purpose of procedure: for sputum aspiration, assessment, tissue biopsy, or removal of foreign body.

5. Reviewed health care orders for preprocedure medication.

6. Assessed patient's medical history for inability to tolerate interruption of high-flow oxygen unless intubated.

7. Assessed patient's/family caregiver's health literacy.

8. Performed hand hygiene. Obtained baseline VS, pulse oximetry (SpO_2) and end-tidal CO_2 values.

9. Assessed type of cough, sputum produced, and heart and lung sounds.

10. Asked whether patient was allergic to local anesthetic used for spraying throat.

11. Assessed time patient last ingested food/fluids or medications.

12. Assessed patient's knowledge, prior experience with bronchoscopy, and feelings about procedure.

PLANNING

1. Determined expected outcomes following completion of procedure.

2. Provided privacy and explained procedure to patient.

3. Organized and set up any equipment needed to perform procedure.

4. In procedure room, draped patient for privacy. In patient room, closed room door or drapes.

	S	U	NP	Comments

5. Administered atropine, opioid, or antianxiety agent 30 minutes before procedure.

6. Removed and safely stored patient's dentures and/or eyeglasses.

IMPLEMENTATION

1. Performed hand hygiene. Assessed current IV access or established new IV access with large-bore cannula.

2. Organized and opened any equipment needed using sterile technique.

3. Helped patient assume position desired by physician.

4. Took time-out to verify patient's name, type of procedure, and procedure site with patient and health care team.

5. Health team members assisting with procedure performed hand hygiene and applied PPE. Nurse prepared by positioning tip of suction catheter for easy access to patient's mouth.

6. Physician sprayed nasopharynx and oropharynx with topical anesthetic as needed.

7. Instructed patient not to swallow local anesthetic; provided emesis basin for expectorating it.

8. Another physician or staff member attached bronchoscope to machine light source.

9. Physician applied goggles, mask, and sterile gloves; introduced bronchoscope into mouth to pharynx; and passed it through glottis and into trachea and bronchi. Used more anesthetic spray as needed to prevent cough reflex. For intubated patients' flexible bronchoscope was introduced via endotracheal tube.

10. Physician suctioned mucus and performed bronchial washing with cytological specimens taken with wire brush or curette. Obtained biopsy specimens as needed.

11. Helped patient through procedure by providing explanations, verbal reassurance, and support.

12. Assessed patient's VS, SpO_2, end-tidal CO_2, and breathing capacity during procedure; observed degree of restlessness, capillary refill, and color of nail beds.

	S	U	NP	Comments

13. Noted characteristics of suctioned material. Expected small amount of blood mixed with aspirate because of tissue trauma.

14. Using gloved hand, wiped patient's mouth and nose to remove lubricant after bronchoscope was removed.

15. Instructed patient not to eat or drink until tracheobronchial anesthesia had worn off and gag reflex had returned, usually in 2 hours. Used tongue depressor to touch pharynx to test for presence of gag reflex.

16. Disposed of all contaminated supplies in appropriate receptacle; removed and disposed of gloves and other PPE.

17. Helped patient to a comfortable postprocedure position.

18. Raised side rails (as appropriate) and lowered bed to lowest position, locking in position.

19. Placed nurse call system in an accessible location within patient's reach.

20. Performed hand hygiene.

EVALUATION

1. Monitored vital signs, SpO_2, and end-tidal CO_2.

2. Observed character and amount of sputum. Conducted serial sputum collection if ordered.

3. Observed respiratory status closely; palpated for facial or neck crepitus.

4. Assessed for return of gag reflex.

5. Used Teach-Back. Revised instruction if patient or family caregiver was not able to teach back correctly.

DOCUMENTATION

1. Documented procedure(s) performed; character of sputum; duration of procedure, patient's tolerance and, if any, complications; and the collection and disposition of specimen(s). Documented time of gag reflex return.

2. Documented evaluation of patient and family caregiver learning.

HAND-OFF REPORTING

1. Reported bleeding or respiratory distress following the procedure or any changes in VS beyond patient's normal limits to physician immediately. Reported results of procedure to appropriate health care personnel.

Student _____ Date _____

Instructor _____ Date _____

PERFORMANCE CHECKLIST SKILL 8.5 **CARE OF A PATIENT UNDERGOING ENDOSCOPY**

	S	U	NP	Comments
ASSESSMENT				
1. Identified patient using at least two identifiers.	___	___	___	_____
2. Verified type of procedure scheduled and procedure site with patient and EHR.	___	___	___	_____
3. Verified that informed consent was obtained before administering sedation.	___	___	___	_____
4. Determined purpose of procedure: biopsy, examination, or coagulation of bleeding sites.	___	___	___	_____
5. Assessed patient's/family caregiver's health literacy.	___	___	___	_____
6. Performed hand hygiene. Determined if GI bleeding was present. Applied gloves if at risk for body fluid exposure. Observed character of emesis, stool, and nasogastric (NG) tube drainage for frank blood or material that looks like coffee grounds.	___	___	___	_____
7. Obtained VS and SpO_2/end-tidal CO_2 values.	___	___	___	_____
8. Verified that patient was on nothing-by-mouth (NPO) status for at least 8 h for endoscopy of upper GI tract.	___	___	___	_____
9. For lower GI studies, verified that patient followed clear liquid diet for 2 days and had completed any ordered bowel-cleansing regimen.	___	___	___	_____
10. Assessed patient's knowledge, prior experience with GI endoscopy, and feelings about procedure.	___	___	___	_____
PLANNING				
1. Determined expected outcomes following completion of procedure.	___	___	___	_____
2. Prepared patient:	___	___	___	_____
a. Provided privacy and explained procedure and sensations to expect.	___	___	___	_____
b. Organized and set up any equipment needed to perform procedure.	___	___	___	_____
c. Administered pain medication or preprocedure medication.	___	___	___	_____

126

	S	U	NP	Comments

IMPLEMENTATION

1. Performed hand hygiene and applied PPE. ___ ___ ___ _____

2. Removed patient's eyeglasses, dentures, or other dental appliances. ___ ___ ___ _____

3. Organized and opened equipment using sterile technique. ___ ___ ___ _____

4. Took time-out to verify patient's name, type of procedure, and procedure site with patient and health care team. ___ ___ ___ _____

5. Ensured that IV line was patent and administered IV sedation as ordered if certified. ___ ___ ___ _____

6. Helped patient assume proper position for procedure and applied appropriate drape. ___ ___ ___ _____

7. Physician performed hand hygiene and put on PPE. ___ ___ ___ _____

8. Upper GI procedures:

   a. Helped physician spray nasopharynx and oropharynx with local anesthetic. ___ ___ ___ _____

   b. Administered atropine if ordered. ___ ___ ___ _____

   c. Positioned tip of suction catheter for easy access in patient's mouth. ___ ___ ___ _____

9. Lower GI procedures:

   a. Prepared lubricant for fiberoptic endoscope. ___ ___ ___ _____

10. Physician lubricated endoscope and slowly passed it into mouth or through anus to view esophagus, stomach, colon, or rectum and advanced to desired depth while visualizing lining of structures. ___ ___ ___ _____

11. Physician insufflated air through endoscope into upper GI tract or carbon dioxide into lower GI tract in case of colonoscopy. ___ ___ ___ _____

12. Assisted patient throughout procedure. ___ ___ ___ _____

   a. Anticipated needs and promoted comfort. ___ ___ ___ _____

   b. Told patient what was happening as each part of procedure was carried out. ___ ___ ___ _____

   c. For upper GI procedures, suctioned if there were excessive oral secretions or vomitus. ___ ___ ___ _____

13. Placed tissue specimens in proper laboratory containers or on proper slides. Sealed as needed. Dated, timed, and initialed all specimen containers before sending to laboratory. ___ ___ ___ _____

14. Helped patient return to comfortable position. ___ ___ ___ _____

	S	U	NP	Comments

15. Disposed of all contaminated supplies in appropriate receptacle; removed and disposed of gloves and other PPE.   ___ ___ ___ _____

16. In recovery, after sedation resolved, informed patient not to eat or drink until gag reflex returned.   ___ ___ ___ _____

17. Helped patient to a comfortable postprocedure position.   ___ ___ ___ _____

18. Raised side rails (as appropriate) and lowered bed to lowest position, locking into position.   ___ ___ ___ _____

19. Placed nurse call system in an accessible location within patient's reach.   ___ ___ ___ _____

20. Performed hand hygiene.   ___ ___ ___ _____

EVALUATION

1. Monitored VS and oxygen saturation according to agency policy.   ___ ___ ___ _____

2. Assessed for levels of sedation and consciousness.   ___ ___ ___ _____

3. Asked patient to describe pain acuity using pain scale of 0 to 10. Observed for pain.   ___ ___ ___ _____

4. Evaluated emesis or aspirated for frank or occult blood. If a lower endoscopy was completed, monitored the abdomen for increased size.   ___ ___ ___ _____

5. Assessed for return of gag reflex. Provided oral hygiene when gag reflex returned.   ___ ___ ___ _____

6. Used Teach-Back. Revised instruction if patient or family caregiver was not able to teach back correctly.   ___ ___ ___ _____

DOCUMENTATION

1. Documented the procedure, duration, VS and pulse oximetry, patient's tolerance, complications and interventions, and collection and disposition of specimen.   ___ ___ ___ _____

2. Documented evaluation of patient and family caregiver learning.   ___ ___ ___ _____

HAND-OFF REPORTING

1. Reported onset of bleeding, abdominal pain, dyspnea, and VS changes to physician.   ___ ___ ___ _____

Student _____   Date _____

Instructor _____   Date _____

PERFORMANCE CHECKLIST SKILL 9.1   **HAND HYGIENE**

	S	U	NP	Comments

ASSESSMENT

1. Inspected surface of hands for breaks or cuts in skin or cuticles. Covered any skin lesions with a dressing before providing care. If lesions were too large to cover, might have been restricted from direct patient care. ___ ___ ___ _____

2. Inspected hands for visible soiling. ___ ___ ___ _____

3. Inspected condition of nails. Ensured fingernails were short, filed, and smooth. ___ ___ ___ _____

PLANNING

1. Determined expected outcomes following completion of procedure. ___ ___ ___ _____

IMPLEMENTATION

1. Pushed wristwatch and long uniform sleeves above wrists. Avoided wearing rings. If worn, removed during hand hygiene. ___ ___ ___ _____

2. Antiseptic hand rub:

   a. According to manufacturer directions, dispensed ample amount of product into palm of one dry hand. ___ ___ ___ _____

   b. Rubbed hands together, covering all surfaces of hands and fingers with antiseptic. ___ ___ ___ _____

   c. Rubbed hands together until alcohol was dry. Allowed hands to dry completely before applying gloves. ___ ___ ___ _____

3. Handwashing using regular or antimicrobial soap:

   a. Stood in front of sink, keeping hands and uniform away from sink surface. ___ ___ ___ _____

   b. Turned on water, pushed knee pedals laterally, or pressed pedals with foot to regulate flow and temperature. ___ ___ ___ _____

   c. Avoided splashing water against uniform. ___ ___ ___ _____

   d. Regulated flow of water so temperature was warm. ___ ___ ___ _____

   e. Wet hands and wrists thoroughly under running water. Kept hands and forearms lower than elbows during washing. ___ ___ ___ _____

	S	U	NP	Comments

f. Applied the amount of antiseptic soap recommended by the manufacturer and rubbed hands together to thoroughly lather hands.

g. Performed hand hygiene using plenty of lather and friction for at least 20 seconds. Interlaced fingers and rubbed palms and back of hands with circular motion at least 5 times each. Kept fingertips down to facilitate removal of microorganisms.

h. Cleaned areas underlying fingernails with fingernails of other hand and additional soap or with disposable nail cleaner.

i. Rinsed hands and wrists thoroughly, keeping hands down and elbows up.

j. Dried hands thoroughly from fingers to wrists with paper towel or single-use cloth.

k. If used, discarded paper towel in proper receptacle.

l. To turn off hand faucet, used clean, dry paper towel; avoided touching handles with hands. Turned off water with foot or knee pedals, if applicable.

m. If hands were dry or chapped, used small amount of lotion or barrier cream dispensed from individual-use container.

EVALUATION

1. Inspected surface of hands for obvious signs of dirt or other contaminants.

2. Inspected hands for dermatitis or cracked skin.

3. Used Teach-Back. Revised instruction if patient or family caregiver was not able to teach back correctly.

Student _____ Date _____

Instructor _____ Date _____

PERFORMANCE CHECKLIST SKILL 9.2 **CARING FOR PATIENTS UNDER ISOLATION PRECAUTIONS**

	S	U	NP	Comments

ASSESSMENT

1. Identified patient using two identifiers according to agency policy.

2. Assessed patient's medical history for possible indications for isolation.

3. Reviewed laboratory test results.

4. Reviewed precautions for specific isolation system, including appropriate barriers to apply. Considered types of care measures to be performed in patient's room.

5. Assessed patient's/family caregiver's knowledge, experience, and health literacy.

6. Assessed whether patient had known latex allergy. If allergy was present, referred to agency policy and resources available to provide full latex-free care. Applied allergy arm band.

7. Assessed patient's knowledge, prior experience with isolation, and feelings about isolation. Reviewed nursing care plan notes or conferred with colleagues regarding patient's emotional state and reaction/adjustment to isolation.

8. Assessed patient's goals or preferences for how isolation was to be performed or what patient expected.

PLANNING

1. Determined expected outcomes following completion of procedure.

2. Explained purpose of isolation and precautions for patient and family caregiver to take. Offered opportunity to ask questions.

3. Closed room door.

IMPLEMENTATION

1. Performed hand hygiene.

2. Prepared all equipment to be taken into patient's room.

3. Prepared for entrance into isolation room. Ideally, before applying PPE, stepped into patient's room and stayed by door. Introduced self and explained care. If this was not possible, or patient was on airborne precautions, applied PPE outside of the room.

    a. Applied gown, being sure that it fully covered torso from neck to knees and from arms to end of wrist and wrapped around the back, covering all outer garments. Pulled sleeves down to wrist. Tied securely at neck and waist.

    b. Applied either surgical mask or fitted respirator. Secured ties or elastic band at middle of head and neck. Fit flexible band to nose bridge. Ensured mask or respirator fit snugly to face and below chin. Fit-checked respirator.

    c. If needed, applied eyewear or goggles snugly around face and eyes. If prescription glasses were worn, wore side shields as indicated.

    d. Applied clean gloves. Brought glove cuffs over edge of gown sleeves.

4. Entered patient's room. Arranged supplies and equipment.

5. If patient was on TB precautions, instructed to cover mouth with tissue when coughing and to wear disposable surgical mask when leaving room.

6. Assessed vital signs.

    a. If patient was infected or colonized with resistant organism, equipment remained in room.

    b. If stethoscope was to be reused, cleaned earpieces and diaphragm or bell with 70% alcohol or agency-approved germicide. Set aside on clean surface.

    c. Used individual or disposable thermometers and BP cuffs when available.

7. Administered medications.

    a. Gave oral medication in wrapper or cup.

    b. Disposed of wrapper or cup in plastic-lined receptacle.

    c. Continued wearing gloves when administering an injection.

    d. Discarded needleless syringe or safety sheathed needle into designated sharps container.

	S	U	NP	Comments

8. Administered hygiene and encouraged patient to ask any questions or express concerns about isolation. Provided informal teaching. ___ ___ ___ _____

   a. Avoided allowing isolation gown to become wet; carried wash basin outward away from gown; avoided leaning against wet tabletop. ___ ___ ___ _____

   b. Helped patient remove own gown; discarded in leak-proof linen bag. ___ ___ ___ _____

   c. Removed linen from bed; avoided contact with isolation gown. Placed in leak-proof linen bag. ___ ___ ___ _____

   d. Provided clean bed linen. ___ ___ ___ _____

   e. Changed gloves and performed hand hygiene if gloves became excessively soiled and further care was necessary. Re-gloved. ___ ___ ___ _____

9. Collected specimens. ___ ___ ___ _____

   a. Placed specimen container on clean paper towel in patient's bathroom. ___ ___ ___ _____

   b. Followed agency procedure for collecting specimen of body fluids. ___ ___ ___ _____

   c. Transferred specimen to container without soiling outside of container. Placed container in plastic bag and placed label on outside of bag or per agency policy. Labeled specimen in front of patient. Performed hand hygiene and re-gloved if additional procedures were needed. ___ ___ ___ _____

   d. Checked label on specimen for accuracy. Sent to laboratory. Labeled containers of blood or body fluids with biohazard sticker. ___ ___ ___ _____

10. Disposed of linen, trash, and disposable items. ___ ___ ___ _____

   a. Used sturdy moisture-impervious bags to contain soiled articles. Used double bag if necessary, for heavily soiled linen or heavy wet trash. ___ ___ ___ _____

   b. Tied bags securely at top in knot. ___ ___ ___ _____

11. Removed all reusable pieces of equipment. Cleaned any contaminated surfaces with hospital-approved disinfectant. ___ ___ ___ _____

12. Resupplied room as needed. Had staff colleague hand in new supplies. Helped patient to a comfortable position. ___ ___ ___ _____

	S	U	NP	Comments

13. Left isolation room. Removed PPE worn in room before leaving room. _____ _____ _____ _____

   a. Removed gloves. Removed one glove by grasping cuff and pulling glove inside out over hand. Held removed glove in gloved hand. Slid fingers of ungloved hand under remaining glove at wrist. Peeled glove off over first glove. Discarded gloves in proper waste container. _____ _____ _____ _____

   b. Removed eyewear, face shield, or goggles. Handled by headband or earpieces. Discarded in proper waste container. _____ _____ _____ _____

   c. Removed gown. Untied neck strings and then untied back strings of gown. Allowed gown to fall from shoulders; touched inside of gown only. Removed hands from sleeves without touching outside of gown. Held gown inside at shoulder seams and folded inside out into bundle; discarded in proper waste container. _____ _____ _____ _____

   d. Removed mask. If mask secured over ears, removed elastic from ears and pulled mask away from face. For tie-on mask, untied bottom mask string and then top strings, pulled mask away from face, and dropped into proper waste container. (Did not touch outer surface of mask.) _____ _____ _____ _____

   e. Performed hand hygiene. If patient was being treated for *C. difficile* infection, cleaned hands with soap and water. _____ _____ _____ _____

   f. Retrieved wristwatch and stethoscope (unless items were to remain in room). _____ _____ _____ _____

   g. Explained to patient when return to room was planned. Asked whether patient required any personal care items. Offered books, magazines, and audiotapes. _____ _____ _____ _____

   h. Raised side rails (as appropriate) and lowered bed to lowest position, locking into position. _____ _____ _____ _____

   i. Placed nurse call system in an accessible location within patient's reach. _____ _____ _____ _____

   j. Disposed of all contaminated supplies and equipment properly. Performed hand hygiene. _____ _____ _____ _____

   k. Left room and closed door if necessary. Closed door if patient was on airborne precautions or in negative-airflow room. _____ _____ _____ _____

EVALUATION

1. Observed patient's and family caregiver's use of isolation precautions when visiting. _____ _____ _____ _____

	S	U	NP	Comments

2. While in room, asked if patient had sufficient chance to discuss health problems, course of treatment, or other topics important to patient.   ___ ___ ___ _____

3. Used Teach-Back. Revised instruction if patient or family caregiver was not able to teach back correctly.   ___ ___ ___ _____

DOCUMENTATION

1. Documented procedures performed and patient's response to social isolation. Also documented any patient or family caregiver education performed and reinforced.   ___ ___ ___ _____

2. Documented type of isolation in use and the microorganisms (if known).   ___ ___ ___ _____

HAND-OFF REPORTING

1. Shared type of isolation precautions and how patient had been responding to social isolation.   ___ ___ ___ _____

2. Shared any related infectious disease testing results.   ___ ___ ___ _____

Student _____ Date _____

Instructor _____ Date _____

PERFORMANCE CHECKLIST SKILL 10.1 **APPLYING AND REMOVING CAP, MASK, AND PROTECTIVE EYEWEAR**

	S	U	NP	Comments

ASSESSMENT

1. Reviewed type of sterile procedure to be performed and consulted agency policy for use of mask/caps/protective eyewear. ___ ___ ___ _____

2. Avoid participating in procedure or applied a mask if self or other health care providers had symptoms of a respiratory infection. ___ ___ ___ _____

3. Assessed patient's risk for infection. ___ ___ ___ _____

PLANNING

1. Determined expected outcomes following completion of procedure. ___ ___ ___ _____

2. Prepared equipment and inspected packaging for integrity and exposure to sterilization. ___ ___ ___ _____

IMPLEMENTATION

1. Performed hand hygiene. ___ ___ ___ _____

2. Option: when assisting with a procedure at a patient's bedside, applied a clean gown if there was a risk of splatter or soiling. Applied the gown with opening to the back. Ensured that it covered all outer garments. Pulled sleeves down to wrist. Tied securely at neck and wrist. ___ ___ ___ _____

3. Prepared to apply a cap. ___ ___ ___ _____

   a. If hair was long, combed back behind ears and secured. ___ ___ ___ _____

   b. Secured hair in place with pins. ___ ___ ___ _____

   c. Applied cap over head like a hairnet. Ensured that all hair fit under edges of cap. ___ ___ ___ _____

4. Applied a mask. ___ ___ ___ _____

   a. Found top edge of mask with thin metal strip along edge. ___ ___ ___ _____

   b. Held mask by top two strings or loops and kept top edge above bridge of nose. ___ ___ ___ _____

   c. Tied two top strings at top of back of head, over cap (if worn), with strings above ears. Alternatively, placed loops over ears. ___ ___ ___ _____

	S	U	NP	Comments

d. Tied two lower ties snugly around neck with mask well under chin. ___ ___ ___ _____

e. Gently pinched upper metal band around bridge of nose. ___ ___ ___ _____

5. Applied protective eyewear. ___ ___ ___ _____

   a. Applied protective glasses, goggles, or face shield comfortably over eyes and checked that vision was clear. ___ ___ ___ _____

   b. Ensured that face shield fit snugly around forehead and face. ___ ___ ___ _____

6. If performing a sterile procedure, applied sterile gown. After applying cap, mask, and eyewear, applied clean gloves for nonsterile procedures and sterile gloves for sterile procedures. Pulled up clean gloves to cover each wrist. Provided a latex-free environment if patient or health care worker had a latex allergy. ___ ___ ___ _____

7. Removed protective barriers. ___ ___ ___ _____

   a. Removed gloves first if worn. Removed gloves by grasping cuff and pulling glove inside out over hand. Held removed glove in hand. Slid fingers of ungloved hand under remaining glove at wrist. Peeled glove off over first glove. Discarded gloves in proper container. ___ ___ ___ _____

   b. Removed eyewear. Avoided placing hands over soiled lens. NOTE: If wearing a face shield, removed it before removing mask. ___ ___ ___ _____

   c. Removed gown by unfastening neck ties and pulling away from neck and shoulders. Touching only inside of gown, turned gown inside out, rolled or folded into a bundle, and discarded. ___ ___ ___ _____

   d. Untied bottom strings of mask. First held strings, untied top strings, and pulled mask away from face while holding strings. Removed mask from face and discarded in proper receptacle. ___ ___ ___ _____

   e. Grasped outer surface of cap and lifted from hair. ___ ___ ___ _____

   f. Discarded cap in proper receptacle and performed hand hygiene. ___ ___ ___ _____

EVALUATION

1. Following the procedure, assessed patient for signs of systemic infections or local area of body treated for drainage, tenderness, edema, or redness. ___ ___ ___ _____

2. Used Teach-Back. Revised instruction if patient or family caregiver was not able to teach back correctly. ___ ___ ___ _____

DOCUMENTATION

1. No documentation is required for using PPE.   ___ ___ ___ _____

HAND-OFF REPORTING

1. No reporting is required for using PPE.   ___ ___ ___ _____

Student _____ Date _____

Instructor _____ Date _____

PERFORMANCE CHECKLIST SKILL 10.2 **PREPARING A STERILE FIELD**

	S	U	NP	Comments

ASSESSMENT

1. Identified patient using at least two identifiers. ___ ___ ___ _____

2. Assessed for latex allergies. ___ ___ ___ _____

3. Verified in agency policy and procedure manual that procedure required surgical aseptic technique. ___ ___ ___ _____

4. Assessed patient/family caregiver's health literacy. ___ ___ ___ _____

5. Assessed patient's comfort, positioning, oxygen requirements, and elimination needs before preparing for procedure. ___ ___ ___ _____

6. Instructed patient and family caregiver not to touch work surface or equipment during procedure. ___ ___ ___ _____

7. Checked sterile package integrity for punctures, tears, discoloration, moisture, or any other signs of contamination. Checked expiration date if applicable. If using commercially packaged supplies or those prepared by agency, checked for sterilization indicator. ___ ___ ___ _____

8. Anticipated number and variety of supplies needed for procedure. ___ ___ ___ _____

9. Assessed patient's knowledge, prior experience with a sterile field, and feelings about procedure. ___ ___ ___ _____

PLANNING

1. Asked visitors to step out briefly during procedure. Instructed staff helping with procedure not to move. ___ ___ ___ _____

2. Determined expected outcomes following completion of procedure. ___ ___ ___ _____

3. Completed all other nursing interventions before beginning procedure. ___ ___ ___ _____

4. Arranged equipment at bedside. ___ ___ ___ _____

5. Provided privacy. Positioned patient comfortably for specific procedure to be performed. If a body part was to be examined or treated, positioned patient so area was accessible. Had AP help with positioning as needed. ___ ___ ___ _____

	S	U	NP	Comments

6. Explained to patient purpose of procedure and importance of sterile technique.

IMPLEMENTATION

1. Performed hand hygiene

2. Applied PPE as needed.

3. Selected a clean, flat, dry work surface above waist level.

4. Prepared sterile work surface.

   a. Used sterile commercial kit or pack containing sterile items.

     (1) Placed sterile kit or pack on the dry and clean work surface.

     (2) Opened outside cover and removed package from dust cover. Placed on work surface.

     (3) Grasped outer surface of tip of outermost flap.

     (4) Opened outermost flap away from body, keeping arm outstretched and away from sterile field

     (5) Grasped outside surface of edge of first side flap.

     (6) Opened side flap, pulling to side, allowing it to lie flat on table surface. Kept arm to side and not over sterile surface.

     (7) Repeated Step 4a(6) for second side flap.

     (8) Grasped outside border of last and innermost flap. Stood away from sterile package and pulled flap back, allowing it to fall flat on table.

   b. Opened sterile linen-wrapped package.

     (1) Placed package on clean, dry, flat work surface above waist level.

     (2) Removed sterilization tape seal and unwrapped both layers following same steps (see Steps 4a [2] through 4a [8]) as for sterile kit.

     (3) Used opened package wrapper as sterile field.

   c. Prepared sterile drape.

     (1) Placed pack containing sterile drape on flat, dry surface and opened as described (see Steps 4a [2] through 4a[8]) for sterile package.

	S	U	NP	Comments

(2) Applied sterile gloves (per agency policy). Only touched outer 2.5-cm (1-inch) border of drape when not wearing gloves.

(3) Using fingertips of one hand, picked up folded top edge of drape along 2.5 cm (1-inch) border. Gently lifted drape up from its wrapper without touching any object. Discarded wrapper with other hand.

(4) With other hand, grasped an adjacent corner of drape and held it straight up and away from body. Allowed drape to unfold, kept it above waist and work surface and away from body. Discarded wrapper with other hand.

(5) Holding drape, positioned bottom half over top half of intended work surface.

(6) Allowed top half of drape to be placed over bottom half of work surface.

5. Added sterile items to sterile field.

   a. Opened sterile item while holding outside wrapper in nondominant hand.

   b. Carefully peeled wrapper over nondominant hand.

   c. Ensured that the wrapper did not fall down onto the sterile field. Placed the item onto the field at an angle. Did not hold arms over sterile field.

   d. Disposed of outer wrapper.

6. Poured sterile solutions.

   a. Verified contents and expiration date of solution.

   b. Placed receptacle for solution near table/work surface edge.

   c. Removed sterile seal and cap from bottle in upward motion.

   d. With solution bottle held away from field and bottle lip 2.5–5 cm (1–2 inches) above inside of sterile receiving container, slowly poured needed amount of solution into container. Held bottle with label facing palm of hand.

7. Helped patient to a comfortable position.

8. Placed nurse call system in an accessible location within patient's reach.

	S	U	NP	Comments

9. Raised side rails (as appropriate) and lowered bed to lowest position, locking into position. ___ ___ ___ _____

10. Removed and disposed of supplies and gloves and performed hand hygiene. ___ ___ ___ _____

EVALUATION

1. Observed for breaks in sterile field. ___ ___ ___ _____

2. Used Teach-Back. Revised instruction if patient or family caregiver was not able to teach back correctly. ___ ___ ___ _____

DOCUMENTATION

1. No documentation is required. ___ ___ ___ _____

HAND-OFF REPORTING

1. No reporting is required. ___ ___ ___ _____

Student _____ Date _____

Instructor _____ Date _____

PERFORMANCE CHECKLIST SKILL 10.3 **STERILE GLOVING**

	S	U	NP	Comments
ASSESSMENT				
1. Considered the type of procedure to be performed and consulted agency policy on use of sterile gloves.	___	___	___	_____
2. Considered patient's risk for infection.	___	___	___	_____
3. Selected correct size and type of gloves, and examined glove package to determine if it was dry and intact with no water stains.	___	___	___	_____
4. Used nonpowdered gloves.	___	___	___	_____
5. Inspected condition of hands for cuts, hangnails, open lesions, or abrasions.	___	___	___	_____
6. Assessed patient for risk factors before applying latex gloves.	___	___	___	_____
7. Assessed patient's/family caregiver's health literacy.	___	___	___	_____
8. Assessed patient's knowledge, prior experience with sterile gloving, and feeling about procedure.	___	___	___	_____
PLANNING				
1. Determined expected outcomes following completion of procedure.	___	___	___	_____
IMPLEMENTATION				
1. Applied sterile gloves.	___	___	___	_____
a. Performed thorough hand hygiene. Placed glove package near work area.	___	___	___	_____
b. Removed outer glove package wrapper by carefully separating and peeling apart sides.	___	___	___	_____
c. Grasped inner package and laid on clean, dry, flat surface at waist level. Opened package, keeping gloves on inside surface of wrapper.	___	___	___	_____
d. Identified right and left glove. Gloved dominant hand first.	___	___	___	_____
e. With thumb and first two fingers of nondominant hand, grasped glove for dominant hand by touching only inside surface of cuff.	___	___	___	_____

		S	U	NP	Comments

f. Carefully pulled glove over dominant hand, leaving a cuff and being sure that cuff did not roll up wrist. Ensured that thumb and fingers were in proper spaces.
    —   —   —   _____

g. With gloved dominant hand, slipped fingers underneath cuff of second glove.
    —   —   —   _____

h. Carefully pulled second glove over fingers of nondominant hand.
    —   —   —   _____

i. After second glove was on, interlocked hands together and held away from body above waist level until beginning procedure.
    —   —   —   _____

2. Performed procedure.
    —   —   —   _____

3. Removed gloves.
    —   —   —   _____

a. Grasped outside of one cuff with other gloved hand; avoided touching wrist.
    —   —   —   _____

b. Pulled glove off, turned it inside out, and placed it in gloved hand.
    —   —   —   _____

c. Took fingers of bare hand and tucked inside remaining glove cuff. Peeled glove off inside out and over previously removed glove. Discarded both gloves in receptacle.
    —   —   —   _____

d. Performed thorough hand hygiene.
    —   —   —   _____

4. Helped patient to a comfortable position.
    —   —   —   _____

5. Placed nurse call system in an accessible location within patient's reach.
    —   —   —   _____

6. Raised side rails (as appropriate) and lowered bed to lowest position, locking into position.
    —   —   —   _____

EVALUATION

1. Assessed patient for signs of infection, focusing on area treated.
    —   —   —   _____

2. Assessed patient for signs of latex allergy.
    —   —   —   _____

3. Used Teach-Back. Revised instruction if patient or family caregiver was not able to teach back correctly.
    —   —   —   _____

DOCUMENTATION

1. It was not necessary to document application of gloves. Documented specific procedure performed and patient's response and status.
    —   —   —   _____

2. In the event of a latex allergy reaction, documented patient's response. Noted type of response and patient's reaction to emergency treatment.
    —   —   —   _____

	S	U	NP	Comments

HAND-OFF REPORTING

1. Reported specific reason for procedure, patient's response to procedure, and response to education. ____ ____ ____ _____

2. In the event of a patient latex allergy, reported the patient response and reaction to emergency treatment. ____ ____ ____ _____

Student _____ Date _____

Instructor _____ Date _____

PERFORMANCE CHECKLIST SKILL 11.1 **USING SAFE AND EFFECTIVE TRANSFER TECHNIQUES**

	S	U	NP	Comments

ASSESSMENT

1. Identified patient using two identifiers according to agency policy. ___ ___ ___ _____

2. Referred to patient's electronic health record (EHR) for most recent documented weight and height for patient. ___ ___ ___ _____

3. Reviewed history for previous fall and if patient had a fear of falling. ___ ___ ___ _____

4. Used EHR to assess previous mode of transferring to bed or chair (if applicable). ___ ___ ___ _____

5. Reviewed EHR for presence of neuromuscular deficits, motor weakness or incoordination, calcium loss from bone, cognitive and visual dysfunction, and altered balance. ___ ___ ___ _____

6. Assessed patient's/family caregiver's health literacy. ___ ___ ___ _____

7. Assessed patient's cognitive status. ___ ___ ___ _____

8. Performed hand hygiene. ___ ___ ___ _____

9. Assessed the patient's mobility: administered the Banner Mobility Assessment Tool (BMAT). ___ ___ ___ _____

10. While assessing mobility, noted any weakness, dizziness, or risk for orthostatic hypotension (OH). ___ ___ ___ _____

11. Assessed activity tolerance, noting fatigue during sitting and standing. ___ ___ ___ _____

12. Assessed sensory status. ___ ___ ___ _____

13. Assessed level of comfort and measured level of pain using scale of 0 to10. Offered prescribed analgesic 30 min before transfer. Provided assistance to patient when analgesic was given. ___ ___ ___ _____

14. Assessed patient's level of motivation. ___ ___ ___ _____

15. Assessed previous mode of transfer in home setting (if applicable). ___ ___ ___ _____

16. Assessed patient's vital signs (VS) just before transfer. ___ ___ ___ _____

146

	S	U	NP	Comments

17. Analyzed assessment data and referred to mobility status and safe-handling algorithms to determine if a lift device or mechanical transfer device was needed and the number of people needed to help with transfer. Did not start procedure until all required caregivers were available.   ___ ___ ___ _____

18. Assessed patient's knowledge, prior experience with transfer, and feelings about procedure.   ___ ___ ___ _____

PLANNING

1. Determined expected outcomes following completion of procedure.   ___ ___ ___ _____

2. Closed room door and bedside curtain. Prepared environment; removed any obstacles impeding transfer.   ___ ___ ___ _____

3. Obtained and organized equipment/lift device for transfer at bedside. Performed hand hygiene.   ___ ___ ___ _____

4. Explained preparations for transfer technique and safety precautions used to patient. Explained benefits and reasons for getting up in a chair.   ___ ___ ___ _____

IMPLEMENTATION

1. Assisted patient from lying to sitting position on edge of bed.   ___ ___ ___ _____

   a. With patient in supine position in bed, raised head of bed 30 to 45 degrees and lowered bed, level with hips. Raised upper side rail on side where patient would exit bed. Applied non-skid shoes or socks.   ___ ___ ___ _____

   b. If patient was fully mobile, allowed to sit on side of bed independently, using side rails to raise up.   ___ ___ ___ _____

   c. If patient needed assistance to sit on side of bed, turned patient onto side facing self while standing on side of bed where patient would sit.   ___ ___ ___ _____

   (1). Stood opposite patient's hips. Turned diagonally to face patient and far corner of foot bed.   ___ ___ ___ _____

   (2). Placed own feet apart in wide base of support with foot closer to head of bed in front of other foot.   ___ ___ ___ _____

   (3). Placed own arm nearer to head of bed under patient's lower shoulder, supporting head and neck. Placed other arm over and under patient's thighs.   ___ ___ ___ _____

   (4). Moved patient's lower legs and feet over side of bed as patient used side rail to push and raise upper body. Pivoted weight onto own rear leg and allowed patient's upper legs to swing downward. Did not lift legs. At same time, continued to shift weight to own rear leg and guided patient in elevating trunk into upright position.   ___ ___ ___ _____

2. Lowered bed so that patient could sit on the side of the bed with feet on floor for 2 to 3 min. Had patient alternately flex and extend feet and move lower legs up and down without touching floor. Asked if patient felt dizzy; if so, checked blood pressure. Had patient relax and take a few deep breaths until dizziness subsided and balance was gained. If dizziness lasted more than 60 seconds or if systolic BP had dropped at least 20 mm Hg within 3 minutes of sitting upright, returned patient to bed. Rechecked BP.

3. Transferred patient from bed to chair (Option: Used seated transfer aid or powered stand-assist device):

   a. Applied clean gloves if bed linen was soiled. Had chair in position at 45-degree angle with one side against bed, facing foot of bed.

   b. Ensured patient's feet were comfortably flat on the floor with the hip and knees at a 90-degree angle. Helped patient apply stable, nonskid shoes/socks.

   c. If patient could bear weight fully during transfer:

      (1) Stood by bedside and allowed patient to transfer independently.

   d. If patient had partial weight bearing or unreliable standing balance, was cooperative and had upper extremity strength and sitting balance:

      (1) Applied gait belt correctly. Belt fit snugly so two fingers fit between the belt and patient's body, with buckle in front of body. Did not place belt over any intravenous lines, wounds, drains, or tubes. Adjusted belt once patient stood as needed.

      (2) Placed patient's weight-bearing or strong leg under the patient and the weak or non-weight bearing foot forward.

      (3) Held the gait belt with both hands and fingers pointing up, along patient's sides. Did not push, pull, lift, or catch patient with use of gait belt.

      (4) Spread own feet apart. Flexed hips and knees, aligning knees with patient's knees.

      (5) Rocked patient up to standing position on count of three while straightening hips and legs and keeping knees slightly flexed. While rocking patient in back-and-forth motion, made sure that own body weight was moving in the same direction as the patient's. Unless contraindicated, instructed patient to use hands to push up if applicable.

148

	S	U	NP	Comments

(6) Maintained stability of patient's weaker leg with own knee, as needed. ____ ____ ____ _____

(7) Pivoted on stronger foot near chair while bearing weight. ____ ____ ____ _____

(8) Instructed patient to use armrests on chair for support and ease into chair. ____ ____ ____ _____

(9) Flexed hips and knees while lowering patient into chair. ____ ____ ____ _____

(10) Assisted patient to assume proper alignment in sitting position. Provided support for weakened extremity (as needed). Used sling or lap board to support an injured or flaccid arm. ____ ____ ____ _____

(11) Ensured proper alignment for sitting position, thighs paralleled and in horizontal plane, both feet supported flat on floor and ankles comfortably flexed. Maintained a 2.5- to 5-cm (1- to 2-inch) space between edge of seat and popliteal space on posterior surface of knee. ____ ____ ____ _____

(12) To return patient to bed from wheelchair, followed steps in Procedural Guideline 11.1, Step 7. ____ ____ ____ _____

e. Transferred patient from bed to chair. If patient was limited cognitively, was uncooperative, or had weight-bearing precautions with upper body strength, or required caregiver to lift more than 15.9 kg (35 lb), used a full body sling lift with two or three caregivers. Followed manufacturer lift guidelines to apply sling correctly. ____ ____ ____ _____

(1) Brought mechanical floor lift to bedside or lowered ceiling lift and positioned properly. ____ ____ ____ _____

(2) Ensured chair was available along one side of bed, facing foot of bed. Allowed adequate space to maneuver the lift. ____ ____ ____ _____

(3) Raised bed to safe working height with mattress flat. Lowered side rail on side near chair. ____ ____ ____ _____

(4) Had second nurse positioned at opposite side of bed. ____ ____ ____ _____

(5) Rolled patient on side away from self. ____ ____ ____ _____

(6) Placed hammock or canvas strips under patient to form sling. With two canvas pieces, lowered edge fits under patient's knees (wide piece), and upper edge fits under patient's shoulders (narrow piece). Placed sling under patient's center of gravity and greatest part of body weight. ____ ____ ____ _____

	S	U	NP	Comments

(7) Rolled patient back toward self as second nurse pulled hammock (straps) through.

(8) Returned patient to supine position. Ensured that hammock or straps were smooth over bed surface. Ensured that sling extended from shoulders to knees to support patient's body weight equally.

(9) Removed patient's glasses if worn.

(10) Rolled the horseshoe base of floor lift under patient's bed (on side with chair).

(11) Lowered horizontal bar to sling level by following manufacturer's directions. Locked valve if required.

(12) Attached hooks on strap (chain) to holes in sling. Short chains or straps hooked to top holes of sling; longer chains hooked to bottom of sling.

(13) Elevated head of bed to Fowler position and had patient fold arms over chest.

(14) If the lift was electric, pushed the button to raise the patient off the bed. If the lift was a nonelectric lift, pumped the hydraulic handle using long, slow, even strokes until patient was raised off bed. For ceiling lift, turned on control device to move lift.

(15) Used lift to raise patient off bed and used steering handle to pull lift from bed as self and another nurse maneuvered patient to chair. Had second nurse alongside patient.

(16) Rolled base of lift around chair with one nurse guiding patient's legs. Released check valve slowly or pushed the button down and lowered patient into chair.

(17) Closed check valve, if needed, as soon as patient was down in chair and straps could be released. Newer lifts may not need this.

(18) Removed straps and rolled mechanical/hydraulic lift out of patient's path.

(19) Checked patient's sitting alignment and corrected if necessary. Kept lift straps in place.

4. Performed lateral transfer from bed to stretcher:

a. If patient could assist (refer to last documented patient weight).

	S	U	NP	Comments

(1) A caregiver stood by for safety, with stretcher and bed locked in flat position, as patient moved to stretcher. Surface of stretcher was ½ inch lower for lateral move. ___ ___ ___ _____

b. If patient was not able to independently transfer and was <91 kg (200 lb), used a friction-reducing device and/or lateral transfer board. ___ ___ ___ _____

(1) Lateral transfer FRD or air assisted device:

    i. Applied clean gloves if there was risk of soiling. Lowered head of bed as much as patient could tolerate, then raised bed to comfortable working height. Was sure to lock bed brakes. ___ ___ ___ _____

    ii. Crossed patient's arms on chest. ___ ___ ___ _____

    iii. Lowered side rails. To place transfer device (slide board) or deflated air-assisted mattress under patient, positioned two nurses on side of bed toward which patient would be turned. Positioned third nurse on other side of bed. ___ ___ ___ _____

    iv. Fanfolded drawsheet on both sides. ___ ___ ___ _____

    v. On count of three, logrolled patient onto side toward the two nurses. Turned patient as one unit with smooth, continuous motion. ___ ___ ___ _____

    vi. Placed slide board or option: deflated mattress of air assisted device under drawsheet. Spread out deflated mattress on bed under patient similar to spreading out a new sheet. ___ ___ ___ _____

    vii. Warned that patient would be rolling over hard or irregular surface. Asked patient to roll toward the nurse on other side of bed staying aligned. Rolled out deflated mattress. Gently turned patient onto supine position to center over FRD. ___ ___ ___ _____

    viii. Ensured board and mattress were centered under patient. Secured patient to air-assisted mattress. ___ ___ ___ _____

    ix. Lined up stretcher so that surface was ½ inch lower than bed mattress. Locked brakes on stretcher. Instructed patient not to move. ___ ___ ___ _____

    x. Option: Inflated the mattress. Secured safety straps over patient (if air-assisted mattress used). ___ ___ ___ _____

	S	U	NP	Comments

xi. Two nurses positioned themselves on side of stretcher while third nurse positioned self on side of bed without stretcher. All three nurses placed feet widely apart with one foot slightly in front of the other and grasped friction-reducing device. ___ ___ ___ _____

xii. Holding the edges of slide board or air inflated mattress with one nurse counting to three, and the two nurses slid board or mattress to stretcher, positioning patient onto stretcher. The third nurse guided slide board or mattress in place. ___ ___ ___ _____

xiii. Positioned patient in center of stretcher. Turned patient to side to remove slide board. Air mattress alright to remain in place deflated. Raised head of stretcher if not contraindicated. Raised stretcher side rails. Covered patient with blanket. ___ ___ ___ _____

c. If patient was not able to independently transfer and was >91kg (200lb), used a ceiling lift or full body-lifting device with seated or supine sling with a minimum of three caregivers.

5. After transferring patient to bed, chair, or stretcher, ensured patient was positioned comfortably. ___ ___ ___ _____

6. Placed nurse call system in an accessible location within patient's reach. ___ ___ ___ _____

7. Raised side rails (as appropriate) and lowered and locked bed into lowest position. ___ ___ ___ _____

8. Removed and disposed of gloves (if used) and performed hand hygiene. ___ ___ ___ _____

EVALUATION

1. Monitored vital signs. Asked if patient felt dizzy or tired and to rate pain on pain scale of 0 to 10. ___ ___ ___ _____

2. Noted patient's behavioral response to transfer. ___ ___ ___ _____

3. Checked condition of patient's skin after each transfer. ___ ___ ___ _____

4. Used Teach-Back. Revised instruction if patient or family caregiver was not able to teach-back correctly. ___ ___ ___ _____

DOCUMENTATION

1. Documented procedure, including pertinent observations: weakness, level of pain, ability to follow directions, weight-bearing ability, balance, strength, ability to pivot, length of time to perform activity, number of personnel needed to help, assist device used, and patient's response. ___ ___ ___ _____

152

	S	U	NP	Comments

2. Documented evaluation of patient and family caregiver learning.

HAND-OFF REPORTING

1. Reported transfer ability, patient response, and help needed to next shift or other caregivers.

2. Reported progress or remission to rehabilitation staff.

Student _____ Date _____

Instructor _____ Date _____

PERFORMANCE CHECKLIST PROCEDURAL GUIDELINE 11.1 **WHEELCHAIR TRANSFER TECHNIQUES**

	S	U	NP	Comments

STEPS

1. Identified patient using at least two identifiers according to agency policy.

2. Reviewed electronic health record (EHR) to assess patient's weight, height, and strength; cognition; level of pain; and balance during previous transfer.

3. Assessed patient's healthy literacy level, knowledge, and experience with wheelchair transfers.

4. Performed hand hygiene. Completed a full assessment, including the Banner Mobility Assessment Tool (BMAT) for functional ability to determine patient's ability to tolerate and help with transfer.

5. Checked wheelchair locks, wheels, and footplates for proper functioning before use.

6. Explained the steps of the transfer procedure to the patient.

7. Transferred patient from a wheelchair to bed (if patient was cooperative and partially weight bearing) using pivot technique:

   a. Adjusted the height of the bed to the level of the seat of the wheelchair (when possible).

   b. Positioned wheelchair with one wheel against the side of the bed midway between the head and foot of the bed, with the wheelchair facing toward the foot of the bed. Removed the armrest nearest the side of the bed.

   c. Locked both wheels of the wheelchair by pushing forward on the handles above the rims of the wheels.

   d. Raised the footplates.

   e. Placed a gait belt on patient completely and snuggly around patient's waist, not over intravenous lines, incisions, drains, or tubes.

   f. Had patient place hands on armrests and stood by as patient moved to the front of the wheelchair.

   g. Stood slightly in front of patient to guard and protect throughout the transfer.

154

h. Placed both hands (palms up) under patient's gait belt, bent knees, and instructed patient to stand at a count of three.

    ____   ____   ____   _____

i. Allowed patient to stand a few seconds ensuring the patient was not dizzy and had good balance. Pivoted with patient while turning to face away from the side of the bed. Then had patient sit on the edge of the mattress. Ensured patient was firmly sitting, and not slipping off edge of bed.

    ____   ____   ____   _____

j. Raised head of bed to 45 degrees. With patient sitting on the edge of the bed, placed own arm nearest the head of the bed under the patient's shoulder while supporting the head and neck. Placed other arm under patient's knees. Bent own knees and kept own back straight.

    ____   ____   ____   _____

k. Told patient to help lift legs when movement began. On a count of three, stood with a wide base of support, raised patient's legs, pivoting the body and lowered the shoulders onto the bed. Remembered to keep own back straight.

    ____   ____   ____   _____

l. Helped patient return to bed, lower head and assume a comfortable position.

    ____   ____   ____   _____

8. Transferred patient from a wheelchair to bed (patient was non–weight bearing and unable to stand but was cooperative and had upper body strength) using transfer board:

    ____   ____   ____   _____

a. Followed steps 7a though 7f.

    ____   ____   ____   _____

b. Ensured seat of the wheelchair was level with the top of the bed mattress. Positioned a transfer board by placing it across the bed to the chair so patient could slide across it. Ensured the board overlapped the chair and mattress so that it would not slip out of place. Then had patient use hands on wheelchair arms to raise hips up and placed the other part of the board under the patient's buttock that was closest to the bed.

    ____   ____   ____   _____

c. Stood in front of patient. Had patient lift and move to the front of the wheelchair.

    ____   ____   ____   _____

d. Placed own legs on the outside of patient's legs. Ensured patient's feet were on the floor. Grasped the gait belt (palms up) along both of patient's sides. Had patient place one hand on the slide board and the other on the mattress surface.

    ____   ____   ____   _____

e. Bent own knees and on a count of three had patient use arms to slide across the board from the chair to the bed.

    ____   ____   ____   _____

	S	U	NP	Comments

f. Had patient sit on edge of bed, slightly above where the bed bends when elevated.

g. Assisted patient by raising the legs while pivoting the patient's body moving legs back onto mattress and positioning comfortably.

9. Placed nurse call system in reach; instructed patient in use.

10. Raised side rails (as appropriate), lowered and locked bed to lowest position. Performed hand hygiene.

11. Monitored vital signs after patient had been transferred. Asked if patient felt dizzy, fatigued or in pain.

12. Noted patient's behavioral response to transfer.

13. Used Teach-Back. Revised instruction if patient or family caregiver was not able to teach back correctly.

14. Documented patient's ability to tolerate transfer and level of assistance required.

15. Hand-off reporting: Reported any intolerance to transfer to next nurse caring for patient.

Student _____ Date _____

Instructor _____ Date _____

PERFORMANCE CHECKLIST SKILL 11.2 **MOVING AND POSITIONING PATIENTS IN BED**

	S	U	NP	Comments

ASSESSMENT

1. Identified patient using two identifiers according to agency policy.

2. Referred to electronic health record (EHR) for most recent documented weight and height for patient.

3. Checked health care provider's orders for any restrictions in movement before positioning patient.

4. Assessed patient's/family caregiver's health literacy.

5. Performed hand hygiene.

6. Assessed patient's range of motion (ROM) and current body alignment while patient was lying down.

7. Examined patient to assess for risk factors that contribute to complications of immobility.

8. Assessed patient's level of consciousness.

9. Assessed patient for presence of pain; rated on scale of 0 to 10.

10. Performed a thorough assessment of condition of patient's skin, especially over bony prominences. Knew patient's Braden score and level of risk for developing a pressure injury.

11. Assessed patient's vision and hearing.

12. Applied clean gloves (as needed) to assess for presence of incisions, drainage tubes, and equipment. Emptied drainage bags before positioning. Removed and disposed of gloves. Performed hand hygiene.

13. Assessed motivation of patient and ability of family caregivers to anticipate in moving and positioning if patient is to be discharged home.

PLANNING

1. Determined expected outcomes following completion of procedure.

2. If patient perceived level of pain to be enough to avoid movement, offered an analgesic 30 minutes (if ordered) before repositioning.

3. Got additional caregivers and/or necessary lift or transfer device to perform positioning.

	S	U	NP	Comments

4. Closed room door or bedside curtains. Explained positioning procedure to patient and what was expected of them.

    _____ _____ _____ _____

IMPLEMENTATION

1. Performed hand hygiene.

    _____ _____ _____ _____

2. Raised level of bed to comfortable working height, level with own elbows. Removed all pillows and any devices used in previous position.

    _____ _____ _____ _____

3. Assisted patient to move up in bed:

    _____ _____ _____ _____

  a. If patient could fully assist:

    (1) Stood at bedside to help with positioning of tubing and equipment as patient moved.

    _____ _____ _____ _____

    (2) Had patient place feet flat on mattress, grasp either side rails or overhead trapeze and, on a count of three, lift hips up and push legs so body moved up in bed.

    _____ _____ _____ _____

    (3) Positioned for comfort.

    _____ _____ _____ _____

  b. If patient could not independently assist:

    (1) Had patient use a repositioning aid such as an FRD or air-assisted lateral transfer or lifting device.

    _____ _____ _____ _____

    (2) If patient weighed <91 kg (200 lb): used FRD and two to three caregivers.

    _____ _____ _____ _____

    (3) If patient weighed >91 kg (200 lb): used FRD and at least three caregivers.

    _____ _____ _____ _____

      i. Using an FRD with three nurses, positioned patient supine with head of bed flat. A nurse stood on each side of bed.

    _____ _____ _____ _____

      ii. Removed pillow from under head and shoulders and placed it at head of bed.

    _____ _____ _____ _____

      iii. Turned patient side to side to place FRD under drawsheet on bed, with device extending from shoulders to thighs or ankles.

    _____ _____ _____ _____

      iv. Returned patient to supine position.

    _____ _____ _____ _____

      v. Had two caregivers grasp draw sheet (one on each side of bed) firmly and had third nurse hold FRD at end of bed.

    _____ _____ _____ _____

      vi. Placed feet apart with forward-backward stance. Flexed knees and hips. On count of three, shifted weight from back to front leg and moved patient and drawsheet to desired position up in bed. Did not lift patient.

    _____ _____ _____ _____

  c. If patient was unable to assist:

	S	U	NP	Comments

(1) Used ceiling lift with supine sling or floor-based lift and two or more nurses to move and position patient up in bed. ___ ___ ___ _____

4. Positioned patient in bed in one of the following positions while ensuring correct body alignment. In all cases protected pressure areas. ___ ___ ___ _____

a. Determined if patient could assist. ___ ___ ___ _____

b. For a patient who could assist fully, began by having patient lie supine and move up in bed following Steps 3a (1)–(3).
For a patient unable to assist independently, followed Step 3b. ___ ___ ___ _____

c. Supported semi-Fowler or Fowler position (two nurses):

(1) With patient lying supine, position pillows using two caregivers. ___ ___ ___ _____

(2) Rested head against mattress or on small pillow. ___ ___ ___ _____

(3) Placed pillows under and along patient's left and right hip and back. Logrolled patient slightly to position pillow on each side. ___ ___ ___ _____

(4) Used pillows to support arms and hands if patient did not have voluntary control of use of hands and arms. ___ ___ ___ _____

(5) Placed pillows lengthwise under each leg (mid-thigh to ankle) to support the knee in slight flexion and allow the heels to float. ___ ___ ___ _____

(6) Raised head of bed 45 to 60 degrees if not contraindicated. ___ ___ ___ _____

d. Hemiplegic patient positioned in supported semi-Fowler or Fowler position (two nurses):

(1) With patient lying supine, positioned pillows using two caregivers. ___ ___ ___ _____

(2) Positioned head on small pillow with chin slightly forward. If patient was totally unable to control head movement, avoided hyperextension of neck. ___ ___ ___ _____

(3) Placed pillows under and along patient's left and right hip and back, being sure patient was as anatomically straight as possible. Logrolled patient slightly to position pillow on each side. ___ ___ ___ _____

(4) Provided support for involved arm and hand by placing arm away from patient's side and supporting elbow with pillow. ___ ___ ___ _____

	S	U	NP	Comments

(5) Placed rolled blanket (trochanter roll) or pillows firmly alongside patient's legs to help prevent the patient from leaning towards the affected side.

(6) Supported feet in dorsiflexion with therapeutic boots or splints.

(7) Elevated 30 to 60 degrees according to patient's tolerance.

e. Patient positioned in supported supine position (two nurses):

(1) With patient laying supine and head of bed flat, used two caregivers to position pillows.

(2) Placed pillow under upper shoulders, neck and head.

(3) Placed pillows under and along patient's left and right hip and back. Logrolled patient slightly to position pillow on each side.

(4) Placed pillows lengthwise under each leg (mid-thigh to ankle) to support the knee in slight flexion (avoiding hyperextension) and allowed the heels to float.

(5) Option: Placed patient's feet in therapeutic boots or splints.

(6) Placed pillows under pronated forearms, keeping upper arms parallel to patient's body.

(7) Option: Placed hand rolls in patient's hands. Considered physical therapy referral for use of hand splints.

f. Hemiplegic patient positioned in supine position (two nurses):

(1) With patient lying supine and head of bed flat, used two caregivers to position.

(2) Placed folded towel or small pillow under shoulder of affected side.

(3) Kept affected arm away from body with elbow extended and palm up. Positioned affected hand in one of recommended positions for flaccid or spastic hand. (Alternatively, placed arm out to side, with elbow bent and hand toward head of bed.).

(4) Placed folded towel under hip of involved side.

(5) Flexed affected knee 30 degrees by supporting it on elongated pillow or folded blanket.

160

	S	U	NP	Comments

    (6) Supported feet with soft pillows placed against sole of feet at right angle to leg. Option: Used soft foot boot.).

g. Patient positioned in 30-degree lateral (side-lying) position (two nurses):

    (1) With patient lying in supine, lowered head of bed completely or as low as patient could tolerate. Once nurse on each side of bed.

    (2) Lowered side rails. Alternatively turned patient side to side to place FRD underneath patient's drawsheet. Then positioned patient by having one nurse pull drawsheet toward side of bed in opposite direction patient was to be turned. Aligned patient straight, then rolled side to side and removed FRD.

    (3) Flexed patient's leg straight on side patient was to lay after being turned. Kept foot on mattress. Nurse on side to which patient was to be turned, placed one hand on patient's upper bent knee and other hand on patient's shoulder.

    (4) Using knee and hip for leverage, nurse rolled patient onto side toward self.

    (5) Placed pillow under patient's head and neck.

    (6) Nurse facing patient's back, placed hands under patient's dependent shoulder and brough shoulder blade forward.

    (7) Positioned both of patient's arms in slightly flexed position. Supported upper arm with pillow level with shoulder; supported other arm against mattress or small pillow.

    (8) Nurse facing patient's back placed hands under dependent hip and realigned hip so angle from hip to mattress was approximately 30 degrees.

    (9) Placed small tuck-back pillow behind patient's back.

    (10) Placed pillow under semiflexed upper leg level at hip from groin to foot.

    (11) Option: Placed pillows or sandbags (if available) parallel against plantar surface of dependent foot. Also may have used ankle-foot orthotic on feet if available.

h. Logrolled patient (three nurses):

    (1) With patient lying supine, placed small pillow between patient's knees.

	S	U	NP	Comments

(2) Crossed patient's arms on chest.

(3) Positioned two nurses on side toward which patient was to be turned and one nurse on side where pillows were to be placed behind patient's back. This nurse also supported patient's neck as needed.

(4) Fanfolded drawsheet along backside of patient.

(5) With one nurse grasping drawsheet at lower hips and thighs and the other nurse grasping drawsheet at patient's shoulders and lower back, rolled patient as one unit in a smooth, continuous motion on count of three.

(6) Nurse on opposite side of bed placed pillows along length of patient for support.

(7) Gently leaned patient as a unit back toward pillows for support. Placed patient's feet in therapeutic boots or splints.

5. Ensured patient felt comfortable in new position.

6. Raised side rails (as appropriate), lowered and locked bed into lowest position.

7. Placed nurse call system within patient's reach.

8. Performed hand hygiene.

EVALUATION

1. Assessed patient's respiratory status, body alignment, position, and level of comfort on an ongoing basis. Patient's body was supported by adequate mattress, and vertebral column was without observable curves.

2. Observed for changes in joint ROM.

3. Observed for areas of erythema or breakdown involving skin, especially in dependent areas.

4. Used Teach-Back. Revised instruction on spot or developed a plan for revised patient/family caregiver teaching if patient or family caregiver was not able to teach back correctly.

DOCUMENTATION

1. Documented positioning change, time of change, FRD used and observations.

2. Documented evaluation of patient learning.

HAND-OFF REPORTING

1. Reported observations of patient's tolerance of position changes to nurse at change of shift.

2. Reported skin or joint complications to health care provider.

162

Student _____ Date _____

Instructor _____ Date _____

PERFORMANCE CHECKLIST SKILL 12.1   **PROMOTING EARLY ACTIVITY AND EXERCISE**

	S	U	NP	Comments

ASSESSMENT

1. Identified patient using at least two identifiers.

2. Reviewed patient's electronic health record (EHR) for conditions that could influence or contraindicate mobility/exercise.
   Inpatient: Reviewed health care provider's order for early mobility or exercise program.
   Outpatient: Obtained health care provider clearance for outpatient exercise.

3. Assessed patient's/family caregiver's health literacy.

4. Performed hand hygiene. Gathered baseline assessment of vital signs (VS) and oxygen saturation (if available).

5. Assessed character of patient's pain; asked patient to rate pain on a scale of 0 to 10.

6. Determined patient's age and calculated target heart rate range. Conformed with health care provider desired target range (as appropriate).

7. Assessed patient's beliefs, values and knowledge regarding current health status and confidence in being capable of performing exercise (including fear of falling).

8. Inpatient Early Progressive Mobility Interventions— begun in intensive care unit (ICU).

9. Outpatient assessment.

   a. Identified patient's activity/exercise history.

   b. Determined if patient had social support from peers, family, or spouse.

   c. Assessed if patient had access to facility or area to exercise.

   d. Considered patient's age, income level, time, available to exercise, rural resident, overweight or obesity, being disabled.

   e. Had patient rate level of quality of life based on current activity level.

	S	U	NP	Comments

PLANNING

1. Determined expected outcomes following completion of procedure. ___ ___ ___ _____

2. Inpatient: Consulted with physical therapist (PT) regarding role in protocol to provide planned active resistance exercise for patients. If PT was available in home health, consulted on types of exercises suited for outpatient's mobility restrictions. ___ ___ ___ _____

3. Inpatient: Explained precautions that would be taken to prevent falls during ambulation. ___ ___ ___ _____

4. Inpatient: As patient progressed to ambulating, tried to schedule ambulation around patient's other activities. ___ ___ ___ _____

5. All patients: Explained benefits and reasons for activity/exercise. Did so in a way that matched patient's beliefs and values regarding recovery or maintaining health. ___ ___ ___ _____

IMPLEMENTATION

1. Implemented Inpatient Early Progressive Mobility Interventions. Each patient's medical status and ability to participate in mobility dictated the start level. Worked closely with interprofessional team to coordinate a plan. The following levels were an example to use: ___ ___ ___ _____

Level 1
- Initiated passive range of motion (ROM) exercises TID (three times a day). ___ ___ ___ _____
- Turned patient at least every 2 hours or more frequently based on assessment for risk of pressure injury. ___ ___ ___ _____
- Helped patient to sitting position in bed and maintained for 20 minutes TID. ___ ___ ___ _____
- Obtained a PT consultation for active resistance exercise. ___ ___ ___ _____

Level 2
- Continued passive ROM exercises TID. ___ ___ ___ _____
- Turned patient at least every 2 hours. ___ ___ ___ _____
- Helped patient to sitting position in bed and maintained for 20 minutes TID. ___ ___ ___ _____
- Initiated sitting patient on edge of bed or lifted patient to chair. ___ ___ ___ _____
- Active resistance exercise by PT. ___ ___ ___ _____

Level 3
- Continued passive ROM exercises TID. ___ ___ ___ _____
- Turned at least every 2 hours. ___ ___ ___ _____
- Helped patient to sitting position in bed and maintained for 20 minutes TID; sat on edge of bed unsupported (but supervised). ___ ___ ___ _____
- Performed active transfer to chair with the goal of the patient sitting up in chair 20 minutes TID. ___ ___ ___ _____
- Active resistance exercise by PT. ___ ___ ___ _____

164

	S	U	NP	Comments

Level 4
- Continued passive ROM TID.
- Turned at least every 2 hours.
- Performed active transfer to chair with patient sitting up in chair 20 minutes TID sitting on edge of bed unsupported (but supervised).
- PT continued with active resistance strengthening program.
- Initiated ambulation. Applied gait belt (if needed). Had patient ambulate. NOTE: Ambulation time/distance increased daily during hospitalization.

2. Promoted outpatient exercise and activity.

   a. Initiated an exercise program that contained at least a warm-up (5 to 10 minutes), balance exercise, and endurance exercises.

   b. Recommended strength training for adults.

   c. Promoted the United States Department of Health and Human Services's (2018) and American Hospital Association (2023a; 2023b) recommended aerobic exercise of at least 150 minutes per week of moderate exercise or 75 minutes per week of vigorous exercise (or combination of moderate and vigorous activity), including activities.

   d. Recommended balance exercises for older adults to decrease risk of falls. Ensured patient had something sturdy nearby on which to hold (wall or chair) if unsteady.

   e. As person progressed, added strengthening exercises such as use of weights or resistance bands. Started by using light weights, then gradually added more. Preformed at least 2 days per week, but did not exercise the same muscle group on any 2 days in a row.

   f. Recommend patient preform cool-down (5 minutes) after exercising.

EVALUATION
1. Measured vital signs and oxygen saturation during activity/exercise and compared findings with baseline and target heart rate range.

2. Evaluated patient's pain severity using 0-to-10 pain scale.

3. Monitored number of steps or estimated distance during walking.

4. After patient had reached level 4 of inpatient mobility protocol or after outpatient had been exercising over 2 to 3 months, evaluated level of confidence in performing exercises.

	S	U	NP	Comments

5. Used Teach-Back. Revised instruction or developed a plan for revised patient/caregiver teaching if patient or family caregiver was not able to teach back correctly.

    ____ ____ ____ _____

DOCUMENTATION

1. Documented results of patient screening, type of exercise implemented, preexercise and postexercise assessments, and patient's tolerance.

    ____ ____ ____ _____

2. Documented evaluation of patient and family caregiver learning.

    ____ ____ ____ _____

HAND-OFF REPORTING

1. Reported to health care provider any signs or symptoms indicative of exercise intolerance.

    ____ ____ ____ _____

Student _____ Date _____

Instructor _____ Date _____

PERFORMANCE CHECKLIST PROCEDURAL GUIDELINE 12.1   **PERFORMING RANGE-OF-MOTION EXERCISES**

	S	U	NP	Comments

STEPS

1. Identified patient using at least two identifiers. ___ ___ ___ _____

2. Reviewed patient's electronic health record (EHR) for physical assessment findings that could affect the performance; health care provider's orders, medical diagnosis, medical history, and progress. ___ ___ ___ _____

3. Assessed patient's/family caregiver's health literacy. ___ ___ ___ _____

4. Assessed patient's current level of fatigue and ability to cooperate with exercises. ___ ___ ___ _____

5. Preformed hand hygiene. Assessed patient's baseline joint function. Observed for obvious limitations in joint mobility, redness over joints; palpate for warmth over joint, joint tenderness, and presence of deformities or edema. Noted baseline ROM for affected joints. ___ ___ ___ _____

6. Assessed character of patient's pain or discomfort including rating pain severity from 0 to 10 before exercises. Determined if patient would benefit from pain medication before beginning ROM exercises; then administered analgesic 30 minutes before exercise. ___ ___ ___ _____

7. Determined patient's or family caregiver's knowledge, experience, and readiness to learn. Explained in plain language reason for the ROM exercises and described and demonstrated exercises to be performed. ___ ___ ___ _____

8. Performed hand hygiene and applied clean gloves if wound drainage or skin lesions were present. ___ ___ ___ _____

9. Helped patient to a comfortable position, preferably sitting or lying down. ___ ___ ___ _____

10. When performing passive ROM exercises, supported joint by holding or cradling distal part of extremity or using cupped hand to support joint. ___ ___ ___ _____

11. Completed exercises in head-to-toe sequence. Repeated each movement 5 times during an exercise session with sessions performed up to 6 times a day. Did not perform during sleeping hours. Informed patient how these exercises can be incorporated into ADLs. ___ ___ ___ _____

	S	U	NP	Comments

12. Once exercises were completed, helped patient to comfortable position. ___ ___ ___ _____

13. Placed nurse call system in an accessible location within patient's reach., raised side rails (as appropriate), lowered and locked bed into lowest position. ___ ___ ___ _____

14. Performed hand hygiene. ___ ___ ___ _____

15. For active ROM, observed patient preform each exercise. Option: Measured joint motion using a goniometer to determine level of improvement. ___ ___ ___ _____

16. Asked patient while exercising to describe any discomfort and rate pain on a pain scale. ___ ___ ___ _____

17. Used Teach-Back. Revised instruction or developed a plan for revised patient/family caregiver teaching if patient or family caregiver was not able to teach back correctly. ___ ___ ___ _____

18. Documented exercises preformed and patient's tolerance in a chart. ___ ___ ___ _____

19. Reported any new onset of pain in a joint or reduction in ROM to health care provider. ___ ___ ___ _____

Student _____ Date _____

Instructor _____ Date _____

PERFORMANCE CHECKLIST PROCEDURAL GUIDELINE 12.2 **APPLYING GRADUATED COMPRESSION (ELASTIC) STOCKINGS AND SEQUENTIAL COMPRESSION DEVICE**

	S	U	NP	Comments

STEPS

1. Identified patient using at least two identifiers. _____ _____ _____ _____

2. Reviewed electronic health record (EHR) for order for sequential compression devices (SCDs)/mobile compression devices (MCDs) or graduated compression stockings. _____ _____ _____ _____

3. Reviewed electronic health record (EHR) to assess patient for risk factors for developing deep vein thrombosis (DVT) such as by using the Wells score. _____ _____ _____ _____

4. Assessed patient's/family caregiver's health literacy. _____ _____ _____ _____

5. Performed hand hygiene. Assessed for contraindications for use of elastic stockings or compression devices. _____ _____ _____ _____

6. Assessed condition of patient's skin and circulation to the legs. Palpated pedal pulses, noted any palpable veins, and inspected skin over lower extremities for edema, skin discoloration, warmth, or presence of lesions. _____ _____ _____ _____

7. Assessed patient's or family caregiver's knowledge or experience regarding previous use of elastic compression stockings or compression devices. _____ _____ _____ _____

8. Explained procedure and reason for applying elastic stockings/SCD/MCD to prevent DVT. _____ _____ _____ _____

9. Closed room curtains or door to provide privacy. Positioned patient in supine position. _____ _____ _____ _____

10. Performed hand hygiene. Bathed patient's legs as needed. Dried thoroughly. Performed hand hygiene. _____ _____ _____ _____

11. Applied graduated compression stocking: _____ _____ _____ _____

    a. Used tape measure to measure patient's leg to determine proper elastic stocking size (followed package directions). _____ _____ _____ _____

    b. Option: Applied a small amount of powder or cornstarch to legs provided patient did not have sensitivity. _____ _____ _____ _____

	S	U	NP	Comments

c. Turned elastic stocking inside out: placed one hand into stocking, holding heel of stocking. Took other hand and pulled stocking inside out until reaching the heel

d. Placed patient's toes into foot of elastic stocking up to the heel and made sure that stocking was smooth.

e. Slid remaining portion of stocking over patient's foot and made sure that toes were covered. Made sure that foot fit into toe and heel position of stocking, with stocking right side out.

f. Slid stocking up over patient's calf until sock was completely extended. Ensured that stocking was smooth and that no ridges or wrinkles were present.

g. Instructed patient not to roll stockings partially down, avoid wrinkles, avoided crossing legs and elevated legs while sitting.

12. Applied SCD sleeve(s):

a. Removed SCD sleeves from plastic cover; unfolded and flattened onto bed.

b. Arranged SCD sleeve under patient's leg according to leg position indicated on inner lining of sleeve.

c. Placed patient's leg on SCD sleeve, lining up the back of the patient's ankle with the ankle marking on the inner lining of the sleeve.

d. Positioned back of knee with popliteal opening on inner sleeve.

e. Wrapped SCD sleeve securely around patient's leg. Checked fit of SCD sleeve by placing two fingers between patient's leg and sleeve.

f. Attached SCD sleeve connector to plug on mechanical unit and lined up the arrows on the connector with the arrows on the plug from the mechanical unit.

g. Turned the mechanical unit on and looked for a green light as an indication that the unit was functioning. Monitored functioning SCD through one full cycle of inflation and deflation.

13. Applied MCD sleeve:

a. Applied cotton stockinettes along with the calf sleeves over the patient's calves.

b. Wrapped the sleeve smoothly around the patient's calf and fastened it beginning at the top, moving towards the bottom.

170

	S	U	NP	Comments

c. Placed two fingers between patient's calf and sleeve to be sure it was snug but not too tight. ___ ___ ___ _____

d. Used either end of the extension tube to connect to the sleeve or device pump. ___ ___ ___ _____

   (1) Connected one end of the extension tube to the sleeve connector. Ensured the white arrows were pointed towards each other. ___ ___ ___ _____

   (2) Connected the other end of the extension tube to the device pump; ensured the white arrow was facing upwards. ___ ___ ___ _____

e. Pressed the power switch located at the back of the device to ON position so that the Configuration Setup Screen was shown on the LCD screen, and the sleeves immediately started to inflate from the bottom to the top. ___ ___ ___ _____

f. Waited 60 seconds for the automatic operation of the device. The device automatically identified which sleeves were connected, selected the suitable treatment mode, and displayed information on the main LCD screen. ___ ___ ___ _____

14. Positioned patient comfortably, then placed nurse call system in an accessible location within patient's reach. Allowed patient wearing MCD sleeves to walk with device in place. ___ ___ ___ _____

15. Raised side rails (as appropriate) lowered and locked bed into lowest position. Performed hand hygiene. ___ ___ ___ _____

16. Removed compression stockings or SCD/MCD sleeves at least once per shift. Ensured compression stockings and devices were only worn during daytime activities and were removed for resting and at night. ___ ___ ___ _____

17. Evaluated skin integrity and circulation to patient's lower extremities as ordered. ___ ___ ___ _____

18. Used Teach-Back. Revised instruction or developed a plan for revised patient/family caregiver teaching if patient or family caregiver was not able to teach back correctly. ___ ___ ___ _____

19. Documented condition of lower extremities, application of stockings/SCDs/MCDs and patient response to education. ___ ___ ___ _____

20. Hand-off reporting: Reported to health care provider or nurse in charge any signs that indicated formation of DVT. ___ ___ ___ _____

Student _____ Date _____

Instructor _____ Date _____

PERFORMANCE CHECKLIST PROCEDURAL GUIDELINE 12.3 **ASSISTING WITH AMBULATION (WITHOUT ASSISTIVE DEVICES)**

	S	U	NP	Comments
STEPS				
1. Identified patient using at least two identifiers.	___	___	___	_____
2. Reviewed electronic health record (EHR) for patient's most recent activity history, including distance ambulated, use of assist device, activity tolerance, balance, and gait. Noted history of orthostatic hypotension and any medications, chronic illnesses, gait alterations, or a history of falling.	___	___	___	_____
3. Reviewed most recently documented weight for patient and any report describing patient's ability to stand and bear weight.	___	___	___	_____
4. Reviewed health care provider's order for ambulation; noted any mobility, ROM, or weight-bearing restrictions.	___	___	___	_____
5. Assessed patient's or family caregiver's health literacy level.	___	___	___	_____
6. Performed hand hygiene. Assessed patient's physical readiness to ambulate:	___	___	___	_____
a. Assessed baseline resting heart rate, blood pressure, oxygen saturation (when available), and respirations.	___	___	___	_____
b. If patient's strength and endurance had been affected by illness or deconditioning, assessed ROM and muscle strength of lower extremities while patient was in bed.	___	___	___	_____
c. Asked if patient felt excessively tired or was currently experiencing any pain. Assessed character of pain and had patient rate pain severity on a pain scale from 0 to 10. Offered an analgesic 30 minutes before ambulation to improve patient's tolerance to exercise.	___	___	___	_____
d. Assessed the patient's mobility: ability to sit up or stand by using the Banner Mobility Assessment Tool.	___	___	___	_____
7. Assessed patient's response to commands and ability to cooperate during ambulation.	___	___	___	_____

172

	S	U	NP	Comments

8. Applied patient's BMAT score to a safe-handling algorithm to determine if patient needed to walk with assist of a movable lift. Did not start procedure until all required caregivers were available. ___ ___ ___ _____

9. Assessed patient for any hearing or visual deficits to ensure he or she could see walking path and hear instructions. ___ ___ ___ _____

10. Checked patient's environment for any barriers or safety If in hospital or rehabilitation center, guided patient to walk in an area where handrails were on the walls and chairs were near. ___ ___ ___ _____

11. Assessed patient's or family caregiver's knowledge and experience regarding ambulation with assistance and patient's goals for ambulating. ___ ___ ___ _____

12. Determined the best time to ambulate; considered all scheduled activities. ___ ___ ___ _____

13. If this was the first time ambulating or if patient had been unsteady in the past, had a chair or wheelchair positioned close to path you choose for ambulation. Option: Had patient push a wheelchair for stability or use a rollator. Moved patient quickly into a safe sitting position if patient became unstable. ___ ___ ___ _____

14. Provided privacy. Organized equipment. ___ ___ ___ _____

15. Removed SCDs from patient's legs if present. Exception: Allowed patient to wear mobile compression devices while walking. ___ ___ ___ _____

16. Explained to patient in simple language preparation for ambulation. Discussed benefits of walking and risk prevention to reduce chance of falling. ___ ___ ___ _____

17. If hands became soiled during assessment, performed hand hygiene. ___ ___ ___ _____

18. Assisted patient from supine position to sitting position on edge of bed: ___ ___ ___ _____

   a. With patient in supine position in bed, raised head of bed 30 to 45 degrees and placed bed in low position, level with own hips. Raised upper side rail on side where patient would exit bed. Applied nonskid shoes or socks. If patient was fully mobile, allowed to sit up on side of bed independently, using side rail to raise up. ___ ___ ___ _____

   b. If patient needed assistance to sit on side of bed, turned patient sideways facing self while standing on side of bed where patient would sit. ___ ___ ___ _____

   c. Stood opposite patient's hips. Turned diagonally to face patient and far corner of foot of bed. ___ ___ ___ _____

	S	U	NP	Comments

d. Placed own feet apart in wide base of support with foot closer to head of bed in front of other foot.

＿＿＿ ＿＿＿ ＿＿＿ ＿＿＿＿＿＿＿＿＿＿＿

e. Placed own arm nearer to head of bed under the patient's lower shoulder, supporting the head and neck. Placed the other arm over and around patient's thighs.

＿＿＿ ＿＿＿ ＿＿＿ ＿＿＿＿＿＿＿＿＿＿＿

f. Moved patient's lower legs and feet over side of bed as patient used side rail to push and raise the upper body. Pivoted weight onto own rear leg as the patient's upper legs swung downward. Did not lift legs. At same time, continued to shift weight to own rear leg and guided patient in elevating the trunk into upright position.

＿＿＿ ＿＿＿ ＿＿＿ ＿＿＿＿＿＿＿＿＿＿＿

19. Allowed patient to sit on the side of the bed with feet on floor for 2 to 3 minutes. Had patient alternately flex and extend feet and moved lower legs up and down without touching floor. Asked if patient felt dizzy; if so, checked blood pressure. Had patient relax and take a few deep breaths until dizziness subsided and balance was gained. If dizziness lasted more than 60 seconds or if systolic blood pressure had dropped at least 10 mm Hg within 3 minutes of sitting upright, returned patient to bed. Rechecked blood pressure.

＿＿＿ ＿＿＿ ＿＿＿ ＿＿＿＿＿＿＿＿＿＿＿

20. Applied gait belt. Ensured that it completely encircled a patient's waist below the belly button. Ensured that belt fit snugly and two fingers could fit between the belt and the patient's body. Avoided placing belt over any intravenous lines, incisions, or drainage tubes. Adjusted belt once patient stood as needed.

＿＿＿ ＿＿＿ ＿＿＿ ＿＿＿＿＿＿＿＿＿＿＿

21. If patient was alert and could bear weight and balance while standing, allowed to stand independently. Assisted by holding gait belt to offer balance assistance.

＿＿＿ ＿＿＿ ＿＿＿ ＿＿＿＿＿＿＿＿＿＿＿

22. If patient could not bear weight or balance to stand independently but was stable to attempt ambulation, used an ambulation lift or ceiling lift with gait harness if available. Allowed patient to walk with support of this mechanical device.

＿＿＿ ＿＿＿ ＿＿＿ ＿＿＿＿＿＿＿＿＿＿＿

23. Confirmed with patient distance to ambulate.

＿＿＿ ＿＿＿ ＿＿＿ ＿＿＿＿＿＿＿＿＿＿＿

24. If patient had an intravenous (IV) line, placed the IV pole on the same side as the site of infusion and instructed patient where to hold and push the pole while ambulating. Ideally, another caregiver pushed the IV pole.

＿＿＿ ＿＿＿ ＿＿＿ ＿＿＿＿＿＿＿＿＿＿＿

	S	U	NP	Comments

25. If a Foley catheter was present, carried the bag below the level of the bladder and prevented tension on the tubing. ___ ___ ___ _____

26. For orthopedic patients, stood on patient's unaffected side. For patients with neurologic deficits, stood on the affected side. For all other patients requiring assistance to maintain balance while weight bearing, stood on involved side. ___ ___ ___ _____

27. Grasped belt firmly with one hand, palm facing down. Took a few steps, guiding patient with one hand grasping the gait belt and the other hand placed under the elbow of the patient's flexed arm. ___ ___ ___ _____

28. When ambulating in a hallway, positioned patient between self and the wall. Encouraged patient to use handrails if available. ___ ___ ___ _____

29. Observed how patient walked and determined distance patient could safely continue walking. Measured pulse and respirations as needed. ___ ___ ___ _____

30. Returned patient to bed or chair (via independent transfer or use of mechanical lift) and assisted patient to assume a comfortable position. Ensured the nurse call system was accessible within patient's reach. ___ ___ ___ _____

31. Raised side rails (as appropriate), lowered and locked bed into lowest position. Performed hand hygiene. ___ ___ ___ _____

32. Performed Teach-Back. Revised instruction or developed a plan for revised patient/family caregiver teaching if patient/family caregiver was not able to teach back correctly. ___ ___ ___ _____

33. Documented time or distance ambulated, any changes in vital signs, and patient's tolerance. ___ ___ ___ _____

34. Reported to health care provider any incident of orthostatic hypotension or patient's unexpected intolerance to exercise. ___ ___ ___ _____

Student _____ Date _____

Instructor _____ Date _____

PERFORMANCE CHECKLIST SKILL 12.2 **ASSISTING WITH USE OF CANES, WALKERS, AND CRUTCHES**

	S	U	NP	Comments

ASSESSMENT

1. Identified patient using at least two identifiers.

2. Completed assessment steps in Procedural Guideline 12.3, Steps to 12.

3. Determined patient's or family caregiver's prior experience and knowledge of type of device to be used in ambulating.

4. Assessed degree of physical assistance that patient needs in alignment with PT recommendation.

PLANNING

1. Determined expected outcomes following completion of procedure.

2. Explained to patient preparation for ambulation. Explained benefits and reasons for activity/exercise in a way that matches patient's educational level and beliefs and values regarding recovery or maintaining health.

3. Explained and demonstrated specific gait technique to patient or family caregiver.

4. Checked for appropriate height and fit of assist device. If PT saw patient, the device was at the appropriate height. NOTE: This was usually done when patient was standing at side of bed and was stable.

5. Made sure that ambulation device had rubber tips and functional brakes as applicable.

IMPLEMENTATION

1. Performed hand hygiene.

2. If using crutches, had patient report any tingling or numbness in upper torso while ambulating.

3. Helped patient from lying position to side of bed or up from chair.

4. Allowed patient to sit on edge of bed for a few minutes. Had patient alternately flex and extend feet and move lower legs. Asked if patient felt dizzy. Had patient relax and take a few deep breaths until dizziness subsided and balance was gained.

176

	S	U	NP	Comments

5. Applied gait belt completely and snuggly around patient's waist below the belly button. Ensured two fingers could fit between the belt and the patient's body. Avoided placing belt over any intravenous lines, incisions, or drainage tubes. Adjusted belt once patient stood as needed.

6. Helped patient to stand at bedside. Held under gait belt along patient's back with palms facing up. Reassessed height of assist device to make sure that it was correct size. Had patient stand fully erect with shoulders back and look ahead (not at floor). Assessed patient's ability to bear weight and balance.

7. If patient was unsteady, positioned in chair or returned to bed immediately.

8. Confirmed with patient how far to ambulate.

9. Implemented ambulation around patient's other activities.

10. Helped patient to walk with cane.

   a. Had patient hold cane on strong/unaffected side. Directed patient to place cane forward and slightly to the side of the foot, keeping body weight on good foot. Allowed approximately 15- to 30-degree elbow flexion.

   b. To begin, had patient move cane and weak/affected leg forward together about 15 to 25 centimeters (6 to 10 inches). The cane and weak/affected leg swung and struck the ground at the same time.

   c. With patient's weight supported on both the cane and weak leg, had patient advance strong/unaffected leg even with the cane.

   d. Repeated sequences as patient tolerated. Once comfortable, had patient advance cane and weak/affected leg together and then advance the stronger/unaffected leg 15 to 25 centimeters (6 to 10 inches) past the cane.

11. Helped patient to crutch walk by using appropriate crutch gait as determined by PT.

   a. Four-point gait:

      (1) Began in tripod position. Had patient lean slightly forward, placing the crutch tips about 15 centimeters (6 inches) to the side and in front of each foot. Had patient place weight on good foot and handgrips, not under arms.

	S	U	NP	Comments

(2) Moved right crutch tip forward 10 to 15 centimeters (4 to 6 inches).

(3) Began step as if patient were going to use the weaker foot or leg but, instead, shifted weight to the crutch. Had patient move left foot forward to level of left crutch.

(4) Moved left crutch forward 10 to 15 centimeters (4 to 6 inches).

(5) Moved right foot forward to level of right crutch.

(6) Repeated above sequence. As patient became stronger, distance to advance crutches increased to 30 centimeters [12 inches]).

b. Three-point gait:

(1) Began in tripod position with patient standing on strong weight-bearing foot.

(2) Advanced both crutches 15 centimeters (6 inches) and weak/affected leg, keeping foot of weak leg off floor.

(3) Moved weight-bearing strong leg forward, stepping on floor.

(4) Repeated sequence.

c. Two-point gait:

(1) Began in tripod position.

(2) Moved left crutch and right foot forward.

(3) Moved right crutch and left foot forward.

(4) Repeated sequence.

d. Swing-to gait:

(1) Began in tripod position.

(2) Moved both crutches forward.

(3) Lifted and swung both legs to crutches, letting crutches support body weight.

(4) Repeated two previous steps.

e. Swing-through gait:

(1) Began in tripod position. Support on strongest leg.

(2) Advanced the left and right crutch, then advanced the left and right legs.

(3) Lifted and swung legs up to the crutches.

(4) Repeated previous steps.

178

	S	U	NP	Comments

12. Helped patient to ascend stairs with a railing with crutches (partial weight bearing, one leg): ___ ___ ___ _____

   a. Had patient begin in tripod position while standing on strong weight-bearing leg and on crutch. ___ ___ ___ _____

   b. Had the patient hold the handrail for support with one hand (strong leg next to railing if possible). Carried the crutch positioned next to the handrail as the patient placed the other crutch under the axilla of weak/affected side. ___ ___ ___ _____

   c. Stayed behind the patient holding onto the gait belt. Then had the patient place weight on the crutches and step up with the strong weight-bearing foot, holding handrail. ___ ___ ___ _____

   d. Had patient straighten strong knee, push down on crutches, and lift body weight, bringing the weak/affected leg and then the crutch up the stair. Ensured the crutch tip was completely on the stair. ___ ___ ___ _____

   e. Repeated sequence of steps , instructed patient to climb one stair at a time until patient reached top of stairs. Observed patient's balance and level of fatigue. ___ ___ ___ _____

   f. Option: Went up stairs without crutches, using patient's seat. Had patient sit on the lower stair. Had patient (or caregiver) place crutches as far up the stairs as possible. Then had patient move them to the top while progressing up the stairs. ___ ___ ___ _____

      (1) In the seated position, had patient reach behind with both arms, then use arms and strong weight-bearing foot / leg to lift up one step. ___ ___ ___ _____

      (2) Repeated this process one step at a time (moved crutches further up if there were additional stairs) until the patient reached the top of the stairs. ___ ___ ___ _____

13. Helped patient to descend stairs with a railing with crutch (partial weight bearing, one leg): ___ ___ ___ _____

   a. Had patient begin in tripod position while bearing weight on strong/unaffected leg and crutch. ___ ___ ___ _____

   b. Had the patient stand close to the edge of the top step. Then had the patient hold the handrail with one hand (strong leg next to railing if possible). Carried the crutch positioned next to the handrail as the patient placed the other crutch under the axilla of the weak/affected side. Stood in front of the patient to be able to guide during a possible fall. Did not hold patient's hand. ___ ___ ___ _____

	S	U	NP	Comments

c. Had the patient bend the strong knee while lowering the crutch down to the step below and then moving the weak/affected leg down a step. ___ ___ ___ _____

d. Patient then supported body weight evenly between handrail, strong leg, and crutch. Ensured that patient had good balance. ___ ___ ___ _____

e. Cautioned patient not to hop while descending stair. ___ ___ ___ _____

f. Option: Went down stairs without crutches using patient's seat. Had patient sit on the top step. Placed crutches down the stairs by sliding them to the lowest possible point on the stairway. Then continued to move them down as patient progressed down the stairs. ___ ___ ___ _____

(1) In the seated position, had patient reach behind with both arms, and then use arms and strong weight-bearing foot/leg to lift bottom down step. ___ ___ ___ _____

(2) Repeated this process one step at a time (moved crutches down if there were additional stairs), until reaching bottom of stairs. ___ ___ ___ _____

14. Helped patient to ambulate with walker: ___ ___ ___ _____

a. Had patient stand straight in center of walker and grasp handgrips on upper bars. Did not allow patient to lean over walker. ___ ___ ___ _____

b. Had patient move walker comfortable distance forward, about 15 to 20 centimeters (6 to 8 inches). Patient then took step forward with weak/affected leg first and followed through with strong/unaffected leg into walker. Instructed patient not to advance leg past the front bar of walker. ___ ___ ___ _____

c. If patient was unable to bear weight on weak leg, had patient slowly hop to center of walker using strong leg, supporting weight on hands. Caution: Did not hop using a rollator. ___ ___ ___ _____

d. Instructed patient not to try to climb stairs with walker unless he or she had specific walker for steps. ___ ___ ___ _____

15. After ambulation, helped patient back to bed or chair and helped assume comfortable position. ___ ___ ___ _____

16. Placed nurse call system in an accessible location within patients reach. ___ ___ ___ _____

17. Raised side rails (as appropriate), lowered and locked bed into lowest position. ___ ___ ___ _____

18. Performed hand hygiene. ___ ___ ___ _____

180

	S	U	NP	Comments

EVALUATION

1. After ambulation, obtained patient's vital signs, observe skin color, and evaluated comfort and energy levels.

2. Evaluated patient's subjective statements regarding experience.

3. Evaluated patient's gait pattern: observed body alignment in standing position and balance during gait.

4. Used Teach-Back. Revised instruction or developed a plan for revised patient/family caregiver teaching if patient or family caregiver was not able to teach back correctly.

DOCUMENTATION

1. Documented assessment findings, type of assist device and gait patient used, amount of help required, distance walked, and activity tolerance.

2. Documented evaluation of patient and family caregiver learning.

HAND-OFF REPORTING

1. Immediately reported any injury sustained during attempts to ambulate, alteration in vital signs, or inability to ambulate to nurse in charge or health care provider.

Student _____ Date _____

Instructor _____ Date _____

PERFORMANCE CHECKLIST SKILL 12.3   **CARE OF A PATIENT WITH AN IMMOBILIZATION DEVICE**

	S	U	NP	Comments
ASSESSMENT				
1. Identified patient using two identifiers.	___	___	___	_____
2. Reviewed patient's electronic health record (EHR), previous and current activity level, description of the condition requiring immobilization, and medical order for device.	___	___	___	_____
3. Performed hand hygiene. Inspected area of skin in contact with immobilization device or area that would be covered by a newly applied device. Applied clean gloves when risk of contacting body fluids.	___	___	___	_____
4. Palpated temperature, pulse, and sensation of extremity distal to where device was to be applied. Performed hand hygiene.	___	___	___	_____
5. Assessed patient's/family caregiver's health literacy.	___	___	___	_____
6. Assessed patient's/family caregiver's knowledge and experience with immobilization devices.	___	___	___	_____
7. Assessed patient's discomfort. If pain was present, assessed character and rate severity on a scale of 0 to 10.	___	___	___	_____
8. Referred to occupational or physical therapy to determine type of device to be used, desired position, and amount of activity and movement permitted.	___	___	___	_____
PLANNING				
1. Determined expected outcomes following completion of procedure.	___	___	___	_____
2. Provided privacy by closing room curtains or doors and prepared environment.	___	___	___	_____
3. Explained to patient and family caregiver purpose of device and how it would be applied.	___	___	___	_____
IMPLEMENTATION				
1. Performed hand hygiene. Assisted patient to a comfortable position: applied upper extremity brace/splint/sling with patient sitting upright; applied lower extremity brace with patient lying down.	___	___	___	_____

182

	S	U	NP	Comments

2. Applied clean gloves when there was a risk of contacting body fluids. Prepared skin that would be enclosed in brace/splint/sling by having cleaned skin with soap and water; rinsed, patted dry, and changed any dressings (if present). If applying a back brace, put a thin cotton shirt or gown on patient. Ensured that there were no wrinkles to cause pressure. ____ ____ ____ _____

3. Inspected device for wear, damage, or rough edges. ____ ____ ____ _____

4. Applied brace/splint/sling as directed by health care provider, orthotist, PT, or occupational therapist. Ensured application provided for the alignment and support indicated in the order. ____ ____ ____ _____

    a. Applied even tension on any bandage or gauze padding that was ordered to be applied against skin, wrapped distal to proximal. ____ ____ ____ _____

    b. Prevented padding from gathering or bunching. ____ ____ ____ _____

    c. Supported joints when positioning and applying the device. ____ ____ ____ _____

5. Applied commercial sling: ____ ____ ____ _____

    a. Ensured correct size was chosen. Placed elbow into close side of sling, aligning arm into sling and slipping wrist and hand through open side of sling or through separate Velcro enclosure. ____ ____ ____ _____

    b. Enclosed Velcro strap around arm, placed strap around patient's neck and tightened buckle until it fit snugly. ____ ____ ____ _____

    c. Positioned arm so that the hand and forearm were higher than the elbow. ____ ____ ____ _____

6. Removed and disposed of gloves. Performed hand hygiene. ____ ____ ____ _____

7. Taught patient and family caregiver the prescribed schedule of wear and activities while in device as directed by health care provider, physical therapist, or occupational therapist. ____ ____ ____ _____

8. Reinforced instruction regarding signs to report to health care provider: skin breakdown, painful pressure, or rubbing. ____ ____ ____ _____

9. Taught patient/family caregiver how to care for brace/splint/sling: ____ ____ ____ _____

    a. When not in use, stored metal braces upright in a safe but easily accessible location. ____ ____ ____ _____

    b. Stored splints of molded materials away from heat. ____ ____ ____ _____

    c. Treated any leather material with leather preservative. ____ ____ ____ _____

	S	U	NP	Comments

d. Kept brace clean, dry, and in good working order. Cleaned plastic parts with a damp cloth and thoroughly dried. Cleaned metal brace joints with a pipe cleaner and oiled weekly. Removed rust with steel wool, and cleaned metal parts with a solvent. ___ ___ ___ _____

10. Assisted patient in ambulating with brace/splint/sling in place. ___ ___ ___ _____

11. Observed patient or family caregiver apply and remove brace/splint/sling. ___ ___ ___ _____

12. Helped patient to comfortable position. ___ ___ ___ _____

13. Placed nurse call system in an accessible location within patient's reach. ___ ___ ___ _____

14. Raised side rails (as appropriate), lowered and locked bed into lowest position. ___ ___ ___ _____

15. Disposed of supplies or dirty linen. Performed hand hygiene. ___ ___ ___ _____

EVALUATION

1. Inspected area of skin underneath device for redness or skin breakdown. If allowed, removed device briefly to assess skin thoroughly. ___ ___ ___ _____

2. Palpated temperature, pulse, and sensation of extremity distal to device. Checked capillary refill by pressing on a toe or finger. ___ ___ ___ _____

3. Inspected alignment of the limb after application of device. ___ ___ ___ _____

4. Asked patient to describe any discomfort, then evaluated character of pain and had patient rate severity on a pain scale after device application. ___ ___ ___ _____

5. Used Teach-Back. Revised instruction or developed a plan for revised patient/family caregiver teaching if patient or family caregiver was not able to teach back correctly. ___ ___ ___ _____

DOCUMENTATION

1. Documented assessments of skin integrity, neurovascular status, application of and type of device, schedule of wear, activity level, movement permitted, patient's tolerance of procedure, and instructions given to patient and family caregiver. ___ ___ ___ _____

2. Documented observations about patient's or family caregiver's ability to apply device, ambulate, and remove device. ___ ___ ___ _____

3. Documented evaluation of patient learning. ___ ___ ___ _____

HAND-OFF REPORTING

1. Reported to health care provider any unexpected outcomes. ___ ___ ___ _____

184

Student _____   Date _____

Instructor _____   Date _____

PERFORMANCE CHECKLIST PROCEDURAL GUIDELINE 13.1   **SELECTION OF A PRESSURE-REDISTRIBUTION SUPPORT SURFACE**

	S	U	NP	Comments

STEPS

1. Identified patient using at least two identifiers according to agency policy.

2. Checked agency policy regarding implementing a support surface.

   a. Obtained a health care provider's order.

   b. Consulted with health care agency case manager or social worker to help with patient's financial eligibility and terms and length of third-party reimbursement for the surface.

   c. Consulted with agency home care or discharge planning services if the device was anticipated for long-term use.

3. Reviewed patient's electronic health record (EHR) for weight, weight distribution and risk factors/comorbidities.

4. Assessed patient's/family caregiver's health literacy.

5. Performed hand hygiene. Applied clean gloves if drainage or open wound present.

6. Assessed patient's risk for skin breakdown using a risk assessment tool. Included mobility and ability to reposition.

7. Assessed patient's risks for medical adhesive-related skin injury (MARSI). Inspected skin under any adhesive or securing devices for nasogastric tubes, urinary catheters, and wound dressings.

8. Assessed patient's existing and past pressure injuries (PIs) including location, condition of skin and stage, areas of blistering, abnormal reactive hyperemia, and abrasion.

9. Assessed the presence of medical devices. Determined patient's risk for medical device-related pressure injuries (MDRPIs). Removed and disposed of gloves. Preformed hand hygiene.

10. Assessed character of patient's pain, and rated acuity on pain scale of 0 to 10.

	S	U	NP	Comments

11. Determined the need for a pressure-reduction surface from assessment data. _____ _____ _____ _____

12. Identified patient factors when selecting an appropriate surface. _____ _____ _____ _____

13. Chose the appropriate surface. Placed at-risk patients on a pressure reduction surface or high-specification foam mattress, and not on a standard hospital mattress. _____ _____ _____ _____

14. Provided privacy and explained procedure to patient or family caregiver. _____ _____ _____ _____

15. Assessed patient's/family caregiver's knowledge, prior experience with PI or support surfaces, and expectations if support surface is to be used at home. _____ _____ _____ _____

16. Applied appropriate support surface to patient's bed. Followed manufacturer's directions. _____ _____ _____ _____

17. Preformed hand hygiene. Applied clean gloves. Regularly inspected condition of skin and existing PIs for evidence of healing according to agency policy to evaluate changes in skin and effectiveness of therapy. _____ _____ _____ _____

18. Removed and disposed of gloves. Preformed hand hygiene. _____ _____ _____ _____

19. Observed for side effects associated with specific pressure-reducing surface. _____ _____ _____ _____

20. Helped patient into a comfortable position. _____ _____ _____ _____

21. Raised side rails (as appropriate), lowered and locked bed into lowest position. _____ _____ _____ _____

22. Placed nurse call system in an accessible location within patient's reach. _____ _____ _____ _____

23. Used Teach-Back. Revised instructions or developed a plan for revised patient/family caregiver teaching if patient/family caregiver was not able to teach back correctly. _____ _____ _____ _____

24. Documented PI risk assessment and skin assessment, type of support surface selected, and patient response to the specific support surface. _____ _____ _____ _____

25. Hand-off report: Notified health care provider of any changes to the patient's skin or existing PIs. _____ _____ _____ _____

Student _____ Date _____

Instructor _____ Date _____

PERFORMANCE CHECKLIST SKILL 13.1 **CARE OF THE PATIENT ON A SUPPORT SURFACE**

	S	U	NP	Comments

ASSESSMENT

1. Identified patient using two identifiers according to agency policy.

2. Reviewed patient's electronic health record (EHR), including health care provider's order.

3. Assessed patient's / family caregiver's health literacy.

4. Performed hand hygiene. Applied clean gloves if open wound present. Determined patient's risk for pressure injury (PI)formation or progression of an existing injury using a valid assessment tool and assessed for risk factors for PIs.

5. Performed skin assessment. Inspected condition of skin, especially over dependent sites, at bony prominences, and under and near medical devices. Removed and disposed of gloves (if worn). Performed hand hygiene.

6. Assessed for dehydration, malnutrition, exposure to radiation, and underlying chronic conditions. Observed skin for edema and under existing dressings, securement devices, and anywhere adhesive was used to secure device, dressing, and so on. Determined risk for and presence of medical adhesive- related skin injury (MARSI).

7. Assessed character of patient's pain and rated acuity on a pain scale of 0 to 10.

8. Assessed patient's knowledge, prior experience with support surfaces, and feelings about procedure.

PLANNING

1. Determined expected outcomes following completion of procedure.

2. Provided privacy and explanation on purpose of mattress and method of application to patient and family caregiver.

3. Organized and set up any specific equipment for support surface.

4. Arranged for extra personnel to help as necessary.

	S	U	NP	Comments

IMPLEMENTATION

1. Performed hand hygiene. Applied clean gloves (if linens are soiled or wet). Transferred patient to chair or stretcher, depending on mobility and type of device being applied. ___ ___ ___ _____

2. Applied support surface to bed or prepared alternative bed. Kept sharp objects away from air mattress or air-surface bed. ___ ___ ___ _____

2. a. Replaced mattress appropriately: ___ ___ ___ _____

   (1) Applied mattress to bedframe after removing standard hospital mattress. ___ ___ ___ _____

   (2) Applied one sheet over mattress. Kept linens between surfaces to a minimum. ___ ___ ___ _____

  b. Prepared an air mattress/overlay: ___ ___ ___ _____

   (1) Applied deflated mattress flat over surface of bed mattress. ___ ___ ___ _____

   (2) Brought any plastic strips or flaps around corners of bed mattress. ___ ___ ___ _____

   (3) Attached connector on air mattress to inflation device. Inflated mattress to proper air pressure using a manual air pump or electric blower. ___ ___ ___ _____

   (4) Placed one sheet over air mattress, being sure to eliminate all wrinkles. ___ ___ ___ _____

   (5) Checked air pumps to be sure that pressure cycle alternated. ___ ___ ___ _____

  c. Installed an air-surface bed: ___ ___ ___ _____

   (1) Obtained and placed linen on bed. ___ ___ ___ _____

   (2) Placed switch in "prevention" mode. ___ ___ ___ _____

3. Used available personnel and helped patient transfer into bed. ___ ___ ___ _____

4. Positioned patient comfortably as desired over support surface. Repositioned routinely. ___ ___ ___ _____

5. Removed and disposed of gloves and performed hand hygiene. ___ ___ ___ _____

6. Raised side rails (as appropriate), lowered and locked bed into lowest position. ___ ___ ___ _____

7. Ensured nurse call system was in an accessible location within patient's reach. ___ ___ ___ _____

8. Performed hand hygiene. ___ ___ ___ _____

EVALUATION

1. Reassessed patient's risk for PI formation at routine intervals; followed agency policy. ___ ___ ___ _____

188

	S	U	NP	Comments

2. Assessed "bottoming out" of support surface. Observed for at least 2.5 centimeters (1 inch) of space between the support surface and patient's skin surface. Less than 2.5 centimeters (1 inch) indicated bottoming out. ____ ____ ____ _____

3. Inspected and compared condition of patient's skin according to agency policy to determine changes in skin integrity, PI status, and effectiveness of support surface. ____ ____ ____ _____

4. Asked patient to describe character of pain and rate acuity on a scale of 0 to 10. ____ ____ ____ _____

5. Evaluated functioning of support surface periodically. ____ ____ ____ _____

6. Used Teach-Back. Revised instruction or developed a plan for revised patient/family caregiver's teaching if patient or family caregiver was not able to teach back correctly. ____ ____ ____ _____

DOCUMENETATION

1. Documented type of support surface applied, extent to which patient tolerated procedure, and condition of patient's skin. ____ ____ ____ _____

2. Documented evaluation of patient and family caregiver learning. ____ ____ ____ _____

HAND-OFF REPORTING

1. Reported evidence of new PI formation or worsening of existing PI to nurse in charge, health care provider, or WOCN. ____ ____ ____ _____

Student _____ Date _____

Instructor _____ Date _____

PERFORMANCE CHECKLIST SKILL 13.2　CARE OF THE PATIENT ON A SPECIAL BED

	S	U	NP	Comments

ASSESSMENT

1. Identified patient using two identifiers according to agency policy.

2. Reviewed patient's electronic health record (EHR), including health care provider's order.

3. Reviewed patient's serum electrolyte levels if available.

4. Assessed patient's/family caregiver's health literacy.

5. Determined if patient needed frequent weights.

6. Performed hand hygiene. Applied clean gloves. Determined patient's risk for pressure injury (PI) formation using a valid assessment tool. Assessed for risk factors for PIs.

7. Inspected condition of skin, especially over dependent sites and bony prominences and areas exposed to medical adhesives, which increase risk for medical adhesive-related skin injury (MARSI). Noted appearance of existing PI and determined stage of injury. Removed and disposed of gloves. Performed hand hygiene.

8. Assessed character of patient's pain and rated acuity on a pain scale of 0 to 10.

9. Assessed risk of complications from air-fluidized beds.

10. Assessed patient's knowledge, prior experience with support surfaces, and feelings about procedure.

PLANNING

1. Determined expected outcomes following completion of procedure.

2. Provided privacy and explained purpose of bed and method of application to patient and family caregiver.

3. Organized and set up any specific equipment for bed.

4. Reviewed instructions provided by manufacturer.

5. Obtained additional personnel needed to transfer patient to bed.

	S	U	NP	Comments

6. For patients with moderate to severe pain, premedicated approximately 30 minutes before transfer to bed.

IMPLEMENTATION

1. Performed hand hygiene. Applied clean gloves (if linens were soiled or wet).

2. Transfered patient to bed using appropriate transfer techniques. Did not attempt to transfer without help.

3. Once patient had been transfered, turned bed on by depressing switch; regulated temperature.

4. Positioned patient and preformed rang-of-motion exercises as appropriate.

5. To turn patient, position bedpans, or preform other therapies, turned on appropriate bed setting. Once the procedure was completed, returned bed to the previous setting.

6. Used special features of bed as needed.

7. Removed and disposed of gloves and performed hand hygiene.

8. Helped patient to a comfortable position.

9. Raised side rails (as appropriate), lowered and locked into lowest position.

10. Placed nurse call system in an accessible location within patient's reach.

11. Performed hand hygiene.

EVALUATION

1. Reassessed patient's risk for PI formation at routine intervals.

2. Assessed "bottoming out" of pressure-relief mattress or seat cushion. Observed for at least 2.5 centimeters (1 inch) between the support surface and the patient's skin surface. Less than 2.5 centimeters (1 inch) indicated bottoming out.

3. Inspected and compared condition of patient's skin every 8 hours or according to agency policy to determine changes in skin integrity, PI status, and effectiveness of support surface.

4. Asked patient to describe pain and rate any discomfort on a scale of 0 to 10.

5. Reviewed fluid and electrolyte status.

6. Evaluated functioning of support surface periodically.

	S	U	NP	Comments

7. Used Teach-Back. Revised instruction or developed a plan for revised patient / family caregiver teaching if patient or family caregiver was not able to teach back correctly. ___ ___ ___ _____

DOCUMENTATION

1. Documented transfer of patient to bed, amount of help needed for transfer, tolerance of procedure, and condition of skin. ___ ___ ___ _____

2. Documented evaluation of patient and family caregiver learning. ___ ___ ___ _____

HAND-OFF REPORTING

1. Reported changes in condition of skin, level of orientation, nausea, and electrolyte levels to health care provider. ___ ___ ___ _____

Student _____ Date _____

Instructor _____ Date _____

PERFORMANCE CHECKLIST SKILL 14.1 **FALL PREVENTION IN HEALTH CARE SETTINGS**

	S	U	NP	Comments
ASSESSMENT				
1. Identified patient using at least two identifiers.	___	___	___	_____
2. Reviewed electronic health record (EHR) and determined if patient had a recent history of a fall and risks for injury (ABCs).	___	___	___	_____
3. Assessed patient's/family caregiver'a health literacy.	___	___	___	_____
4. Performed hand hygiene. Assessed for fall risks using a validated fall risk assessment tool. Computed fall risk score.	___	___	___	_____
5. Continued with a comprehensive individualized patient assessment and consider patient's unique intrinsic fall risks. Performed a fall risk assessment in general acute care settings on admission, on transfer from one unit to another, with a significant change in a patient's condition, or after a fall.	___	___	___	_____
6. Performed the Banner Mobility Assessment Tool (BMAT) or the Timed Up and Go (TUG) test if patient was able to ambulate. At a minimum, observed an ambulatory patient walking in room (with or without help).	___	___	___	_____
7. Assessed patient's pain severity (used rating scale ranging from 0 to 10).	___	___	___	_____
8. Asked patient or family caregiver if patient had a history of recent falls or other injuries within the home. Assessed previous falls using the acronym SPLATT.	___	___	___	_____
9. Reviewed patient's medications (including over-the-counter [OTC] medications and herbal products) for drugs that create risk for falls. Compared those drugs with ones on the Beers Criteria® lists.	___	___	___	_____
10. Assessed for polypharmacy.	___	___	___	_____
11. Assessed patient's fear of falling using the Falls Efficacy Scale (FES-1) or the Activities-specific Balance Confidence (ABC) scale.	___	___	___	_____
12. Assessed for orthostatic hypotension (OH) in patients who were 65 and older, had a history of a fall, and/or took multiple medications.	___	___	___	_____

	S	U	NP	Comments

13. Assessed condition of any assistive devices or equipment used by patient. ____ ____ ____ _____

14. If patient was in a wheelchair, assessed level of comfort, fatigue, boredom, mental status, and level of engagement with others. ____ ____ ____ _____

15. Used patient-centered approach to determine what patient already knew about risks for falling. Showed patient and family caregiver results of fall risk assessment and explained significance of risk factors. Explained how a plan for fall prevention would be developed. ____ ____ ____ _____

16. Assessed patient's knowledge, prior experience with fall prevention, and feelings about these measures. ____ ____ ____ _____

17. Assessed patient's goals or preferences for how to implement fall prevention strategies. ____ ____ ____ _____

18. If patient had a fall risk, applied color-coded wristband/sign on door/socks or gowns as applicable. ____ ____ ____ _____

PLANNING

1. Determined expected outcomes following completion of procedure. ____ ____ ____ _____

2. Provided privacy by closing room curtains or door. Ensured patient was comfortable. ____ ____ ____ _____

3. Performed hand hygiene. Prepared equipment at bedside, making sure all was functional. ____ ____ ____ _____

4. Explained safety measures to be taken as they pertained to patient's specific fall risks. Also planned for time to discuss fall prevention in the home. Option: Used a patient acknowledgment form for patients to personally acknowledge their fall risks. ____ ____ ____ _____

5. Educated patients and family caregivers on medication side effects that increased risk for falls. ____ ____ ____ _____

IMPLEMENTATION

1. Conducted hourly purposeful rounds on all patients to determine status of pain, was proactive in offering assist to toilet, assessed comfort of position, and assessed need to relocate personal items for easy reach; provided pain-relief intervention. ____ ____ ____ _____

2. Implemented early mobility protocols within health care agency. Followed protocols to ensure patient increased level of mobility progressively. Considered use of accelerometers. ____ ____ ____ _____

3. Implemented Universal Fall Precautions. ____ ____ ____ _____

   a. Adjusted bed to low position with wheels locked. ____ ____ ____ _____

	S	U	NP	Comments

b. Encouraged use of properly fitted skid-proof footwear.   ____ ____   _____

c. Oriented patient to surroundings. Explained nurse call system and routines to expect in plan of care.   ____ ____ ____ _____

   (1) Provided patient's hearing aid and glasses. Ensured that each was functioning and clean. If patient complained of visual or hearing problems, referred to appropriate health care provider.   ____ ____ ____ _____

   (2) Placed nurse call system in an accessible location within patient's reach. Explained and demonstrated how to use system at bedside and in bathroom. Had patient perform return demonstration.   ____ ____ ____ _____

   (3) Explained to patient/family member when and why to use nurse call system. Provided clear instructions regarding mobility restrictions.   ____ ____   _____

d. Used side rails safely.   ____ ____ ____ _____

   (1) Explained to patient and family caregiver reason for patient to use side rails.   ____ ____ ____ _____

   (2) Checked agency policy regarding side rail use.   ____ ____ ____ _____

e. Made patient's environment safe: ____ ____ ____ _____

   (1) Removed excess equipment, supplies, and furniture from rooms and halls.   ____ ____ ____ _____

   (2) Kept floors free of clutter and obstacles.   ____ ____ ____ _____

   (3) Coiled and secured excess cords or tubing.   ____ ____ ____ _____

   (4) Cleaned all spills on floors promptly. Posted sign indicating wet floor. Removed sign when floor was dry.   ____ ____ ____ _____

   (5) Ensured adequate glare-free lighting; used a night-light at night.   ____ ____ ____ _____

   (6) Had assistive devices on exit side of bed. Had chair back of a bedside commode placed against wall of room if possible.   ____ ____ ____ _____

   (7) Arranged personal items within patient's easy reach and in logical way.   ____ ____ ____ _____

   (8) Secured locks on beds, stretchers, and wheelchairs.   ____ ____ ____ _____

4. Used a proper-size mattress or mattress with raised foam edges.   ____ ____ ____ _____

  a. Reduced the gaps between the mattress and side rails.   ____ ____ ____ _____

	S	U	NP	Comments

5. Provided comfort measures; offered ordered analgesics for patients experiencing pain, preferably around-the-clock. ___ ___ ___ _____

6. Interventions for patients at moderate to high risk for falling (based on fall risk assessment):

   a. Prioritized call-light responses to patients at high risk; used a team approach. All staff knew responsibility to respond. ___ ___ ___ _____

   b. Established elimination schedule, used bedside commode when appropriate. ___ ___ ___ _____

   c. Stayed with patient during toileting (stood outside bathroom door). Increased availability and use of raised toilet seats and toilet safety frames/grab bars. ___ ___ ___ _____

   d. Placed patient in a geri chair or wheelchair. Used wheelchair only for transport, not for sitting an extended time. Consulted with therapy services when considering the use of a wedge cushion. ___ ___ ___ _____

   e. Provided hip protectors, worn over or in place of underwear. ___ ___ ___ _____

   f. Considered use of a low bed that has lower height than standard hospital bed. Applied nonskid floor mats. ___ ___ ___ _____

   g. Activated a bed alarm or surveillance system. ___ ___ ___ _____

   h. Conferred with physical therapist about gait training, strength and balance training, and regular weight-bearing activities. ___ ___ ___ _____

   i. Used sitters or restraints only when alternatives were exhausted. ___ ___ ___ _____

   j. Considered having patient wear head protective gear. ___ ___ ___ _____

7. When ambulating patient, had patient wear a gait belt or use a walking sling, and walked alongside patient. ___ ___ ___ _____

8. Safe use of wheelchair:

   a. Ensured wheelchair was correct fit for patient: Ensured patient thighs were level while sitting, feet flat on floor, back of chair came up to mid-shoulder, elbows rested on armrests without leaning over or tucking arms in, and that two finger widths of space fit between patient and side of chair. ___ ___ ___ _____

   b. Transferred patient to wheelchair using safe handling techniques. ___ ___ ___ _____

	S	U	NP	Comments

  c. Backed wheelchair into and out of elevator or door, leading with large rear wheels first. ___ ___ ___ _____

  d. Managed patient's pain and did not allow patient to sit in wheelchair for an extended amount of time; provided alternative sitting option. ___ ___ ___ _____

9. Scheduled oral medication administration for at least 2 hours prior to "bedtime." ___ ___ ___ _____

10. After implementing safety strategies, helped patient to comfortable position. ___ ___ ___ _____

11. Raised side rails (as appropriate), lowered and locked bed into lowest position. ___ ___ ___ _____

12. Placed nurse call system in an accessible location within patient's reach. ___ ___ ___ _____

13. Removed and disposed of supplies and performed hand hygiene. ___ ___ ___ _____

EVALUATION

1. Asked patient/family caregiver to identify patient's fall risks. ___ ___ ___ _____

2. Asked patient/family caregiver to describe fall prevention interventions to implement. ___ ___ ___ _____

3. Evaluated patient's ability to use assistive devices at different times during the day. ___ ___ ___ _____

4. Evaluated for changes in motor, sensory, and cognitive status and reviewed if any falls or injuries occurred. ___ ___ ___ _____

5. Evaluated patient's character and level of pain using a pain rating scale. ___ ___ ___ _____

6. Evaluated patient adherence with fall prevention interventions. ___ ___ ___ _____

7. Continued hourly purposeful rounding. ___ ___ ___ _____

8. Used Teach-Back. Revised or developed a plan for revised patient/family caregiver teaching if patientf/family caregiver was not able to teach back correctly. ___ ___ ___ _____

DOCUMENTATION

1. Documented in the plan of care specific fall prevention interventions. Used whiteboards in patient rooms to communicate patient fall risks to all staff. ___ ___ ___ _____

2. Documented what patient was able to explain or not explain about fall risks and interventions taken. ___ ___ ___ _____

3. If fall occurred, completed an agency safety event or incident report, noting objective details of a fall. Did not place the report in patient's EHR. ___ ___ ___ _____

	S	U	NP	Comments

4. Documented overvaluation of patient/family caregiver learning and adherence to the plan of care. ___ ___ ___ _____

HAND-OFF REPORTING

1. Used a hand-off communication tool that included specific patient risks for falls and falls with injury between caregivers (included assistive personnel). Discussed patient-specific interventions taken. ___ ___ ___ _____

2. Reported immediately to the health care provider if patient sustained a fall or an injury. ___ ___ ___ _____

Student _____ Date _____

Instructor _____ Date _____

PERFORMANCE CHECKLIST SKILL 14.2 **DESIGNING A RESTRAINT-FREE ENVIRONMENT**

	S	U	NP	Comments

ASSESSMENT

1. Identified patient using two identifiers. ___ ___ ___ _____

2. Reviewed patient's electronic health record (EHR) for history of for memory impairment and underlying causes of agitation and cognitive impairment. Also assessed for the following: considered dangerous to self or others, gravely disabled as result of mental disorder, lack of cognitive ability (either permanently or temporarily) to make relevant decisions, alcohol or substance withdrawal, fluid and electrolyte imbalance, physical limitations that increase risk. ___ ___ ___ _____

3. In patients with known dementia, assessed for signs of restlessness: pacing, fidgeting, repetitive motor movements or questioning. ___ ___ ___ _____

4. Reviewed patient's medications for over-the-counter (OTC) and prescribed medications that pose risk for falling (compared with medications on Beers Criteria® lists). Assessed for interactions and untoward effects. ___ ___ ___ _____

5. Performed hand hygiene. Assessed patient's behavior, balance, gait, vision, hearing, bowel/bladder routine, level of pain, electrolyte and blood count values, and presence of orthostatic hypotension. ___ ___ ___ _____

6. For patients who wander or have known dementia, assessed for cognitive decline using a validated patient assessment tool, such as the General Practitioner Assessment of Cognition (GPCOG), the Memory Impairment Screen (MIS), or the Mini-Cog™. Assessed patient during time of day when cognition normally decreases. ___ ___ ___ _____

7. Assessed degree of wandering behavior using Algase Wandering Scale (Version 2) (AWS-V2). ___ ___ ___ _____

8. Assessed patient's and family caregiver's health literacy. ___ ___ ___ _____

9. Assessed patient's or family caregiver's knowledge of condition and risks for falls or wandering. ___ ___ ___ _____

	S	U	NP	Comments

10. For patients with dementia, asked family about their usual communication style and cues to indicate pain, fatigue, hunger, and need to urinate or defecate. ___ ___ ___ _____

11. Inspected condition of any therapeutic medical devices. ___ ___ ___ _____

12. Assessed daily to determine if a medical device is necessary or can be discontinued. Considered alternative therapy when possible. ___ ___ ___ _____

PLANNING

1. Determined expected outcomes following completion of procedure. ___ ___ ___ _____

2. Provided privacy, ensured patient was comfortable, and prepared room environment. ___ ___ ___ _____

3. Explained procedure to patient and family caregiver. ___ ___ ___ _____

4. Performed hand hygiene and gathered necessary supplies. ___ ___ ___ _____

IMPLEMENTATION

1. Oriented patient and family caregiver to surroundings, introduced to staff, and explained all treatments and procedures. Ensured patient could read name badge. ___ ___ ___ _____

2. Assigned same staff to care for patient as often as possible. Encouraged family and friends (and volunteers as applicable) to stay with patient. ___ ___ ___ _____

3. Placed patient in room that was easily accessible to care providers and close to nurses' station. ___ ___ ___ _____

4. Followed all Universal Fall Precautions to create a safe environment. ___ ___ ___ _____

5. Ensured that patient was wearing glasses, functioning hearing aid, or other sensory-aid devices were all functioning. ___ ___ ___ _____

6. Provided visual and auditory stimuli meaningful to patient. ___ ___ ___ _____

7. Anticipated patient's basic needs as quickly as possible; conducted hourly rounds. ___ ___ ___ _____

8. Provided scheduled ambulation, chair activity, and toileting. Organized treatments so patient had uninterrupted periods throughout the day. Considered using a bedside commode for patients who were weak, unsteady, or unsafe to ambulate to the bathroom (insisted that patient be assisted out of bed). ___ ___ ___ _____

	S	U	NP	Comments

9. Positioned intravenous (IV) catheters, urinary catheters, and tubes/drains out of patient view. Used commercial tube holders, camouflage by wrapping IV site with bandage or stockinette and used long-sleeved robes and commercial sleeves over arms. Placed undergarments on patient with urinary catheter or cover abdominal feeding tubes/drains with loose abdominal binder.   ___ ___ ___ _____

10. Implemented strategies to decrease wandering: ___ ___ ___ _____

   a. Eliminated stressors from environment.   ___ ___ ___ _____

   b. Used stress-reduction techniques.   ___ ___ ___ _____

   c. Used activity-based interventions and the integration of purposeful activities such as chores and crafts. Ensured those activities were of patient interest. Involved family caregiver (if appropriate).   ___ ___ ___ _____

11. Positioned patient comfortably in chair or wheelchair with a wraparound safety belt.   ___ ___ ___ _____

12. Used motion or bed occupancy alarm system for unsteady patients who forget or do not call for assistance when getting out of bed or chair. Referred to manufacturer's directions and agency policy. Option: Used chair pad with alarm.   ___ ___ ___ _____

   a. Explained use of device to patient and family caregiver.   ___ ___ ___ _____

   b. When in chair, positioned pad so it was correctly positioned under patient's buttocks.   ___ ___ ___ _____

   c. Tested alarm by applying and releasing pressure.   ___ ___ ___ _____

13. Used available locating technology for patients who wander. Followed manufacturer's directions.   ___ ___ ___ _____

14. Minimized invasive treatments as much as possible.   ___ ___ ___ _____

15. Assisted patient to a comfortable position.   ___ ___ ___ _____

16. Raised side rails (as appropriate), lowered and locked bed into lowest position.   ___ ___ ___ _____

17. Placed nurse call system in an accessible location within patient's reach.   ___ ___ ___ _____

18. Disposed of supplies and performed hand hygiene.   ___ ___ ___ _____

EVALUATION

1. Monitored patient's behavior routinely and checked condition of medical devices.   ___ ___ ___ _____

2. Observed patient for any injuries.   ___ ___ ___ _____

	S	U	NP	Comments

3. Observed patient's behavior toward staff, visitors, and other patients.

4. Used Teach-Back. Revised instruction or developed a plan for revised family caregiver teaching if family caregiver was not able to teach back correctly.

DOCUMENTATION

1. Documented all behaviors that related to cognitive status and ability to maintain safety and follow directions, mood and emotional status, understanding of condition and treatment plan, medication effects related to behaviors, restraint alternatives used, and patient response to interventions.

2. Documented evaluation of patient/family caregiver learning.

HAND-OFF REPORTING

1. Reported to other health care providers all interventions being used to prevent agitation or wandering, and any occurrences of wandering or other behavior that placed the patient at risk for injury.

2. Reported any patient injury from a fall to health care provider immediately.

Student _____ Date _____

Instructor _____ Date _____

PERFORMANCE CHECKLIST SKILL 14.3 **APPLYING PHYSICAL RESTRAINTS**

	S	U	NP	Comments

ASSESSMENT

1. Identified patient using two identifiers.

2. Reviewed electronic health record (EHR) to assess for underlying cause(s) of agitation and cognitive impairment that may lead to patient-initiated medical device removal.

   a. If there was abrupt change in perception, attention, or level of consciousness, performed hand hygiene. Assessed for respiratory and neurological alterations, fever and sepsis, hypoglycemia and hyperglycemia, alcohol or substance withdrawal, and fluid and electrolyte imbalance.

   b. Notified health care provider of change in mental status and compromised physiological status.

3. Obtained baseline or premorbid cognitive function from family caregivers.

4. Established whether patient has history of wandering behavior, dementia or depression.

5. Reviewed medications that can cause risk for falling and changes in mental status.

6. Reviewed EHR for current laboratory values.

7. Assessed patient's current behavior. Did patient create a risk to other patients?

8. If restraint alternatives failed earlier, conferred with health care provider. Reviewed agency policies and state laws regarding restraints. Obtained current health care provider's order for restraint, including purpose, type, location, and time or duration of restraint. Determined if signed consent for use of restraint is necessary (long-term care). For nonviolent/non-self-destructive patients, orders were renewed per hospital policy.

9. Reviewed manufacturer instructions for restraint application. Determined most appropriate size restraint. Was familiar with all devices.

10. Assessed patient and family caregiver health literacy.

11. Assessed patient's/family caregiver's knowledge, prior experience with restraints, and feelings about their use.

	S	U	NP	Comments

PLANNING

1. Determined expected outcomes following completion of procedure.

2. Performed hand hygiene. Prepared restraint, ensuring it was intact.

3. Provided patient privacy and draped as appropriate for comfort.

4. Explained to patient and family caregiver the choice of restraint and why it was needed, how it would be applied, length of time it would be used, procedure for ongoing assessment, and criteria for discontinuation.

IMPLEMENTATION

1. Adjusted bed to proper height and lowered side rail on side of patient contact. Ensured that patient was comfortable and in proper body alignment.

2. Inspected area where restraint was to be placed. Noted if there was any nearby tubing or device. Assessed condition of skin, sensation, adequacy of circulation, and range of joint motion.

3. Padded skin and bony prominences (as necessary) that would be under restraint.

4. Applied proper-size restraint per manufacturer directions.

   a. Mitten restraint: Placed hand in mitten; ensured that Velcro strap was around wrist and not forearm.

   b. Elbow restraint (freedom splint): Centered splint over elbow with opening facing away from patient. Secured splint by threading hook and loop strap through buckle and back onto self. Ensured Velcro straps were positioned away from the patient.

   c. Self- releasing roll belt restraint:

      (1) While patient was out of bed, centered belt on bed at patient's waist level with belt label facing head of bed.

      (2) Positioned the long straps so they hung off each side of mattress. Attached straps to each side of the bed frame by using quick-release ties or a quick-release buckle.

      (3) Reconnected the QR buckle and pulled on the strap end and tightened strap to bed; repeated on other side of bed.

	S	U	NP	Comments

(4) Attached belt to patient by having opened the QR buckle and the belt; placed patient on bed with belt at waist level. Brought belt around patient waist and secured hook and loop fastener and QR buckle.

(5) Ensured belt was snug but did not restrict breathing. Ensured bed frame straps were snug to the mattress and would not slide or move if bed was adjusted.

d. Option: Placed patient in an enclosure bed.

e. Soft extremity (ankle or wrist) restraint: Wrapped limb restraint around wrist or ankle with soft part toward skin and secured snugly (not tightly) in place by Velcro strap. Inserted two fingers under secured restraint.

5. Attached restraint straps to part of bedframe that moved when raising or lowering head of bed. Ensured that straps were secure. Did not attach to side rails. Attached restraint to chair frame for patient in chair or wheelchair, ensured that buckle was out of patient's reach. (Exception: Freedom restraint not secured to bed frame).

6. Secured restraints on bedframe with quick-release buckle. Did not tie strap in a knot. Ensured that buckle was out of patient reach.

7. Double-checked and inserted two fingers under secured restraint. Assessed proper placement of restraint, including skin integrity, pulses, skin temperature and color, and sensation of restrained body part. Raised side rails (as appropriate). Placed bed in lowest position after restraint(s) applied.

8. Performed hand hygiene. Followed agency policies regarding frequency of restraint removal, monitoring and assessment, and assessment content. Depending on type of restraint used, cognitive status, and individual needs of the patient, more frequent monitoring was used. Repositioned patient, provided comfort and toileting measures, and evaluated patient condition each time. If patient was agitated, violent, or nonadherent, removed one restraint at a time and/or had staff assist while removing restraints.

9. Placed nurse call system within patient's reach.

10. Left bed or chair with wheels locked. Raised side rails (as appropriate), lowered and locked bed into lowest position.

11. Removed and disposed of any supplies. Performed hand hygiene.

	S	U	NP	Comments

EVALUATION

1. After restraint application, evaluated patient's response to restraints:

   a. Nonviolent patients: Conducted evaluation for signs of injury, behavior and psychological status, and readiness for discontinuation.

   b. Violent/self-destructive patients: Conducted same evaluation per agency policy. Performed visual checks if patient was too agitated to approach.

2. Evaluated patient's need for toileting, nutrition and fluids, hygiene, and elimination, and released restraint at least every 2 hours.

3. Evaluated patient for any complications of immobility.

4. Renewal of restraints:

   a. Nonviolent patients may have had renewal of restraints based on hospital policy. Discontinued restraint at the earliest possible time, regardless of the scheduled expiration of the order.

   b. Violent/self-destructive patients may have had restraints renewed within the required limits. Orders may have been renewed according to the time limits for a maximum of 24 consecutive hours.

5. Observed IV catheters, urinary catheters, and drainage tubes to determine that they were positioned correctly and that therapy remained uninterrupted.

6. Used Teach-Back. Revised instruction or developed a plan for revised family caregiver teaching if family caregiver was not able to teach back correctly.

DOCUMENTATION

1. Documented restraint alternatives used and patient's response, patient's current behavior and medical condition, level of orientation, and patient or family member's statement of understanding of the purpose of restraint and consent for application (if required by agency).

2. Documented placement and purpose for restraint, type and location of restraint, time applied, time restraint ended, and all routine assessments.

	S	U	NP	Comments

3. Documented patient's behavior after restraint application. Documented times patient was assessed, attempts to use alternatives to restraint and patient's response, times restraint was released (temporarily and permanently), and patient's response when restraint was removed. ___ ___ ___ _____

4. Documented evaluation of patient's/family caregiver's learning. ___ ___ ___ _____

HAND-OFF REPORTING

1. Reported any injury resulting from a restraint to registered nurse in charge and health care provider immediately. ___ ___ ___ _____

2. During hand-off report, noted the location and type of restraint, last time assessment was conducted, and findings. ___ ___ ___ _____

Student _____ Date _____

Instructor _____ Date _____

PERFORMANCE CHECKLIST PROCEDURAL GUIDELINE 14.1 **FIRE, ELECTRICAL, AND CHEMICAL SAFETY**

	S	U	NP	Comments

STEPS

1. Reviewed agency policies for rapid response to fire, electrical, and chemical emergency. Knew responsibilities such as initiating fire alarm and patient evacuation. ___ ___ ___ _____

2. Knew the location of fire alarms, emergency equipment, safety data sheet (SDS) forms, emergency eyewash stations, and emergency exit routes on work unit. ___ ___ ___ _____

3. Was alert to situations that increased the risk of fire. Regularly checked a patient room for electrical or fire hazards. ___ ___ ___ _____

4. Knew which patients were on oxygen. Was aware of location and who has access to the oxygen shut-off valve. ___ ___ ___ _____

5. Inspected equipment for current maintenance sticker. Checked electrical equipment for basic safety features. Knew agency process for tagging and reporting broken or unsafe equipment. ___ ___ ___ _____

6. Knew the patient's mental status and ability to ambulate, transfer, or move so that if a fire occurred nurse could anticipate the procedures needed for evacuation. ___ ___ ___ _____

7. Fire safety:

   a. Followed the acronym RACE. ___ ___ ___ _____

      (1) Rescued patient from immediate injury by removing from area or shielding from fire to avoid burns. ___ ___ ___ _____

      (2) Activated fire alarm immediately. Followed agency policy for alerting staff to respond. (Often preformed simultaneously as Step (1) by using call system to alert staff while patients at risk were helped.) ___ ___ ___ _____

      (3) Contained the fire: ___ ___ ___ _____

         (a) Closed all doors and windows. ___ ___ ___ _____

         (b) Turned off oxygen and electrical equipment. ___ ___ ___ _____

         (c) Placed wet towels along base of doors. ___ ___ ___ _____

	S	U	NP	Comments

(4) Evacuated patients: ___ ___ ___ _____

  (a) Directed ambulatory patients to walk by themselves to a safe area. Knew the fire exits and emergency evacuation route. ___ ___ ___ _____

  (b) If patient was on life support, maintained respiratory status manually (Ambu bag) until nurse removed patient from fire area. ___ ___ ___ _____

  (c) Moved bedridden patients by stretcher, bed, or wheelchair. ___ ___ ___ _____

  (d) For patients who could not walk or ambulate: ___ ___ ___ _____

    (i) Placed on blanket and dragged patient out of area of danger. ___ ___ ___ _____

    (ii) Used two-person swing: Placed patient in sitting position and had two staff members form a seat by clasping forearms together. Lifted patient into "seat" and carried out of area of danger. ___ ___ ___ _____

  (e) If fire department personnel were on the scene, they helped with evacuation of patients. ___ ___ ___ _____

b. Extinguished fire using appropriate fire extinguisher: type A for ordinary combustibles, type B for flammable liquids, type C for electrical equipment, type ABC for any type of fire. Followed the acronym PASS. ___ ___ ___ _____

  (1) Pulled the pin. ___ ___ ___ _____

  (2) Aimed nozzle at base of fire. ___ ___ ___ _____

  (3) Squeezed extinguisher handles. ___ ___ ___ _____

  (4) Swept from side to side to coat area evenly. ___ ___ ___ _____

c. Fire doors were not blocked. ___ ___ ___ _____

8. Once patient was evacuated, made the patient comfortable. Kept locks on wheelchairs or beds locked. Performed hand hygiene. ___ ___ ___ _____

9. Electrical safety:

a. If patient received an electrical shock, immediately turned off power to electrical source and assessed for presence of a pulse. Caution: When disengaging electrical source, checked for presence of water on floor. ___ ___ ___ _____

b. Once the source of electricity was disconnected, provided appropriate assistance. If patient was pulseless, instituted emergency resuscitation. ___ ___ ___ _____

c. Notified emergency personnel and patient's health care provider. ___ ___ ___ _____

d. If patient had a pulse and remained alert and oriented, obtained vital signs and assessed the skin for signs of thermal injury. ___ ___ ___ _____

10. Chemical safety for liquid hazardous drugs (HD):

a. Referred to health care agency specific policies and/or SDS once cleaning up an HD spill. Obtained an HD spill kit if available. ___ ___ ___ _____

b. If self or a work colleague was exposed to an HD/chemotherapy drug:

   (1) Removed both sets of contaminated gloves and/or clothing immediately. ___ ___ ___ _____

   (2) Disposed of gloves and clothing in hazardous drug waste bag for placement in container designated for hazardous drugs. ___ ___ ___ _____

   (3) Washed hands thoroughly with soap and water for at least 15 minutes. ___ ___ ___ _____

   (4) If contamination of skin or eyes was suspected, sought medical attention as soon as possible. ___ ___ ___ _____

   (5) Treated chemical splashes to the eyes immediately. Flushed eyes with water using clean, lukewarm tap water for 15 to 20 minutes. Removed contact lenses if flushing did not remove them. ___ ___ ___ _____

   (6) Treated skin exposure by standing under a shower or placed exposed area under faucet with running lukewarm tap water for 15 to 20 minutes. ___ ___ ___ _____

c. Notified people in the immediate area of a spill and evacuated all nonessential personnel from area. ___ ___ ___ _____

d. Referred to SDS; if spilled material was flammable, turned off electrical and heat sources. ___ ___ ___ _____

e. Avoided breathing vapors of spilled material; applied appropriate respirator. ___ ___ ___ _____

f. Disposed of any materials used in cleanup as hazardous waste. ___ ___ ___ _____

	S	U	NP	Comments
11. Documentation: Documented as a sentinel event report and not in electronic health record (EHR).	___	___	___	_____
12. Hand-off reporting; Followed agency policy for reporting a sentinel event.	___	___	___	_____

211

Student _____ Date _____

Instructor _____ Date _____

PERFORMANCE CHECKLIST SKILL 14.4 **SEIZURE PRECAUTIONS**

	S	U	NP	Comments

ASSESSMENT

1. Identified patient using two identifiers.

2. Reviewed electronic health record (EHR) for medical and surgical conditions that might contribute to or be a cause of a seizure and for any bleeding tendencies.

3. Assessed EHR for patient's seizure history, previous precipitating factors, frequency of seizures, presence and type of aura, symptoms during a seizure, and phases of seizure events known. Used a family caregiver as resource if needed.

4. Assessed patient's/family caregiver's health literacy.

5. Assessed medication history. Asked patient about adherence to anticonvulsants and reviewed therapeutic drug levels if laboratory test results were available.

6. Inspected patient's environment for potential safety hazards. Kept bed in low position with side rails up at head of bed.

7. Assessed patient's individual and cultural perspective about the meaning of seizures/epilepsy and treatment.

8. Assessed patient's knowledge, prior experience with seizure precautions, and feelings about these measures.

PLANNING

1. Determined expected outcomes following completion of procedure.

2. Performed hand hygiene and prepared equipment.

3. Ensured patient was in a comfortable position. Reduced lighting in room and tried to control for any sudden, loud, unexpected noise.

212

	S	U	NP	Comments

4. Informed patient and appropriate family caregiver that patient was on seizure precautions and what these precautions entailed. Discussed the possible triggers that result in patient's seizure activity. Included discussion of approaches to adopt seizure precautions in the patient's home environment. ____ ____ ____ _____

IMPLEMENTATION

1. For patients with history of seizures, kept bed in lowest position with side rails up (according to agency policy). Padded rails if patient was at risk for head injury and optionally offered protective head gear. Had oral suction and oxygen equipment ready for use. ____ ____ ____ _____

2. Placed patient with history of seizures in room close to nurse's station or room with video monitor (if available). ____ ____ ____ _____

3. Focal/partial or general seizure response:

   a. Positioned patient safely. ____ ____ ____ _____

      (1) Guided a patient who was standing or sitting to the floor, and protected head by cradling in lap or placed pillow under head. Positioned patient so as to keep head tilted to maximize breathing (if able). Tried to position patient on side but did not force. Did not lift patient from floor to bed during seizure. ____ ____ ____ _____

      (2) If patient was in bed, turned onto side (did not force) and raised side rails. ____ ____ ____ _____

   b. Noted time the seizure began, stayed with the patient and called for help immediately to have staff member bring emergency cart to bedside and clear surrounding area of furniture. Provided airway protection and gas exchange by positioning head. Had health care provider and Rapid Response Team notified immediately. ____ ____ ____ _____

   c. Kept patient in side-lying position (if possible), supporting head and keeping it flexed slightly forward. ____ ____ ____ _____

   d. Did not restrain patient; if patient was flailing limbs, held them loosely. Loosened restrictive clothing/gown to aid breathing. ____ ____ ____ _____

   e. Never forced any object into patient's mouth when teeth were clenched. ____ ____ ____ _____

   f. If possible, provided privacy. Had staff control flow of visitors in area. ____ ____ ____ _____

	S	U	NP	Comments

g. Observed sequence and timing of seizure activity. Noted type of seizure activity; whether more than one type of seizure occurred; sequence of seizure progression; level of conscientiousness; character of breathing; presence of incontinence; presence of autonomic signs of lip smacking; mastication, and grimacing; rolling of eyes.   ____ ____ ____ _____

h. As patient regained consciousness, assessed vital signs and reoriented and reassured. Explained what happened and answered patient's questions. Stayed with patient until fully awake.   ____ ____ ____ _____

4. Status epilepticus (medical emergency):

a. Followed Steps 3a to 3e to protect patient, and called Rapid Response Team.   ____ ____ ____ _____

b. Assisted health care provider with oropharyngeal or nasopharyngeal airway insertion if oxygen saturation was compromised or if seizure lasted greater or equal to 30 minutes. (Note: Applied clean gloves if timing allowed.) Physician on team intubated patient when jaw was relaxed (between seizure activity).   ____ ____ ____ _____

c. Accessed and administered oxygen; turned on suction equipment; kept airway patent with oral suctioning (if possible).   ____ ____ ____ _____

d. Had another nurse on team measure blood pressure, heart rate, respirations, and oxygen saturation immediately and then every 2 minutes, and had team member perform fingerstick to check blood glucose.   ____ ____ ____ _____

e. Member of team prepared for and inserted IV catheter (if one was not in place) with 0.9% sodium chloride infusing and administered IV antiseizure medications.   ____ ____ ____ _____

f. As seizure subsided, suctioned patient's airway if secretions accumulated. If oral airway was inserted, ensured that it remained in correct position. Continued oxygen administration.   ____ ____ ____ _____

g. Kept patient in side-lying position of comfort in bed with side rails up and bed in lowest position and locked into place.   ____ ____ ____ _____

5. As patient regained consciousness, reoriented and reassured. Explained what happened and provided quiet, nonstimulating environment.   ____ ____ ____ _____

	S	U	NP	Comments

6. Placed nurse call system in an accessible location within patient's reach. Instructed patient not to get out of bed without help.

   ____ ____ ____ _____

7. Cleaned up patient care area; disposed of used supplies. Performed hand hygiene.

   ____ ____ ____ _____

EVALUATION

1. Checked vital signs and oxygen saturation every 15 minutes during postictal phase and maintained patent airway.

   ____ ____ ____ _____

2. Rechecked blood glucose per health care provider order or agency protocol.

   ____ ____ ____ _____

3. Examined patient for injury, including oral cavity and extremities.

   ____ ____ ____ _____

4. Evaluated patient's mental status after seizure. Encouraged patient to verbalize feelings and describe an awareness of seizure triggers.

   ____ ____ ____ _____

5. Helped health care provider conduct neurological examination of patient and collected any ordered blood test specimens.

   ____ ____ ____ _____

6. After patient has returned to level of consciousness where patient could be attentive, used Teach-Back. Revised instruction or developed a plan for revised patient/family caregiver teaching if patient or family caregiver was not able to teach back correctly.

   ____ ____ ____ _____

DOCUMENTATION

1. Documented in nurses' notes observations before, during, and after seizure. Provided detailed description of the type of seizure activity and sequence of events.

   ____ ____ ____ _____

2. Documented treatments administered for the seizure, establishment of IV line, fluid infusing, and stabilization of airway.

   ____ ____ ____ _____

3. Documented evaluation of patient/family caregiver learning.

   ____ ____ ____ _____

HAND-OFF REPORTING

1. Once a patient has had a seizure, reported to oncoming staff a detailed description of seizure and patient's response to therapy.

   ____ ____ ____ _____

2. Alerted health care provider immediately as seizure began.

   ____ ____ ____ _____

PERFORMANCE CHECKLIST SKILL 15.1   **CARE OF A PATIENT AFTER BIOLOGICAL EXPOSURE**

	S	U	NP	Comments
ASSESSMENT				
1. Performed hand hygiene. Donned proper PPE.	___	___	___	_____
2. Identified patient using two identifiers according to agency policy.	___	___	___	_____
3. Conducted focused health history and physical examination. Reviewed history of patient's presenting symptoms and determined if pattern existed.	___	___	___	_____
4. Measured patient's vital signs (including SpO_2) and included assessment of pain on a scale of 1 to 10.	___	___	___	_____
5. Assessed patient's/family caregiver's health literacy.	___	___	___	_____
6. Reviewed results of diagnostic tests and consulted with health care provider.	___	___	___	_____
7. Assessed patient for health risks that complicate effects of exposure to a biological agent.	___	___	___	_____
8. Stayed calm. Listened and assessed patient's immediate psychological response after exposure, including dissociative symptoms.	___	___	___	_____
9. Identified and gathered all patient contacts before the patient left the emergency department (ED).	___	___	___	_____
10. Identified agency resources available.	___	___	___	_____
PLANNING				
1. Determined expected outcomes following completion of procedure.	___	___	___	_____
2. Provided timely and accurate information: accurate description of agent to which patient was exposed and implications for patient and family.	___	___	___	_____
3. Assembled necessary supplies.	___	___	___	_____
4. Closed door to room or bedside curtain.	___	___	___	_____
IMPLEMENTATION				
1. Continued wearing PPE applied before assessment. Followed transmission-based isolation precautions. Used strict isolation with smallpox. Used Airborne Precautions, Contact Precautions, and a negative-pressure room for patients suspected of having smallpox.	___	___	___	_____

	S	U	NP	Comments

2. Decontaminated. If anthrax was suspected, had patient remove clothing and placed it in labeled plastic biohazard bag. Did not pull over patient's head; instead, cut garments off. Instructed patient to shower thoroughly with soap and water.

3. Administered appropriate antibiotics and/or anti-toxins.

4. Administered immunizations (in the event of smallpox).

5. Administered fluid and nutrition therapy.

6. Administered oxygen therapy.

7. Provided supportive care.

8. Counseled patient and family about acute and potential long-term psychological effects of exposure. Offered access to trained counselors. Supported survivors of a disaster by identifying resources available.

9. When leaving patient's room, raised side rails as appropriate and lowered and locked bed into lowest position.

10. Disposed of any used supplies in appropriate receptacle.

11. Placed nurse call system in an accessible location within patient's reach.

12. After leaving patient area, removed most heavily contaminated items first. Peeled off gown and gloves, rolled them inside out, and disposed of them. Performed hand hygiene. Removed face shield from behind and disposed of safely. Removed goggles and mask from behind. Placed goggles in container for reprocessing; disposed of mask safely. Performed hand hygiene.

EVALUATION

1. Observed for improved airway maintenance, breathing, circulation, level of consciousness (LOC), and neurological functioning.

2. Evaluated vital signs and character of pain.

3. Inspected condition of patient's skin; noted character of remaining lesions.

4. Used Teach-Back. Revised instruction or developed a plan for revised patient/family caregiver teaching if patient or family caregiver was not able to teach back correctly.

	S	U	NP	Comments

DOCUMENTATION

1. Used disaster checklists to quickly record specific data regarding patient status, treatment administered, and response to treatment/or comfort measures. Documented patient/family caregiver's response to instruction.

    ___ ___ ___ _____

HAND-OFF REPORTING

1. Reported any unexpected outcome to health care provider in charge.

    ___ ___ ___ _____

2. Reported suspected cases of a biological incident to health care provider or ED officer.

    ___ ___ ___ _____

Student _____ Date _____

Instructor _____ Date _____

PERFORMANCE CHECKLIST SKILL 15.2   **CARE OF A PATIENT AFTER CHEMICAL EXPOSURE**

	S	U	NP	Comments

ASSESSMENT

1. Performed hand hygiene. Donned proper PPE.

2. Identified patient using at least two identifiers according to agency policy.

3. Conducted focused physical assessment. Observed for presence of liquid on patient's skin, mucous membranes, or clothing and odor, assessing the condition of skin to determine severity of exposure.

4. Measured patient's vital signs (including SpO_2) and include assessment of pain severity on a scale of 0 to 10.

5. Assessed patient's/family caregiver's health literacy.

6. Assessed patient for preexisting medical conditions that would complicate effects of toxic chemical exposure.

7. Remained calm. Listened and assessed patient's immediate psychological response after exposure, including dissociative symptoms.

8. Identified agency resources available.

PLANNING

1. Determined expected outcomes following completion of procedure.

2. Provided privacy. Explained care to patient and family caregivers, including decontamination and treatment. Explained own role, oriented to location and activities to perform, explained what patient had experienced, and asked, "How are you feeling right now?" Assured them that a medical professional would see them shortly.

3. Obtained and organized equipment for decontamination.

IMPLEMENTATION

1. Continued wearing PPE applied during assessment. Prepared for decontamination.

2. Decontaminated patient.

   a. Acted quickly; avoided touching contaminated parts of clothing as much as possible.

	S	U	NP	Comments

b. Removed all of patient's clothing. Did not pull clothing over patient's head; instead, cut garments off.

         ___ ___ ___ _____

c. Used large amounts of soap and water to wash patient thoroughly.

         ___ ___ ___ _____

d. If eyes were burning or vision was blurred, rinsed eyes with plain water for 10 to 15 minutes. If patient wore contacts, removed and placed with contaminated clothing; did not re-insert in eyes. Washed eyeglasses with soap and water; reapplied when completed.

         ___ ___ ___ _____

3. Disposed of patient's contaminated clothing in appropriate biohazard bag and seal. Placed bag in another plastic bag and sealed.

         ___ ___ ___ _____

4. Initiated treatment for chemical agent using appropriate chemical agent protocol.

         ___ ___ ___ _____

5. Established airway if needed; administered oxygen therapy.

         ___ ___ ___ _____

6. Controlled bleeding.

         ___ ___ ___ _____

7. Established intravascular access. Administered fluid and nutrition therapy.

         ___ ___ ___ _____

8. Provided supportive care.

         ___ ___ ___ _____

9. Counseled patient and family on both acute and potential long-term psychological effects of exposure. Offered access to trained counselors.

         ___ ___ ___ _____

10. When leaving room, raised side rails (as appropriate) and lowered and locked bed into lowest position.

         ___ ___ ___ _____

11. Disposed of any used supplies in appropriate receptacle.

         ___ ___ ___ _____

12. Placed nurse call system in an accessible location within patient's reach.

         ___ ___ ___ _____

13. Removed most heavily contaminated items first. Peeled off gown and gloves, rolled inside out, and disposed of them. Performed hand hygiene. Removed face shield from behind and disposed of safely. Removed goggles and mask from behind. Placed goggles in container for reprocessing; disposed of mask safely. Performed hand hygiene.

         ___ ___ ___ _____

EVALUATION

1. Observed status of airway maintenance, breathing, circulation, LOC, and neurological functioning. Assessed vital signs.

         ___ ___ ___ _____

2. Asked patient to rate pain acuity on a scale of 0 to 10.

         ___ ___ ___ _____

3. Inspected condition of skin; noted extent of blistering.

         ___ ___ ___ _____

	S	U	NP	Comments

4. Evaluated patient's level of orientation, ability to problem solve, and perception of condition.

5. Used Teach-Back. Revised instruction or developed a plan for revised patient/family caregiver teaching if patient or family caregiver was not able to teach back correctly.

DOCUMENTATION

1. Documented patient's status, decontamination and treatment procedures, and response to treatment and/or comfort measures. Documented patient/family's response to instruction.

HAND-OFF REPORTING

1. Reported any unexpected outcome to health care provider in charge.

2. Reported suspected cases of a toxic chemical event to health care provider or emergency officer.

Student _____ Date _____

Instructor _____ Date _____

PERFORMANCE CHECKLIST SKILL 15.3   **CARE OF A PATIENT AFTER RADIATION EXPOSURE**

	S	U	NP	Comments
ASSESSMENT				
1. Performed hand hygiene. Donned proper PPE.	___	___	___	_____
2. Identified patient using two identifiers according to agency policy.	___	___	___	_____
3. Assessed patient's symptoms by performing a focused physical examination.	___	___	___	_____
4. Measured patient's vital signs (including SpO_2) and included assessment of the character of pain on a scale of 0 to 10.	___	___	___	_____
5. Assessed patient's/family caregiver's health literacy.	___	___	___	_____
6. Assessed patient for preexisting medical conditions that would complicate effects of the radiological exposure.	___	___	___	_____
7. Reviewed results of diagnostic tests and consulted with health care provider.	___	___	___	_____
8. Determined patient's allergies, specifically allergy to iodine. Ensured patient had an allergy identification wrist band.	___	___	___	_____
9. Assessed individual psychological response to a radiological event, including dissociative symptoms. Asked patient, "How do you feel now?" Determined level of orientation and ability to follow conversation.	___	___	___	_____
10. Identified agency resources available.	___	___	___	_____
PLANNING				
1. Determined expected outcomes following completion of procedure.	___	___	___	_____
2. Provided privacy and explained care to patient and family. Explained own role, oriented patient to location and activities to preform, explained what patient had experienced, and asked, "How are you feeling now?" Assured them that medical personnel would see them shortly.	___	___	___	_____
3. Obtained and organized decontamination equipment.	___	___	___	_____
IMPLEMENTATION				
1. Performed hand hygiene. Applied clean gloves.	___	___	___	_____

222

	S	U	NP	Comments

2. Continued wearing personal protective equipment (PPE) applied during assessment. Prepared for decontamination. _____ _____ _____ _____

3. Decontaminated patient: _____ _____ _____ _____

   a. Removed patient's clothing. _____ _____ _____ _____

   b. Washed patient's skin thoroughly with water and soap, taking care not to abrade or irritate the skin. _____ _____ _____ _____

   c. Used tepid decontamination water. Covered wounds with waterproof dressings. _____ _____ _____ _____

   d. Had radiation technician resurvey patient after washing using dosimeter. Rewashed as necessary. _____ _____ _____ _____

   e. Isolated and covered any area of skin that was still positive for radiation by using a plastic bag or wrap. _____ _____ _____ _____

4. Bagged and tagged patient's contaminated clothing for further evaluation and placed in appropriate biohazard container. _____ _____ _____ _____

5. Prepared for possibly obtaining a complete blood count (CBC), urinalysis, fecal specimen, and swabs of body orifices. _____ _____ _____ _____

6. Treated symptoms according to ordinary treatment practices: provided intravenous fluid support, antidiarrheal therapies, antiemetic medications, and potassium iodide tablets. _____ _____ _____ _____

7. Counseled patient and family on both acute and potential long-term psychological effects of exposure. Offered access to trained counselors. _____ _____ _____ _____

8. When leaving patient room raised side rails (as appropriate) and lowered and locked bed to lowest position. _____ _____ _____ _____

9. Disposed of any used supplies in appropriate receptacle. _____ _____ _____ _____

10. Placed nurse call system in an accessible location within patient's reach. _____ _____ _____ _____

11. Removed most heavily contaminated items first. Peeled off gown and gloves, rolled inside out, and disposed. Performed hand hygiene. Removed face shield from behind and disposed of safely. Removed goggles and mask from behind. Placed goggles in container for reprocessing; disposed of mask safely. Performed hand hygiene. _____ _____ _____ _____

	S	U	NP	Comments

EVALUATION

1. Observed skin integrity, fluid balance, respiratory and gastrointestinal (GI) status, LOC, and neurological functioning. Looked for improvement of other radiological agent-specific symptoms. Evaluated vital signs.

2. Monitored CBC and other laboratory tests.

3. Evaluated patient's LOC, orientation, and ability to relate events. Asked if patient remembers what has occurred; observed affect.

4. Used Teach-Back. Revised instruction or developed a plan for revised patient/family caregiver teaching if patient or family caregiver was not able to teach back correctly.

DOCUMENTATION

1. Documented treatments provided and patient's physical and psychological response. Documented patient and family caregiver response to instruction.

HAND-OFF REPORTING

1. Reported presence of open wound and any suspected radioactive fragment to health care provider in charge immediately.

2. Reported any unexpected outcomes to health care provider.

Student _____ Date _____

Instructor _____ Date _____

PERFORMANCE CHECKLIST SKILL 15.4 **CARE OF A PATIENT AFTER A NATURAL DISASTER**

	S	U	NP	Comments

ASSESSMENT

1. Performed hand hygiene. Donned proper PPE.

2. Identified patient using two identifiers according to agency policy.

3. Conducted focused health history and physical examination depending on area of injury. Reviewed history of patient's presenting symptoms and determined if a pattern exists.

4. Measured patient's vital signs and included assessment of character of pain on a scale of 0 to 10.

5. Assessed patient's/family caregiver's health literacy.

6. Assessed patient for health risks that complicate effects of exposure to the natural disaster.

7. Reviewed results of diagnostic tests and consulted with health care provider.

8. Stayed calm. Listened and assessed patient's immediate psychological response after exposure, including dissociative symptoms.

9. Identified agency resources available.

PLANNING

1. Determined expected outcomes following completion of procedure.

2. Dispensed timely and accurate information: accurate description of the disaster to which patient was exposed and implications to patient and family caregiver.

3. Provided for patient privacy.

4. Obtained and organized equipment for decontamination.

IMPLEMENTATION

1. Continued wearing PPE applied before assessment. Followed transmission-based isolation precautions.

2. Administered appropriate antibiotics as indicated.

3. Administered fluid and nutrition therapy.

4. Administered appropriate wound care.

5. Provided supportive care.

	S	U	NP	Comments

6. Counseled patient and family caregiver about acute and potential long-term psychological effects of experiencing a disaster. Offered access to trained counselors. Supported survivors of a disaster by identifying resources available.

_____ _____ _____ _____

7. When leaving patient room, raised side rails (as appropriate) and lowered and locked bed into lowest position.

_____ _____ _____ _____

8. Disposed of any used supplies in appropriate receptacle.

_____ _____ _____ _____

9. Placed nurse call system in an accessible location within patient's reach.

_____ _____ _____ _____

10. After leaving patient area, removed most heavily contaminated items first. Peeled off gown and gloves, rolled inside out, and disposed. Performed hand hygiene. Removed face shield from behind and disposed of safely. Removed goggles and mask from behind. Placed goggles in container for reprocessing; disposed of mask safely. Performed hand hygiene.

_____ _____ _____ _____

EVALUATION

1. Observed for improved airway maintenance, breathing, circulation, LOC, and neurological functioning.

_____ _____ _____ _____

2. Evaluated vital signs and level of pain.

_____ _____ _____ _____

3. Inspected condition of patient's skin; noted character of any wounds.

_____ _____ _____ _____

4. Queried patient, "Tell me how you feel right now." Checked level of orientation and ability to conduct conversation.

_____ _____ _____ _____

5. Used Teach-Back. Revised instruction or developed a plan for revised patient/family caregiver teaching if patient or family caregiver was not able to teach back correctly.

_____ _____ _____ _____

DOCUMENTATION

1. Documented patient's status, treatments provided, and response. Documented patient and family caregiver response to teaching.

_____ _____ _____ _____

HAND-OFF REPORTING

1. Reported presence of new wounds and injuries to health care provider in charge.

_____ _____ _____ _____

2. Reported any unexpected outcomes to health care provider.

_____ _____ _____ _____

Student _____ Date _____

Instructor _____ Date _____

PERFORMANCE CHECKLIST SKILL 16.1   **PAIN ASSESSMENT AND BASIC COMFORT MEASURES**

	S	U	NP	Comments
ASSESSMENT				
1. Identified patient using two identifiers.	___	___	___	_____
2. Obtained data from patient's electronic health record (EHR).	___	___	___	_____
3. Assessed patient's/family caregiver's health literacy.	___	___	___	_____
4. Assessed patient's knowledge, prior experience with pain management, and feelings about procedure.	___	___	___	_____
5. If patient could self-report, asked if the patient was in pain. Asked family caregivers if they believed the patient was in pain. Selected pain measures according to the patient's ability to communicate. Used a comprehensive approach for patients who were nonverbal. Used terms, such as hurt or discomfort, or used a professional interpreter if language difference existed.	___	___	___	_____
6. Performed hand hygiene and applied gloves. Had patient point to area of discomfort. Examined area: inspected for discoloration, swelling, or drainage; palpate for change in temperature, area of altered sensation, painful area, or areas that trigger pain; assess range of motion (ROM) of involved joints. When assessing abdomen, always auscultated first and then inspected and palpated.	___	___	___	_____
7. When patient self-reported pain, assessed physical, behavioral, and emotional signs and symptoms, including nonverbal indicators of pain.	___	___	___	_____
8. Assessed for decreased gastrointestinal (GI) motility, constipation, nausea, and vomiting.	___	___	___	_____
9. Assessed for insomnia, anorexia, and fatigue.	___	___	___	_____
10. Assessed the character of pain (acute or chronic), location(s) of the pain, pain history, pain quality, pain type, pain duration (intermittent, constant, or breakthrough), and pain intensity. Followed agency policy regarding frequency of assessment. Used of the PQRSTU pain assessment guides in collecting complete information about a patient's pain experience.	___	___	___	_____

a. Provocative/palliative factors: Considered patient's experience with over-the-counter (OTC) drugs (including herbals, marijuana and topicals) or exercises, and cognitive behavioral therapies that have helped to reduce pain in the past.

b. Quality: Used open-ended questions.

c. Region/radiation: Had patient use finger (if possible) to point out areas of pain.

d. Severity: Used valid pain rating scale appropriate to patient's age, language skills, developmental level, and comprehension. Asked patient to rate pain at rest, before any intervention, and when moving or engaged in care activity. In the case of patients with dementia, those who have no verbal skills, or patients who were sedated or intubated, used observational pain assessment scales.

e. Timing: Asked patient how long pain has been present and how often it occurred.

f. U: Asked how pain affected patient's activities of daily living (ADLs), work, relationships, and enjoyment of life.

11. Assessed patient's response to previous pharmacological interventions, especially ability to function. Determined if any analgesic side effects were likely based on medication and patient's previous responses.

12. Assessed for allergies to medications, with focus on medications. Applied allergy band if an allergy was identified.

PLANNING

1. Determined expected outcomes following completion of procedure.

2. Set pain-intensity goal with patient (when appropriate).

3. Provided privacy by closing room door or bedside curtains.

4. Prepared patient's environment.

5. Explained procedures to be used for pain relief and how patient could be involved.

6. Provided educational materials to patient and family caregiver.

IMPLEMENTATION

1. Performed hand hygiene and applied clean gloves (if indicated).

2. Taught patient how to use appropriate pain rating scale. Explained range of intensity scores and how they related to measuring pain. ___ ___ ___ _____

3. Prepared and administered appropriate pain-relieving medications per health care provider's order. ___ ___ ___ _____

4. Removed or reduced painful stimuli: ___ ___ ___ _____

   a. Helped patient to turn and repositioned to comfortable position in good body alignment. ___ ___ ___ _____

   b. Smoothed wrinkles in bed linens. ___ ___ ___ _____

   c. Loosened constrictive bandages (if appropriate to purpose of bandage) or loosened or removed devices. ___ ___ ___ _____

   d. Repositioned underlying tubes or equipment. ___ ___ ___ _____

   e. Used pillows as needed for alignment and positioning support. ___ ___ ___ _____

5. Taught patient how to splint over painful site using either a pillow or hand. ___ ___ ___ _____

   a. Explained purpose of splinting. ___ ___ ___ _____

   b. Placed pillow or blanket over site of discomfort and helped patient place hands firmly over area of discomfort. Option: splinted using hands only. ___ ___ ___ _____

   c. Had patient splint area firmly while coughing, deep breathing, and turning. ___ ___ ___ _____

6. Reduced or eliminated emotional factors that increase pain experiences. Used biopsychosocial treatments. ___ ___ ___ _____

   a. Offered information that reduced anxiety. ___ ___ ___ _____

   b. Offered patient opportunity to pray or read spiritual writings (if appropriate). ___ ___ ___ _____

   c. Spent time to allow patient to talk about pain and answer questions. Listened attentively. ___ ___ ___ _____

7. Before leaving, made sure patient was in a comfortable position. ___ ___ ___ _____

8. Raised side rails (as appropriate) and lowered and locked bed into lowest position. ___ ___ ___ _____

9. Placed nurse call system in an accessible location within patient's reach. ___ ___ ___ _____

10. If used, removed and disposed of gloves. Performed hand hygiene. ___ ___ ___ _____

EVALUATION

1. Based on agency reassessment criteria, reassessed patient's pain after comfort measures. ___ ___ ___ _____

2. Compared patient's current pain with personally set pain intensity goal. ___ ___ _____

3. Compared patient's ability to function and perform ADLs before and after pain interventions. Initiated a nurse-patient dialogue about the effect of pain-relieving interventions on function and ability to perform ADLs. ___ ___ _____

4. Observed patient's nonverbal behaviors after pain interventions. Implemented validated observational pain-assessment tool with patients who were unable to self-report. ___ ___ _____

5. Used Teach-Back. Revised instruction or developed a plan for revised patient/family caregiver teaching if patient or family caregiver was not able to teach back correctly. ___ ___ _____

DOCUMENTATION

1. Documented character of pain before and after an intervention, the pain-relief therapies used, whether pain relief was achieved, patient or family education provided, and patient response to interventions. ___ ___ _____

2. Documented evaluation of patient learning. ___ ___ _____

HAND-OFF REPORTING

1. Reported inadequate pain relief, a reduction in patient function, and side effects and adverse effects of both pharmacological and nonpharmacological pain interventions. ___ ___ _____

Student _____ Date _____

Instructor _____ Date _____

PERFORMANCE CHECKLIST SKILL 16.2   **NONPHARMACOLOGICAL PAIN MANAGEMENT**

	S	U	NP	Comments

ASSESSMENT

1. Identified patient using two identifiers.

2. Assessed patient's and/or family caregiver's health literacy.

3. Assessed patient's knowledge, prior experience with nonpharmacological pain management, and feelings about procedure.

4. Identified descriptive terms to be used when guiding patient through relaxation or guided imagery.

5. Performed hand hygiene. Performed complete pain assessment.

6. Assessed character of patient's respirations.

7. Reviewed health care provider's orders for pain relief (if required by agency).

8. Assessed patient's understanding of pain and willingness to receive nonpharmacological pain-relief measures.

9. Assessed preferred patient pastime activities.

10. Assessed type of image patient would prefer to use in guided imagery.

11. Reviewed any restrictions in patient's mobility or positioning.

PLANNING

1. Determined expected outcomes following completion of procedure.

2. Provided privacy by closing room door or bedside curtains.

3. Performed hand hygiene. Organized equipment at bedside.

4. Explained purpose of nonpharmacological technique and what was expected of patient during activity. Explained how to use pain rating scale.

5. Set mutual pain-intensity goal with patient (when able) for rest and during routine care activities.

6. Planned time to perform technique when patient could concentrate.

	S	U	NP	Comments

7. Administered an ordered analgesic 30 minutes before implementing a nonpharmacological therapy. ___ ___ ___ _____

8. Positioned the patient and drape if needed. ___ ___ ___ _____

9. Prepared environment: Made room temperature suited to patient. Controlled level of sound and lighting. Minimized interruptions and coordinated care activities; allowed time for rest. ___ ___ ___ _____

IMPLEMENTATION

1. Performed hand hygiene. ___ ___ ___ _____

2. Performed massage:

   a. Placed patient in comfortable position such as prone or side lying. Had patients with difficulty breathing lie on side of bed with head of bed elevated. ___ ___ ___ _____

   b. Adjusted bed to comfortable position; lowered upper side rail on working side. Draped patient to expose only area being massaged. ___ ___ ___ _____

   c. Turned on music to patient's preference. ___ ___ ___ _____

   d. Ensured that patient was not allergic to lotion and accepted using it; warmed lotion in hands or in basin of warm water. If head and scalp massaged, delayed use of lotion until completed. ___ ___ ___ _____

   e. Chose stroke technique based on desired effect or body part. Asked patient to identify the type of touch preferred. ___ ___ ___ _____

   f. Encouraged patient to breathe deeply in and out (consciously allowing pelvic muscles to relax) during massage. ___ ___ ___ _____

   g. Stood behind patient, and stimulated scalp and temples. ___ ___ ___ _____

   h. Supporting patient's head, used own fingers to apply gentle friction to rub muscles at base of head. ___ ___ ___ _____

   i. Repositioned if needed. With patient in supine position, massaged hands and arms as appropriate. ___ ___ ___ _____

      (1) Supported hand, and gently applied friction to palm using both thumbs. ___ ___ ___ _____

      (2) Supported base of finger and worked each finger in corkscrewlike motion, then massaged back of hand. ___ ___ ___ _____

      (3) Used pétrissage over (kneaded) muscles of forearm and upper arm between thumb and forefinger. ___ ___ ___ _____

232

	S	U	NP	Comments

j. After determining that patient had no neck injury or condition that contraindicates neck manipulation, massaged neck as appropriate: ___ ___ ___ _____

  (1) Placed patient prone unless contraindicated. Otherwise, used side-lying position. ___ ___ ___ _____

  (2) Used pétrissage over each neck muscle between thumb and forefinger. ___ ___ ___ _____

  (3) Gently stretched neck by placing one hand on top of shoulders and other at base of head. Gently moved hands away from one another. ___ ___ ___ _____

k. Massaged back as appropriate: ___ ___ ___ _____

  (1) Assisted patient to prone position unless contraindicated; side-lying position as an option. ___ ___ ___ _____

  (2) Did not allow hands to leave patient's skin. ___ ___ ___ _____

  (3) Applied hands first to sacral area; and used effleurage (massaged in circular motion). Stroked upward from buttocks to shoulders. Massaged over scapulae with smooth, firm stroke. Continued in one smooth stroke to upper arms and laterally along sides of back down to iliac crest. Continued massage pattern for 3 minutes. ___ ___ ___ _____

  (4) Used effleurage (long, gliding or circular massage strokes) along muscles of spine in upward and outward motion. ___ ___ ___ _____

  (5) Used pétrissage on muscles of each shoulder toward front of patient. ___ ___ ___ _____

  (6) Used palms in upward and outward circular motion from lower buttocks to neck. ___ ___ ___ _____

  (7) Kneaded muscles of upper back and shoulder. ___ ___ ___ _____

  (8) Used both hands to knead muscles up one side of back and then the other. ___ ___ ___ _____

  (9) Ended massage with long, stroking effleurage movements. ___ ___ ___ _____

l. Massaged feet as appropriate: ___ ___ ___ _____

  (1) Placed patient in supine position. ___ ___ ___ _____

  (2) Held foot firmly. Supported ankle with one hand or supported sides of foot with each hand while performing massage. ___ ___ ___ _____

  (3) Made circular motions with thumb and fingers around bones of ankle and top of foot. ___ ___ ___ _____

  (4) Massaged sides and top of each toe. ___ ___ ___ _____

  (5) Used friction (firm and focused rubbing) to make circular motions on bottom of foot. ___ ___ ___ _____

(6) Kneaded sides of foot between index finger and thumb.   ___ ___ ___ _____

(7) Concluded with firm, sweeping motions over top and bottom of foot.   ___ ___ ___ _____

m. Told patient that the massage was ending.   ___ ___ ___ _____

n. When procedure was complete, instructed patient to inhale deeply and exhale. Cautioned patient to move slowly after resting a few minutes.   ___ ___ ___ _____

o. Wiped excess lotion or oil from patient's body with bath towel.   ___ ___ ___ _____

3. Progressive relaxation with slow, deep breathing:

a. Had patient assume comfortable sitting position: sit with feet uncrossed or lie in supine position with small pillow under head.   ___ ___ ___ _____

b. Instructed patient to take several slow, deep breaths, relaxing lower pelvic muscles. Option to have patient close their eyes.   ___ ___ ___ _____

c. Explained as follows: "Let the air coming in through your nose move downward into your lower belly. Let your belly expand fully. Now breathe out through your mouth (or your nose, if that feels more natural). Let the muscles in your pelvis and lower belly relax. Alternate normal and deep breaths several times. Pay attention to how you feel when you breathe in and breathe out normally and when you breathe deeply. Notice how shallow breathing can make you feel tense and constricted, while deep breathing can help you relax."   ___ ___ ___ _____

d. Continued the exercise: "To practice, put one hand on your abdomen, just below your belly button. Feel your hand rise about an inch each time you breathe in and fall about an inch each time you breathe out. Your chest will rise slightly, too, along with your belly. Remember to relax your belly so that each time you breathe in, it expands fully. As you breathe out slowly, let yourself sigh out loud."   ___ ___ ___ _____

e. Observed patient and cautioned against hyperventilation.   ___ ___ ___ _____

f. Coached patient to locate any area of muscle tension and alternate tightening and relaxing all muscle groups for 6 to 7 seconds, beginning at feet and working upward toward head.   ___ ___ ___ _____

(1) Instructed patient to tighten muscles during inhalation and relax muscles during exhalation.   ___ ___ ___ _____

	S	U	NP	Comments

(2) As each muscle group relaxed, asked patient to enjoy relaxed feeling and allow mind to drift and think how nice it is to be relaxed. Had patient breathe deeply. ___ ___ ___ _____

(3) Calmly explained during exercise that patient may feel sensations of tingling, heaviness, floating, or warmth as relaxation occurs. ___ ___ ___ _____

(4) Had patient continue slow, deep breaths throughout exercise. ___ ___ ___ _____

(5) When finished, had patient inhale deeply, exhale, and then initially move about slowly after resting a few minutes. ___ ___ ___ _____

4. Guided imagery:

   a. Directed patient through exercise by having the patient focus on an image: ___ ___ ___ _____

      (1) Instructed patient to imagine that inhaled air is a ball of healing energy. ___ ___ ___ _____

      (2) Imagine that inhaled air travels to area of pain. ___ ___ ___ _____

   b. Alternatively, directed imagery: ___ ___ ___ _____

      (1) Asked patient to imagine a pleasant place such as a beach or mountains. Gave examples, but made sure that it was an image and experience that the patient chose. ___ ___ ___ _____

      (2) Directed patient to experience all sensory aspects of the restful place. ___ ___ ___ _____

      (3) Directed patient to continue deep, slow, rhythmic breathing. ___ ___ ___ _____

      (4) Directed patient to count to three, inhale, and open eyes. Suggested that patient move about slowly initially. ___ ___ ___ _____

      (5) Provided patient time to practice exercise without interruption. ___ ___ ___ _____

5. Distraction:

   a. Directed patient's attention away from pain by involving patient in a distraction technique. ___ ___ ___ _____

   b. Music: Played selection for approximately 30 minutes in location where patient was comfortable. Set volume or loudness at comfortable level. Used music of patient's choosing. Emphasized listening to rhythm and adjusted volume as pain increases or decreases. ___ ___ ___ _____

   c. Directed patient to give detailed account of an event or story; described pleasant memories. ___ ___ ___ _____

	S	U	NP	Comments

d. Provided activity at time when patient was relaxed.

e. Engaged patient in meaningful conversation; encouraged participation of family members and visitors.

6. Helped patient to a comfortable position.

7. Raised side rails (as appropriate) and lowered and locked bed into lowest position.

8. Appropriately disposed of supplies and equipment. Removed and disposed of gloves, and performed hand hygiene.

9. Placed nurse call system in an accessible location within patient's reach.

EVALUATION

1. Observed character of respirations, body position, facial expression, tone of voice, mood, mannerisms, and verbalization of discomfort.

2. Asked patient to describe character of pain using pain rating scale to rate comfort level; compare with patient's goal.

3. Observed patient perform pain-control measures.

4. Used Teach-Back. Revised instruction or developed plan for revised patient/family caregiver learning if patient or family caregiver was not able to teach back correctly.

DOCUMENTATION

1. Documented patient's assessment findings before and after procedure, nonpharmacological technique(s) used, preparation and instruction given to patient, patient's response to procedure or technique, change in pain character and intensity, and further comfort needs required. Incorporated pain-relief technique into nursing care plan.

2. Documented evaluation of patient and family caregiver learning.

HAND-OFF REPORTING

1. Reported any unusual responses to techniques to nurse in charge or health care provider.

2. Reported inadequate pain relief, a reduction in patient function, and side effects or adverse effects from pain interventions to health care provider.

3. Reported patient's response to nonpharmacological interventions to the staff at change of shift and in care planning meetings.

Student _____ Date _____

Instructor _____ Date _____

PERFORMANCE CHECKLIST SKILL 16.3 **PHARMACOLOGICAL PAIN MANAGEMENT**

	S	U	NP	Comments

ASSESSMENT

1. Reviewed electronic health record (EHR) for medical and medication history, including history of allergies. ___ ___ ___ _____

2. Assessed patient's risks for receiving analgesics. ___ ___ ___ _____

3. Identified patient using two identifiers. ___ ___ ___ _____

4. Assessed patient's/family caregiver's health literacy. ___ ___ ___ _____

5. Assessed patient's knowledge, prior experience with pharmacological pain management, and feelings about procedure. ___ ___ ___ _____

6. Performed hand hygiene and completed a thorough pain assessment, including patient's previous response to ordered analgesic. ___ ___ ___ _____

7. For patients going into surgery or undergoing procedure requiring sedation, completed an assessment of patient's risk for obstructive sleep apnea (OSA) by using the STOP- Bang screening tool. ___ ___ ___ _____

8. Assessed the anticipated time of onset, time to peak effect, duration of action, and side effects of analgesic to be administered (reviewed pharmacology reference). ___ ___ ___ _____

9. Considered the type of activities patient was scheduled to undergo. ___ ___ ___ _____

10. Checked last time medication was administered (including dose and route) and degree of relief experienced. Verified the appropriateness of the dose and dosing interval for the current situation. Consulted with health care provider about an around-the-clock (ATC) dose. ___ ___ ___ _____

11. Assessed patient's respiratory rate and sedation level (as appropriate) by using the Pasero Opioid Sedation Scale (POSS). ___ ___ ___ _____

12. Knew the comparative potencies of analgesics given by different routes. Referred to an equianalgesic chart or pharmacist. ___ ___ ___ _____

PLANNING

1. Determined expected outcomes following completion of procedure. ___ ___ ___ _____

	S	U	NP	Comments

2. Talked with patient and determined an individualized pain-management strategy with a pain-relief goal that was agreeable to the patient. Used the wipe-off whiteboard in patient's room to write the plan for administration times. Identified strategies.   ___ ___ ___ _____

3. Provided privacy by closing room door or bedside curtain.   ___ ___ ___ _____

4. Set up equipment at bedside.   ___ ___ ___ _____

5. Positioned and draped patient if needed.   ___ ___ ___ _____

6. Explained medication to be administered, anticipated effects, and what patient should report.   ___ ___ ___ _____

7. Provided educational information to patient and family caregiver. If the patient needed opioid therapy at home, education and a prescription for naloxone and training in the administration of naloxone were given.   ___ ___ ___ _____

IMPLEMENTATION

1. Checked accuracy and completeness of each medication administration record (MAR) or computer printout with health care provider's written medication order. Checked patient's name, medication name and dosage, route of administration, and frequency or time of administration. Reprinted any portion of MAR that was difficult to read.   ___ ___ ___ _____

2. Performed hand hygiene. Prepared selected analgesic, following the "seven rights" for medication administration.   ___ ___ ___ _____

3. Rechecked patient's identity at bedside using two identifiers according to agency policy. Compared identifiers with information on the patient's MAR or electronic health record (EHR).   ___ ___ ___ _____

4. At the bedside, compared MAR or computer printout with the name of the medication on the medication label and patient name (armband). Rechecked and asked if patient had allergies.   ___ ___ ___ _____

5. Reassessed patient's pain/sedation level and respiratory status before administering the medication.   ___ ___ ___ _____

6. Performed hand hygiene and applied gloves (if needed based on route of medication).   ___ ___ ___ _____

7. Prepared analgesic and then administered following guidelines: ___ ___ ___ _____

   a. Administered as soon as pain occurred, or ATC as ordered.   ___ ___ ___ _____

   b. Administered prn or one-time dose 30 to 60 minutes before pain-producing procedures or activities.   ___ ___ ___ _____

	S	U	NP	Comments

8. Provided basic and nonpharmacological comfort measures in addition to analgesics.

9. Administered nursing care measures during times of peak effects of analgesics. Explained the plan for care after giving medication. Considered duration of action of analgesics when planning activities.

10. Helped patient to a comfortable position.

11. Raised side rails (as appropriate) and lowered and locked bed into lowest position.

12. Removed and disposed of gloves (if used) and performed hand hygiene.

13. Placed nurse call system in an accessible location within patient's reach.

EVALUATION

1. Had patient self-report PQRSTU aspects of pain and pain intensity using appropriate pain scales both at rest and with activity. Used nonverbal scale as needed.

2. Monitored for adverse medication effect and performed vital sign (VS) measurement, noted signs of opioid-induced sedation and respiratory depression (OSRD).

3. Observed patient's position; mobility; relaxation; and ability to rest, sleep, eat, and participate in usual activities.

4. When opioids were used, evaluated for opioid-induced constipation (OIC).

5. Used Teach-Back. Revised instruction or developed a plan for revised patient/family caregiver teaching if patient or family caregiver was not able to teach back correctly.

DOCUMENTATION

1. Documented patient's pain rating (15 to 30 minutes before and after intravenous (IV) medication and 30 to 60 minutes before and after oral medication), other self-report descriptions, behavioral and physiological response to analgesic, and additional comfort measures given. Incorporated pain-relief techniques in nursing care plan.

2. Documented medication, indication for the medication, dose, route, and time given in MAR or computer printout.

3. Documented evaluation of patient and family caregiver learning.

HAND-OFF REPORTING

1. Reported unsuccessful or untoward patient response to analgesics to health care provider.

Student _____ Date _____

Instructor _____ Date _____

PERFORMANCE CHECKLIST SKILL 16.4   **PATIENT-CONTROLLED ANALGESIA**

	S	U	NP	Comments

ASSESSMENT

1. Reviewed electronic health record (EHR) to assess patient's medical and medication history, including drug allergies.

2. Reviewed medication information in drug reference manual or consulted with pharmacist if uncertain about any patient-controlled analgesia (PCA) medications to be administered.

3. Identified patient using two identifiers and compared identifiers with information on patient's medication administration record (MAR) or EHR.

4. Assessed patient's/family caregiver's health literacy.

5. Assessed patient's knowledge, prior experience with previous pain-management strategies, including PCA, and feelings about procedure.

6. Assessed patient's ability to manipulate PCA control and cognitive status for ability to understand purpose of PCA and how to use control device.

7. Assessed environment for factors that could contribute to pain.

8. Assessed for presence of known, untreated, or unknown obstructive sleep apnea syndrome (OSAS). Used the STOP-Bang questionnaire to assess the patient for OSAS.

9. Performed hand hygiene. Applied clean gloves. Assessed patency of IV access and surrounding tissue for inflammation or swelling. Removed and disposed of gloves; performed hand hygiene.

PLANNING

1. Determined expected outcomes following completion of procedure.

2. Talked with patient, and determine a mutual pain-relief goal.

3. Provided privacy by closing room door or bedside curtains.

4. Organized equipment at bedside.

	S	U	NP	Comments

5. Positioned and draped patient comfortably if needed. ___ ___ ___ _____

6. Provided patient and family caregiver with individually tailored education, including information on procedure for administration and treatment options for management of postoperative pain with PCA. If the patient would need opioid therapy at home, provided education and a prescription for naloxone and training in the administration of naloxone. ___ ___ ___ _____

IMPLEMENTATION

1. Checked accuracy and completeness of each MAR or computer printout with health care provider's written medication order. Checked patient's name, medication name and dosage, route of administration, lockout period, and frequency of medication (demand, continuous, or both). Reprinted any portion of MAR that was difficult to read. ___ ___ ___ _____

2. Performed hand hygiene. Followed the "seven rights" for medication administration. Obtained PCA analgesic in module prepared by pharmacy. Checked label of medication two times: when removed from storage and when preparing for assembly. ___ ___ ___ _____

3. Rechecked patient's identity at bedside, using at least two identifiers. Compared identifiers with information on patient's MAR or EHR. ___ ___ ___ _____

4. At bedside, compared MAR or computer printout with name of medication on drug cartridge. Had second registered nurse (RN) confirm health care provider's order and correct setup of PCA independently, not just looking at existing setup. ___ ___ ___ _____

5. Before initiating analgesia: ___ ___ ___ _____

   a. Explained again the purpose of PCA and demonstrated function of PCA to patient and family caregiver. Gave verbal and written instruction warning against anyone other than the patient pressing the PCA button. ___ ___ ___ _____

   b. Explained type of medication and method of delivery. ___ ___ ___ _____

   c. If background basal rate was used, explained that device would safely administer continuous medication, but a self-initiated on-demand small, frequent amount of medication would be administered for unrelieved pain when patient pushed the PCA button. ___ ___ ___ _____

   d. Explained that self-dosing was desirable as it aids patient in repositioning, walking, and coughing or deep breathing. ___ ___ ___ _____

e. Explained that device was programmed to deliver ordered type and dose of pain medication, lockout interval, and 1- to -4-hour dosage limits. Explained how lockout time prevented overdose.

    ___ ___ ___ _____

f. Demonstrated to patient how to push medication demand button. Instructed family caregiver to not push PCA button to give medication.

    ___ ___ ___ _____

g. Instructed patient to notify nurse for possible side effects: problems gaining pain relief, changes in severity or location of pain, alarm sounding, or questions.

    ___ ___ ___ _____

6. Applied clean gloves. Checked infuser and patient-control module for accurate labeling or evidence of leaking.

    ___ ___ ___ _____

7. Positioned patient to be sure that venipuncture or central-line site was accessible.

    ___ ___ ___ _____

8. Inserted drug cartridge into infusion device and primed tubing.

    ___ ___ ___ _____

9. Attached needleless adapter to tubing adapter of patient-controlled module.

    ___ ___ ___ _____

10. Wiped injection port of maintenance IV line vigorously with antiseptic swab for 15 seconds and allowed to dry.

    ___ ___ ___ _____

11. Inserted needleless adapter into injection port nearest patient (at Y-site of peripheral IV, port on saline lock or port on central line). Ensured no chance to use PCA tubing for administering IV push with another drug.

    ___ ___ ___ _____

12. Secured connection and anchored PCA tubing onto patient's arm with tape. Labeled PCA tubing.

    ___ ___ ___ _____

13. Programed computerized PCA pump as ordered to deliver prescribed medication dose and lockout interval. Had second nurse check setting. (NOTE: Rechecked with oncoming RN during shift hand-off to ensure line reconciliation.)

    ___ ___ ___ _____

14. Administered loading dose of analgesia as prescribed. Manually gave one-time dose or turned on pump and programmed dose into pump.

    ___ ___ ___ _____

15. Removed and discarded gloves and used supplies in appropriate containers. Disposed of empty cassette or syringe in compliance with institutional policy. Performed hand hygiene.

    ___ ___ ___ _____

16. If experiencing pain, had patient demonstrate use of PCA system; if not, had patient repeat instructions given earlier.

    ___ ___ ___ _____

	S	U	NP	Comments

17. Ensured that IV access site was protected, and rechecked infusion rate before leaving patient.   ___ ___ ___ _____

18. Assisted patient into comfortable position.   ___ ___ ___ _____

19. Raised side rails (as appropriate) and lowered and locked bed into lowest position.   ___ ___ ___ _____

20. Placed nurse call system in an accessible location within patient's reach.   ___ ___ ___ _____

21. To discontinue PCA:

   a. Identified patient using at lest two identifiers. Checked health care provider order for discontinuation. Obtained necessary PCA information from pump for documentation; note date, time, amount infused, and amount of drug wasted and reason for wastage.   ___ ___ ___ _____

   b. Performed hand hygiene and applied clean gloves. Turned off pump. Disconnected PCA tubing from primary IV line but maintained IV access.   ___ ___ ___ _____

   c. Disposed of empty cartridge, tubing, and soiled supplies according to agency policy. Removed and disposed of gloves and performed hand hygiene.   ___ ___ ___ _____

   d. Helped patient to a comfortable position.   ___ ___ ___ _____

   e. Raised side rails (as appropriate) and lowered and locked bed into lowest position.   ___ ___ ___ _____

   f. Placed nurse call system in an accessible location within patient's reach.   ___ ___ ___ _____

EVALUATION

1. Asked patient if pain was relieved. Then used pain rating scale to evaluate patient's pain intensity following ambulation, treatments, and procedures according to agency policy.   ___ ___ ___ _____

2. Observed patient for nausea or pruritus.   ___ ___ ___ _____

3. Monitored patient's level of sedation using Pasero Opioid Sedation Scale (POSS) with VS, pulse oximerty, and capnography. Monitored every 1 to 2 hours for first 12 hours for the 24-hour period after surgery. Monitored more often at start, during first 24 hours, and at night.   ___ ___ ___ _____

4. Had patient demonstrate dose delivery.   ___ ___ ___ _____

5. According to agency policy, evaluated number of attempts (number of times patient pushed button), delivery of demand doses (number of times drug actually given and total amount of medication delivered in particular time frame), and basal dose if ordered.   ___ ___ ___ _____

	S	U	NP	Comments

6. Observed patient initiate self-care.

7. Used Teach-Back. Revised instruction or developed a plan for patient/family caregiver teaching if patient or family caregiver was not able to teach back correctly.

DOCUMENTATION

1. Recorded on MAR appropriate drug, concentration, dose (basal and demand), time started, lockout time, and amount of solution infused and remaining per agency policy.

2. Documented assessment of patient's response to analgesic. Also included VS, oximetry and capnography results, sedation status, and status of vascular access device.

3. Calculated and documented infused dose: added demand and continuous doses together.

4. Documented evaluation of patient learning.

HAND-OFF REPORTING

1. Hand-off report included information regarding VS, pulse oximetry and capnography, pain-assessment scores, STOP-Bang score for OSAS if done, POSS sedation scores, level of consciousness, anxiety level, and activity level.

2. During a hand-off report, the oncoming and outgoing nurse inspected and agreed with PCA pump programming as a means of medication reconciliation.

3. Reported signs of oversedation to health care provider immediately.

244

Student _____ Date _____

Instructor _____ Date _____

PERFORMANCE CHECKLIST SKILL 16.5 **EPIDURAL ANALGESIA**

	S	U	NP	Comments

ASSESSMENT

1. Identified patient using at least two identifiers. Compared identifiers with information on patient's medical administration record (MAR) or electronic health record (EHR). ___ ___ ___ _____

2. Reviewed EHR to assess patient's medical and medication history, including drug allergies. ___ ___ ___ _____

3. Checked EHR to see if patient was receiving anticoagulants. NOTE: This was checked by a health care provider before catheter insertion: ___ ___ ___ _____

   a. Obtained dosage, route, date, and time of last anticoagulant administration. ___ ___ ___ _____

   b. Reviewed coagulation lab results. ___ ___ ___ _____

   c. Consulted with provider regarding how long to withhold anticoagulants before planned insertion. ___ ___ ___ _____

4. Assessed Patient's/family caregiver's health literacy. ___ ___ ___ _____

5. Assessed if patient routinely took herbal medications; documented complete list. ___ ___ ___ _____

6. Assessed patient for presence of any allergies or history of reactions to opioids or anesthetics. Had patient describe allergic response. ___ ___ ___ _____

7. Performed hand hygiene and completed a pain assessment. ___ ___ ___ _____

8. Assessed patient's sedation level by using Pasero Opioid Sedation Scale (POSS), assessed level of wakefulness or alertness, ability to follow commands, and level of drowsiness/responsiveness. ___ ___ ___ _____

9. Assessed rate, pattern, and depth of respirations; pulse oximetry, or capnography; blood pressure; and temperature. ___ ___ ___ _____

10. Assessed initial motor and sensory function of lower extremities. Tested sensation to touch in lower extremities. Had patient flex both feet and knees and raise each leg off bed. Paid special attention to patients with preexisting sensory or motor abnormalities. ___ ___ ___ _____

	S	U	NP	Comments

11. Applied clean gloves. Inspected epidural catheter insertion site for redness, warmth, tenderness, swelling, and drainage. Applied a sterile, clean, and dry semipermeable transparent dressing over insertion site in a way that was intact and secure (as needed). ____ ____ ____ _____

12. Followed epidural catheter tubing and verified that catheter was secured to patient's skin from back, side, or front. ____ ____ ____ _____

13. Checked condition of any peripheral IV site and patency of IV tubing. ____ ____ ____ _____

14. Removed and disposed of gloves. Performed hand hygiene. ____ ____ ____ _____

15. Assessed patient's knowledge, prior experience with epidural analgesia, and feelings about procedure. ____ ____ ____ _____

PLANNING

1. Determined expected outcomes following completion of procedure. ____ ____ ____ _____

2. Talked with patient and determined a mutual pain-relief goal. ____ ____ ____ _____

3. Placed patients receiving epidural analgesia close to nurses' station. ____ ____ ____ _____

4. Provided privacy by closing room door or bedside curtains. ____ ____ ____ _____

5. Set up equipment. ____ ____ ____ _____

6. Educated patient and family caregiver with individually tailored education: purpose of epidural and treatment options such as PCEA. If needing opioid therapy at home, provided education and a prescription for naloxone and training in the administration of naloxone. ____ ____ ____ _____

IMPLEMENTATION

1. Checked accuracy and completeness of each MAR or computer printout with health care provider's written medication order. Checked patient's name, medication name and dosage, route of administration, and frequency or time of administration. Reprinted any portion of MAR that was difficult to read. ____ ____ ____ _____

2. Performed hand hygiene and followed the "seven rights" for medication administration. NOTE: Pharmacy prepared medication for pump. Checked label of medication carefully with MAR or computer printout two times. ____ ____ ____ _____

246

3. Rechecked patient's identity at bedside using at least two identifiers according to agency policy if preparing infusion. Compared identifiers with information on patient's MAR or EHR.

    ____　____　____　_____

4. At the bedside, compared MAR or computer printout with name of medication on drug cassette/container. Performed an independent double check with another qualified RN, pharmacist, or physician prior to administration (including when syringe/medication container, rate, and/or concentration was changed).

    ____　____　____　_____

5. Applied clean gloves. Maintained infusion and gave boluses after anesthesia provider started or administered first dose.

    ____　____　____　_____

  a. Continuous epidural infusion (CEI):

    (1) Infusion pump: Inserted cassette/container of diluted preservative-free medication into pump. Then connected pump to NRFit infusion tubing and primed tubing.

      ____　____　____　_____

    (2) Inserted NRFit tubing into infusion pump and attached distal end of tubing to antibacterial filter; then wiped off hub of epidural catheter thoroughly with antiseptic swab, then dried. Used aseptic technique, connected end of NRFit tubing to hub of catheter.

      ____　____　____　_____

    (3) Checked infusion pump for proper calibration, setting, and operation.

      ____　____　____　_____

    (4) Taped tubing and hub connections. Epidural infusion system between pump and patient was considered closed, with no injection or Y-ports. Epidural infusions were labeled "For Epidural Use Only." Started infusion.

      ____　____　____　_____

  b. Bolus dose via infusion pump:

    (1) While helping anesthesia provider, performed Steps 5a (1) to (4) above. Adjusted infusion pump setting for preset limit for maximum bolus size and interval. Initiated pump to deliver ordered bolus.

      ____　____　____　_____

  c. PCEA bolus dose on demand:

    (1) While helping anesthesia provider, performed Steps 5a (1) to (4) above. Set pump for bolus size and lockout time (as ordered).

      ____　____　____　_____

	S	U	NP	Comments

(2) Had patient initiate demand dose as needed to relieve pain.

6. Assessed and monitored patients after initiating or restarting an epidural infusion for at least the first 24 hours; assessed every 1 to 2 hours until stable, then every 4 hours or with each home visit. Explained procedure to patient and instructed patient on signs or problems to report to nurse.

7. Helped patient to a comfortable position.

8. Raised side rails (as appropriate) and lowered and locked bed into lowest position.

9. Disposed of supplies and equipment.

10. Removed and disposed of gloves. Performed hand hygiene.

11. Placed nurse call system in an accessible location within patient's reach.

12. Postanalgesia:

    a. Kept a peripheral IV line patent for 24 hours after epidural analgesia ended.

    b. Before removal of epidural catheter, consulted with provider regarding how long to withhold therapeutic anticoagulants before the planned procedure. Checked agency policy for removal of epidural catheter and extra precautions if patient was receiving anticoagulation therapy.

EVALUATION

1. Evaluated patient's pain character and measured severity using a pain rating scale of 0 to 10. Compared with patient's desired goal.

2. Evaluated blood pressure and heart rate; respiratory rate, rhythm, depth, and pattern; pulse oximetry or capnography; and sedation level based on patient's clinical condition. Measured more frequently in first 12 hours of infusions, after bolus infusions or changes of infusion rate, and in periods of cardiovascular or respiratory instability.

3. Evaluated catheter insertion site every 2 to 4 hours for redness, warmth, tenderness, swelling, or drainage. Noted character of drainage.

4. Inspected epidural site for disruption or displacement of catheter.

248

	S	U	NP	Comments

5. Observed for pruritus, especially of face, head, neck, and torso. Informed patient that this was a side effect but was often not an allergic response. ___ ___ ___ _____

6. Observed for nausea and vomiting and presence of headache. Noted any nonverbal signs of headache. Monitored for patient sensing a metallic taste in mouth. ___ ___ ___ _____

7. Monitored intake and output. Evaluated for bladder distention and urinary frequency or urgency. Consulted with health care provider for possible need for intermittent catheterization. ___ ___ ___ _____

8. Evaluated for motor weakness or numbness and tingling of lower extremities (paresthesias). ___ ___ ___ _____

9. Used Teach-Back. Revised instruction or developed plan for revised patient/family caregiver teaching if patient or family caregiver was not able to teach back correctly. ___ ___ ___ _____

DOCUMENTATION

1. Documented drug name, dose, method of infusion (bolus, demand, or continuous), and time given (if bolus) or time begun and ended (if continuous or demand infusion) on appropriate MAR. Specified concentration and diluent. ___ ___ ___ _____

2. With continuous or demand infusion, obtained and documented pump readout hourly for first 24 hours after infusion began and then every 4 hours. ___ ___ ___ _____

3. Documented regular periodic assessments of patient's status including VS, SpO2 or end-tidal carbon dioxide, intake and output (I&O), sedation level, pain character and severity, neurological status, appearance of epidural site, presence or absence of side effects or adverse reactions to medication, and presence or absence of complications. ___ ___ ___ _____

4. Documented evaluation of patient and family caregiver learning. ___ ___ ___ _____

HAND-OFF REPORTING

1. Reported the patient's pain-management plan, changes in infusion, patient, responses, and most recent doses to aid in reducing medication errors. ___ ___ ___ _____

2. The oncoming and outgoing RNs inspected and agreed with infusion pump programming/settings as a means of medication reconciliation. ___ ___ ___ _____

3. Reported detailed information regarding VS, pulse oximetry and capnography, pain-assessment, STOP-Bang score for obstructive sleep apnea syndrome (OSAS) if appropriate, POSS sedation scores, level of consciousness, anxiety level, and activity level. ___ ___ ___ _____

Student _____ Date _____

Instructor _____ Date _____

PERFORMANCE CHECKLIST SKILL 16.6   **LOCAL ANESTHETIC INFUSION PUMP FOR ANALGESIA**

	S	U	NP	Comments

ASSESSMENT

1. Identified patient using two identifiers. Compared identifiers with information on patient's medication administration record (MAR) or electronic health record (EHR).

2. Reviewed surgeon's operative report for position of catheter.

3. Assessed patient's/family caregiver's health literacy.

4. Assessed patient's knowledge, prior experience with local infusion pump for analgesia, and feelings about procedure.

5. Performed hand hygiene, applied clean gloves, and assessed surgical dressing and site of catheter insertion. Ensured dressing was dry and intact.

6. Ensured catheter tubing was correctly labeled. Assessed catheter connection, ensuring it was secure. If catheter became detached, did not reattach or reinsert; instead, notified surgeon immediately.

7. Assessed for presence of blood backing up in tubing. If blood was present, stopped infusion and notified health care provider. Removed and disposed of gloves and performed hand hygiene.

8. Performed a complete pain assessment.

9. Read medication label on device and compared with MAR or health care provider's orders.

10. Determined level of activity that patient could perform per health care provider's orders.

11. Confirmed patient's allergies. Assessed for early signs of local anesthetic toxicity: tinnitus, blurred vision, dizziness, tongue paresthesias, and circumoral numbness.

PLANNING

1. Determined expected outcomes following completion of procedure.

250

	S	U	NP	Comments

2. Talked with patient and determined a mutual pain relief goal.

3. Provided privacy by closing door or bedside curtains. Set up equipment.

4. Positioned and draped patient as needed so that catheter insertion site was visible.

5. Instructed patients on purpose and pain relief function of infusion pump. In cases of bolus delivery, instructed patient on how and when to use. Instructed family members to not deliver a bolus to patient. Let patients know they might still require a safe oral analgesic.

IMPLEMENTATION

1. Performed hand hygiene.

2. While patient was still an inpatient, routinely checked:
   - Pump functioning
   - Catheter insertion site in wound
   - Effects of the nerve block
   - Patient's self-report of pain control
   - Overall skin condition
   - Muscle strength

3. Used caution when repositioning or ambulating patient. Did not pull on catheter.

4. Prepared patient for discharge: Depending on type of pump, connected the catheter to a smaller pump for use at home. Referenced manufacturer's directions.

5. Taught the patient or family caregiver what to observe and how to remove catheter at home (may also be done by home health nurse). Provided educational materials. Instructions for removal:

   a. Explained how to perform hand hygiene and apply clean gloves.

   b. Had patient assume relaxed position in bed or chair with lower extremity in normal alignment.

   c. Applied clean gloves. Had patient or family caregiver gently lift adhesive dressing covering catheter insertion site and removed any remaining tape.

   d. Directed the patient or family caregiver to place 4 × 4–inch gauze over site, grasp catheter as close as possible to where it enters skin, and gently pull it out with steady motion.

		S	U	NP	Comments

e. Had patient or family caregiver look for mark on end of catheter tip and hold new sterile gauze using pressure over the site for at least 2 minutes. ___ ___ ___ _____

f. Washed skin to remove any surgical soap or adhesive near the site. Applied clean adhesive bandage. ___ ___ ___ _____

g. Placed catheter in plastic bag using Standard Precautions. Reminded patient to bring to health care provider's office at first follow-up visit. Removed and disposed of gloves; performed hand hygiene. ___ ___ ___ _____

h. Explained to patient that any remaining numbness should go away within 24 hours after catheter removal. ___ ___ ___ _____

6. Reminded patient or family caregiver of follow-up appointment with surgeon. ___ ___ ___ _____

7. Discharged per health care provider order and agency policy. ___ ___ ___ _____

EVALUATION

1. Inpatient setting:

   a. Asked patient to describe character of pain and rate severity using a pain scale both at rest and with activity. ___ ___ ___ _____

   b. Observed for signs of adverse drug reaction. ___ ___ ___ _____

   c. Observe patient's position, mobility and strength, relaxation, participation in ADLs, and any nonverbal behaviors. ___ ___ ___ _____

   d. Inspected condition of skin and surgical dressing. ___ ___ ___ _____

2. During follow-up visit, inspected catheter exit site. ___ ___ ___ _____

3. Used Teach-Back. Revised instruction or developed a plan for revised patient/family caregiver teaching if patient or family caregiver was not able to teach back correctly. ___ ___ ___ _____

DOCUMENTATION

1. Documented drug, concentration, dose administered, type of demand feature, additional analgesics needed to control pain, and any side effects or adverse reactions to epidural opioid or local anesthetic.

	S	U	NP	Comments

2. Documented location of catheter, patient's pain character and rating, condition of insertion site and dressing, response to anesthetic, additional comfort measures, and date of catheter removed (if still inpatient). ___ ___ ___ _____

3. Documented evaluation of patient and family caregiver learning. ___ ___ ___ _____

HAND-OFF REPORTING

1. Reported damp dressing or displaced catheter to surgeon. ___ ___ ___ _____

2. Reported to oncoming nurse the location of catheter, type of pump, type of medication, concentration, dose and time local analgesia initiated, patient bolus administration history, patient response, and any side effects or adverse reactions to local anesthetic. ___ ___ ___ _____

3. Reported patient's pain-management plan, including additional comfort measures. ___ ___ ___ _____

PERFORMANCE CHECKLIST SKILL 16.7   **MOIST AND DRY HEAT APPLICATIONS**

	S	U	NP	Comments

ASSESSMENT

1. Identified patient using two identifiers.

2. Referred to health care provider's order for type of heat application, location and duration of application, and desired temperature. Checked agency policies regarding temperature.

3. Referred to patient's electronic health record (EHR) for history of unstable cardiac conditions; experienced side effect of cardiac, antihypertensive, or vasoactive medications; active bleeding; receiving nitroglycerin or other therapeutic medicinal skin patch; acute inflammatory reactions; recent (<72 hours) musculoskeletal injury; vascular disease; paralysis; peripheral neuropathy; multiple sclerosis; with patient sensitive to heat; and skin conditions such as eczema.

4. Reviewed EHR for history of diabetes mellitus with neuropathy and for history of and open skin lesions; especially active shingles and/or postherpetic neuralgia.

5. Assessed patient's/family caregiver's health literacy.

6. Assessed patient's knowledge, prior experience with moist or dry heat application, and feelings about procedure.

7. Performed hand hygiene, applied gloves, and assessed condition of skin around area to be treated. Performed neurovascular assessments for sensitivity to temperature and pain by measuring light touch, pinprick, and temperature sensation.

8. When treating a wound (see implementation Step 2c), assessed it for size, color, drainage type and volume, and odor. Removed and discarded gloves; performed hand hygiene.

9. Assessed patient's level of consciousness and responsiveness.

10. Asked patient to describe pain character and intensity on pain scale of 0 to 10.

11. Assessed patient's blood pressure and pulse.

12. Assessed patient's mobility: ROM, ability to align extremity for aquathermia pad application and ability to position self in sitz bath and sit up from bath.

	S	U	NP	Comments

13. Checked electrical plugs and cords of aquathermia pad for obvious fraying or cracking. ___ ___ ___ _____

PLANNING

1. Determined expected outcomes following completion of procedure. ___ ___ ___ _____

2. Talked with patient and determined a mutual pain-relief goal. ___ ___ ___ _____

3. Provided privacy by closing room door or bedside curtain. ___ ___ ___ _____

4. Prepared and organized equipment at bedside. ___ ___ ___ _____

5. Positioned patient in bed, keeping affected body part in proper alignment. Exposed body part to be covered with heat application and drape patient with bath blanket or towel as needed. ___ ___ ___ _____

6. Placed waterproof pad under patient (Exception: did not do this with sitz bath or commercial heat pad). ___ ___ ___ _____

7. Explained steps of procedure and purpose to patient. Described sensation that patient will feel, such as warmth and wetness. Explained precautions to prevent burning. ___ ___ ___ _____

8. Provided patient and family caregiver education materials regarding heat therapy. ___ ___ ___ _____

IMPLEMENTATION

1. Performed hand hygiene and applied clean gloves. ___ ___ ___ _____

2. Applied moist sterile compress: ___ ___ ___ _____

   a. Heated prescribed solution to desired temperature by immersing closed bottle of solution in basin of warm water. Did not use a microwave to warm solution. ___ ___ ___ _____

   b. Prepared aquathermia pad if it was to be placed over compress. ___ ___ ___ _____

   c. Removed any existing dressing covering wound. Inspected condition of wound and surrounding skin. Removed and placed gloves and soiled dressing in biohazard bag and disposed per agency policy. ___ ___ ___ _____

   d. Performed hand hygiene. ___ ___ ___ _____

   e. Moistened compress. ___ ___ ___ _____

     (1) Poured warmed solution into container. If sterile asepsis was required, used sterile container. ___ ___ ___ _____

     (2) Opened gauze. If applying sterile technique, opened and laid on sterile wrapper. Then immersed sterile gauze into sterile solution. ___ ___ ___ _____

	S	U	NP	Comments

(3) If sterile technique was not required, immersed gauze into container of solution using clean aseptic technique.

(4) If using commercially prepared compress, followed manufacturer instructions for warming.

f. Applied sterile gloves if compress was sterile; otherwise applied clean gloves.

g. Picked up one layer of immersed gauze, wrung out any excess solution, and applied it lightly to wound; avoided unaffected skin. Option: Applied commercial compress or heat pack over wound only; used only with clean wounds.

h. After a few seconds, lifted edge of gauze to assess for skin redness or other injuries.

i. If patient tolerated compress, packed gauze snugly against wound. Ensured covering of all wound surfaces with warm compress.

j. Covered moist compress with dry sterile dressing and bath towel. If necessary, pinned or tied in place. Removed and disposed of gloves and performed hand hygiene.

k. Option: Applied aquathermia, commercial heat pack, or waterproof heating pad over towel. Kept it in place for desired duration of application.

l. Left compress in place for 15 to 20 minutes or less (per order or agency policy), and changed warm compress using sterile technique every 5 to 10 minutes (observing condition of skin) or as ordered during duration of therapy.

m. After prescribed time, performed hand hygiene and applied clean gloves. Removed pad, towel, and compress. Evaluated wound and condition of skin and replaced dry sterile dressing (using sterile gloves) as ordered.

3. Sitz bath or warm soak:

a. Removed any existing dressing covering wound. Inspected condition of wound and surrounding skin. Paid particular attention to suture line.

b. Removed and disposed of gloves and dressings in proper receptacle and performed hand hygiene.

c. When exudate or drainage was present, applied a new pair of clean gloves and cleaned intact skin around open area with clean cloth and soap and water. Sterile gloves and gauze used as needed to clean open wound (checked agency policy). Removed and disposed of gloves and performed hand hygiene.

	S	U	NP	Comments

d. Fill sitz bath or bathtub in bathroom with warmed solution. Checked temperature (checked agency policy). Option: If using bag of normal saline, warmed per agency policy.

e. Assisted patient to bathroom to immerse body part in sitz bath, bathtub, or basin. Covered patient with bath blanket or towel once position was achieved.

f. Assessed heart rate. Made sure that patient did not feel light-headed or dizzy and that nurse call system was within reach. Checked every 5 minutes for patient tolerance.

g. Applied clean gloves. After 15 to 20 minutes, removed patient from soak or bath; dried body parts thoroughly.

h. Assisted patient to preferred comfortable position.

i. Drained solution from basin or tub. Cleaned and placed in proper storage area according to agency policy. Disposed of soiled linen. Removed and discarded gloves; performed hand hygiene.

4. Aquathermia heating pad for dry application:

a. Covered or wrapped area to be treated with single layer of bath towel or enclose pad with pillowcase.

b. Placed pad over affected area and secured with tape, tie, or gauze as needed.

c. Turned on aquathermia unit and checked temperature setting. NOTE: Agency's bioengineering department set temperature of unit. Removed gloves and performed hand hygiene.

d. Monitored condition of skin over site every 5 minutes, and asked patient about sensation of burning.

e. After no more than 20 minutes (or time ordered by health care provider), performed hand hygiene, applied clean gloves, and removed pad and store.

5. Applied commercially prepared heat pack:

a. Broke pouch inside larger pack (followed manufacturer guidelines). Applied to affected area.

b. Monitored condition of skin over site every 5 minutes, observed underlying skin for injury, and asked patient about any sensation of burning. Removed gloves and performed hand hygiene.

S   U   NP   Comments

   c. After no more than 20 minutes (or time ordered by health care provider), performed hand hygiene, applied new pair of clean gloves, and removed pad and stored.

  6. Removed and disposed of any remaining equipment and gloves; performed hand hygiene.

  7. Helped patient return to preferred comfortable position.

  8. Raised side rails (as appropriate) and lowered and locked bed into lowest position.

  9. Placed nurse call system in an accessible location within patient's reach.

EVALUATION

1. Inspected condition of body part or wound; observed skin integrity, color, and temperature, and noted any dryness, edema, blistering, drainage or sensitivity to touch. In case of sitz bath, inspected perineal area.

2. Obtained blood pressure and pulse; compared with baseline.

3. Asked patient to describe character and severity of pain using a pain scale. Asked about any sensation of burning following treatment.

4. Evaluated ROM of affected body part.

5. Used Teach-Back. Revised instruction or developed a plan for revised patient/family caregiver learning if patient or family caregiver was not able to teach back correctly.

DOCUMENTATION

1. Documented type of application (compress, pad, or pack); location and duration of application; condition of body part, wound, or skin before and after treatment; and patient's response to therapy.

2. Documented evaluation of patient and family caregiver learning.

HAND-OFF REPORTING

1. During hand-off to next shift, reported the location and type of heat therapy, medication used (if ordered), duration and time of therapy, skin assessment, VS, pain assessment before and after therapy, patient response to therapy, and any adverse reactions.

2. Reported patient's heat therapy management plan to oncoming nurse.

258

Student _____ Date _____

Instructor _____ Date _____

PERFORMANCE CHECKLIST SKILL 16.8 **COLD APPLICATION**

	S	U	NP	Comments

ASSESSMENT

1. Identified patient using two identifiers. ___ ___ ___ _____

2. Referred to health care provider's order for type, location, and duration of application. ___ ___ ___ _____

3. Considered time elapsed since injury occurred. If an acute injury, followed the principles Protect, Rest, Ice, Compress, and Elevate. ___ ___ ___ _____

4. Reviewed electronic health record (EHR) for any contraindications or precautionary conditions. ___ ___ ___ _____

5. Assessed patient's/family caregiver's health literacy. ___ ___ ___ _____

6. Performed hand hygiene and applied clean gloves. Inspected condition of injured or affected part. Gently palpated area for edema (applied clean gloves if there was a risk of exposure to body fluids). ___ ___ ___ _____

7. Performed neurovascular check and inspected surrounding skin for integrity, circulation (presence of pulses), color, temperature, and sensitivity to touch. Removed and disposed of gloves. Performed hand hygiene. ___ ___ ___ _____

8. Assessed patient's level of consciousness and responsiveness. ___ ___ ___ _____

9. Asked patient to describe character of pain and rate severity on a valid pain scale. Assessed range of motion (ROM) of affected extremity. ___ ___ ___ _____

10. Assessed patient's knowledge, prior experience with cold application, and feelings about procedure. ___ ___ ___ _____

PLANNING

1. Determined expected outcomes following completion of procedure. ___ ___ ___ _____

2. Talked with patient and determined a mutual pain-relief goal. ___ ___ ___ _____

3. Provided privacy by closing room door or curtain. ___ ___ ___ _____

	S	U	NP	Comments

4. Performed hand hygiene. Prepared equipment at bedside.

5. Positioned patient in bed, keeping affected body part in proper alignment. Exposed body part to be covered with cold application, and draped other body parts with bath blanket or towel as needed.

6. Explained procedure and precautions.

7. Provided patient and family caregiver with educational materials regarding how to use cold therapy safely at home.

IMPLEMENTATION

1. Performed hand hygiene and applied clean gloves.

2. Placed towel or absorbent pad under area to treat.

3. Applied cold compress:

   a. Placed ice and water in basin, and tested temperature on inner aspect of own arm.

   b. Submerged gauze into basin filled with cold solution; wrung out excess moisture.

   c. Applied compress to affected area, molding it gently over site.

   d. Removed, remoistened, and reapplied to maintain temperature as needed for a total time of 15 to 20 minutes.

4. Applied ice pack or bag:

   a. Filled bag with water, secured cap, and inverted.

   b. Emptied water and filled bag two-thirds full with small ice chips and water.

   c. Expressed excess air from bag, secured bag closure, and wiped bag dry.

   d. Squeezed or kneaded commercial ice pack according to manufacturer's directions.

   e. Wrapped pack or bag with single layer of towel, pillowcase, or stockinette. Applied over injury. Secured with tape as needed. Placed a barrier between cooling device and the patient's skin to avoid tissue injury.

5. Applied commercial gel pack:

   a. Removed from freezer.

   b. Wrapped pack with towel, pillowcase, or stockinette. Applied pack directly over injury.

260

	S	U	NP	Comments

c. Secured with gauze, cloth tape, or ties as needed. Kept in place 15 to 20 minutes. Repeated 4 to 8 times daily or as ordered. ___ ___ ___ _____

6. Applied electronically controlled cooling device: ___ ___ ___ _____

a. Prepared device following manufacturer's directions. For gravity-fed devices, manually filled with ice water. ___ ___ ___ _____

b. Made sure that all connections were intact and temperature, if adjustable, was set (following agency policy). ___ ___ ___ _____

c. Wrapped cool-water flow pad in single layer of towel or pillowcase. ___ ___ ___ _____

d. Wrapped cool pad around body part. ___ ___ ___ _____

e. Turned device on and checked correct temperature. (NOTE: Temperature often preset in health care settings [checked agency policy]). ___ ___ ___ _____

f. Secured with elastic wrap bandage, gauze roll, or ties. Kept in place 15 to 20 minutes. Repeated 4 to 8 times daily or as ordered. ___ ___ ___ _____

7. Removed and disposed of gloves in proper container. Performed hand hygiene. ___ ___ ___ _____

8. Checked condition of skin every 5 minutes for duration of application. ___ ___ ___ _____

a. If area was edematous, used extra caution during cold therapy and assessed site more often. ___ ___ ___ _____

b. Stopped treatment when patient complained of burning sensation or increased sensation of numbness in the area of treatment. ___ ___ ___ _____

9. After 15 to 20 minutes (or as ordered by health care provider), performed hand hygiene, applied clean gloves, removed cold application, and gently dried off any moisture. ___ ___ ___ _____

10. Assisted patient to comfortable position. ___ ___ ___ _____

11. Raised side rails (as appropriate), and lowered and locked bed into lowest position. ___ ___ ___ _____

12. Disposed of soiled linen, supplies, and equipment. Removed gloves and performed hand hygiene. ___ ___ ___ _____

13. Placed nurse call system within reach. ___ ___ ___ _____

EVALUATION

1. Inspected affected area for integrity, color, temperature, and sensitivity to touch. Reevaluated 30 minutes after procedure. ___ ___ ___ _____

	S	U	NP	Comments

2. Applied clean gloves. Palpated affected area gently, and noted any edema, bruising, and bleeding. Removed and disposed of gloves; performed hand hygiene.

3. Asked patient to report pain level and rate severity on a pain rating scale.

4. Measured ROM of affected body part.

5. Used Teach-Back. Revised instruction or developed a plan for revised patient/family caregiver learning if patient or family caregiver was not able to teach back correctly.

DOCUMENTATION

1. Documented location of treatment site; pain level; appearance and condition of skin before and after treatment; type, location, and duration of application; and patient's response to therapy.

2. Documented evaluation of patient and family caregiver learning.

HAND-OFF REPORTING

1. Reported any sensations of burning, numbness, or unrelieved pain or skin color changes to health care provider.

2. During hand-off to next shift, reported the location and type of cold therapy, medication used (if ordered), duration and time of therapy, skin assessment, VS, pain assessment before and after therapy, patient response to therapy, and any adverse reactions.

3. Reported patient's cold therapy management plan and patient and family caregiver's understanding of therapy.

Student _____ Date _____

Instructor _____ Date _____

PERFORMANCE CHECKLIST SKILL 17.1 **SUPPORTING PATIENTS AND FAMILIES IN GRIEF**

	S	U	NP	Comments
ASSESSMENT				
1. Identified patient using two identifiers according to agency policy.	___	___	___	_____
2. Sat near patient in a quiet, private location. Centered self and established a quiet presence. Established eye contact, if culturally appropriate.	___	___	___	_____
3. Considered the influence of patient's cultural background on communication. Applied principles of plain language and health literacy during assessment.	___	___	___	_____
4. Assessed patient's/family caregiver's health literacy.	___	___	___	_____
5. Listened carefully to patient's story. Observed patient responses. Used open communication. Encouraged questions.	___	___	___	_____
6. Determined meaning of the loss to patient: its type, suddenness, and when it occurred. Used open-ended questions.	___	___	___	_____
7. Combined knowledge of grief theory with observation of patient behaviors. Validated observations by sharing them with patient; paraphrased, clarified, or summarized.	___	___	___	_____
8. Encouraged patient to describe the loss and its impact on daily life.	___	___	___	_____
9. Asked patient to describe the coping strategies that he or she used most often in difficult times.	___	___	___	_____
10. Assessed family caregivers' unique needs and resources. Noted if patient received care at home and who gave the care.	___	___	___	_____
11. Assessed patient's spiritual needs, beliefs, and resources. Focused on needs such as trust, life purpose, faith / belief, and hope.	___	___	___	_____
PLANNING				
1. Determined expected outcomes following completion of procedure.	___	___	___	_____
2. Closed room door and bedside curtain.	___	___	___	_____

IMPLEMENTATION

	S	U	NP	Comments

1. Showed an empathic understanding of patient's strengths and needs.

2. Offered information about patient's illness and treatment. Clarified misunderstandings or misinformation. Used culturally appropriate language, simple terms, and appropriate instructional material.

3. Encouraged patient to sustain relationships with others to help maintain independence and receive necessary help. Included patient-identified family caregivers and support people in discussions.

4. Helped patient achieve short-term goals.

5. Provided frequent opportunities for patient and family caregivers to express their fears and concerns. Was attentive to expressions of intense emotions.

6. Educated and supported patient and family caregivers. Discussed procedures, plan of care, and anticipated changes. Used interdisciplinary team to support patient's needs and preferences.

7. Instructed patient in relaxation strategies: mindfulness-based stress reduction, guided imagery, meditation, hand massage, healing touch.

8. Encouraged visits with loved ones, life review with stories or photographs, or projects such as organizing photo albums or journal writing.

9. Facilitated patient's religious / spiritual practices and connections with religious community. Used prayer or music and provide a listening presence. Made a referral to a spiritual care provider if appropriate.

10. At end of discussion, helped patient to comfortable position.

11. Placed nurse call system in an accessible location within patient's reach.

12. Raised side rails (as appropriate) and lowered and locked bed to lowest position.

EVALUATION

1. Noted patient descriptions of relationships and activities with others.

2. Observed patient's behaviors during ongoing interactions.

3. Elicited patient perceptions of benefit or outcomes gained from use of coping interventions.

264

	S	U	NP	Comments

4. Discussed progress toward performing routine activities at home.

5. Used Teach-Back. Revised instruction or developed a plan for revised patient/caregiver teaching if patient or family caregiver was not able to teach back correctly.

DOCUMENTATION

1. Documented interventions used to support patient coping and note patient's verbal and nonverbal responses.

HAND-OFF REPORTING

1. Reported patient's grief reactions to members of the interdisciplinary team, noting behaviors that affect health outcomes such as treatment refusals or prolonged inactivity.

Student _____ Date _____

Instructor _____ Date _____

PERFORMANCE CHECKLIST SKILL 17.2 **SYMPTOM MANAGEMENT AT THE END OF LIFE**

	S	U	NP	Comments
ASSESSMENT				
1. Identified patient using two identifiers according to agency policy.	___	___	___	_____
2. Assessed patient's and family caregiver's health literacy, level of understanding, and experience with symptoms.	___	___	___	_____
3. Asked patients to describe symptoms in their own words. Used open-ended prompts.	___	___	___	_____
4. Allowed sufficient time for patients to describe their symptoms and encouraged them to say more.	___	___	___	_____
5. Assessed patient's emotional health. Used standardized tool to assess anxiety if available.	___	___	___	_____
6. Assessed patient's pain severity on a pain scale of 0 to 10. If patient could not self-report pain, observed for symptoms.	___	___	___	_____
7. Performed hand hygiene. Applied clean gloves.	___	___	___	_____
8. Assessed for feeling of breathlessness, respiratory rate, breathing patterns, and lung sounds. Assessed for presence of airway secretions.	___	___	___	_____
9. Observed condition of skin, especially dependent areas such as the back, heels, and buttocks.	___	___	___	_____
10. Inspected patient's oral cavity, including mucosa, tongue, and teeth.	___	___	___	_____
11. Assessed bowel function.	___	___	___	_____
a. Determined usual bowel elimination pattern (frequency, character, usual time of day) and effectiveness of usual bowel management routines.	___	___	___	_____
b. If patient was passing liquid stool, assessed for presence of fecal impaction. Removed and disposed of gloves, performed hand hygiene, and reapplied clean gloves.	___	___	___	_____
c. Reviewed medication regimens, prescriptions, and over-the-counter drugs known to cause constipation.	___	___	___	_____
d. Identified typical food and fluid intake over 1 week and patient's activity levels.	___	___	___	_____

266

	S	U	NP	Comments

12. Assessed urinary elimination and ability to control urination. If incontinent, assessed for skin breakdown around perineum and dependent areas and for patient discomfort. ___ ___ ___ _____

13. Removed and disposed of gloves. Performed hand hygiene. ___ ___ ___ _____

14. Assessed patient's appetite, ability to swallow, and for presence of nausea or vomiting. Used standardized tool for assessment if available. ___ ___ ___ _____

15. Assessed daily food and fluid intake in relation to patient's condition and preferences. ___ ___ ___ _____

16. Used descriptive scale to assess fatigue. Asked if fatigue limited patient's ability to perform desired activities. ___ ___ ___ _____

17. Assessed for terminal delirium in patient near death. ___ ___ ___ _____

   a. Considered if patient had pain, nausea, dyspnea, full bladder or bowel, poor sleep patterns, anxiety, or joint pain from immobility. ___ ___ ___ _____

   b. Reviewed electronic health record (EHR) for hypercalcemia, hypoglycemia, hyponatremia, or dehydration. ___ ___ ___ _____

   c. Reviewed patient's medications. ___ ___ ___ _____

   d. Determined if patient had unresolved emotional or spiritual issues. ___ ___ ___ _____

18. Assessed patient's or family caregiver's goals for symptom management. ___ ___ ___ _____

PLANNING

1. Determined expected outcomes following completion of procedure. ___ ___ ___ _____

2. Closed room door and bedside curtain. ___ ___ ___ _____

3. Obtained and organized equipment at bedside. ___ ___ ___ _____

4. Arranged for extra personnel as needed. ___ ___ ___ _____

IMPLEMENTATION

1. Performed hand hygiene. ___ ___ ___ _____

2. Provided pain relief. Used multimodal interventions. ___ ___ ___ _____

   a. Administered ordered analgesics and adjuvants. Conferred with health care provider and recommended an around-the-clock (ATC) dosing schedule, especially if pain was anticipated for majority of day. ___ ___ ___ _____

   b. Provided nonpharmacological interventions. ___ ___ ___ _____

	S	U	NP	Comments

c. Provided patient and family education on causes and patterns of pain and safety of opioid use and explained interventions.

    _____ _____ _____ _____

d. Reassessed patient's pain 1 hour after administration of pain medication or alternative therapy. If pain medication was administered via IV push route, reassessed in 15–30 minutes.

    _____ _____ _____ _____

3. Provided general comfort measures.

    _____ _____ _____ _____

   a. Provided bath and skin care based on patient's preferences and hygiene needs.

    _____ _____ _____ _____

   b. Provided eye care and use artificial tears in patients with decreased consciousness.

    _____ _____ _____ _____

   c. Repositioned frequently; did not position on tubes or other objects.

    _____ _____ _____ _____

4. Provided oral hygiene after meals and at bedtime while awake and more frequently in mouth-breathing or unconscious patients.

    _____ _____ _____ _____

   a. Used antifungal oral rinses as prescribed or sodium bicarbonate or normal saline rinses.

    _____ _____ _____ _____

   b. Moistened lips with nonpetroleum balm.

    _____ _____ _____ _____

5. Initiated bowel management regimen to reduce risk for constipation or diarrhea.

    _____ _____ _____ _____

   a. Gave patient whatever fluids were enjoyable if medically tolerated. Did not force fluid intake if near end of life.

    _____ _____ _____ _____

   b. Encouraged regular physical activity if desired or tolerated.

    _____ _____ _____ _____

   c. Administered daily stool softener or laxative, especially in patients using opioids for pain management.

    _____ _____ _____ _____

   d. In case of diarrhea, provided low-residue diet; treated infections or discontinued medications if possible. Administered antidiarrheal medications. If patient had chronic diarrhea, implemented rigorous skin care to promote comfort.

    _____ _____ _____ _____

6. Managed urinary incontinence with intervention appropriate for patient's conditions.

    _____ _____ _____ _____

7. Offered patient favorite foods in amount and at times desired. Did not overly encourage patient to eat.

    _____ _____ _____ _____

   a. Treated nausea by administering antiemetics intravenously or rectally as prescribed. As nausea subsided, offered clear liquids and ice chips if able to swallow. Avoided caffeinated liquids, milk, and fruit juices.

    _____ _____ _____ _____

268

	S	U	NP	Comments

8. Managed fatigue. ___ ___ ___ _____

   a. Helped patient identify valued or desired tasks and preferred time of day to perform tasks. Determined how to conserve energy for only those tasks. Helped with activities of daily living. Eliminated extra steps in activities. ___ ___ ___ _____

   b. Explained care activities before performing and included patient in setting daily schedule. ___ ___ ___ _____

   c. Discussed with patient easy ways to incorporate gentle movement into daily activities. ___ ___ ___ _____

9. Supported patient's breathing efforts. ___ ___ ___ _____

   a. Positioned for comfort in semi-Fowler or Fowler position. ___ ___ ___ _____

   b. Elevated head to facilitate postural drainage. Turned from side to side to mobilize and drain secretions. Suctioned only if necessary. ___ ___ ___ _____

   c. Provided ordered antimuscarinic medications. ___ ___ ___ _____

   d. Stayed with patients experiencing dyspnea or air hunger. Used interventions that patients perceive as relieving their shortness of breath (choice of oxygen-delivery modes, fan near face, body position). Administered opioids or anxiolytics as prescribed. Kept room cool with low humidity. ___ ___ ___ _____

10. Managed restlessness. ___ ___ ___ _____

   a. Kept patient's room quiet with soft lighting and at comfortable temperature. Offered family members opportunities to maintain close contact. Encouraged use of soft music, prayer, or reading from patient's favorite book. ___ ___ ___ _____

   b. Used least-sedating pharmacological options to control restlessness. Consulted with interprofessional team about titrating a medication. Discontinued all nonessential medication. Used subcutaneous, transdermal, sublingual, or rectal medication delivery routes. ___ ___ ___ _____

11. Managed anxiety. ___ ___ ___ _____

   a. Provided counseling and supportive therapy. Consulted with prescribing health care provider for benzodiazepines, the drugs of choice. Offered available counseling services. ___ ___ ___ _____

12. Removed and disposed of gloves. Performed hand hygiene. ___ ___ ___ _____

13. Raised side rails (as appropriate) and lowered and locked bed into lowest position. ___ ___ ___ _____

	S	U	NP	Comments

14. Ensured nurse call system was in an accessible location within patient's reach. ___ ___ ___ _____

15. Performed hand hygiene. ___ ___ ___ _____

EVALUATION

1. Asked patient to rate pain on scale of 0 to 10 and evaluated for change in pain characteristics. Assessed behavior in nonverbal patients. ___ ___ ___ _____

2. Asked patient to describe mouth comfort and inspected oral cavity. ___ ___ ___ _____

3. Evaluated frequency of defecation; after patient defecates, inspected feces. ___ ___ ___ _____

4. Observed skin condition. ___ ___ ___ _____

5. Asked patient to rate fatigue (scale from none to moderate to severe) and compared with baseline. Observed for fatigue or shortness of breath when patient performed activities. ___ ___ ___ _____

6. Observed patient's respiratory patterns and asked if breathing was easy and comfortable. ___ ___ ___ _____

7. Observed patient's behavior or asked family to report on it. Noted level of restlessness. ___ ___ ___ _____

8. Used Teach-Back. Revised instruction or developed a plan for revised patient / family caregiver learning if patient or family caregiver was not able to teach back correctly. ___ ___ ___ _____

DOCUMENTATION

1. Documented detailed description of patient symptoms, related interventions, and patient response. Used consistent descriptors for comparison over time. ___ ___ ___ _____

2. Documented evaluation of patient and family caregiver learning. ___ ___ ___ _____

3. Documented successful symptom interventions in the care plan. ___ ___ ___ _____

HAND-OFF REPORTING

1. Reported unexpected new symptoms or uncontrolled existing symptoms to health care provider. ___ ___ ___ _____

PERFORMANCE CHECKLIST SKILL 17.3 **CARE OF THE BODY AFTER DEATH**

	S	U	NP	Comments

ASSESSMENT

1. Identified patient using two identifiers according to agency policy.

2. Asked health care provider to establish time of death and determine if an autopsy was requested. If an autopsy was planned or a possible crime was involved, used special precautions to preserve evidence.

3. Determined if family members or significant others were present and if they had been informed of the death. Identified patient's surrogate.

4. Determined if patient's surrogate had been asked about organ and tissue donation and validated that donation request form had been signed. Notified organ request team per agency policy.

5. Provided family caregivers and friends a private place to gather. Allowed them time to ask questions (including those about medical care) or discuss grief.

6. Asked family members if they had requests for preparation or viewing of the body. Determined if they wished to be present or help with care of the body.

7. Contacted support person to stay with family caregivers not helping to prepare the body. Implemented in timely manner a bereavement care plan after patient's death when family remained the focus of care.

8. Consulted health care providers' orders for special care directives or specimens that were to be collected.

9. Performed hand hygiene; applied clean gloves, gown, or protective barriers.

10. Assessed general condition of the body and noted presence of dressings, tubes, and medical equipment.

PLANNING

1. Determined expected outcomes following completion of procedure.

	S	U	NP	Comments

2. Positioned patient supine in bed, arms at side, in a private room if possible. If patient had a roommate, explained and moved this person to another location temporarily. Removed and disposed of gloves and other PPE and performed hand hygiene.

3. As soon as possible, notified someone in authority to "pronounce" the death.

4. Directed AP to gather needed equipment and arrange at bedside.

IMPLEMENTATION

1. Helped family members notify others of the death. Promptly notified the chosen mortuary and discussed plans for postmortem care.

2. If patient made tissue donation, consulted agency policy for guidelines regarding care of the body.

3. Prepared body. Performed hand hygiene; applied clean gloves, gown, or other PPE. Closed room door.

4. Removed indwelling devices. Disconnected and capped off (no need to remove) intravenous lines. Did not remove indwelling devices in cases of autopsy.

5. Cleaned the mouth and cleaned and replaced dentures as soon as possible. If dentures could not be replaced, sent them with body in clearly labeled denture cup and transported with body to mortuary. If culturally appropriate, closed mouth with rolled-up towel under chin.

6. Placed small pillow under head or positioned according to cultural preferences. Did not tie hands together on top of body. Checked agency policy regarding need to secure hands and feet. Used only circular gauze bandaging on body.

7. Closed eyes by applying light pressure for 30 seconds (if culturally appropriate). Used saline-moistened gauze if corneal or eye donation was to take place.

8. Groomed and arranged hair into preferred style, if known. Removed any clips, hairpins, or rubber bands. Did not shave patient.

9. Washed soiled body parts, if culturally appropriate.

10. Removed soiled dressings and replaced with clean dressings, using paper tape or circular gauze bandaging.

11. Placed absorbent pad under buttocks.

12. Placed clean gown on body, per agency policy.

272

	S	U	NP	Comments

13. Identified personal belongings that stay with body and those to be given to family.

14. If family caregivers requested viewing, respected individual cultural practices. Otherwise, placed clean sheet over body up to chin with arms outside covers. Removed medical equipment from room. Provided soft lighting and chairs.

15. Allowed family time alone with body and encourage them to say goodbye with religious rituals and in a culturally appropriate manner. Did not rush any grieving process.

16. After viewing, removed linens and gown per agency policy. Placed body in shroud provided by the agency.

17. Placed identification label on outside of shroud if required by agency policy. Followed agency policy for marking a body that posed an infectious risk to others. Removed and disposed of personal protective equipment and performed hygiene.

18. Arranged prompt transportation of body to the mortuary. If a delay was anticipated, transported body to the morgue.

EVALUATION

1. Observed family caregivers' friends', and significant others' response to the loss.

2. Noted appearance and condition of patient's skin during preparation of the body.

DOCUMENTATION

1. Documented time of death described any resuscitative measures taken (if applicable), and noted the name of the professional certifying the death.

2. Documented any special preparation of the body for autopsy or organ/tissue donation. Noted who was called and who made the request for organ/tissue donation.

3. Documented name of mortuary and names of family caregivers notified at the time of death and their relationship to the deceased.

4. Documented on appropriate form personal articles left on the body, jewelry taped to skin, or tubes and lines left in place. Noted how valuables and personal belongings were handled and who received them. Secured signatures as required by agency policy.

5. Documented time the body was transported and its destination. Noted the location of body identification tags.

Student _____ Date _____

Instructor _____ Date _____

PERFORMANCE CHECKLIST SKILL 18.1 **COMPLETE OR PARTIAL BED BATH**

	S	U	NP	Comments

ASSESSMENT

1. Identified patient using at least two identifiers. ___ ___ ___ _____

2. Reviewed patient's electronic health record (EHR) for orders for specific precautions concerning patient's movement or positioning and whether there was an order for a therapeutic bath. ___ ___ ___ _____

3. Reviewed patient's EHR for allergy or sensitivity to CHG. ___ ___ ___ _____

4. Reviewed prior nurses' notes to determine patient's tolerance for bathing: activity tolerance, comfort level, musculoskeletal function, and presence of shortness of breath. ___ ___ ___ _____

5. Reviewed EHR to determine patient's risk for developing a medical adhesive–related skin injury (MARSI): using adhesive devices or tape on skin, moisture-associated skin damage (MASD), and incontinence-associated dermatitis (IAD). ___ ___ ___ _____

6. Assessed patient's/family caregiver's health literacy. ___ ___ ___ _____

7. Noted and confirmed with patient any allergies or sensitivities to bath products. ___ ___ ___ _____

8. Assessed patient's fall risk status (if partial bathing out of bed or self-bath was to be performed). ___ ___ ___ _____

9. Assessed patient's cognitive (Mini-Mental State Examination) and functional status. For patients with suspected dementia, observed for agitation and changes in behavior, especially after telling patient it was bath time. ___ ___ ___ _____

10. Performed hand hygiene and applied clean gloves (for body fluid contact). Assessed patient's visual status, ability to sit without support, hand grasp, and ROM of extremities. ___ ___ ___ _____

11. Assessed for presence and position of external medical device/equipment. Inspected condition of skin under devices. ___ ___ ___ _____

12. Assessed patient's bathing preferences. ___ ___ ___ _____

13. Asked if patient had noticed any problems related to condition of skin and genitalia. ___ ___ ___ _____

	S	U	NP	Comments

14. Identified risks for skin impairment. Option: Used a pressure injury assessment tool.   _____ _____ _____ _____

15. Before or during bath, assessed condition of patient's skin.   _____ _____ _____ _____

16. Removed and disposed of gloves (if worn) and performed hand hygiene.   _____ _____ _____ _____

17. Assessed character of patient's pain (if present) and had patient rate pain severity on a 0-to-10 pain scale.   _____ _____ _____ _____

18. Assessed patient's knowledge and prior experience with skin hygiene in terms of its importance, preventive measures to take, and common problems and feelings about procedure.   _____ _____ _____ _____

PLANNING

1. Determined expected outcomes following completion of procedure.   _____ _____ _____ _____

2. Provided privacy, explained procedure, and asked patient for suggestions on how to prepare supplies. If partial bath, asked how much of bath patient wished to complete.   _____ _____ _____ _____

3. Adjusted room temperature and ventilation, closed room doors and windows, and drew room divider curtain.   _____ _____ _____ _____

4. Organized and prepared equipment on bedside table. If it was necessary to leave room, ensured that nurse call system was within patient's reach, bed was in low position, and wheels were locked.   _____ _____ _____ _____

IMPLEMENTATION

1. Performed hand hygiene and applied clean gloves. Offered bedpan or urinal. Provided toilet tissue and disposed of any excrement properly. Disposed of gloves and performed hand hygiene. Provided patient towel and moist washcloth.   _____ _____ _____ _____

2. If patient had nonintact skin or skin was soiled with drainage, excretions, or body secretions, applied new pair of clean gloves before beginning bath.   _____ _____ _____ _____

3. Raised bed to comfortable working height. Lowered side rail closest to nurse and helped patient assume comfortable supine position, maintaining body alignment. Brought patient toward side closest to nurse (stayed supine).   _____ _____ _____ _____

4. Placed bath blanket over patient. Had patient hold top of bath blanket and removed top sheet from under bath blanket without exposing patient. Placed soiled linen in laundry bag.   _____ _____ _____ _____

5. Removed patient's gown or pajamas.   _____ _____ _____ _____

   a. If gown had snaps on sleeves, unsnapped and removed gown without pulling IV tubing (if present).

   b. If gown had no snaps and if an extremity was injured or had reduced mobility, began removal from unaffected side first.

   c. If patient had an IV line and gown with no snaps at shoulders and sleeve, removed gown from arm without IV line first. Then removed gown from arm with IV line. Paused IV fluid infusion by pressing appropriate sensor on IV pump. Removed IV tubing from pump; used regulator to slow IV infusion. Removed IV bag from pole and slid IV bag and tubing through arm of patient's gown. Rehung IV bag, reconnected tubing to pump, opened regulator clamp, and restarted IV fluid infusion by pressing appropriate sensor on IV pump. If IV fluids were infusing by gravity, checked IV flow rate and regulated if necessary. Did not disconnect IV tubing to remove gown.

6. Raised side rail. Lowered bed temporarily to lowest position and raised on return after filling wash basin two-thirds full with warm water. Placed basin along with supplies on over-bed table and positioned over patient's bed. Checked water temperature and had patient place fingers in water.

7. Lowered side rail. Removed pillow (if tolerated). Raised head of bed 30 to 45 degrees if allowed. Placed bath towel under patient's head. Placed second bath towel over patient's chest.

8. Washed face.

   a. Asked if patient was wearing contact lenses. Removed if necessary/desired.

   b. Formed a mitt with washcloth; immersed in water and wrung thoroughly.

   c. Washed patient's eyes with plain warm water, using a clean area of cloth for each eye and bathing from inner to outer canthus. Soaked any crusts on eyelid for 2 to 3 minutes with warm, damp cloth before attempting removal. Dried around eyes thoroughly but gently.

   d. Asked if patient preferred to use soap on face. Otherwise washed, rinsed, and dried forehead, cheeks, nose, neck, and ears without using soap. Asked patient if they wanted to be shaved.

   e. Provided eye care for unconscious patient.

	S	U	NP	Comments

(1) Instilled eyedrops or ointment per health care provider's order.

(2) In the absence of blink reflex, kept eyelids closed. Closed eye gently, using back of fingertip, before placing eye patch or shield. Placed tape over patch or shield. Did not tape eyelid.

9. Washed upper extremities and trunk. Option: Changed bath water at this time. Obtained new 6-quart basin and mixed contents of a 4-ounce bottle of 4% CHG with warm water.

   a. Removed bath blanket from patient's arm that was closest to nurse. Placed bath towel lengthwise under arm using long, firm strokes from distal to proximal.

   b. Raised and supported arm above head (if possible) to wash axilla, rinsed, and dried thoroughly. Applied deodorant to underarms as needed or desired.

   c. Moved to other side of bed and repeated steps with other arm.

   d. Covered patient's chest with bath towel and folded bath blanket down to umbilicus. Bathed chest with long, firm strokes. Took special care with skin under patient's breasts, lifting breast upward if necessary while bathing underneath breast. Rinsed if using soap and water and dried well.

10. Washed hands and nails.

   a. Folded bath towel in half and laid it on bed beside patient. Placed basin on towel. Immersed patient's hand in water. Allowed hand to soak for 3 - 5 minutes before cleaning fingernails. Repeated for other hand.

11. Checked temperature of bath water and changed water if necessary; otherwise continued. Note: If using CHG solution in bath water, did not discard water.

12. Washed abdomen.

   a. Placed bath towel lengthwise over chest and abdomen; used two towels if necessary. Folded bath blanket down to just above pubic region. Bathed, rinsed, and dried abdomen with special attention to umbilicus and skinfolds of abdomen and groin. Kept abdomen covered between washing and rinsing. Dried well.

   b. Applied clean gown or pajama top by dressing affected side first. Option: This step may be omitted until completion of bath.

	S	U	NP	Comments

13. Washed lower extremities.

   a. Covered chest and abdomen with top of bath blanket. Exposed near leg by folding blanket toward midline. Ensured that other leg and perineum remain draped. Placed bath towel under leg as nurse supported patient's knee and ankle.

   b. Washed leg using long, firm strokes from ankle to knee and knee to thigh. Assessed condition of extremities. Rinsed and dried well. Removed and discarded towel.

   c. Cleaned foot, making sure to bathe between toes. Cleaned and filed nails as needed (checked agency policy). Dried toes and feet completely.

   d. Raised side rail; removed towel; moved to opposite side of bed, lowered side rail, placed dry towel under second leg, and repeated Steps 13b and c for other leg and foot. Applied light layer of moisturizing lotion to both feet. When finished, removed used towel.

   e. Covered patient with bath blanket, raised side rail, removed and disposed of soiled gloves, and performed hand hygiene. Changed bath water and/or CHG solution and water.

14. Washed back.

   a. Applied clean gloves (if not already applied). Lowered side rail. Helped patient assume prone or side-lying position, using safe patient-handling techniques (as applicable). Placed towel lengthwise along patient's side.

   b. If fecal material was present, enclosed in fold of underpad or toilet tissue and removed with disposable wipes.

   c. Kept patient draped by sliding bath blanket over shoulders and thighs during bathing. Washed, rinsed, and dried back from neck to buttocks with long, firm strokes. Paid special attention to folds of buttocks and anus.

   d. Cleaned buttocks and anus, washing front to back. Cleaned, rinsed, and dried area thoroughly. If needed, placed clean, absorbent pad under patient's buttocks. Removed and disposed of gloves. Performed hand hygiene.

15. While patient was supine, provided perineal care. Performed hand hygiene.

16. Massaged back if patient desired.

17. Applied body lotion to skin and topical moisturizing agents to dry, flaky, reddened, or scaling areas.

278

	S	U	NP	Comments

18. Helped patient to a comfortable position.

19. Helped patient complete grooming.

20. Checked function and position of external devices.

21. Replaced top bed linen by pulling sheet and bedspread from foot of bed to cover patient before removing bath blanket. Applied clean gloves if linen was soiled. Option: Made occupied bed at this time.

22. Raised side rails (as appropriate) and lowered bed to lowest position, locking into position.

23. Placed nurse call system in an accessible location within patient's reach.

24. Applied clean gloves and disinfected/rinsed and dried bed basin according to agency policy. This is especially important if CHG solution was used. Removed and disposed of gloves and performed hand hygiene.

EVALUATION

1. Observed skin; paid particular attention to areas that were previously soiled, reddened, flaking, scaling, or cracking or that showed early signs of breakdown. Inspected areas normally exposed to pressure.

2. Observed how patient moved extremities during bathing. If necessary, asked patient to move specific extremities.

3. Asked patient if pain relieved (when appropriate) and asked patient to rate level of comfort (on a scale of 0 to 10).

4. Asked if patient felt tired (on a scale of 0 to 10).

5. Used Teach-Back: Revised instruction if patient/family caregiver could not teach back correctly.

RECORDING

1. Documented procedure, observations, level of patient participation, and how the patient tolerated procedure.

2. Documented evaluation of patient and family caregiver learning.

HAND-OFF REPORTING

1. Reported evidence of alterations in skin integrity, break in suture line, or increased wound secretions to nurse in charge or health care provider.

Student _____ Date _____

Instructor _____ Date _____

PERFORMANCE CHECKLIST PROCEDURAL GUIDELINE 18.1 **PERINEAL CARE**

	S	U	NP	Comments

PROCEDURAL STEPS

1. Identified patient using at least two identifiers. ___ ___ ___ _____

2. Assessed environment for safety. ___ ___ ___ _____

3. Assessed patient's/family caregiver's health literacy. ___ ___ ___ _____

4. Assessed patient's knowledge, prior experience with perineal care, and feelings about procedure. ___ ___ ___ _____

5. Provided privacy and explained procedure and importance in preventing infection. ___ ___ ___ _____

6. Gathered and organized supplies needed for procedure. ___ ___ ___ _____

7. Performed hand hygiene. Applied clean gloves. Placed basin with warm water and cleansing solution on over-bed table. ___ ___ ___ _____

8. Perineal care for a female:

   a. If patient was able to maneuver and handle washcloth, allowed to clean perineum on own. ___ ___ ___ _____

   b. If patient had limited mobility, helped to assume dorsal recumbent position. Noted restrictions or a limitation in patient's positioning. Positioned waterproof pad under patient's buttocks. ___ ___ ___ _____

   c. Draped patient with bath blanket placed in shape of a diamond. ___ ___ ___ _____

   d. Folded both outer corners of bath blanket up around patient's legs onto abdomen and under hip. Lifted lower tip of bath blanket when ready to expose the perineum. ___ ___ ___ _____

   e. Inspected buttock and entire perineum for signs of IAD from urine or stool. ___ ___ ___ _____

   f. Inspected perineum for any urethral or vaginal discharge. If catheter present, observed for any discharge on the catheter. ___ ___ ___ _____

   g. Washed and dried patient's upper thighs. (Note: If agency uses CHG solution for perineal care, did not rinse; allowed to dry.) ___ ___ ___ _____

	S	U	NP	Comments

h. Washed labia majora. Used nondominant hand to gently retract labia from thigh. Used dominant hand to wash carefully in skinfolds. Wiped in direction from perineum to rectum (front to back). Repeated on opposite side using separate section of washcloth or new washcloth. Rinsed and dried area thoroughly.

i. Gently separated labia with nondominant hand to expose urethral meatus and vaginal orifice. With dominant hand, washed downward from pubic area toward rectum in one smooth stroke. Used separate section of cloth for each stroke. Cleaned thoroughly over labia minora, clitoris, and vaginal orifice. Avoided tension on indwelling catheter if present, and cleaned area around it thoroughly.

j. Rinsed and dried area thoroughly using front-to-back method.

k. If patient used bedpan, poured warm water over perineal area and dried thoroughly. (Exception: did not rinse if using CHG.)

l. Folded lower corner of bath blanket back between patient's legs and over perineum. Asked patient to lower legs and assume comfortable position.

9. Perineal care for a male:

a. If patient was able to maneuver and handle washcloth, allowed to clean perineum on own.

b. Helped patient to supine position. Noted restriction in mobility.

c. Folded lower half of bath blanket up to expose upper thighs. Washed and dried thighs.

d. Covered thighs with bath towels. Raised bath blanket to expose genitalia. Gently raised penis and placed bath towel underneath. Gently grasped shaft of penis. If patient was uncircumcised, retracted foreskin. If patient had an erection, deferred procedure until later.

e. Inspected the perineum. Observed for any drainage or irritation. Inspected buttock and entire perineum for signs of IAD from urine or stool.

f. Washed tip of penis at urethral meatus first. Using circular motion, cleaned from meatus outward. Discarded washcloth and repeated with clean cloth until penis was clean. Rinsed and dried gently and thoroughly. (Exception: did not rinse if using CHG.)

g. Returned foreskin to its natural position.

	S	U	NP	Comments

h. Took a new washcloth and gently cleaned shaft of penis and scrotum by having patient abduct legs. Paid special attention to underlying surface of penis. Lifted scrotum carefully and washed underlying skinfolds. Rinsed and dried thoroughly. (Exception: did not rinse if using CHG.) ___ ___ ___ _____

i. Folded bath blanket back over patient's perineum and helped him to comfortable position. ___ ___ ___ _____

10. For all patients, avoided placing tension on an indwelling catheter, if present, and cleaned around it thoroughly during procedure. ___ ___ ___ _____

11. Observed perineal skin for any irritation, redness, or drainage that persisted after perineal hygiene. ___ ___ ___ _____

12. Removed and disposed of gloves and used supplies in proper receptacles and performed hand hygiene. ___ ___ ___ _____

13. Helped patient to comfortable position. ___ ___ ___ _____

14. Raised side rails (as appropriate) and lowered bed to lowest position, locking into position. ___ ___ ___ _____

15. Placed nurse call system in an accessible location within patient's reach. ___ ___ ___ _____

16. Used Teach-Back. Revised instruction if patient/family caregiver could not teach back correctly. ___ ___ ___ _____

17. Documented perineal skin assessment and patient tolerance of procedure. ___ ___ ___ _____

18. Provided hand-off report to health care provider for changes in perineal skin integrity. ___ ___ ___ _____

Student _____ Date _____

Instructor _____ Date _____

PERFORMANCE CHECKLIST PROCEDURAL GUIDELINE 18.2

BATHING WITH USE OF CHLORHEXIDINE CHLORIDE GLUCONATE (CHG) DISPOSABLE WASHCLOTHS, TUB, OR SHOWER

	S	U	NP	Comments

PROCEDURAL STEPS

1. Identified patient using at least two identifiers.   ___ ___ ___ _____

2. Assessed environment for safety and provided privacy.   ___ ___ ___ _____

3. Assessed degree of help patient needed for bathing, risk for falling, patient's risk for skin breakdown, and presence of allergy or sensitivity to bathing solution.   ___ ___ ___ _____

4. Assessed patient's/family caregiver's health literacy.   ___ ___ ___ _____

5. Assessed patient's knowledge, prior experience with bathing, and feelings about procedure.   ___ ___ ___ _____

6. Provided privacy and explained procedure.   ___ ___ ___ _____

7. Arranged supplies and toiletry items at bedside if using CHG-impregnated cloths; otherwise, prepared supplies and equipment in patient's bathroom or a shower room.   ___ ___ ___ _____

8. Performed hand hygiene and applied clean gloves.   ___ ___ ___ _____

9. Bathing cloths:

   a. Adjusted room temperature and ventilation, closed room doors and windows, and drew room divider curtain.   ___ ___ ___ _____

   b. Positioned patient supine or in a position of comfort. Used a bath blanket to drape areas of body not being cleaned as bath proceeded.   ___ ___ ___ _____

   c. Helped patient remove old gown.   ___ ___ ___ _____

   d. Option: Warmed package of bathing cloths in a microwave, following package directions. Did not use a microwave used for food preparation. Checked the amount of cloths before beginning.   ___ U NP _____

   e. Washed patient's face and eyes with plain warm water.   ___ ___ ___ _____

   f. Used all six bathing cloths in the following order, positioning and using drapes as described in Skill 18.1:   ___ ___ ___ _____

	S	U	NP	Comments

(1) Cloth 1: Neck, shoulders, and chest   ___ ___ ___ _____

(2) Cloth 2: Both arms, both hands, web spaces, and axilla   ___ ___ ___ _____

(3) Cloth 3: Abdomen and groin/perineum   ___ ___ ___ _____

(4) Cloth 4: Right leg, right foot, and web spaces   ___ ___ ___ _____

(5) Cloth 5: Left leg, left foot, and web spaces   ___ ___ ___ _____

(6) Cloth 6: Back of neck, back, and buttocks.   ___ ___ ___ _____

g. Firmly cleansed skin with CHG cloth. Told patient that the skin might feel sticky for a few minutes.   ___ ___ ___ _____

h. Ensured thorough cleaning of soiled areas, such as the neck, skinfolds, and perineal areas.   ___ ___ ___ _____

i. Did not rinse, wipe off, or dry with another cloth. Allowed to air dry.   ___ ___ ___ _____

j. After application of cloth to each body site, used separate cloths for cleaning tubing from Foleys, drains, G-tube/J-tubes, rectal tubes, or chest tubes within 6 inches of the patient.   ___ ___ ___ _____

k. Told patient skin might feel sticky for a few minutes.   ___ ___ ___ _____

l. If additional moisturizer was needed, used only CHG-compatible products, per agency policy.   ___ ___ ___ _____

m. Disposed of leftover cloths, helped patient to comfortable position, and assisted in applying clean gown.   ___ ___ ___ _____

10. Tub bath or shower:

a. Scheduled use of shower or tub.   ___ ___ ___ _____

b. Checked tub or shower for cleanliness. Used cleaning techniques outlined in agency policy. Placed rubber mat on tub or shower bottom. Placed skid-proof disposable bathmat or towel on floor in front of tub or shower.   ___ ___ ___ _____

c. Placed hygiene and toiletry items within easy reach of tub or shower.   ___ ___ ___ _____

d. Helped patient to bathroom if necessary. Had patient wear robe and skid-proof slippers to bathroom.   ___ ___ ___ _____

e. Demonstrated how to use nurse call signal for help. Placed "occupied" sign on bathroom door. Closed door.   ___ ___ ___ _____

	S	U	NP	Comments

f. Filled bathtub halfway with warm water. Checked temperature of bath water, had patient test it, and adjusted it if it was too warm or too cold. Explained which faucet controls hot water. ___ ___ ___ _____

g. If patient was taking shower, turned shower on and adjusted water temperature before patient entered shower stall. Used shower seat or tub chair if available. ___ ___ ___ _____

h. Explained that patient could not remain in tub longer than 20 minutes. Checked on patient every 5 minutes. Removed and disposed of gloves; performed hand hygiene. ___ ___ ___ _____

i. Applied clean gloves. Returned to bathroom when patient signaled and knocked before entering. ___ ___ ___ _____

j. For patient who was unsteady, drained tub of water before patient attempted to get out. Placed bath towel over patient's shoulders. Helped patient get out of tub as needed and helped with drying. If possible, had a shower chair available for patient to sit. ___ ___ ___ _____

k. Helped patient as needed to don clean gown or pajamas, slippers, and robe. (In home, extended care, or rehabilitation setting, encouraged patient to wear regular clothing.) ___ ___ ___ _____

l. Helped patient to room and to comfortable position in bed or chair. ___ ___ ___ _____

m. If patient was in bed, raised side rails (as appropriate) and lowered bed to lowest position, locking into position. ___ ___ ___ _____

n. Placed nurse call system in an accessible location within patient's reach. ___ ___ ___ _____

o. Cleaned tub or shower according to agency policy. Removed soiled linen and placed in dirty laundry bag. Discarded disposable equipment in proper receptacle. Placed "unoccupied" sign on bathroom door. Returned supplies to storage area. ___ ___ ___ _____

p. Removed and disposed of gloves and used supplies in proper receptacles and performed hand hygiene. ___ ___ ___ _____

11. Observed condition of patient's skin. Paid attention to areas that were previously soiled, reddened, flaking, scaling, or showing signs of breakdown. ___ ___ ___ _____

12. Asked patient to rate level of fatigue and comfort. ___ ___ ___ _____

	S	U	NP	Comments

13. Used Teach-Back: Revised instruction if patient/family caregiver could not teach back correctly. ___ ___ ___ _____

14. Documented the type of bathing and patient tolerance and any changes to the patient's skin. ___ ___ ___ _____

15. Provided hand-off report about any changes in skin integrity to health care provider. ___ ___ ___ _____

Student _____ Date _____

Instructor _____ Date _____

PERFORMANCE CHECKLIST SKILL 18.2 **ORAL HYGIENE**

	S	U	NP	Comments

ASSESSMENT

1. Identified patient using at least two identifiers.

2. Reviewed patient's EHR, including health care provider's order and nurses' notes, and identified presence of common oral hygiene problems.

3. Reviewed EHR and assessed patient's risk for oral hygiene problems.

4. Assessed patient's/family caregiver's health literacy.

5. Asked patient about routine oral hygiene practices.

6. Assessed patient's ability to grasp and manipulate toothbrush.

7. Performed hand hygiene and applied clean gloves.

8. Using tongue depressor and penlight, inspected integrity of lips, teeth, buccal mucosa, gums, palate, and tongue; also, assessed for gag reflex and ability to swallow. Removed and disposed of gloves and performed hand hygiene.

9. Assessed patient's knowledge, prior experience with oral hygiene, and feelings about procedure.

PLANNING

1. Determined expected outcomes following completion of procedure.

2. Provided privacy and explained procedure to patient and discussed preferences regarding use of hygiene aids.

3. Organized and set up any equipment and supplies at bedside.

4. Raised bed to comfortable working height. Raised HOB to at least semi-Fowler position (unless contraindicated) and lowered side rail. Moved patient or helped patient move close to side from which nurse chose to work.

IMPLEMENTATION

1. Placed towel over patient's chest.

2. Performed hand hygiene. Applied clean gloves.

	S	U	NP	Comments

3. Applied toothpaste to brush bristles. Held brush over emesis basin. Poured small amount of water over toothpaste.

4. Allowed patient to help by brushing. Held toothbrush bristles at 45-degree angle to gum line. Ensured that tips of bristles rested against and penetrated under gum line. Brushed inner and outer surfaces of upper and lower teeth by brushing from gum to crown of each tooth. Cleaned biting surfaces of teeth by holding top of bristles parallel with teeth and brushing gently back and forth. Brushed sides of teeth by moving bristles back and forth.

5. Had patient hold brush at 45-degree angle and lightly brushed over surface and sides of tongue. Avoided initiating gag reflex.

6. Allowed patient to rinse mouth thoroughly with water by taking several sips of water (could use straw), swishing water across all tooth surfaces, and spitting into emesis basin. Used this time to observe patient's brushing technique and taught importance of brushing teeth twice a day.

7. Had patient rinse teeth with antiseptic mouthwash for 30 seconds. Then had patient spit rinse into emesis basin.

8. Helped to wipe patient's mouth.

9. Option: Allowed patient to floss. Flossed between all teeth. Held floss against tooth while moving it up and down sides of teeth. Instructed patient in importance of daily flossing.

10. Wiped off bedside table, discarded soiled linen in dirty laundry bag, and returned equipment to proper place.

11. Helped patient to comfortable position.

12. Raised side rails (as appropriate) and lowered bed to lowest position, locking into position.

13. Removed and disposed of supplies and gloves and performed hand hygiene.

14. Placed nurse call system was in an accessible location within patient's reach.

EVALUATION

1. Asked patient if any area of oral cavity felt uncomfortable or irritated.

2. Applied clean gloves and inspected condition of oral cavity. Removed and disposed of gloves and performed hand hygiene.

288

	S	U	NP	Comments

3. Observed patient brushing and flossing.

4. Used Teach-Back. Revised instruction if patient/ family caregiver could not teach back correctly.

RECORDING

1. Document procedure on basic care checklist.

2. Documented condition of oral cavity.

3. Documented evaluation of patient and family caregiver learning.

HAND-OFF REPORTING

1. Reported bleeding, pain, or presence of lesions to nurse in charge or health care provider.

Student _____ Date _____

Instructor _____ Date _____

PERFORMANCE CHECKLIST PROCEDURAL GUIDELINE 18.3 **CARE OF DENTURES**

	S	U	NP	Comments

PROCEDURAL STEPS

1. Identified patient using at least two identifiers.

2. Assessed environment for safety.

3. Assessed patient's/family caregiver's health literacy.

4. Assessed patent's knowledge, prior experience with denture care and feelings about procedure.

5. Performed hand hygiene.

6. Asked patient whether dentures fit and whether there was any gum or mucous membrane tenderness or irritation. Asked patient about denture care and product preferences.

7. Determined whether patient had necessary dexterity to clean dentures independently or required help.

8. Lowered side rail. Positioned patient comfortably sitting up in bed or helped patient walk from bed to chair placed in front of sink.

9. Filled emesis basin with tepid water. (If using sink, placed washcloth in bottom of sink and filled sink with approximately 2.5 cm [1 inch] of water.)

10. Performed hand hygiene again and applied clean gloves.

11. Asked patient to remove dentures. If patient was unable to do this independently, grasped upper plate at front with thumb and index finger wrapped in gauze and pulled downward. Gently lifted lower denture from jaw and rotated one side downward to remove from patient's mouth. Placed dentures in emesis basin or sink lined with washcloth and 2.5 cm (1 inch) of water.

12. Inspected oral cavity, paying attention to gums, tongue, and upper palate. Observed for lesions, plaques, and areas of irritation. Palpated areas as needed.

	S	U	NP	Comments

13. Applied cleaning agent to brush and brushed surfaces of dentures. Held dentures close to water. Held brush horizontally and used back-and-forth motion to clean biting surfaces. Used short strokes from top of denture to biting surfaces to clean outer teeth surfaces. Held brush vertically and used short strokes to clean inner teeth surfaces. Held brush horizontally and used back-and-forth motion to clean undersurface of dentures. ___ ___ ___ _____

14. Rinsed thoroughly in tepid water. ___ ___ ___ _____

15. If necessary, applied a thin layer of denture adhesive to undersurface before inserting. ___ ___ ___ _____

16. Reinserted dentures as soon as possible. If patient needed help with inserting dentures, moistened upper denture and pressed firmly to seal it in place. Inserted moistened lower denture (if applicable). Asked whether denture(s) felt comfortable. ___ ___ ___ _____

17. If patient wanted to store dentures, stored in tepid water in enclosed, labeled denture cup. Kept denture cup in a secure place labeled with patient's name. ___ ___ ___ _____

18. Used Teach-Back: Revised instruction if patient/family caregiver could not teach back correctly. ___ ___ ___ _____

19. Returned patient to comfortable position. Raised side rails (as appropriate) and lowered bed to lowest position, locking into position. ___ ___ ___ _____

20. Removed and disposed of supplies and gloves (if worn) and performed hand hygiene. ___ ___ ___ _____

21. Placed nurse call system in an accessible location within patient's reach. ___ ___ ___ _____

22. Documented and reported any abnormalities noted involving oral mucosa. ___ ___ ___ _____

23. Provided hand-off report to health care provider regarding any oral lesions, or poor-fitting dentures. ___ ___ ___ _____

Student _____ Date _____

Instructor _____ Date _____

PERFORMANCE CHECKLIST SKILL 18.3   **PERFORMING MOUTH CARE FOR AN UNCONSCIOUS OR DEBILITATED PATIENT**

	S	U	NP	Comments
ASSESSMENT				
1. Identified patient using at least two identifiers.	___	___	___	_____
2. Reviewed patient's EHR, including health care provider's order and nurses' notes. Noted condition of oral cavity, previous suctioning, and any antiseptic solutions used.	___	___	___	_____
3. Reviewed patient's EHR to assess patient's risk for oral hygiene problems.	___	___	___	_____
4. Assessed patient's/family caregiver's health literacy.	___	___	___	_____
5. Performed hand hygiene and applied clean gloves.	___	___	___	_____
6. Assessed for presence of gag reflex by placing tongue blade on back half of tongue.	___	___	___	_____
7. Inspected condition of oral cavity. Inspected lips, teeth, gums, buccal mucosa, palate, and tongue, using tongue blade and penlight if necessary.	___	___	___	_____
8. Assessed patient's respirations or oxygen saturation.	___	___	___	_____
9. Removed and disposed of gloves. Performed hand hygiene.	___	___	___	_____
10. Assessed patient's or family caregiver's knowledge, prior experience with mouth care, and feelings about procedure.	___	___	___	_____
PLANNING				
1. Determined expected outcomes following completion of procedure.	___	___	___	_____
2. Provided privacy and explained procedure to patient or family caregiver if present.	___	___	___	_____
3. Gathered equipment and supplies and organized at bedside. Had AP assist if needed.	___	___	___	_____
IMPLEMENTATION				
1. Performed hand hygiene and applied clean gloves.	___	___	___	_____

292

	S	U	NP	Comments

2. Placed towel on over-bed table and arranged equipment. If needed, turned on suction machine and connected tubing to suction catheter. ___ ___ ___ _____

3. Raised bed to appropriate working height; lowered side rail. ___ ___ ___ _____

4. Unless contraindicated, positioned patient in side-lying position. Turned patient's head toward mattress in dependent position with HOB elevated at least 30 degrees. ___ ___ ___ _____

5. Placed second towel under patient's head and emesis basin under chin. ___ ___ ___ _____

6. Removed dentures or partial plates if present. ___ ___ ___ _____

7. If patient was uncooperative or having difficulty keeping mouth open, inserted an oral airway. Inserted upside down and turned airway sideways and over tongue to keep teeth apart. Inserted when patient was relaxed if possible. Did not use force. ___ ___ ___ _____

8. Cleaned mouth using brush moistened in water. Applied toothpaste or used antibacterial solution to loosen crusts. Held toothbrush bristles at 45-degree angle to gum line. Ensured that tips of bristles rested against and penetrated under gum line. Brushed inner and outer surfaces of upper and lower teeth by brushing from gum to crown of each tooth; cleaned biting surfaces of teeth by holding top of bristles parallel with teeth and brushing gently back and forth. Brushed sides of teeth by moving bristles back and forth. Used toothette sponge if patient had bleeding tendency or use of toothbrush was contraindicated. Suctioned any accumulated secretions. Moistened brush with clear water or CHG solution to rinse. Cleaned lips and mucosa with toothette. Used brush or toothette to clean roof of mouth, gums, and inside cheeks. Gently brushed tongue but avoided stimulating gag reflex (if present). Repeated rinsing several times and used suction to remove secretions. Used towel to dry off lips. ___ ___ ___ _____

9. Applied thin layer of water-soluble moisturizer to lips. ___ ___ ___ _____

10. Informed patient that procedure was completed. Helped patient to a comfortable position. ___ ___ ___ _____

11. Cleaned equipment and returned to its proper place. Placed soiled linen in dirty laundry bag. ___ ___ ___ _____

	S	U	NP	Comments

12. Removed and disposed of supplies and gloves and performed hand hygiene.

13. When suction equipment was used, ensured a clean suction catheter was ready and attached to the suction source.

14. Raised side rails (as appropriate) and lowered bed to lowest position, locking into position.

15. Placed nurse call system in an accessible location within patient's reach.

EVALUATION

1. Applied clean gloves and used tongue blade and penlight to inspect oral cavity.

2. Asked alert, debilitated patient if mouth felt clean.

3. Used Teach-Back: Revised instruction if patient/family caregiver could not teach back correctly.

RECORDING

1. Documented procedure, appearance of oral cavity, presence of gag reflex, and patient's response to procedure.

2. Documented evaluation of patient and family caregiver learning.

HAND-OFF REPORTING

1. Reported any unusual findings to nurse in charge or health care provider.

294

Student _____ Date _____

Instructor _____ Date _____

PERFORMANCE CHECKLIST PROCEDURAL GUIDELINE 18.4   **HAIR CARE—COMBING AND SHAVING**

	S	U	NP	Comments

PROCEDURAL STEPS

1. Identified patient using at least two identifiers. ____ ____ ____ _____

2. Reviewed patient's EHR to determine that there were no contraindications to procedure. Checked agency policy for health care provider order as needed. ____ ____ ____ _____

3. Assessed patient's/family caregiver's health literacy. ____ ____ ____ _____

4. Assessed patient's hair care and shaving product preferences. ____ ____ ____ _____

5. Assessed if patient had bleeding tendency. Reviewed medical history, medications, and laboratory values. ____ ____ ____ _____

6. Assessed patient's knowledge, prior experience with hair care, and feelings about procedure. ____ ____ ____ _____

7. Assessed patient's ability to manipulate comb, brush, or razor. ____ ____ ____ _____

8. Provided privacy and explained your intent to provide hair/beard care. Asked patient to explain during the procedure the steps used to comb hair and/or shave. Asked patient to indicate if there was any discomfort during procedure. ____ ____ ____ _____

9. Gathered equipment and arranged supplies at patient's bedside. ____ ____ ____ _____

10. Positioned patient sitting in chair or up in bed with head elevated 45 to 90 degrees (as tolerated). ____ ____ ____ _____

11. Performed hand hygiene. Inspected condition of hair and scalp. Inspected for presence of any infestation. Inspected head for drainage from any head wounds. Note: Applied clean gloves if drainage or infestation suspected. Applied a gown if infestation suspected. ____ ____ ____ _____

12. Performed hand hygiene, disposed of gloves (if worn), and applied clean gloves if necessary. ____ ____ ____ _____

13. Combed and brushed hair: ____ ____ ____ _____

    a. Parted hair into two sections and then separated it into two more sections. ____ ____ ____ _____

		S	U	NP	Comments

b. Brushed or combed from scalp toward hair ends.

c. Moistened hair lightly with water, conditioner, or alcohol-free detangle product before combing.

d. Moved fingers through hair to loosen any larger tangles.

e. Using a wide-tooth comb, started on either side of head and inserted comb with teeth upward to hair near scalp. Combed through hair in circular motion by turning wrist while lifting up and out. Continued until all hair was combed through and combed into place to shape and style.

14. Shaved with disposable razor:

a. Placed bath towel over patient's chest and shoulders.

b. Ran warm water in washbasin. Checked water temperature.

c. Placed washcloth in basin and wrung out thoroughly. Applied cloth over patient's entire face for several seconds.

d. Applied approximately 1/4 inch shaving cream or soap to patient's face. Smoothed cream evenly over sides of face, on chin, and under nose.

e. Held razor in dominant hand at 45-degree angle to patient's skin. Began by shaving across one side of patient's face using short, firm strokes in direction of hair growth. Used nondominant hand to gently pull skin taut while shaving. Asked if patient felt comfortable.

f. Dipped razor blade in water because shaving cream accumulated on edge of blade.

g. After all facial hair was shaved, rinsed face thoroughly with warm, moistened washcloth.

h. Dried face thoroughly and applied aftershave lotion if desired. Removed towel.

15. Shaved with electric razor:

a. Placed bath towel over patient's chest and shoulders.

b. Applied skin conditioner or preshave preparation.

c. Turned razor on and began by shaving across side of face. Gently held skin taut while shaving over surface of skin. Used gentle downward stroke of razor in direction of hair growth.

296

	S	U	NP	Comments

d. After completing shave, removed towel and applied aftershave lotion as desired unless contraindicated.

16. Mustache and beard care:

   a. Placed bath towel over patient's chest and shoulders.

   b. If necessary, gently combed mustache or beard.

   c. Allowed patient to use mirror and direct areas to trim with scissors.

   d. After completing, removed towel.

17. Discarded soiled linen in dirty laundry bag. Removed and disposed of gloves. Performed hand hygiene.

18. Helped patient to a comfortable position.

19. Raised side rails (as appropriate) and lowered and locked bed into position.

20. Returned reusable equipment to proper place.

21. Inspected condition of shaved area and skin underneath beard or mustache. Looked for areas of localized bleeding from cuts and areas of dryness. If there was an area of bleeding, took a tissue and applied direct pressure for a minute.

22. Asked patient how hair and scalp felt, and if patient was shaved, asked if face felt clean and comfortable.

23. Placed nurse call system in an accessible location within patient's reach.

24. Used Teach-Back: Revised instruction if patient/family caregiver could not teach back correctly.

25. Documented procedure and patient tolerance of procedure.

26. Provided hand-off report to health care provider for an intolerance to procedure or bleeding that continued over a minute.

Student _____ Date _____

Instructor _____ Date _____

PERFORMEDANCE CHECKLIST PROCEDURAL GUIDELINE 18.5 **HAIR CARE—SHAMPOOING USING DISPOSABLE DRY SHAMPOO CAP**

	S	U	NP	Comments

PROCEDURAL STEPS

1. Identified patient using at least two identifiers. ___ ___ ___ _____

2. Reviewed patient's EHR to ensure there were no contraindications to procedure. Made sure that a patient's condition did not contraindicate neck hyperextension. Checked agency policy for health care provider order as needed. ___ ___ ___ _____

3. Assessed patient's/family caregiver's health literacy. ___ ___ ___ _____

4. Assessed patient's knowledge, prior experience with a disposable shampoo cap, and feelings about procedure. ___ ___ ___ _____

5. Performed hand hygiene and applied clean gloves. Inspected condition of hair and scalp before beginning shampoo. In trauma patients, inspected for draining head wounds. If lice were present, wore disposable gown in addition to gloves. Removed and disposed of gloves. Performed hand hygiene. ___ ___ ___ _____

6. Provided privacy and explained procedure and what the patient needed to do during the procedure. ___ ___ ___ _____

7. Gathered and assembled equipment at bedside, including pitcher with warm water, shampoo, and extra towels. ___ ___ ___ _____

8. Raised bed to comfortable working height and lowered side rail on nurse's working side. ___ ___ ___ _____

9. Shampooed with disposable shampoo product using a cap: ___ ___ ___ _____

   a. Positioned patient supine with head and shoulders at top edge of bed or had patient sit on chair or in bed. Applied clean gloves. ___ ___ ___ _____

   b. Combed hair to remove any tangles or debris. ___ ___ ___ _____

   c. Opened package, applied cap, and secured all hair beneath cap. ___ ___ ___ _____

   d. Massaged head through cap. Checked fitting around head to maintain correct fit. ___ ___ ___ _____

	S	U	NP	Comments
e. Massaged 2 to 4 minutes according to directions on package; used additional time as required for longer hair or hair matted with blood.	___	___	___	_____
f. Discarded cap in trash.	___	___	___	_____
g. If patient desired, towel dried hair. Placed patient in a comfortable position to brush or comb patient's hair.	___	___	___	_____
10. Removed and disposed of gloves and used supplies in proper receptacles and performed hand hygiene. Stored reusable supplies.	___	___	___	_____
11. Inspected condition of hair and scalp.	___	___	___	_____
12. Raised side rails (as appropriate) and lowered bed to lowest position, locking into position.	___	___	___	_____
13. Placed nurse call system in an accessible location within patient's reach.	___	___	___	_____
14. Used Teach-Back: Revised instruction if patient/ family caregiver could not teach back correctly.	___	___	___	_____
15. Documented procedure and patient's tolerance on appropriate checklist or nurses' notes.	___	___	___	_____
16. Reported to health care provider any episodes of extreme dizziness or discomfort in the neck during shampooing.	___	___	___	_____

Student _____ Date _____

Instructor _____ Date _____

PERFORMANCE CHECKLIST SKILL 18.4   **PERFORMING NAIL AND FOOT CARE**

	S	U	NP	Comments
ASSESSMENT				
1. Identified patient using at least two identifiers.	___	___	___	_____
2. Reviewed patient's EHR, including health care provider's order and nurses' notes. Verified health care provider's order for cutting nails (checked agency policy).	___	___	___	_____
3. Reviewed EHR for patient's risk for foot or nail problems.	___	___	___	_____
4. Assessed environment for safety.	___	___	___	_____
5. Assessed patient's/family caregiver's health literacy.	___	___	___	_____
6. Assessed patient's foot and nail care practices for existing foot problems. Used this time to instruct patients about foot care.	___	___	___	_____
7. Assessed type of home remedies that patient used for existing foot problems.	___	___	___	_____
8. Asked patient whether they used nail polish and polish remover frequently.	___	___	___	_____
9. Assessed type of footwear patient wears.	___	___	___	_____
10. If possible, observed patients walking to assess gait.	___	___	___	_____
11. Performed hand hygiene. Applied clean gloves if drainage present. Inspected all surfaces of fingers, toes, feet, and nails. Paid particular attention to areas of dryness, inflammation, or cracking. Also inspected areas between toes, heels, and soles of feet.	___	___	___	_____
12. Assessed color and temperature of toes, feet, and fingers. Assessed capillary refill of nails. Palpated radial and ulnar pulse of each hand and dorsalis pedis pulse of foot; noted character of pulses. Removed and disposed of gloves (if worn). Performed hand hygiene.	___	___	___	_____
13. Assessed patient or family caregiver's ability to care for nails or feet.	___	___	___	_____
14. Assessed patient's knowledge, prior experience with nail and foot care, and feelings about procedure.	___	___	___	_____

	S	U	NP	Comments

PLANNING

1. Determined expected outcomes following completion of procedure.

2. Provided privacy and explained procedure to patient, including fact that proper soaking of nails on hands requires several minutes in warm water. If patient had diabetes mellitus, did not soak hands or feet.

3. Gathered and organized equipment and supplies at bedside on over-bed table.

IMPLEMENTATION

1. Helped ambulatory patient sit in chair and placed disposable bathmat on floor under patient's feet. Helped bedfast patient to supine position with head of bed elevated 45 degrees and placed waterproof pad on mattress (kept side rail up until ready to begin).

2. Filled wash bin with warm water. Tested water temperature. Placed basin on floor or lowered side rail and placed basin on pad on mattress. Ensured patient could bend knees and placed one foot in basin at a time. If patient had diabetes mellitus, peripheral neuropathy, or PVD, went to Step 11 to begin foot care.

3. Adjusted over-bed table to low position and placed it over patient's lap.

4. Instructed patient to place fingers in emesis basin and arms in comfortable position.

5. Allowed feet and fingernails to soak 3 to 5 minutes. If patient had diabetes mellitus, peripheral neuropathy, or PVD, skipped this step and went straight to Step 11.

6. Performed hand hygiene and applied clean gloves. Cleaned under fingernails with end of plastic applicator stick while fingers were immersed.

7. Used soft cuticle brush or nailbrush to clean around cuticles.

8. Removed emesis basin and dried fingers thoroughly.

9. Filed fingernails straight across and even with tops of fingers. If permitted by agency policy, used nail clippers and clipped fingernails straight across and even with tops of fingers and then smoothed nail using file. Used disposable emery board and filed nail to ensure no sharp corners.

10. Moved over-bed table away from patient.

	S	U	NP	Comments

11. Performed hand hygiene and applied clean gloves. Began foot care by scrubbing callused areas of feet with washcloth. Cleaned between toes with washcloth. _____ _____ _____ _____

12. Dried feet thoroughly and cleaned under toenails. _____ _____ _____ _____

13. Trimmed toenails using procedures in Step 9. Did not file corners of toenails. Checked agency policy for trimming patient's nails. _____ _____ _____ _____

14. Applied lotion to feet and hands. Rubbed in thoroughly. Did not leave excess lotion between toes. _____ _____ _____ _____

15. Helped patient to a comfortable position in bed. _____ _____ _____ _____

16. Raised side rails (as appropriate) and lowered bed to lowest position, locking into position. _____ _____ _____ _____

17. Placed nurse call system in an accessible location within patient's reach. _____ _____ _____ _____

18. Cleaned equipment according to organizational policy and returned equipment to proper place. Removed and disposed of supplies and gloves and performed hand hygiene. _____ _____ _____ _____

EVALUATION

1. Inspected nails, areas between fingers and toes, and surrounding skin surfaces. _____ _____ _____ _____

2. If possible, had patient stand and walk and describe any discomfort. _____ _____ _____ _____

3. Observed patient's walk after foot and nail care. _____ _____ _____ _____

4. Used Teach-Back: Revised instruction if patient/family caregiver could not teach back correctly. _____ _____ _____ _____

RECORDING

1. Documented procedure and observations of condition of nails and skin around nails. _____ _____ _____ _____

2. Documented evaluation of patient and family caregiver learning. _____ _____ _____ _____

HAND-OFF REPORTING

1. Reported any areas of discomfort, breaks in skin, or ulcerations to nurse in charge or health care provider. _____ _____ _____ _____

Student _____ Date _____

Instructor _____ Date _____

PERFORMANCE CHECKLIST PROCEDURAL GUIDELINE 18.6 **MAKING AN OCCUPIED BED**

	S	U	NP	Comments

PROCEDURAL STEPS

1. Reviewed patient's EHR and assessed restrictions in mobility/positioning of patient. ___ ___ ___ _____

2. Organized supplies and closed room door or divider curtain to provide privacy. ___ ___ ___ _____

3. Assessed environment for safety. ___ ___ ___ _____

4. Performed hand hygiene. Applied clean gloves if patient had been incontinent or if drainage was present on linen. ___ ___ ___ _____

5. Explained procedure to patient, noting that patient would be asked to turn over layers of linen. ___ ___ ___ _____

6. Raised bed to a comfortable working height; lowered HOB as tolerated, keeping patient comfortable. Removed nurse call system (if separate from bed rails). ___ ___ ___ _____

7. Lowered side rail on side where nurse was standing. Loosened all top linen. Removed bedspread and blanket separately, leaving patient covered with top sheet. If blanket or spread was soiled, placed in linen bag. If to be reused, folded into square and placed over back of chair. ___ ___ ___ _____

8. Covered patient with clean bath blanket by unfolding it over top sheet. Had patient hold top edge of bath blanket or tuck blanket under shoulders. Grasped top sheet under bath blanket at patient's shoulders and brought sheet down to foot of bed. Removed sheet and discarded in dirty laundry bag. ___ ___ ___ _____

9. Positioned patient on far side of bed, turned onto side and facing away from nurse. Encouraged patient to use side rail to turn. Adjusted pillow under patient's head. ___ ___ ___ _____

10. Assessed to make sure that there was no tension on any external medical devices. ___ ___ ___ _____

11. Loosened bottom linens, moving from head to foot. Fanfolded or rolled any cloth incontinence pads, drawsheet (if present), and bottom sheet (in that order) toward patient. Tucked edges of old linen just under patient's buttocks, back, and shoulders. Did not fanfold mattress pad (if it was to be reused). Removed any disposable pads and discarded in receptacle. ___ ___ ___ _____

12. Cleaned, disinfected, and dried mattress surface if it was soiled or had moisture, per agency policy.

   ____ ____ ____ _____

13. Applied clean linens to the exposed half of bed in separate layers. If needed, started with a new mattress pad by placing it lengthwise with center crease in middle of bed. Fanfolded pad to center of bed alongside patient. Repeated process with bottom sheet.

   ____ ____ ____ _____

14. If bottom sheet was fitted, pulled corners of new sheet smoothly over mattress corner at top and bottom of bed. Folded remaining portion of sheet across bed surface, toward patient's back.

   ____ ____ ____ _____

15. If bottom sheet was flat, placed over mattress. Allowed edge of sheet closest to nurse to hang about 25 cm (10 inches) over mattress edge on side and at HOB. Ensured that lower hem of bottom sheet lay seam down along bottom edge of mattress. Spread remaining portion of sheet over mattress toward patient's back.

   ____ ____ ____ _____

16. If bottom sheet was flat, mitered top corner at HOB.

   ____ ____ ____ _____

   a. Faced HOB diagonally. Placed hand away from HOB under top corner of mattress, near mattress edge, and lifted.

   ____ ____ ____ _____

   b. With other hand, tucked top edge of bottom sheet smoothly under mattress so that side edges of sheet above and below mattress met when brought together.

   ____ ____ ____ _____

   c. To miter a corner, picked up top edge of sheet at about 45 cm (18 inches) from top end of mattress.

   ____ ____ ____ _____

   d. Lifted sheet and laid it on top of mattress to form a neat triangular fold with lower base of triangle even with mattress side edges.

   ____ ____ ____ _____

   e. Tucked lower edge of sheet, which was hanging free below the mattress, under the mattress. Tucked with palms down, without pulling triangular fold.

   ____ ____ ____ _____

   f. Held part of sheet covering side of mattress in place with one hand. With other hand, picked up top of triangular linen fold and brought it down over side of mattress. Tucked under mattress with palms down without pulling fold.

   ____ ____ ____ _____

17. Tucked remaining part of sheet under side of mattress, moving toward foot of bed. Kept linen smooth.

   ____ ____ ____ _____

18. Placed new drawsheet along middle of bed lengthwise. Fanfolded or rolled drawsheet on top of clean bottom sheet. Tucked under patient's buttocks and torso without touching old linen.

   ____ ____ ____ _____

304

	S	U	NP	Comments

19. Added waterproof pad (absorbent side up) over drawsheet with seam side down. Fanfolded toward patient. Continued to keep clean and soiled linen separate. Also kept linen under patient as flat as possible.

20. Explained that the patient would be rolling over a thick layer of linens. Keeping patient covered, asked patient to log roll toward nurse slowly over layers of linen and to not raise hips. Stressed the need to roll while staying aligned.

21. Raised side rail and moved to opposite side of bed. Option: The caregiver helped position patient. Had patient roll away from nurse toward other side of bed, over all the folds of linen. Again, had patient keep hips still.

22. Lowered side rail. Loosened edges of soiled linen from under mattress. Removed soiled linen by folding into a bundle or square.

23. Held linen away from body and placed it in laundry bag.

24. Cleaned, disinfected, and dried other half of mattress as needed.

25. Pulled clean, fanfolded or rolled mattress pad, sheet, drawsheet, and incontinence pad out from beneath patient toward nurse. Smoothed all linen out over mattress from head to foot of bed. Helped patient roll back to supine position and repositioned pillow.

26. If bottom sheet was fitted, pulled corners over mattress edges. Smoothed out sheet.

27. If flat sheet was used, mitered top corner of bottom flat sheet (see Steps 16a-f).

28. Facing side of bed, grasped remaining edge of bottom flat sheet. Leaned back slightly, keeping back straight, and pulled while tucking excess linen under mattress from HOB to foot of bed. Avoided lifting mattress during tucking.

29. Smoothed fanfolded drawsheet over bottom sheet (tucking optional). Smoothed waterproof incontinence pads, making sure that bed surface was wrinkle-free.

30. Placed top sheet over patient with vertical centerfold lengthwise down middle of bed and with seam side of hem facing up. Opened sheet out from head to foot and unfolded over patient. Ensured that top edge of sheet was even with top edge of mattress.

31. Placed clean or reused bed blanket on bed over patient. Made sure that top edge was parallel with top edge of sheet and 15 to 20 cm (6 to 8 inches) from edge of top sheet. Raised side rail.

    ____ ____ ____ _____

32. Went to other side of bed. Lowered side rail. Spread sheet and blanket out evenly.

    ____ ____ ____ _____

33. Had patient hold onto sheet and blanket while nurse removed bath blanket; discarded in linen bag.

    ____ ____ ____ _____

34. Made cuff by turning edge of top sheet down over top edge of blanket.

    ____ ____ ____ _____

35. Made horizontal toe pleat; stood at foot of bed and fanfolded in sheet and blanket 5 to 10 cm (2 to 4 inches) across bed. Pulled sheet and blanket up from bottom to make fold approximately 15 cm (6 inches) from bottom edge of mattress.

    ____ ____ ____ _____

36. Standing at side of bed, tucked in remaining part of sheet and blanket under foot of mattress. Tucked top sheet and blanket together. Ensure that toe pleats were not pulled out.

    ____ ____ ____ _____

37. Made modified mitered corner with top sheet and blanket. (Followed Steps 16a–f.) After making triangular fold, did not tuck tip of triangle.

    ____ ____ ____ _____

38. Went to other side of bed. Repeated Steps 35 and 37.

    ____ ____ ____ _____

39. Changed pillowcase. Had patient raise head. While supporting neck with one hand, removed pillow. Allowed patient to lower head. Removed soiled case and placed in linen bag. Grasped clean pillowcase at center of closed end. Gathered case, turning it inside out over the hand holding it. With the same hand, picked up middle of one end of pillow. Pulled pillowcase down over pillow with other hand. Did not hold pillow against uniform. Ensured that pillow corners fit evenly into corners of case. Repositioned pillow under patient's head.

    ____ ____ ____ _____

40. Helped patient to a comfortable position.

    ____ ____ ____ _____

41. Raised side rails (as appropriate), lowered, and locked bed into lowest position.

    ____ ____ ____ _____

42. Placed nurse call system in an accessible location within patient's reach.

    ____ ____ ____ _____

43. Placed all linen in dirty laundry bag. Removed and disposed of gloves.

    ____ ____ ____ _____

44. Arranged and organized patient's room and performed hand hygiene.

    ____ ____ ____ _____

45. During procedure, inspected skin for areas of irritation. Observed patient for signs of fatigue, dyspnea, pain, or other sources of discomfort.

    ____ ____ ____ _____

Student _____ Date _____

Instructor _____ Date _____

PERFORMANCE CHECKLIST PROCEDURAL GUIDELINE 18.7 **MAKING AN UNOCCUPIED BED**

	S	U	NP	Comments

PROCEDURAL STEPS

1. Performed hand hygiene. If patient had been incontinent or if excess drainage was on linen, applied clean gloves. ___ ___ ___ _____

2. Assessed activity orders or restrictions in mobility in planning whether patient could get out of bed for procedure. Helped patient to bedside chair or recliner. ___ ___ ___ _____

3. Lowered side rails on both sides of bed and raised bed to comfortable working position. ___ ___ ___ _____

4. Removed soiled linen and placed in laundry bag. Avoided shaking or fanning linen. ___ ___ ___ _____

5. Repositioned mattress and wiped off any moisture with a washcloth or paper towel moistened in antiseptic solution. Dried thoroughly. ___ ___ ___ _____

6. Applied all bottom linen on one side of bed (before moving to opposite side): ___ ___ ___ _____

   a. For a fitted sheet, pulled corners over ends of mattress, ensuring it was placed smoothly over mattress. ___ ___ ___ _____

   b. For a flat unfitted sheet, allowed about 25 cm (10 inches) to hang over sides of mattress edges (along sides and HOB). Made sure that lower hem of sheet was seam down, even with bottom edge of mattress. Pulled remaining top part of sheet over top edge of mattress. ___ ___ ___ _____

7. While standing at head of bed, mitered top corner of flat bottom sheet (see Procedural Guideline 18.6, Steps 16a-f). ___ ___ ___ _____

8. Tucked remaining part of unfitted sheet under mattress from head to foot of bed. ___ ___ ___ _____

9. Optional: Applied drawsheet and waterproof incontinence pad, and waterproof incontinence pad laying centerfolds along middle of bed lengthwise. Smoothed drawsheet and pad over mattress and tucked excess edge of drawsheet under mattress, keeping palms down. Centered position of pad over bottom sheet. ___ ___ ___ _____

	S	U	NP	Comments

10. Moved to opposite side of bed and pulled corners of fitted sheet over ends of mattress, and then spread it smoothly over edge of mattress from head to foot of bed.

    S ___ U ___ NP ___   _____

11. For an unfitted sheet, mitered top corner of bottom sheet (see Step 7), making sure that corner was taut.

    ___ ___ ___   _____

12. Grasped remaining edge of unfitted bottom sheet and tucked tightly under mattress while moving from head to foot of bed.

    ___ ___ ___   _____

13. Smoothed folded drawsheet over bottom sheet and tucked under mattress, first at middle, then at top, and then at bottom.

    ___ ___ ___   _____

14. If needed, applied single waterproof pad over bottom sheet or drawsheet.

    ___ ___ ___   _____

15. Placed top sheet over bed with vertical centerfold lengthwise down middle of bed. Opened sheet out from head to foot, ensuring that top edge of sheet was even with top edge of mattress.

    ___ ___ ___   _____

16. Made horizontal toe pleat: stood at foot of bed and made fanfold in sheet 5 to 10 cm (2 to 4 inches) across bed. Pulled sheet up from bottom to make fold approximately 15 cm (6 inches) from bottom edge of mattress.

    ___ ___ ___   _____

17. Tucked in remaining part of sheet under foot of mattress. Placed blanket over bed with top edge parallel to top edge of sheet and 15 to 20 cm (6 to 8 inches) down from edge of sheet. (Optional: Applied additional spread over bed.)

    ___ ___ ___   _____

18. Made cuff by turning edge of top sheet down over top edge of blanket and spread.

    ___ ___ ___   _____

19. Standing on one side at foot of bed, lifted mattress corner slightly with one hand; with other hand, tucked top sheet, blanket, and spread under mattress. Ensure that toe pleats were not pulled out.

    ___ ___ ___   _____

20. Made modified mitered corner with top sheet, blanket, and spread. After making triangular fold, did not tuck tip of triangle (see Procedural Guideline 18.6, Step 37).

    ___ ___ ___   _____

21. Went to other side of bed. Spread sheet, blanket, and bedspread out evenly. Made cuff with top sheet and blanket. Made modified corner at foot of bed.

    ___ ___ ___   _____

22. Applied clean pillowcase.

    ___ ___ ___   _____

	S	U	NP	Comments

23. Placed nurse call system in an accessible location within patient's reach. Returned bed to low position, allowing for patient transfer. Locked wheels. Helped patient to bed to assume a comfortable position. ___ ___ ___ _____

24. Arranged patient's room. Removed and discarded supplies. Performed hand hygiene. ___ ___ ___ _____

Student _____ Date _____

Instructor _____ Date _____

PERFORMANCE CHECKLIST PROCEDURAL GUIDELINE 19.1 **EYE CARE FOR COMATOSE PATIENTS**

	S	U	NP	Comments

PROCEDURAL STEPS

1. Identified patient using at least two identifiers according to agency policy.

2. Reviewed patient's electronic health record (EHR) to identify any preadmission eye conditions and current treatments that may pose a risk for reduced blink reflex.

3. Assessed patient's/family caregiver's health literacy.

4. Performed hand hygiene.

5. Applied clean gloves if drainage was present. Observed patient's eyes for drainage, corneal dullness, irritation, redness of conjunctiva, and lesions.

6. Continually explained each step of the assessment procedure. Had an interpreter available, if possible, if you knew the patient did not speak English.

7. Removed eye patch (if present). Assessed for blink reflex.

8. Examined the pupils; determined if pupils were equal and round and reactive to light and accommodation (PERRLA).

9. Observed patient's eye movements, noting symmetry of movement. Removed and disposed of gloves (if worn) and performed hand hygiene. Applied new pair of gloves.

10. Arranged supplies at bedside. Lowered side rails and placed bed in working position.

11. Provided privacy and explained procedure to patient and family caregivers.

12. Positioned patient in supine position.

13. Used clean washcloth or cotton balls moistened with warm water or sterile saline and gently wiped each eye from inner to outer canthus. Used a separate, clean cotton ball or corner of the washcloth for each eye.

310

	S	U	NP	Comments
14. Applied lubricant to eye.	___	___	___	_____
a. Ointment: Pulled the lower eyelid down with finger and applied the ointment over the top of the lower lid into the gap between the lid and the conjunctiva. Twisted tube slightly to release ointment.	___	___	___	_____
b. Eyedrops: Used eyedropper to instill the prescribed lubricant into conjunctival sac, wiping away any excess lubricant.	___	___	___	_____
15. Ensured the lashes were positioned clear of the cornea to prevent iatrogenic corneal abrasion.	___	___	___	_____
16. If the blink reflex was absent, gently closed patient's eyes and applied eye patches or pads. Secured patch, being careful not to tape a patient's eyes. If eye patches or pads were soiled, replaced with fresh ones to decrease risk of infection.	___	___	___	_____
17. Disposed of used supplies; removed and disposed of gloves, and performed hand hygiene.	___	___	___	_____
18. Helped patient to a comfortable position.	___	___	___	_____
19. Placed nurse call system in an accessible location within patient's reach.	___	___	___	_____
20. Raised side rails (as appropriate) and lowered bed to lowest position, locking into position.	___	___	___	_____
21. Removed eye pads or patches every 4 hours or as ordered, and observed condition of patient's eyes for drainage, irritation, redness, and lesions.	___	___	___	_____
22. Used Teach-Back: Revised instruction if patient/family caregiver could not teach back correctly.	___	___	___	_____
23. Documented eye examination findings, administration of ointment or drops, and family caregiver learning.	___	___	___	_____
24. Notified health care provider about signs of irritation or infection.	___	___	___	_____

Student _____ Date _____

Instructor _____ Date _____

PERFORMANCE CHECKLIST PROCEDURAL GUIDELINE 19.2   **TAKING CARE OF CONTACT LENSES**

	S	U	NP	Comments

PROCEDURAL STEPS

1. Identified patient using at least two identifiers according to agency policy.

2. Assessed patient's/family caregiver's health literacy.

3. Performed hand hygiene. Inspected patient's eyes or asked patient if contact lens was in place.

4. Determined if patient was able to manipulate and hold contact lenses and if glasses were available for periods when contacts were not in use.

5. If patient had worn lenses, assessed knowledge about usual routine for wearing, cleaning, and storing lenses.

6. Asked if patient had experienced any unusual visual signs/symptoms.

7. Reviewed types of medication prescribed for patient.

8. Provided privacy and explained procedure to patient. Prepared equipment at bedside, including any written materials or photo images to complement instruction.

9. Had patient sit in bed or chair with a mirror available.

10. Encouraged patient to keep fingernails short and smooth and instructed to perform hand hygiene before lens care.

11. Had patient verify expiration date of all solutions.

12. Instructed patient on lens removal:

   a. Removal of soft lens: Had patient follow Steps (1) through (6) for each eye.

     (1) Looked at the contact lens in the eye. Shone a penlight or flashlight sideways onto the eye to help locate the position of the lens if needed.

312

	S	U	NP	Comments

(2) Instilled 2 or 3 drops of sterile saline solution into the eye.   ___ ___ ___ _____

(3) Looked straight ahead, retracted the lower eyelid with the nondominant hand, and exposed lower edge of lens.   ___ ___ ___ _____

(4) Used the pad of the index finger of the dominant hand and slid lens off cornea down onto lower sclera.   ___ ___ ___ _____

(5) While pulling the upper eyelid down gently with thumb of nondominant hand, compressed lens lightly between thumb and index finger.   ___ ___ ___ _____

(6) By gently pinching the lens, lifted the lens out without allowing edges to stick together. Placed lens in storage case.   ___ ___ ___ _____

b. Removal of hard lenses: Had patient follow Steps (1) through (6) for each eye.   ___ ___ ___ _____

(1) Looked at the contact lens in the eye. Shone a penlight or flashlight sideways onto the eye to help locate the position of the lens if needed.   ___ ___ ___ _____

(2) Placed index finger of dominant hand on outer corner of the eye and gently drew skin back toward ear.   ___ ___ ___ _____

(3) Blinked while being careful to not release pressure on corner of eye.   ___ ___ ___ _____

(4) If lens did not dislodge, gently retracted eyelid beyond edge of lens. Pressed lower eyelid gently against lower edge of lens to dislodge it.   ___ ___ ___ _____

(5) Allowed both eyelids to close slightly and grasped lens as it rose from the eye. Cupped lens in hand.   ___ ___ ___ _____

(6) Looked at the lens to be sure that it was intact. Placed it in storage container.   ___ ___ ___ _____

13. Cleaning and storage: Typical cleaning and disinfecting of contact lenses (verified specific method for lenses):

a. Discussed with patient the risk for infection if lenses were not properly cleaned on a regular basis and stored between use.   ___ ___ ___ _____

b. Had patient apply 1 or 2 drops of cleaning solution to lens in palm of hand. Using index finger (soft lenses) or little finger (rigid lenses), rubbed lens gently but thoroughly on both sides for 20 to 30 seconds.   ___ ___ ___ _____

	S	U	NP	Comments

c. Held lens over emesis basin, and had patient rinse thoroughly with recommended rinsing solution.

d. Had patient place lens in proper storage case compartment. Placed rigid lenses inside up.

e. Filled the storage case with recommended disinfectant or storage solution.

f. Instructed patient to secure cover(s) over storage case. (If lenses were to be stored at a patient's bedside in health care facility, labeled case with patient's name, identification number, and room number.)

14. Inserting lenses:

a. Inserting a soft lens: Had patient follow Steps (1) through (6) for each eye.

   (1) Removed right lens from storage case and rinsed with recommended rinsing solution; inspected lens for foreign materials, tears, and other damage.

   (2) Held lens on tip of index finger of dominant hand with concave side up.

   (3) Looked at lens from side at eye level to ensure that it was not inverted.

   (4) Took index finger of nondominant hand and retracted upper eyelid until iris was exposed. Then, using thumb of nondominant hand, pulled down lower lid.

   (5) Looked straight ahead and focused on an object in the distance while gently tipping and placing lens directly on cornea and released lids slowly, starting with lower lid.

   (6) Closed the eyes briefly and avoided blinking.

b. Inserting a rigid lens: Had patient follow Steps (1) through (7) for each eye.

   (1) Removed right lens from storage case; tried to lift lens straight up.

   (2) Held lens on tip of index finger of dominant hand with concave side up.

   (3) Looked at the lens to ensure that it was moist, clean, clear, and free of chips or cracks.

314

	S	U	NP	Comments

(4) Wet the lens surfaces with a few drops of prescribed wetting solution. ___ ___ ___ _____

(5) Took index finger of nondominant hand and retracted upper eyelid until iris was exposed. Used thumb of nondominant hand and pulled down lower lid. ___ ___ ___ _____

(6) Looked straight ahead and focused on an object in the distance. Gently placed lens directly on cornea and released lids slowly, starting with lower lid. ___ ___ ___ _____

(7) Closed eyes briefly and avoided blinking. ___ ___ ___ _____

15. Inspected eye to ensure that patient had placed lens on cornea. ___ ___ ___ _____

16. Asked patient to cover other eye with hand and report if vision was clear and lens was comfortable. ___ ___ ___ _____

17. Disposed of supplies in appropriate container and had patient perform hand hygiene. ___ ___ ___ _____

18. Helped patient to comfortable position. ___ ___ ___ _____

19. Placed nurse call system in an accessible location within patient's reach. ___ ___ ___ _____

20. Raised side rails (as appropriate) and lowered bed to lowest position locking into position. Performed hand hygiene. ___ ___ ___ _____

21. Asked patient if lens felt comfortable after removal and reinsertion of lenses. ___ ___ ___ _____

22. Asked patient if there was blurred vision, pain, or foreign body sensation. ___ ___ ___ _____

23. Taught patient to inspect the eyes for redness, pain, or swelling of eyelids or conjunctiva after lens removal. Also looked for discharge or excess tearing. ___ ___ ___ _____

24. Used Teach-Back: Revised instruction if patient/family caregiver could not teach back correctly. ___ ___ ___ _____

Student _____ Date _____

Instructor _____ Date _____

PERFORMANCE CHECKLIST SKILL 19.1   **EYE IRRIGATION**

_____

	S	U	NP	Comments

ASSESSMENT

1. Acute emergent situations: Performed hand hygiene and prepared to use copious amounts of clear, cool water to flush eyes until secretions were cleared. Followed irrigation steps in Implementation section, below.

2. Nonemergent situations: Identified patient using at least two identifiers.

3. Reviewed health care provider's medication order, including solution to be instilled and affected eye(s) (right, left, or both) to receive irrigation.

4. Assessed patient/family caregiver's health literacy.

5. Obtained history of the injury.

6. Performed hand hygiene. Applied gloves if drainage was present. Determined the patient's ability to open the affected eye. If the patient was unable to open eye, held eyelids open manually or with an eye speculum.

7. If time permitted, performed a complete eye examination. Had patient look in all directions to determine if there were any visible foreign bodies.

8. Observed eye for redness, excessive tearing, discharge, and swelling. Asked patient about symptoms of itching, burning, pain, blurred vision, or photophobia. Removed and disposed of gloves; performed hand hygiene.

9. If chemical contamination was suspected, assessed pH of the patient's tears. Inserted a folded end of a universal pH strip into the conjunctival sac and read results after 30 seconds. Compared pH in both eyes.

10. Asked patient to rate level of eye pain. Used scale of 0 to 10.

11. Assessed patient's knowledge, prior experience with eye irrigation, and feelings about procedure.

	S	U	NP	Comments

PLANNING

1. Determined expected outcomes following completion of procedure.

2. Checked accuracy and completeness of each MAR with health care provider's written medication or procedure order. Checked patient's name, irrigation solution name and concentration, route of administration, and time for administration. Compared MAR with label of eye irrigation solution.

3. Provided privacy and explained procedure to patient.

4. Organized and set up any equipment needed to perform procedure.

IMPLEMENTATION

1. Performed hand hygiene. Applied clean gloves.

2. Removed any contact lens if possible. Removed and disposed of gloves after contact lens was removed. Performed hand hygiene and applied new gloves.

3. Explained to patient that eye could be closed periodically and that no object would touch it.

4. With patient in supine or semi-Fowler position in bed, placed towel or waterproof pad under patient's face and curved emesis basin just below patient's cheek on side of affected eye. Turned head toward affected eye. If both eyes were affected, kept patient supine for simultaneous irrigation of both eyes.

5. Using gauze moistened with health care provider's ordered solution (or normal saline), gently cleaned visible secretions or foreign material from eyelid margins and eyelashes, wiping from inner to outer canthus.

6. Explained next steps to patient and encouraged relaxation:

   a. With gloved finger, gently retracted upper and lower eyelids to expose conjunctival sacs.

   b. To hold lids open, applied gentle pressure to lower bony orbit and bony prominence beneath eyebrow. Did not apply pressure over eye.

7. Held irrigating syringe, dropper, or IV tubing approximately 2.5 cm (1 inch) from inner canthus.

8. Asked patient to look in all directions while maintaining irrigation. Gently irrigated with steady stream toward lower conjunctival sac, moving from inner to outer canthus.

	S	U	NP	Comments

9. Reinforced importance of procedure and encouraged patient by using calm, confident, soft voice.

    ___   ___   ___   _____

10. Allowed patient to blink periodically.

    ___   ___   ___   _____

11. Continued irrigation with prescribed solution volume or time, or until secretions are cleared.

    ___   ___   ___   _____

12. Blotted excess moisture from eyelids and face with gauze or towel.

    ___   ___   ___   _____

13. Disposed of soiled supplies; removed and disposed of gloves. Performed hand hygiene.

    ___   ___   ___   _____

14. Helped patient to comfortable position.

    ___   ___   ___   _____

15. Raised side rails (as appropriate) and lowered bed to lowest position locking into position.

    ___   ___   ___   _____

16. Placed nurse call system in an accessible location within patient's reach.

    ___   ___   ___   _____

EVALUATION

1. Observed for verbal and nonverbal signs of anxiety during irrigation.

    ___   ___   ___   _____

2. Assessed patient's comfort level after irrigation.

    ___   ___   ___   _____

3. Inspected eye for movement and determined if pupils were equal, round, and reactive to light and accommodation.

    ___   ___   ___   _____

4. Asked patient about improved visual acuity. Had patient read written material.

    ___   ___   ___   _____

5. Used Teach-Back. Revised instruction if patient/family caregiver could not teach back correctly.

    ___   ___   ___   _____

RECORDING

1. Documented reason for irrigation, condition of eye before and after irrigation, patient's report of pain and visual symptoms, type and amount of irrigation solution, and length of time irrigation performed.

    ___   ___   ___   _____

2. Documented evaluation of patient and family caregiver learning.

    ___   ___   ___   _____

HAND-OFF REPORTING

1. Used agency's standardized hand-off communication to communicate reason for irrigation, type and amount of irrigation solution, and length of time irrigation performed.

    ___   ___   ___   _____

2. Reported patient's condition of eye, symptoms, and tolerance of eye irrigation.

    ___   ___   ___   _____

3. Reported immediately to the health care provider if patient complained of increased pain, blurred vision, or other visual changes.

    ___   ___   ___   _____

Student _____ Date _____

Instructor _____ Date _____

PERFORMANCE CHECKLIST SKILL 19.2 **EAR IRRIGATION**

	S	U	NP	Comments

ASSESSMENT

1. Identified patient at least using two identifiers according to agency policy.

2. Review health care provider's irrigation order, including solution to be instilled and affected ear(s).

3. Reviewed electronic health record for history of diabetes, eczema or other skin problem in the ear canal, a weakened immune system, ruptured tympanic membrane, placement of myringotomy tubes, or surgery of the auditory canal.

4. Assessed patient's/family caregiver's health literacy.

5. Performed hand hygiene and inspected pinna and external auditory meatus for redness, swelling, drainage, abrasions, and presence of cerumen or foreign objects. Applied clean gloves if drainage present.

   a. Always attempted to remove foreign objects in ear by first simply straightening ear canal.

6. Used otoscope to inspect deeper parts of auditory canal and tympanic membrane.

7. Asked if patient was having earache or fullness in the ear, partial hearing loss, tinnitus (ringing in the ear), itching or discharge in ear, or coughing.

8. Using a scale of 0 to 10, asked patient to rate severity of ear discomfort. Removed and disposed of gloves (if worn). Performed hand hygiene.

9. Assessed patient's hearing acuity.

10. Assessed patient's knowledge, prior experience with ear irrigation, and feelings about procedure.

	S	U	NP	Comments

PLANNING

1. Determined expected outcomes following completion of procedure.

2. If patient was found to have impacted cerumen, instilled 1 or 2 drops of cerumen softener into ear twice a day for 2 to 3 days before irrigation.

3. Provided privacy and explained procedure. Informed patients that irrigation may cause sensation of dizziness, ear fullness, and warmth.

4. Organized and set up equipment needed to perform procedure.

5. Assisted patient into a sitting or lying position with head turned toward affected ear. Placed towel under patient's head and ear. When possible, had patient hold emesis basin.

IMPLEMENTATION

1. Performed hand hygiene. Poured warmed water into basin. Checked temperature of solution by pouring small drop on inner forearm. Used sterile basin if sterile irrigating water was used, sterile basin was required.

2. Applied clean gloves. Gently cleaned auricle and outer ear canal with gauze or cotton balls. Did not force drainage or cerumen into ear canal. Removed and disposed of gloves. Performed hand hygiene. Reapplied clean gloves.

3. Filled irrigating syringe with solution (approximately 50 mL).

4. For adults and children over 3 years old, gently pulled pinna up and back. In children 3 years or younger, pulled pinna down and back. Placed tip of irrigating device just inside external meatus. Left space around irrigating tip and canal.

5. Slowly instilled irrigating solution by holding tip of syringe 1 cm (½ inch) above opening to ear canal. Directed fluid toward superior aspect of ear canal. Allowed it to drain out into basin during instillation. Continued until canal was cleaned or solution was used.

	S	U	NP	Comments

6. Maintained flow of irrigation in steady stream until pieces of cerumen or exudate flow from canal.

7. Periodically asked if patient was experiencing pain, nausea, or vertigo.

8. Drained excessive fluid from ear by having patient tilt head toward affected side.

9. Dried outer ear canal gently with cotton ball. Left cotton ball in place for 5 to 10 minutes.

10. Helped patient to comfortable position.

11. Removed and disposed of gloves. Performed hand hygiene.

12. Raised side rails (as appropriate) and lowered bed to lowest position, locking into position.

13. Placed nurse call system in an accessible location within patient's reach.

EVALUATION

1. Asked patient if discomfort was noted during instillation of solution.

2. Asked patient about sensations of light-headedness or dizziness.

3. Reinspected condition of meatus and canal.

4. Assessed patient's level of pain and hearing acuity and assessed for presence of preirrigation symptoms.

5. Used Teach-Back: Revised instruction if patient/family caregiver could not teach back correctly.

RECORDING

1. Documented indication for ear irrigation, symptoms of cerumen buildup or infection, condition of the tympanic membrane and ear canal before and after irrigation, characteristics of cerumen or other material removed, and patient's hearing acuity before and after procedure.

2. Documented the type and amount of solution, time of administration, and the ear receiving the irrigation

3. Documented adverse effects and patient response to ear irrigation.

4. Documented evaluation of patient and family caregiver learning.

	S	U	NP	Comments

HAND-OFF REPORTING

1. Reported indication for ear irrigation, which ear was irrigated, any adverse effects, and any change in hearing acuity. ___ ___ ___ _____

2. Reported patient response to procedure and outcome of irrigation. ___ ___ ___ _____

Student _____ Date _____

Instructor _____ Date _____

PERFORMANCE CHECKLIST SKILL 19.3 **CARE OF HEARING AIDS**

	S	U	NP	Comments

ASSESSMENT

1. Identified patient using two identifiers according to agency policy.

2. Reviewed patient electronic health record for type of hearing aid and patient's hearing acuity.

3. Determined whether patient could hear clearly with hearing aid by talking slowly and clearly in normal tone of voice.

4. Assessed patient's/family caregiver's health literacy.

5. Asked patient to demonstrate (if able) manipulation and holding of hearing aid.

6. Assessed if hearing aid was working by removing from patient's ear. Closed battery case and turned volume slowly to high. Cupped hand over hearing aid to detect feedback. If no sound was heard, replaced batteries and tested again.

7. Determined patient's usual hearing aid–care practices. Option: Observed patient clean hearing aid.

8. Performed hand hygiene. If drainage was present, applied clean gloves. Assessed patient for any unusual physical or auditory signs/symptoms. If hearing was reduced, asked: When did this start? Is it present all the time? Does the quality of hearing acuity change with male versus female voices or adult versus children's voices?

9. Removed gloves (if worn). Performed hand hygiene.

10. Assessed hearing aid for cracks, rough edges, or accumulation of cerumen around aid, which can block sound.

11. Assessed patient's and family caregiver's knowledge, prior experience with cleaning and maintaining hearing aid and feelings about procedure.

	S	U	NP	Comments

PLANNING

1. Determined expected outcomes following completion of procedure. ___ ___ ___ _____

2. Provided privacy and explained procedure with patient and family caregiver (if present). Explained all steps before removing aid. ___ ___ ___ _____

3. Organized and set up any equipment needed to perform procedure. ___ ___ ___ _____

4. Had patient assume supine, side-lying, or sitting position in bed or chair. ___ ___ ___ _____

IMPLEMENTATION

1. Performed hand hygiene. Applied clean gloves if patient had ear drainage. ___ ___ ___ _____

2. Removed and cleaned hearing aid(s): ___ ___ ___ _____

   a. Patient or nurse turned hearing aid(s) volume off. Then grasped aid securely and gently removed device following natural ear contour. ___ ___ ___ _____

   b. Held aid over towel and wiped exterior with tissue to remove cerumen. ___ ___ ___ _____

   c. Inspected ear mold for cracks or rough edges, any fray in cords, or accumulation of cerumen around aid. ___ ___ ___ _____

   d. Inspected all openings in aid for accumulated cerumen. Carefully removed cerumen with wax loop or other device supplied with hearing aid. ___ ___ ___ _____

   e. Opened battery door, placed hearing aid in labeled storage container, and allowed it to air dry. ___ ___ ___ _____

   f. Placed towel beneath patient's ear(s). Washed ear canal(s) with washcloth moistened in soap and water. Rinsed with moistened cloth and then dried. ___ ___ ___ _____

   g. Assessed ear canal for redness, tenderness, discharge, or odor. ___ ___ ___ _____

   h. Repeated procedure for other hearing aid if bilateral. ___ ___ ___ _____

   i. If storing hearing aid(s), placed each in dry storage case with desiccant material. Labeled case with patient's name and room number. If more than one aid, noted right or left. Indicated in patient's electronic health record where aid was stored. ___ ___ ___ _____

324

	S	U	NP	Comments

j. Disposed of towels, removed and disposed of gloves, and performed hand hygiene.

3. Inserted hearing aid(s)

   a. Removed hearing aid(s) from storage case and checked battery. Checked that volume was off.

   b. Identified hearing aid as either right or left.

   c. When possible, allowed patient to insert aid. Otherwise, held hearing aid with thumb and index finger of dominant hand so canal was at bottom. Inserted pointed end of ear mold into ear canal. Followed natural ear contours to guide aid into place.

   d. Anchored any separate pieces, as in case of behind-the-ear (BTE) aid or body aid.

   e. Adjusted or had patient adjust volume gradually to comfortable level for talking to patient in regular voice 3 to 4 feet away. For BTE device, rotated volume control toward nose to increase volume and away from nose to decrease volume.

   f. Repeated insertion for other hearing aid, if bilateral.

   g. Closed and stored case. Removed and disposed of gloves if worn.

   h. Assisted patient to comfortable position.

   i. Raised side rails (as appropriate) and lowered bed to lowest position locking into position.

   j. Placed nurse call system in an accessible location within patient's reach.

   k. Performed hand hygiene.

EVALUATION

1. Asked patient to rate level of comfort after removal or insertion.

2. Observed patient during normal conversation and in response to environmental sounds.

3. Used Teach-Back: Revised instruction if patient/family caregiver could not teach back correctly.

RECORDING

1. Documented appearance of external ear, symptoms of cerumen buildup, and patient's hearing acuity before and after procedure.

	S	U	NP	Comments

2. Documented removal of hearing aid, storage location if not reinserted after cleaning, and patient's preferred communication techniques. If family took aid home, ensured that this information was documented.

3. Documented evaluation of patient and family caregiver learning.

HAND-OFF REPORTING

1. Reported any sudden changes in hearing to health care provider.

PERFORMANCE CHECKLIST SKILL 21.1 **ADMINISTERING ORAL MEDICATIONS**

	S	U	NP	Comments

ASSESSMENT

1. Checked accuracy and completeness of each MAR or computer printout with the health care provider's written medication order. Checked patient's name, medication name and dosage, route of administration, and time of administration. Clarified incomplete or unclear orders with health care provider before administration.

2. Reviewed medication reference for pertinent information related to medication, including action, purpose, normal dose and route, side effects, time of onset and peak action, and nursing implications.

3. Reviewed electronic health record (EHR) for any contraindications to patient receiving oral medication. Notified health care provider if any contraindications present.

4. Assessed patient's medical and medication history and history of allergies. Listed medication allergies on each page of the MAR and prominently displayed on the patient's EHR. When allergies were present, patient wore an allergy bracelet.

5. Checked date of expiration for medication.

6. Assessed patient's/family caregiver's health literacy.

7. Performed hand hygiene and assessed for any contraindications to patient receiving oral medication. Notified health care provider if contraindications were present.

8. Assessed risk for aspiration using a dysphagia screening tool if available. Protected patient from aspiration by assessing swallowing ability.

9. Asked patient to confirm their history of allergies.

10. Gathered and reviewed physical assessment findings and laboratory data that influenced drug administration.

11. Assessed patient's preference for fluids and determined if medications could be given with these fluids. Maintained fluid restrictions as prescribed.

	S	U	NP	Comments

12. Assessed patient's knowledge, prior experience regarding health and medication use, medication schedule, and ability to prepare medications. ___ ___ ___ _____

PLANNING

1. Determined expected outcomes following completion of procedure. ___ ___ ___ _____

2. Provided privacy and explained procedure to patient. Discussed purpose and side effects of each medication. If applicable, taught patient how to report any side effects. Was specific if patient wished to self-administer medications. Allowed sufficient time for patient to ask questions. ___ ___ ___ _____

3. Planned preparation to avoid interruptions. Created a quiet environment. Did not take phone calls or talk with others. Followed agency "No-Interruption Zone (NIZ)" policy. Kept all pages of MARs or computer printouts for one patient together or looked at only one patient's electronic MAR at a time. ___ ___ ___ _____

4. Collected and organized appropriate equipment and MAR. ___ ___ ___ _____

IMPLEMENTATION

1. Performed hand hygiene. Prepared medications for one patient at a time, avoiding distractions. ___ ___ ___ _____

   a. Arranged medication tray and cups in medication preparation area or moved medication cart to a position outside patient's room. ___ ___ ___ _____

   b. Logged on to automated medication dispensing system (AMDS) or unlocked medicine drawer or cart. ___ ___ ___ _____

   c. Prepared medications by following the seven rights of medication administration. Kept all pages of MARs or computer printouts for one patient together or looked at only one patient's medication administration computer screen. ___ ___ ___ _____

   d. Selected correct medication. Compared name of medication on label with MAR or computer printout. Exited AMDS after removing drug(s). ___ ___ ___ _____

   e. Checked or calculated medication dose as needed. Double-checked any calculation. Checked expiration date on all medications and returned outdated medication to pharmacy. ___ ___ ___ _____

   f. If preparing a controlled substance, checked record for previous medication count and compared current count with available supply. ___ ___ ___ _____

   g. Prepared solid forms of oral medications. ___ ___ ___ _____

328

	S	U	NP	Comments

(1) To prepare unit-dose tablets or capsules, placed packaged tablet or capsule directly into medication cup without removing wrapper. Administered medications only from containers with labels that were clearly marked. ___ ___ ___ _____

(2) When using a blister pack, "popped" medications through foil or paper backing into medication cup. ___ ___ ___ _____

(3) When preparing tablet or capsule from a floor stock bottle, poured required number into bottle cap and transferred to medication cup. Did not touch medication with fingers. Returned unused medication to container. ___ ___ ___ _____

(4) If it was necessary to give half the dose of medication, pharmacy should have split, labeled, packaged, and sent medication to unit. If you had to split medication, used clean, gloved hand to cut with clean pill-cutting device. Only cut tablets that were pre-scored by the manufacturer. ___ ___ ___ _____

(5) Placed all tablets or capsules in unit-dose individual packets that patient would receive in one medicine cup, except for those requiring preadministration assessments. Placed those medications in separate additional cups with wrapper intact. ___ ___ ___ _____

(6) If patient had difficulty swallowing and liquid medications were not an option, used a pill-crushing device. Cleaned device before using. Placed medicine between two cups and ground and crushed. Mixed ground tablet in a small amount of soft food. ___ ___ ___ _____

h. Prepared liquids. ___ ___ ___ _____

(1) Used unit-dose container with correct amount of medication. Gently shook container. Administered medication packaged in a single-dose cup directly from the single-dose cup. Did not pour medicine into another cup. ___ ___ ___ _____

(2) Administered medications only in oral use syringes, which in some agencies are prepared by the pharmacy. Did not use hypodermic syringe or syringe with needle or syringe cap. ___ ___ ___ _____

i. Returned stock containers or unused unit-dose medications to shelf or drawer. Labeled medication cups and poured medications with patient's name before leaving medication preparation area. Did not leave drugs unattended. ___ ___ ___ _____

	S	U	NP	Comments

j. Before going to patient's room, compared patient's name and name of medication on label of prepared medications with MAR.   ___ ___ ___ _____

2. Administered medications.   ___ ___ ___ _____

   a. Took medication to patient at correct time, per agency policy. During administration, applied seven rights of medication administration. Performed hand hygiene.   ___ ___ ___ _____

   b. Identified patient using at least two identifiers, per agency policy. Compared identifiers with information on patient's MAR or EHR.   ___ ___ ___ _____

   c. At patient's bedside, again compared MAR or computer printout with names of medications on medication labels and patient name. Asked patient again about any allergies.   ___ ___ ___ _____

   d. Closed curtains or room door. Performed hand hygiene. Performed necessary preadministration assessment for specific medications.   ___ ___ ___ _____

   e. Helped patient to sitting or Fowler position. Used side-lying position if patient was unable to sit. Had patient stay in this position for 30 minutes after administration.   ___ ___ ___ _____

   f. For tablets: Allowed patient to hold solid medications in hand or cup before placing in mouth. Offered water or preferred liquid to help patient swallow medications.   ___ ___ ___ _____

   g. For orally disintegrating formulations (tablets or strips): Removed medication from packet just before use. Did not push tablet through foil. Placed medication on top of patient's tongue. Cautioned against chewing it.   ___ ___ ___ _____

   h. For sublingually administered medications: Had patient place medication under tongue and allowed it to dissolve completely. Cautioned patient against swallowing tablet.   ___ ___ ___ _____

   i. For buccal-administered medications: Had patient place medication in mouth against mucous membranes of cheek and gums until it dissolved.   ___ ___ ___ _____

   j. For powdered medications: Mixed with liquids at bedside and gave to patient to drink.   ___ ___ ___ _____

   k. For crushed medications mixed with food: Gave each medication separately in teaspoon of food.   ___ ___ ___ _____

   l. For lozenge: Cautioned patient against chewing or swallowing lozenges.   ___ ___ ___ _____

   m. For effervescent medication: Added tablet or powder to glass of water. Administered immediately after dissolving.   ___ ___ ___ _____

330

n. If patient was unable to hold medications, placed medication cup or oral syringe to lips and gently introduced each medication into mouth one at a time. Administered each tablet or capsule one at a time. Injected liquid from oral syringe slowly. Did not rush or force medications.   ___ ___ ___ _____

o. Stayed until patient swallowed each medication completely or took it by the prescribed route. Asked patient to open mouth if uncertain whether medication had been swallowed.   ___ ___ ___ _____

p. For highly acidic medications, offered patient a nonfat snack if not contraindicated.   ___ ___ ___ _____

3. Helped patient return to position of comfort.   ___ ___ ___ _____

4. Raised side rails (as appropriate) and lowered bed to lowest position, locking into position.   ___ ___ ___ _____

5. Placed nurse call system in an accessible location within patient's reach.   ___ ___ ___ _____

6. Disposed of all contaminated supplies in appropriate receptacle, removed and disposed of gloves, and performed hand hygiene.   ___ ___ ___ _____

7. Replenished stock such as cups and straws, returned cart to medication room, and cleaned work area.   ___ ___ ___ _____

EVALUATION

1. Returned to bedside to evaluate patient's response to medications at times that correlated with onset, peak, and duration of the medication.   ___ ___ ___ _____

2. Asked patient or family caregiver to identify medication name and explain its purpose, action, dose schedule, and potential side effects.   ___ ___ ___ _____

3. Used Teach-Back. Revised instruction if patient or family caregiver was not able to teach back correctly.   ___ ___ ___ _____

DOCUMENTATION

1. Documented drug, dose, route, and time administered immediately after administration, not before. Included initials or signature.   ___ ___ ___ _____

2. Documented patient's response and any adverse effects to medication.   ___ ___ ___ _____

3. Documented evaluation of patient learning.   ___ ___ ___ _____

4. If drug was withheld, documented reason and followed agency policy for noting withheld doses.   ___ ___ ___ _____

HAND-OFF REPORTING

1. Reported adverse effects/patient response and/or withheld drugs to nurse in charge or health care provider. Depending on medication, notified health care provider immediately.   ___ ___ ___ _____

Student _____ Date _____

Instructor _____ Date _____

PERFORMANCE CHECKLIST SKILL 21.2 **ADMINISTERING MEDICATIONS THROUGH A FEEDING TUBE**

	S	U	NP	Comments

ASSESSMENT

1. Checked accuracy and completeness of MAR or computer printout with health care provider's original medication order. Checked patient's name, medication name and dosage, route of administration, and time of administration. Re-printed on computer any part of MAR that was difficult to read.

2. Reviewed medication reference for pertinent information related to medication, including action, purpose, normal dose and route, side effects, time of onset and peak action, and nursing implications.

   a. Determined if there was any type of interaction between medications delivered via feeding tube and contacted pharmacist if there was any question.

3. Assessed patient's medical and medication history and history of allergies. Listed food and medication allergies on each page of the MAR and prominently displayed on the patient's electronic health record (EHR). If allergies were present, patient wore an allergy bracelet.

4. Reviewed EHR to determine patient's age and history of dehydration, malnutrition, exposure to radiation therapy, underlying chronic conditions, and edema of the skin.

5. Assessed patient's/family caregiver's health literacy.

6. Reviewed EHR for any contraindications to receiving enteral medications.

7. Asked patient to confirm allergies: known allergies and allergic response.

8. For postoperative patient, reviewed postoperative orders for type of enteral tube care.

	S	U	NP	Comments

9. Performed hand hygiene. Gathered and reviewed physical assessment data, observed patient's skin around feeding tube and tape or securement devices for signs of MARSI, and reviewed laboratory data that influence drug administration.   ___ ___ ___ _____

10. Checked with pharmacy for availability of liquid preparation for patient's medications.   ___ ___ ___ _____

11. Avoided complicated medication schedule that interrupted enteral feedings. Checked with health care provider and used an alternative medication route when possible.   ___ ___ ___ _____

   a. Determined where medication was absorbed and ensured that point of absorption was not bypassed by feeding tube.   ___ ___ ___ _____

   b. Determined whether medication interacted with enteral feedings. If there was a risk of interaction, stopped feeding for at least 20 minutes before administering medication, per agency policy.   ___ ___ ___ _____

12. Assessed patient's knowledge, prior experience with enteral medication, and feelings about procedure.   ___ ___ ___ _____

PLANNING

1. Determined expected outcomes following completion of procedure.   ___ ___ ___ _____

2. Provided privacy and explained procedure to patient. Discussed purpose of each medication, indication, action, and possible adverse effects. Allowed patient to ask any questions.   ___ ___ ___ _____

3. Planned preparation to avoid interruptions. Created a quiet environment. Did not take phone calls or talk with others. Followed agency "No-Interruption Zone" policy. Kept all pages of MARs or computer printouts for one patient together or looked at only one patient's electronic MAR at a time.   ___ ___ ___ _____

4. Collected and organized appropriate equipment and MAR for administering enteral medications at bedside.   ___ ___ ___ _____

IMPLEMENTATION

1. Performed hand hygiene. Prepared medications for instillation into feeding tube. Checked medication label against MAR two times. Filled graduated container with 50 to 100 mL of tepid water. Used sterile water for immunocompromised or critically ill patients.   ___ ___ ___ _____

	S	U	NP	Comments

a. Tablets: Crushed each tablet into a fine powder, using a pill-crushing device or two medication cups. Dissolved each tablet into a separate cup of 30 mL of warm water.

    _____   _____   _____   _____

b. Capsules: Ensured that contents of capsule could be expressed from covering (consulted with pharmacist). Performed hand hygiene, applied gloves, and opened capsule or pierced gel cap with a sterile needle and emptied contents into 30 mL of warm water (or solution designated by drug company). Allowed adequate time (15 to 20 minutes) for gel caps to dissolve.

    _____   _____   _____   _____

c. Prepared liquid medication according to Skill 21.1.

    _____   _____   _____   _____

2. Never added medications directly to a container or bag of tube feeding. Held tube feeding as necessary. Verified this and the amount of time to hold a feeding with agency policy.

    _____   _____   _____   _____

3. Took medication(s) to patient at correct time, per agency policy. During administration, applied seven rights of medication administration. Performed hand hygiene.

    _____   _____   _____   _____

4. Identified patient using at least two identifiers, per agency policy. Compared identifiers with information on patient's MAR or EHR.

    _____   _____   _____   _____

5. At patient's bedside, again compared MAR or computer printout with names of medications on medication labels and patient name. Asked patient again about any allergies.

    _____   _____   _____   _____

6. Provided privacy. Assisted patient to sitting position. Elevated head of bed to minimum of 30 degrees (preferably 45 degrees unless contraindicated) or sat patient up in a chair.

    _____   _____   _____   _____

7. If continuous enteral tube feeding was infusing, adjusted infusion pump setting to hold tube feeding.

    _____   _____   _____   _____

8. Performed hand hygiene and applied clean gloves. Auscultated for presence of bowel sounds. Verified placement of feeding tube by observing gastric contents and checking pH of aspirate contents.

    _____   _____   _____   _____

	S	U	NP	Comments

9. Checked for gastric residual volume (GRV). Drew up 10 to 30 mL of air into a 60-mL syringe and connected syringe to feeding tube. Flushed tube with air and pulled back slowly to aspirate gastric contents. Determined GRV using either scale on syringe or a graduate container. Returned aspirated contents to stomach unless a single GRV exceeded 500 mL (per agency policy). If GRV was excessive, held medication and contacted health care provider.   ___ ___ ___ _____

10. Irrigated the tubing.   ___ ___ ___ _____

   a. Pinched or clamped enteral tube and removed syringe. Drew up 30 mL of water into syringe. Reinserted tip of syringe into tube, released clamp, and flushed tubing. Clamped tube again and removed syringe.   ___ ___ ___ _____

   b. Using the appropriate enteral connector, attached to enteral tube.   ___ ___ ___ _____

11. Attached medication syringe to connector port on the enteral feeding tube. Ensured there was an airtight connection between the syringe and enteral tube and administered medication slowly.   ___ ___ ___ _____

12. Option: For a large-bore feeding tube, attached Asepto syringe to ENFit connector. Administered dose liquid or dissolved medication by pouring into syringe. Allowed to flow by gravity.   ___ ___ ___ _____

   a. After giving only one dose of medication, flushed tubing with 30 to 60 mL of water after administration.   ___ ___ ___ _____

   b. To administer more than one medication, gave each separately and flushed between medications with 15 to 30 mL of water.   ___ ___ ___ _____

   c. Followed last dose of medication with 30 to 60 mL of water.   ___ ___ ___ _____

13. Clamped proximal end of a feeding tube if tube feeding was not being administered and capped end of tube.   ___ ___ ___ _____

14. If continuous tube feeding was being administered by infusion pump, disconnected infusion pump and administered medication as ordered, followed by at least 15 mL of water, and then immediately reattached infusion pump. If medications were not compatible with feeding solution, held feeding for an additional 30 to 60 minutes as ordered.   ___ ___ ___ _____

	S	U	NP	Comments

15. Removed and disposed of gloves.

16. Helped patient to a comfortable position and kept head of bed elevated for 1 hour, per agency policy.

17. Raised side rails (as appropriate) and lowered bed to lowest position, locking into position.

18. Placed nurse call system in an accessible location within patient's reach.

19. Disposed of all contaminated supplies in appropriate receptacle and performed hand hygiene.

EVALUATION

1. Observed patient for signs of aspiration.

2. Returned within 30 minutes to evaluate patient's response to medications.

3. Used Teach-Back. Revised instruction if patient or family caregiver was not able to teach back correctly.

DOCUMENTATION

1. Documented method used to check for tube placement, GRV, and pH of aspirate. Documented drug, dose, route, and time administered immediately after administration, not before.

2. Documented evaluation of patient learning.

3. Documented total amount of water used for medication administration.

HAND-OFF REPORTING

1. Reported adverse effects or patient response and withheld drugs to nurse in charge or health care provider.

Student _____ Date _____

Instructor _____ Date _____

PERFORMANCE CHECKLIST SKILL 21.3 **APPLYING TOPICAL MEDICATIONS TO THE SKIN**

	S	U	NP	Comments

ASSESSMENT

1. Checked accuracy and completeness of each MAR or computer printout with health care provider's written medication order. Checked patient's name, medication name and dosage, route of administration, and time of administration. Clarified incomplete or unclear orders with heath care provider before administration. ___ ___ ___ _____

2. Reviewed medication reference information related to medication, including action, purpose, normal dose and route, side effects, time of onset and peak action, and nursing implications. ___ ___ ___ _____

3. Assessed patient's medical and medication history and history of allergies (including latex and topical agent). Listed drug allergies on each page of the MAR and prominently displayed them on the patient's electronic health record, per agency policy. If patient had an allergy, provided allergy bracelet. ___ ___ ___ _____

4. Reviewed EHR to determine patient's age and history of dehydration, malnutrition, exposure to radiation therapy, underlying chronic conditions, and edema of the skin. ___ ___ ___ _____

5. Assessed patient's/family caregiver's health literacy. ___ ___ ___ _____

6. Asked patient to confirm history of allergies: known allergies and allergic response. ___ ___ ___ _____

7. Performed hand hygiene and assessed condition of skin or membrane where medication was to be applied. If there was an open wound or drainage, applied clean gloves. First washed site thoroughly with mild, nondrying soap and warm water; rinsed; and dried. Ensured any previously applied medication or debris was removed. Also removed any blood, body fluids, secretions, or excretions. Assessed for symptoms of skin irritation. Removed gloves when finished. Performed hand hygiene. ___ ___ ___ _____

8. Determined amount of topical agent required for application by assessing skin site, reviewing health care provider's order, and reading application directions carefully. ___ ___ ___ _____

	S	U	NP	Comments

9. Determined if patient or family caregiver was physically able to apply medication by assessing grasp, hand strength, reach, and coordination.   ___ ___ ___ _____

10. Assessed patient's knowledge, prior experience with topical medications, and feelings about the procedure.   ___ ___ ___ _____

PLANNING

1. Determined expected outcomes following completion of procedure.   ___ ___ ___ _____

2. Provided privacy and explained procedure to patient. Discussed purpose and side effects of each medication. If applicable, taught patient how to report any side effects. Was specific if patient wished to self-administer medications. Allowed sufficient time for patient to ask questions.   ___ ___ ___ _____

3. Planned preparation to avoid interruption. Created a quiet environment. Did not take phone calls or talk with others. Followed agency "No-Interruption Zone" policy. Kept all pages of the MAR or computer printout for one patient together or looked only at one patient's electronic MAR at a time.   ___ ___ ___ _____

4. Obtained and organized supplies for topical medication administration at bedside.   ___ ___ ___ _____

IMPLEMENTATION

1. Performed hand hygiene. Prepared medications for application. Checked label of medication against MAR two times. Checked expiration date on container.   ___ ___ ___ _____

2. Took medication(s) to patient at correct time, per agency policy. During administration, applied seven rights of medication administration. Performed hand hygiene.   ___ ___ ___ _____

3. Identified patient using at least two identifiers, per agency policy. Compared identifiers with information on patient's MAR or EHR.   ___ ___ ___ _____

4. At patient's bedside, again compared MAR or computer printout with names of medications on medication labels and patient name. Asked patient again about any allergies.   ___ ___ ___ _____

5. Helped patient to a comfortable position. Organized and arranged supplies at bedside.   ___ ___ ___ _____

6. Performed hand hygiene. If patient's skin was broken, applied sterile gloves. Otherwise, applied clean gloves.   ___ ___ ___ _____

7. Applied topical creams, ointments, and oil-based lotions.   ___ ___ ___ _____

	S	U	NP	Comments

a. Exposed affected area while keeping unaffected areas covered.

b. Washed, rinsed, and dried affected area before applying medication if not done earlier.

c. If skin was excessively dry and flaking, applied topical agent while skin was still damp.

d. After washing, removed gloves, performed hand hygiene, and applied new clean or sterile gloves.

e. Placed required amount of medication in palm of gloved hand and softened by rubbing briskly between hands.

f. Told patient that initial application of agent might feel cold. Once medication was softened, spread it evenly over skin surface, using long, even strokes that followed direction of hair growth. Did not vigorously rub skin. Applied to thickness specified by manufacturer instructions.

g. Explained to patient that skin might feel greasy after application.

8. Applied antianginal (nitroglycerin) ointment.

a. Removed previous dose paper. Folded used paper containing any residual medication with used sides together and disposed of it in biohazard trash container. Wiped off residual medication with tissue.

b. Wrote date, time, and initials on new application paper.

c. Applied desired number of inches of ointment using paper-measuring guide.

d. Selected new application site: Applied nitroglycerin to chest area, back, abdomen, or anterior thigh. Did not apply on nonintact skin or hairy surfaces or over scar tissue.

e. Applied ointment to skin surface by holding edge or back of paper-measuring guide and placing ointment and paper directly on skin. Did not rub or massage ointment into skin.

f. Secured ointment and paper with transparent dressing or strip of tape. Applied dressing or plastic wrap only when instructed by pharmacy.

9. Applied transdermal patches.

a. If old patch was present, removed it and cleaned the area. Checked between skinfolds for patch.

	S	U	NP	Comments

b. Disposed of old patch by folding in half with sticky sides together; cut per agency policy. Disposed of it in biohazard trash bag. Removed and disposed of gloves and performed hand hygiene.   ___ ___ ___   _____

c. Use soft-tip or felt-tip pen to date and initial outer side of new patch before applying it and noted time of administration.   ___ ___ ___   _____

d. Chose a new site that was clean, intact, dry, and free of hair. Followed specific instructions for placement locations, if applicable. Did not apply patch on skin that was oily, burned, cut, or irritated.   ___ ___ ___   _____

e. Applied clean gloves. Carefully removed patch from its protective covering by pulling off liner. Held patch by edge without touching adhesive edges.   ___ ___ ___   _____

f. Applied patch. Held palm of one hand firmly over patch for 10 seconds. Made sure that it stuck well, especially around edges. Applied overlay if provided with patch.   ___ ___ ___   _____

g. Did not apply patch to previously used sites for at least 1 week.   ___ ___ ___   _____

h. Instructed patient that transdermal patches were never to be cut in half; a change in dose would require a prescription for new strength of transdermal medication.   ___ ___ ___   _____

i. Instructed patient to always remove old patch and clean skin before applying new and to not use alternative forms of medication when using patches.   ___ ___ ___   _____

10. Administered aerosol sprays.   ___ ___ ___   _____

a. Shook container vigorously. Read container label for distance recommended to hold spray away from area.   ___ ___ ___   _____

b. Asked patient to turn face away from spray or briefly cover face with towel while spraying neck or chest.   ___ ___ ___   _____

c. Sprayed medication evenly over affected site.   ___ ___ ___   _____

11. Applied suspension-based lotion.   ___ ___ ___   _____

a. Shook container vigorously.   ___ ___ ___   _____

b. Applied small amount of lotion to small gauze dressing or pad and applied to skin by stroking evenly in direction of hair growth.   ___ ___ ___   _____

c. Explained to patient that area would feel cool and dry.   ___ ___ ___   _____

340

	S	U	NP	Comments

12. Applied powder.

   a. Ensured that skin surface was thoroughly dry. With nondominant hand, fully spread apart any skinfolds, such as between toes or under axilla, and dried with a towel.

   b. If area of application was near face, asked patient to turn face away from powder or briefly cover face with a towel.

   c. Dusted skin site lightly with dispenser so that area was covered with fine, thin layer of powder. Option: Covered skin area with dressing if ordered by health care provider.

13. Helped patient to a comfortable position, reapplied gown, and covered with bed linen as desired.

14. Raised side rails (as appropriate) and lowered bed to lowest position, locking into position.

15. Placed nurse call system in accessible location within patient's reach.

16. Disposed of all contaminated supplies in an appropriate receptacle, removed and disposed of gloves, and performed hand hygiene.

EVALUATION

1. Inspected condition of skin between applications.

2. Had patient keep diary of doses taken.

3. Observed patient or family caregiver apply topical medication.

4. Used Teach-Back: Revised instruction if patient or family caregiver was not able to teach back correctly.

DOCUMENTATION

1. Documented drug, dose or strength, site of application, and time administered immediately after administration, not before.

2. Documented evaluation of patient learning.

3. Described condition of skin before each topical application of medication.

HAND-OFF REPORTING

1. Reported adverse effects or changes in appearance and condition of skin lesions to health care provider.

PERFORMANCE CHECKLIST SKILL 21.4 **ADMINISTERING OPHTHALMIC MEDICATIONS**

	S	U	NP	Comments

ASSESSMENT

1. Checked accuracy and completeness of each MAR or computer printout with health care provider's written medication order. Check patient's name, medication name and dosage, route of administration, and time of administration. Clarified incomplete or unclear orders with health care provider before administration.

2. Reviewed medication reference information about medication, including action, purpose, normal dose and route, side effects, time of onset and peak action, and nursing implications.

3. Assessed patient's medical and medication history and history of allergies (including latex). Listed drug allergies on each page of the MAR and prominently displayed on the patient's electronic health record (EHR), per agency policy. If patient had an allergy, provided an allergy bracelet.

4. Assessed patient's/family caregiver's health literacy.

5. Asked patient to confirm history of allergies: known allergies and allergic response.

6. Performed hand hygiene and applied clean gloves (if drainage present). Assessed condition of external eye structures.

7. Determined whether patient had any symptoms of eye discomfort or visual impairment.

8. Assessed patient's level of consciousness (LOC) and ability to follow directions.

9. Assessed patient's and family caregiver's ability to manipulate and hold dropper or ocular disk.

10. Assessed patient's and family caregiver's knowledge, prior experience with eye medications, and feelings about procedure.

PLANNING

1. Determined expected outcomes following completion of procedure.

	S	U	NP	Comments

2. Provided privacy and explained the purpose of each medication, action, indication, and possible adverse effects. Allowed sufficient time for patient to ask any questions. Allowed patients who self-instill medications to give drops under nurse's supervision, per agency policy. ___ ___ ___ _____

3. Planned preparation to avoid interruption. Created a quiet environment. Did not take phone calls or talk with others. Followed agency "No-Interruption Zone" policy. Kept all pages of the MAR or computer printout for one patient together or looked only at one patient's electronic MAR at a time. ___ ___ ___ _____

4. Obtained and organized equipment for ophthalmic medication administration at the bedside. ___ ___ ___ _____

5. If required, took eyedrops out of refrigerator and rewarmed to room temperature before administering to patient. Checked expiration date on container. ___ ___ ___ _____

IMPLEMENTATION

1. Performed hand hygiene. Prepared medications for one patient at a time using aseptic technique and avoiding distractions. Checked label of medication against MAR two times, when removing medication from unit dose or AMDS and before leaving preparation area. ___ ___ ___ _____

2. Took medication(s) to patient at correct time, per agency policy. During administration, applied seven rights of medication administration. Performed hand hygiene. ___ ___ ___ _____

3. Identified patient using at least two identifiers, per agency policy. Compared identifiers with information on patient's MAR or EHR. ___ ___ ___ _____

4. At patient's bedside, again compared MAR or computer printout with names of medications on medication labels and patient name. Asked patient about any allergies. ___ ___ ___ _____

5. Provided privacy and helped patient to a comfortable sitting position. Arranged supplies at bedside. ___ ___ ___ _____

6. Administered eye medications. ___ ___ ___ _____

   a. Performed hand hygiene. Applied clean gloves. Asked patient to lie supine or sit back in a chair with head slightly hyperextended, looking up. ___ ___ ___ _____

   b. If drainage or crusting was present along eyelid margins or inner canthus, gently washed away. Soaked any dried crusts with a warm, damp washcloth or cotton ball over eye for several minutes. Always wiped clean from inner to outer canthus. Removed and disposed of gloves and performed hand hygiene. ___ ___ ___ _____

	S	U	NP	Comments

c. Explained that there might be a temporary burning sensation from drops.

    ___ ___ ___ _____

d. Instilled eyedrops.

    ___ ___ ___ _____

  (1) Applied clean gloves. Held clean cotton ball or tissue in nondominant hand on patient's cheekbone just below lower eyelid.

    ___ ___ ___ _____

  (2) With tissue or cotton ball resting below lower lid, gently pressed downward with thumb or forefinger against bony orbit, exposing conjunctival sac. Never pressed directly against patient's eyeball.

    ___ ___ ___ _____

  (3) Asked patient to look at ceiling. Rested dominant hand on patient's forehead; held filled medication eyedropper approximately 1 to 2 cm (1/4 to 1/2 inch) above conjunctival sac.

    ___ ___ ___ _____

  (4) Dropped prescribed number of drops into lower conjunctival sac

    ___ ___ ___ _____

  (5) If patient blinked or closed eye, causing drops to land on outer lid margins, repeated procedure.

    ___ ___ ___ _____

  (6) When administering drops that may cause systemic effects, applied gentle pressure to patient's nasolacrimal duct with clean tissue for 30 to 60 seconds over each eye, one at a time. Avoided pressure directly against patient's eyeball.

    ___ ___ ___ _____

  (7) After instilling drops, asked patient to close eyes gently.

    ___ ___ ___ _____

e. Instilled ophthalmic ointment.

    ___ ___ ___ _____

  (1) Applied clean gloves. Holding applicator above lower lid margin, applied thin ribbon of ointment evenly along inner edge of lower eyelid on conjunctiva from inner to outer canthus.

    ___ ___ ___ _____

  (2) Had patient close eye and rubbed lid lightly in a circular motion with a cotton ball if not contraindicated. Avoided placing pressure directly against patient's eyeball.

    ___ ___ ___ _____

  (3) If excess medication was on eyelid, gently wiped it from inner to outer canthus.

    ___ ___ ___ _____

  (4) If patient needed an eye patch, applied a clean one by placing it over affected eye so that entire eye was covered. Taped securely without applying pressure to eye.

    ___ ___ ___ _____

f. Inserted intraocular disk.

    ___ ___ ___ _____

	S	U	NP	Comments

(1) Applied clean gloves. Opened package containing disk. Gently pressed fingertip against disk so that it adhered to finger. Positioned convex side of disk on fingertip. ___ ___ ___ _____

(2) With other hand, gently pulled patient's lower eyelid away from eye. Asked patient to look up. ___ ___ ___ _____

(3) Placed disk in a conjunctival sac so that it floated on sclera between iris and lower eyelid. ___ ___ ___ _____

(4) Pulled patient's lower eyelid out and over disk. Repeated if disk was visible. ___ ___ ___ _____

7. After administering eye medications, removed and disposed of gloves and soiled supplies; performed hand hygiene. ___ ___ ___ _____

8. Removed intraocular disk. ___ ___ ___ _____

   a. Performed hand hygiene and applied clean gloves. Gently pulled downward on lower eyelid using nondominant hand. ___ ___ ___ _____

   b. Using forefinger and thumb of dominant hand, pinched disk and lifted it out of patient's eye. ___ ___ ___ _____

   c. Removed and disposed of gloves and performed hand hygiene. ___ ___ ___ _____

9. Helped patient to a comfortable position. ___ ___ ___ _____

10. Raised side rails (as appropriate) and lowered bed to lowest position, locking into position. ___ ___ ___ _____

11. Placed nurse call system in accessible location within patient's reach. ___ ___ ___ _____

12. Performed hand hygiene. ___ ___ ___ _____

EVALUATION

1. Observed response to medication by assessing visual changes, asking if symptoms were relieved, and noting any side effects or discomfort felt. ___ ___ ___ _____

2. Asked patient to discuss purpose of drug, action, side effects, and technique of administration. ___ ___ ___ _____

3. Used Teach-Back. Revised instruction if patient or family caregiver was not able to teach back correctly. ___ ___ ___ _____

DOCUMENTATION

1. Documented drug, concentration, dose or strength, number of drops, site of application, and time of administration immediately after administration, not before. Included initials or signature. ___ ___ ___ _____

	S	U	NP	Comments

2. Documented evaluation of patient learning.   _____ _____ _____ _____

3. Documented objective data related to tissues involved, any subjective data, and patient's response to medications. Noted evidence of any side effects.   _____ _____ _____ _____

HAND-OFF REPORTING

1. Reported adverse effects/patient response and/or withheld drugs to nurse in charge or health care provider. If necessary, notified health care provider immediately.   _____ _____ _____ _____

Student _____ Date _____

Instructor _____ Date _____

PERFORMANCE CHECKLIST SKILL 21.5 **ADMINISTERING EAR MEDICATIONS**

	S	U	NP	Comments

ASSESSMENT

1. Checked accuracy and completeness of each MAR with health care provider's written medication order. Checked patient's name, medication name and dosage, route of administration, and time of administration. Clarified incomplete or unclear orders with health care provider before administration. ___ ___ ___ _____

2. Reviewed medication reference information for pertinent information related to medication, including action, purpose, normal dose and route, side effects, time of onset and peak action, and nursing implications. ___ ___ ___ _____

3. Assessed patient's medical and medication history and history of allergies (including latex). Listed drug allergies on each page of the MAR and prominently displayed on the patient's electronic health record (EHR), per agency policy. If patient had an allergy, provided an allergy bracelet. ___ ___ ___ _____

4. Assessed patient's/family caregiver's health literacy. ___ ___ ___ _____

5. Asked patient to confirm history of allergies: known allergies and allergic response. ___ ___ ___ _____

6. Performed hand hygiene and assessed condition of external ear structures. If drainage was present, applied clean gloves. ___ ___ ___ _____

7. Determined whether patient had any symptoms of ear discomfort or hearing impairment. ___ ___ ___ _____

8. Assessed patient's level of consciousness (LOC) and ability to follow directions. Performed hand hygiene. ___ ___ ___ _____

9. Assessed patient's or family caregiver's ability to manipulate and hold ear dropper. ___ ___ ___ _____

10. Assessed patient's knowledge, prior experience with ear medications, desire to self-administer medication, and feelings about procedure. ___ ___ ___ _____

PLANNING

1. Determined expected outcomes following completion of procedure. ___ ___ ___ _____

	S	U	NP	Comments

2. Provided privacy and explained purpose of each medication, action, indication, and possible adverse effects. Allowed sufficient time for patient to ask any questions. Allowed patients who self-instill medications to give ear medications under nurse's supervision.

3. Planned procedure to avoid interruption. Created a quiet environment. Did not take phone calls or talk with others. Followed agency "No-Interruption Zone" policy. Kept all pages of the MAR or computer printout for one patient together or looked only at one patient's electronic MAR at a time.

4. Obtained and organized equipment for eardrop installation at bedside.

5. If required, took eardrops out of refrigerator and rewarmed to room temperature before administering to patient. Checked expiration date on container.

IMPLEMENTATION

1. Performed hand hygiene. Prepared medications for one patient at a time using aseptic technique and avoiding distractions. Checked label of medication carefully with MAR or computer printout two times when preparing medication.

2. Took medication(s) to patient at correct time, per agency policy. During administration, applied seven rights of medication administration. Performed hand hygiene.

3. Identified patient using at least two identifiers, per agency policy. Compared identifiers with information on patient's MAR or EHR.

4. At patient's bedside, again compared MAR or computer printout with names of medications on medication labels and patient name. Asked patient again about any allergies.

5. Performed hand hygiene. Positioned patient on side (if not contraindicated) with ear to be treated facing up, or had patient sit in a chair or at the bedside. Stabilized patient's head with patient's own hand. Option: Applied clean gloves if ear drainage present.

6. Straightened ear canal by pulling pinna up and back to 10 o'clock position (adult or child older than age 3) or down and back to 6 to 9 o'clock position (child younger than age 3).

	S	U	NP	Comments

7. If cerumen or drainage occluded outermost part of ear canal, wiped out gently with a cotton-tipped applicator. Took care not to force cerumen into canal. ___ ___ ___ _____

8. Instilled prescribed drops holding dropper 1 cm (1/2 inch) above ear canal. ___ ___ ___ _____

9. Asked patient to remain in side-lying position for a few minutes. Applied gentle massage or pressure to tragus of ear with finger. ___ ___ ___ _____

10. If ordered, gently inserted part of cotton ball into outermost part of canal. Did not press cotton into canal. ___ ___ ___ _____

11. Removed cotton after 15 minutes. Helped patient to a comfortable position after drops were absorbed. ___ ___ ___ _____

12. Raised side rails (as appropriate) and lowered bed to lowest position locking into position. ___ ___ ___ _____

13. Placed nurse call system in an accessible location within patient's reach. ___ ___ ___ _____

14. Disposed of all contaminated supplies in appropriate receptacle, removed and disposed of gloves, and performed hand hygiene. ___ ___ ___ _____

EVALUATION

1. Observed response to medication by assessing hearing changes, asking if symptoms were relieved, and noting any side effects or discomfort felt. ___ ___ ___ _____

2. Asked patient to discuss purpose of drug, action, side effects, and technique of administration. ___ ___ ___ _____

3. Used Teach-Back. Revised instruction if patient or family caregiver was not able to teach back correctly. ___ ___ ___ _____

DOCUMENTATION

1. Documented drug, concentration, dose or strength, number of drops, site of application, and time of administration on MAR immediately after administration, not before. Included initials or signature. ___ ___ ___ _____

2. Documented objective data related to tissues involved, any subjective data, and patient's response to medications. Noted any side effects experienced. ___ ___ ___ _____

3. Documented evaluation of patient learning. ___ ___ ___ _____

HAND-OFF REPORTING

1. Reported adverse effects/patient response and/or withheld drugs to nurse in charge or health care provider. If required, notified health care provider immediately. ___ ___ ___ _____

Student _____ Date _____

Instructor _____ Date _____

PERFORMANCE CHECKLIST SKILL 21.6 **ADMINISTERING NASAL INSTILLATIONS**

	S	U	NP	Comments

ASSESSMENT

1. Checked accuracy and completeness of each MAR or computer printout with health care provider's written medication order. Checked patient's name, medication name and dosage, route of administration, and time of administration. Clarified incomplete or unclear orders with health care provider before administration.

2. Reviewed medication reference information for medication action, purpose, normal dose, side effects, time and peak of onset, how slowly to give medication, and nursing implications.

3. Assessed patient's medical history, medication history, and history of allergies. Listed drug allergies on each page of the MAR and prominently displayed on the patient's electronic health record (EHR), per agency policy. If patient had allergy, provided an allergy bracelet.

4. Assessed patient's/family caregiver's health literacy.

5. Asked patient to confirm history of allergies: known allergies and allergic response.

6. Performed hand hygiene. When drainage present, applied clean gloves. Used penlight and inspected condition of nose and sinuses. Palpated sinuses for pain or tenderness. Noted type of drainage if present. Removed gloves and performed hand hygiene.

7. Assessed patient's knowledge, prior experience regarding use of nasal instillations, technique for instillation, willingness to learn self-administration, and feelings about procedure.

PLANNING

1. Determined expected outcomes following completion of procedure.

2. Provided privacy and explained procedure to patient. Discussed purpose and side effects of each medication. If applicable, taught patient how to report any side effects. Was specific if patient wished to self-administer medications. Allowed sufficient time for patient to ask questions.

350

	S	U	NP	Comments

3. Planned preparation to avoid interruption. Created a quiet environment. Did not take phone calls or talk with others. Followed agency "No-Interruption Zone" policy. Kept all pages of the MAR or computer printout for one patient together or looked only at one patient's electronic MAR at a time. ___ ___ ___ _____

4. Obtained and organized equipment for nasal instillation of medication at bedside. ___ ___ ___ _____

5. Removed nasal spray from storage and took to patient's room. Checked expiration date on container. ___ ___ ___ _____

IMPLEMENTATION

1. Performed hand hygiene. Prepared medications for one patient at a time using aseptic technique and avoiding distractions. Checked label of medication carefully with MAR or computer printout two times. ___ ___ ___ _____

2. Took medication(s) to patient at correct time, per agency policy. During administration, applied seven rights of medication administration. Performed hand hygiene. ___ ___ ___ _____

3. Identified patient using at least two identifiers, per agency policy. Compared identifiers with information on patient's MAR or EHR. ___ ___ ___ _____

4. At patient's bedside again compared MAR or computer printout with names of medications on medication labels and patient name. Asked patient again about any allergies. ___ ___ ___ _____

5. Helped patient to a comfortable position. ___ ___ ___ _____

6. Performed hand hygiene. Arranged supplies and medications at bedside. Applied clean gloves if drainage was present. ___ ___ ___ _____

7. Gently rolled or shook container. Instructed patient to clear or blow their nose gently unless contraindicated. ___ ___ ___ _____

8. Administered nose drops. ___ ___ ___ _____

   a. Helped patient to supine position and positioned head properly. ___ ___ ___ _____

     (1) For access to posterior pharynx, tilted patient's head backward. ___ ___ ___ _____

     (2) For access to ethmoid or sphenoid sinus, tilted head back over edge of bed or placed small pillow under patient's shoulder and tilted head back. ___ ___ ___ _____

	S	U	NP	Comments

(3) For access to frontal and maxillary sinus, tilted head back over edge of bed or pillow with head turned toward side to be treated.

    b. Supported patient's head with nondominant hand.

    c. Instructed patient to breathe through mouth.

    d. Held dropper 1 cm (1/2 inch) above nares and instilled prescribed number of drops toward midline of ethmoid bone.

    e. Had patient remain in supine position for 5 minutes.

    f. Offered facial tissue to blot runny nose, but cautioned patient against blowing nose for several minutes.

9. Administered nasal spray.

    a. Helped patient into upright position with head tilted slightly forward.

    b. Instructed or assisted patient to insert tip of nasal spray into appropriate nares and occlude other nostril with finger. Pointed spray tip toward side and away from center of nose.

    c. Had patient spray medication into nose while inhaling. Helped remove nozzle from nose and instructed to breathe out through mouth.

    d. Offered facial tissue to blot runny nose, but cautioned patient against blowing nose for several minutes.

10. Helped patient to a comfortable position after medication was absorbed.

11. Raised side rails (as appropriate) and lowered bed to lowest position, locking into position.

12. Placed nurse call system in an accessible location within patient's reach.

13. Disposed of all contaminated supplies in an appropriate receptacle, removed and disposed of gloves, and performed hand hygiene.

EVALUATION

1. Observed patient for onset of side effects 15 to 30 minutes after administration.

2. Asked if patient was able to breathe through nose after decongestant administration. If necessary, had patient occlude one nostril at a time and breathe deeply.

352

	S	U	NP	Comments

3. Reinspected condition of nasal passages between instillations. ___ ___ ___ _____

4. Asked patient to describe risks of overuse of decongestants and methods for administration. ___ ___ ___ _____

5. Had patient demonstrate self-medication. ___ ___ ___ _____

6. Used Teach-Back. Revised instruction if patient or family caregiver was not able to teach back correctly. ___ ___ ___ _____

DOCUMENTATION

1. Documented drug name, concentration, number of drops, nares into which drug was instilled, and actual time of administration immediately after administration, not before. Included initials or signature. ___ ___ ___ _____

2. Documented patient's response to medication. ___ ___ ___ _____

3. Documented evaluation of patient learning. ___ ___ ___ _____

HAND-OFF REPORTING

1. Reported any unusual systemic or adverse effects/patient response and/or withheld drugs to nurse in charge or health care provider. ___ ___ ___ _____

PERFORMANCE CHECKLIST SKILL 21.7 **USING METERED-DOSE INHALERS (MDIS)**

	S	U	NP	Comments

ASSESSMENT

1. Checked accuracy and completeness of each MAR or computer printout with health care provider's written medication order. Checked patient's name, medication name and dosage, route of administration, and time of administration. Clarified incomplete or unclear orders with health care provider before administration.

2. Reviewed medication reference information for pertinent information related to medication, including action, purpose, normal dose and route, side effects, time of onset and peak action, and nursing implications.

3. Assessed patient's medical and medication history and history of allergies. Listed drug allergies on each page of the MAR and prominently displayed on the patient's electronic health record (EHR), per agency policy. If patient had allergy, provided allergy bracelet.

4. Assessed patient's/family caregiver's health literacy.

5. Asked patient to confirm history of allergies: known allergies and allergic response.

6. Performed hand hygiene and assessed respiratory pattern and auscultated breath sounds. Also assessed exercise tolerance.

7. Measured patient's peak expiratory flow rate using a peak flow meter. Had patient measure if doing so at home. Used patient's peak flow meter if available.

8. Assessed patient's symptoms before initiating medication therapy.

9. Assessed patient's ability to hold, manipulate, and depress canister and inhaler.

10. If patient was previously instructed in self-administration, had patient demonstrate how to use the device. Performed hand hygiene.

11. Assessed patient's readiness and ability to learn.

	S	U	NP	Comments

12. Assessed patient's knowledge, prior experience, understanding of disease and purpose and action of prescribed medications, and feelings about procedure. ___ ___ ___ _____

PLANNING

1. Determined expected outcomes following completion of procedure. ___ ___ ___ _____

2. Provided privacy and explained procedure to patient. Discussed purpose of each medication, action, and possible adverse effects. Allowed patient to ask any questions about the drugs. Explained what a metered dose was and how to administer. Warned about overuse of inhaler and side effects. Was specific if patient wished to self-administer drug. Explained where and how to set up at home. ___ ___ ___ _____

3. Planned preparation to avoid interruption. Created a quiet environment. Did not take phone calls or talk with others. Followed agency "No-Interruption Zone" policy. Kept all pages of the MAR or computer printout for one patient together or looked only at one patient's electronic MAR at a time. ___ ___ ___ _____

4. Organized and set up equipment for MDI administration at bedside. ___ ___ ___ _____

IMPLEMENTATION

1. Performed hand hygiene and prepared medications for inhalation. Checked label of medication against MAR two times. Took inhaler device out of storage and into the patient's room. Checked expiration date on container. ___ ___ ___ _____

2. Took medication(s) to patient at correct time, per agency policy. During administration, applied seven rights of medication administration. Performed hand hygiene. ___ ___ ___ _____

3. Identified patient using at least two identifiers, per agency policy. Compared identifiers with information on patient's MAR or EHR. ___ ___ ___ _____

4. At patient's bedside, again compared MAR or computer printout with names of medications on medication labels and patient name. Asked patient about any allergies. ___ ___ ___ _____

5. Helped patient to sit up in a chair or high-Fowler position if in bed. Allowed adequate time for patient to manipulate inhaler, canister, and spacer device (if provided). Explained and demonstrated how canister fit into the inhaler. ___ ___ ___ _____

6. Performed hand hygiene. Explained and demonstrated steps for administering MDI without spacer. ___ ___ ___ _____

	S	U	NP	Comments

a. Inserted MDI canister into holder. Then removed mouthpiece cover from inhaler. ___ ___ ___ _____

b. Shook inhaler well for 2 to 5 seconds (five or six shakes). ___ ___ ___ _____

c. Held inhaler in dominant hand. ___ ___ ___ _____

d. Had patient stand or sit and instructed how to position inhaler in one of two ways: ___ ___ ___ _____

(1) Had patient place the mouthpiece in the mouth between the teeth and over the tongue, aimed toward back of throat, with lips closed tightly around it. Did not block the mouthpiece with the teeth or tongue. ___ ___ ___ _____

(2) Positioned mouthpiece 2 to 4 cm (1 to 2 inches) in front of widely opened mouth, with opening of inhaler toward back of throat. Lips did not touch inhaler. ___ ___ ___ _____

e. While holding the mouthpiece away from the mouth, had patient take a deep breath and exhale completely. ___ ___ ___ _____

f. With inhaler positioned, had patient hold it with a thumb at mouthpiece and index and middle fingers at top. ___ ___ ___ _____

g. Instructed patient to tilt head back slightly and inhale slowly and deeply through mouth for 3 to 5 seconds while depressing canister fully. ___ ___ ___ _____

h. Had patient hold breath for about 10 seconds. ___ ___ ___ _____

i. Had patient remove MDI from mouth before exhaling and exhale slowly through nose or pursed lips. ___ ___ ___ _____

7. Explained and demonstrated steps to administer MDI using spacer device. ___ ___ ___ _____

a. Removed mouthpiece cover from MDI and mouthpiece of spacer device. ___ ___ ___ _____

b. Shook inhaler well for 2 to 5 seconds (five or six shakes). ___ ___ ___ _____

c. Inserted MDI into end of spacer device. ___ ___ ___ _____

d. Instructed patient to place spacer device mouthpiece in mouth and close lips. Did not insert beyond raised lip on mouthpiece. Avoided covering small exhalation slots with lips. ___ ___ ___ _____

e. Had patient take a deep breath, exhale, and then breathe normally through spacer device mouthpiece. ___ ___ ___ _____

	S	U	NP	Comments

f. Instructed patient to depress medication canister one (1) time, spraying (1) one puff into spacer device. ___ ___ ___ _____

g. Had patient breathe in slowly and fully through the mouth for 5 seconds. ___ ___ ___ _____

h. Instructed patient to hold full breath for 10 seconds. ___ ___ ___ _____

i. Had patient remove MDI and spacer and then exhale. ___ ___ ___ _____

8. Explained steps to administer a DPI. ___ ___ ___ _____

   a. If DPI had an external counter, noted number indicated. ___ ___ ___ _____

   b. Removed mouthpiece cover. Did not shake inhaler. ___ ___ ___ _____

   c. Prepared medication. Followed manufacturer's specific instructions. ___ ___ ___ _____

   d. Had patient take a breath and exhale away from the inhaler. ___ ___ ___ _____

   e. Had patient position mouthpiece of DPI between lips and inhale quickly and deeply through mouth. ___ ___ ___ _____

   f. Had patient hold breath for 5 to 10 seconds. ___ ___ ___ _____

9. Explained steps to administer a soft mist inhaler: ___ ___ ___ _____

   a. Prepared inhaler. Followed package directions. ___ ___ ___ _____

   b. Primed inhaler. Pointed the inhaler toward the ground and pressed the dose-release button before closing the cap. With the cap closed, turned the clear base half a turn in the same direction as the arrows on the label until the base clicked. Then fully opened the cap and once again pointed the inhaler at the ground and pressed the dose-release button. Repeated this process until a cloud of mist was visible. Repeated the process three more times. ___ ___ ___ _____

   c. Loaded one puff of medication by keeping the cap closed and turning the clear base half a turn in the same direction as the arrows on the label until the base clicked. ___ ___ ___ _____

   d. Opened the cap until it snapped fully open. Stood or sat up straight and breathed out slowly and fully. ___ ___ ___ _____

   e. Did not breathe out over the inhaler. ___ ___ ___ _____

	S	U	NP	Comments

f. Sealed lips around the mouthpiece of the inhaler without covering the air vents on the sides and pointed the inhaler toward the back of the throat.

g. Took a slow, deep breath in through the mouthpiece and pressed the dose-release button. Breathed in slowly, then held breath for 10 seconds before slowing exhaling.

h. Repeated the process to deliver the second puff (two puffs equals one dose).

i. Closed the cap and stored inhaler.

10. Instructed patient to wait 20 to 30 seconds between inhalations (if same medication) or 2 to 5 minutes between inhalations (if different medications). Ensured patient inhaled correct number of prescribed puffs.

11. Instructed patient to not repeat inhalations before next scheduled dose.

12. Warned patient that they might feel a gagging sensation in throat caused by droplets of medication on pharynx or tongue.

13. About 2 minutes after last dose, instructed patient to rinse mouth with warm water and spit water out.

14. Instructed patient how to clean the inhaler.

a. Once a day, removed MDI canister and cap from mouthpiece. Did not wash canister or immerse it in water. Ran warm tap water through top and bottom of plastic mouthpiece for 30 to 60 seconds. Made sure that inhaler was completely dry before reusing. Did not get valve mechanism of canister wet.

b. Instructed patient to clean mouthpiece twice a week with mild dishwashing soap, rinse thoroughly, and dry completely before storage.

c. Cleaned SMI once a week by wiping the mouthpiece (inside and outside) with a clean, damp cloth.

15. Asked if patient had any questions.

16. Helped patient to a comfortable position.

17. Raised side rails (as appropriate) and lowered bed to lowest position, locking into position.

18. Placed nurse call system in an accessible location within patient's reach.

	S	U	NP	Comments

19. Disposed of all contaminated supplies in appropriate receptacle, removed and disposed of gloves, and performed hand hygiene. ___ ___ ___ _____

EVALUATION

1. Auscultated patient lungs, listened for abnormal breath sounds, and obtained peak flow measures if ordered. ___ ___ ___ _____

2. Had patient explain and demonstrate steps in use and cleaning of inhaler. ___ ___ ___ _____

3. Asked patient to explain drug schedule and dose of medication. ___ ___ ___ _____

4. Asked patient to describe side effects of medication and criteria for calling health care provider. ___ ___ ___ _____

5. Used Teach-Back. Revised instruction if patient or family caregiver was not able to teach back correctly. ___ ___ ___ _____

DOCUMENTATION

1. Documented drug, dose or strength, number of inhalations, and time administered immediately after administration, not before. Included initials or signature. ___ ___ ___ _____

2. Documented patient's response to MDI, evidence of side effects, and patient's ability to use MDI. ___ ___ ___ _____

3. Documented evaluation of patient learning. ___ ___ ___ _____

HAND-OFF REPORTING

1. Reported any side effects of medication to health care provider. ___ ___ ___ _____

Student _____ Date _____

Instructor _____ Date _____

PERFORMANCE CHECKLIST SKILL 21.8 **USING SMALL-VOLUME NEBULIZERS**

	S	U	NP	Comments

ASSESSMENT

1. Check accuracy and completeness of each MAR or computer printout with health care provider's written medication order. Checked patient's name, medication name and dosage, route of administration, and time of administration. Clarified incomplete or unclear orders with health care provider before administration.

2. Reviewed medication reference for pertinent information related to medication, including diluent, action, purpose, normal dose and route, side effects, time of onset and peak action, and nursing implications.

3. Assessed patient's medical and medication history and history of allergies. Listed medication allergies on each page of the MAR and prominently displayed on the patient's electronic health record (EHR). If allergies were present, patient wore an allergy bracelet.

4. Assessed patient's/family caregiver's health literacy.

5. Asked patient to describe history of allergies: known allergies and allergic response.

6. Performed hand hygiene. Assessed pulse, respirations, breath sounds, pulse oximetry, and peak flow measurement (if ordered) before beginning treatment.

7. Assessed patient's grasp and ability to assemble, hold, and manipulate nebulizer mouthpiece and tubing; identified any mobility restrictions.

8. Assessed patient's knowledge, prior experience with nebulizers and nebulizer medication, and feelings about procedure.

9. Assessed patient's readiness to learn.

PLANNING

1. Determined expected outcomes following completion of procedure.

	S	U	NP	Comments

2. Provided privacy and explained procedure to patient. Was specific if patient wished to self-administer drug. Discussed purpose of each medication, action, and possible adverse effects. Allowed patient to ask any questions about the drugs. Explained how to assemble nebulizer and proper use.

3. Planned preparation to avoid interruption. Created a quiet environment. Did not take phone calls or talk with others. Followed agency "No-Interruption Zone" policy. Kept all pages of MAR or computer printout for one patient together or looked at only one patient's electronic MAR at a time.

4. Organized and set up equipment for nebulizer treatment at bedside.

IMPLEMENTATION

1. Performed hand hygiene and prepared medications for inhalation. Checked label of medication against MAR two times. Took medication vial out of storage and to patient's room. Checked expiration date on container.

2. Took medication(s) to patient at correct time, per agency policy. During administration, applied seven rights of medication administration. Performed hand hygiene.

3. Identified patient using at least two identifiers, per agency policy. Compared identifiers with information on patient's MAR or EHR.

4. At patient's bedside, again compared MAR or computer printout with names of medications on medication labels and patient name. Asked patient again if they had any allergies.

5. Performed hand hygiene and applied clean gloves (if risk of exposure to secretions). Assembled nebulizer equipment per manufacturer directions.

6. Added prescribed medication by pouring medicine into nebulizer cup. (Option: Used a medicine dropper to instill medications.)

7. Attached top to nebulizer cup and ensured that it was secure. Then connected cup to mouthpiece or face mask.

8. Connected tubing to both aerosol compressor and nebulizer cup.

9. Assisted patient to a sitting or semi-Fowler position. Had patient hold mouthpiece between lips with gentle pressure, but ensured lips were sealed.

	S	U	NP	Comments

10. Turned on small-volume nebulizer machine and ensured that a sufficient mist began to flow. ____ ____ ____ _____

11. Instructed patient to take a deep breath, slowly, to a volume slightly greater than normal. Encouraged brief, end-inspiratory pause for about 2 to 3 seconds, and then had patient exhale passively. Option: If needed, used a nose clip so patient breathed only through the mouth. ____ ____ ____ _____

   a. If patient was dyspneic, encouraged holding every fourth or fifth breath for 5 to 10 seconds. ____ ____ ____ _____

   b. Reminded patient to repeat breathing pattern until drug was completely nebulized. ____ ____ ____ _____

     (1) If health care provider instructed, set time limit as length of treatment rather than waiting for medication to completely nebulize. ____ ____ ____ _____

   c. Tapped nebulizer cup occasionally during and toward end of treatment. ____ ____ ____ _____

   d. Monitored patient's pulse during procedure, especially if beta-adrenergic bronchodilators were used. ____ ____ ____ _____

12. When medication was completely nebulized, turned off machine. Rinsed nebulizer cup per agency policy. Dried completely and stored tubing assembly per agency policy. ____ ____ ____ _____

13. If steroids were nebulized, instructed patient to rinse mouth and gargle with warm water after nebulizer treatment. Had patient spit out solution. ____ ____ ____ _____

14. After nebulizer treatment was complete, had patient take several deep breaths and cough to expectorate mucus. ____ ____ ____ _____

15. Helped patient to a comfortable position. ____ ____ ____ _____

16. Raised side rails (as appropriate) and lowered bed to lowest position, locking into position. ____ ____ ____ _____

17. Placed nurse call system in accessible location within patient's reach. ____ ____ ____ _____

18. Disposed of all contaminated supplies in an appropriate receptacle, removed and disposed of gloves, and performed hand hygiene. ____ ____ ____ _____

EVALUATION

1. Assessed patient's respirations, breath sounds, cough effort, sputum production, pulse oximetry, and peak flow measures if ordered. ____ ____ ____ _____

2. Asked patient to explain drug schedule. ____ ____ ____ _____

362

	S	U	NP	Comments
3. Asked patient to describe side effects of medication and criteria for calling health care provider.	——	——	——	————————
4. Used Teach-Back: Revised instruction if patient or family caregiver was not able to teach back correctly.	——	——	——	————————

DOCUMENTATION

	S	U	NP	Comments
1. Documented drug, dose and strength, route, length of treatment, and time administered immediately after administration, not before.	——	——	——	————————
2. Documented patient's response to treatment.	——	——	——	————————
3. Documented evaluation of patient learning.	——	——	——	————————

HAND-OFF REPORTING

	S	U	NP	Comments
1. Reported adverse effects/patient response and/or withheld drugs to nurse in charge or health care provider.	——	——	——	————————

PERFORMANCE CHECKLIST PROCEDURAL GUIDELINE 21.1   **ADMINISTERING VAGINAL MEDICATIONS**

	S	U	NP	Comments

PROCEDURAL STEPS

1. Checked accuracy and completeness of each MAR or computer printout with health care provider's written medication order. Clarified incomplete or unclear orders with health care provider before administration.

2. Reviewed pertinent information related to medication, including action, indication, purpose, normal dose and route, side effects, time of onset and peak action, and nursing implications.

3. Assessed patient's medical and medication history and history of allergies. Listed drug allergies on each page of the MAR and prominently displayed on the patient's electronic health record (EHR), per agency policy. If patient had an allergy, provided an allergy bracelet.

4. Assessed patient's/family caregiver's health literacy.

5. Asked patient to confirm history of allergies: known allergies and allergic response.

6. Asked if patient was experiencing any symptoms of pruritus, burning, or discomfort.

7. Assessed patient's knowledge and prior experience with vaginal suppository insertion.

8. Performed hand hygiene and applied clean gloves. During perineal care, inspected condition of vaginal tissues; noted if irritation or drainage present. Removed gloves and performed hand hygiene.

9. Assessed patient's ability to manipulate applicator, suppository, or irrigation equipment and to properly position self to insert medication.

10. Discussed purpose of each medication, action, and possible adverse effects. Allowed patient to ask any questions.

11. Performed hand hygiene and prepared medication using aseptic technique. Prepared medications for one patient at a time, avoiding distractions. Kept all pages of MARs or computer printouts for one patient together or looked at only one patient's electronic MAR at a time. Checked label of medical carefully with MAR or computer printout two times when preparing medication.

	S	U	NP	Comments

12. Took medication(s) to patient at correct time, per agency policy. During administration, applied seven rights of medication administration. Performed hand hygiene. ___ ___ ___ _____

13. Identified patient using at least two identifiers, per agency policy. Compared identifiers with information on patient's MAR or EHR. ___ ___ ___ _____

14. At patient's bedside, again compared MAR or computer printout with names of medications on medication labels and patient name. Asked patient again about any allergies. ___ ___ ___ _____

15. Closed room door or bedside curtains. Arranged supplies at bedside. Had patient void. Helped patient lie in dorsal recumbent position; patients with restricted mobility in knees or hips were positioned supine with legs abducted. ___ ___ ___ _____

16. Kept abdomen and lower extremities draped. ___ ___ ___ _____

17. Ensured that vaginal orifice was well illuminated by room light or positioned portable gooseneck lamp. ___ ___ ___ _____

18. Performed hand hygiene and applied clean gloves. ___ ___ ___ _____

19. Inserted vaginal suppository. ___ ___ ___ _____

   a. Removed suppository from wrapper and applied liberal amount of water-soluble lubricant to smooth or rounded end. Ensured that suppository was at room temperature. Lubricated gloved index finger of dominant hand. ___ ___ ___ _____

   b. With nondominant gloved hand, gently separated labial folds in front-to-back direction. ___ ___ ___ _____

   c. With dominant gloved hand, inserted rounded end of suppository along posterior wall of vaginal canal the entire length of finger (7.5 to 10 cm [3 to 4 inches]). ___ ___ ___ _____

   d. Withdrew finger and wiped away remaining lubricant from around orifice and labia with tissue or cloth. ___ ___ ___ _____

20. Applied cream or foam. ___ ___ ___ _____

   a. Filled cream or foam applicator following package directions. ___ ___ ___ _____

   b. With nondominant gloved hand, gently separated labial folds. ___ ___ ___ _____

   c. With dominant gloved hand, gently inserted applicator approximately 5 to 7.5 cm (2 to 3 inches). Pushed applicator plunger to deposit medication into vagina. ___ ___ ___ _____

	S	U	NP	Comments

d. Withdrew applicator and placed on paper towel. Wiped off residual cream from labia or vaginal orifice with tissue or cloth.

    ___ ___ ___ _____

21. Administered irrigation or douche.

    ___ ___ ___ _____

    a. Placed patient on bedpan with absorbent pad underneath.

    ___ ___ ___ _____

    b. Ensured that irrigation or douche fluid was at body temperature. Ran fluid through container nozzle.

    ___ ___ ___ _____

    c. Gently separated labial folds and directed nozzle toward sacrum, following floor of vagina.

    ___ ___ ___ _____

    d. Raised container approximately 30 to 50 cm (12 to 20 inches) above level of vagina. Inserted nozzle 7 to 10 cm (3 to 4 inches). Allowed solution to flow while rotating nozzle. Administered all irrigating solution.

    ___ ___ ___ _____

    e. Withdrew nozzle and helped patient to a comfortable sitting position.

    ___ ___ ___ _____

    f. Allowed patient to remain on bedpan for a few minutes. Cleaned perineum with soap and water.

    ___ ___ ___ _____

    g. Helped patient off bedpan. Dried perineal area. Returned patient to a comfortable position.

    ___ ___ ___ _____

22. Instructed patient who received suppository, cream, or tablet to remain on back for at least 10 minutes.

    ___ ___ ___ _____

23. If an applicator was used, washed with soap and warm water, rinsed, air dried, and then stored for future use.

    ___ ___ ___ _____

24. Removed and disposed of gloves and soiled supplies. Performed hand hygiene.

    ___ ___ ___ _____

25. Offered perineal pad when patient resumed ambulation.

    ___ ___ ___ _____

26. Raised side rails (as appropriate) and lowered bed to lowest position, locking into position.

    ___ ___ ___ _____

27. Placed nurse call system in accessible location within patient's reach.

    ___ ___ ___ _____

28. Thirty minutes after administration, returned to patient's room. Performed hand hygiene and applied gloves. Inspected condition of vaginal canal and external genitalia between applications. Assessed vaginal irritation or discharge if present. Removed and disposed of gloves and performed hand hygiene.

    ___ ___ ___ _____

29. Used Teach-Back: Revised instruction if patient/family caregiver was not able to teach back correctly.

    ___ ___ ___ _____

	S	U	NP	Comments

30. Documented drug (or vaginal irrigating solution), dose, type of installation, and time administered. Documented patient response and your evaluation of patient learning.   —— —— —— _____

31. Reported to health care provider if symptoms did not improve or worsened.   —— —— —— _____

Student _____ Date _____

Instructor _____ Date _____

PERFORMANCE CHECKLIST PROCEDURAL GUIDELINE 21.3   **ADMINISTERING RECTAL SUPPOSITORIES**

	S	U	NP	Comments

PROCEDURAL STEPS

1. Checked accuracy and completeness of each MAR or computer printout with health care provider's written medication order. Reprinted on computer any part of MAR that was difficult to read.

2. Reviewed pertinent information related to medication, including action, indication, purpose, normal dose and route, side effects, time of onset and peak action, and nursing implications.

3. Assessed patient's medical and medication history and history of allergies. Listed drug allergies on each page of the MAR and prominently displayed on the patient's electronic health record (EHR), per agency policy. If patient had an allergy, provided an allergy bracelet.

4. Assessed patient's/family caregiver's health literacy.

5. Asked patient to confirm history of allergies: known allergies and allergic response.

6. Reviewed any presenting signs and symptoms of GI alterations.

7. Assessed patient's ability to hold suppository and position self to insert medication.

8. Assessed patient's knowledge and experience with rectal suppository insertion.

9. Discussed purpose of each medication, action, indication, and possible adverse effects. Allowed patient to ask any questions.

10. Performed hand hygiene and prepared medication using aseptic technique. Prepared medications for one patient at a time, avoiding distractions. Kept all pages of MARs or computer printouts for one patient together or looked at only one patient's electronic MAR at a time. Checked label of medication carefully with MAR or computer printout two times when preparing medication.

	S	U	NP	Comments

11. Took medication(s) to patient at correct time, per agency policy. During administration, applied seven rights of medication administration. Performed hand hygiene. ____ ____ ____ _____

12. Identified patient using at least two identifiers, per agency policy. Compared identifiers with information on patient's MAR or EHR. ____ ____ ____ _____

13. At patient's bedside, again compared MAR or computer printout with names of medications on medication labels and patient name. Asked patient if they had any allergies. ____ ____ ____ _____

14. Provided privacy and prepared environment. Performed hand hygiene and applied clean gloves. ____ ____ ____ _____

15. Helped patient assume left side-lying position with upper leg flexed upward. ____ ____ ____ _____

16. If patient had mobility impairment, helped into lateral position. Obtained help to turn patient and used pillows under upper arm and leg. ____ ____ ____ _____

17. Kept patient draped with only anal area exposed. ____ ____ ____ _____

18. Examined condition of anus externally. Option: Palpated rectal walls as needed. If rectal walls palpated, disposed of gloves by turning them inside out and placing them in proper receptacle if they became soiled. Otherwise, kept gloves on hands and proceeded to Step 20. ____ ____ ____ _____

19. If previous gloves were soiled or discarded, performed hand hygiene and applied new pair of clean gloves. ____ ____ ____ _____

20. Removed suppository from foil wrapper and lubricated rounded end with water-soluble lubricant. Lubricated gloved index finger of dominant hand. If patient had hemorrhoids, used liberal amount of lubricant and touched area gently. ____ ____ ____ _____

21. Asked patient to take slow, deep breaths through mouth and relax anal sphincter. ____ ____ ____ _____

22. Retracted patient's buttocks with nondominant hand. With gloved index finger of dominant hand, inserted suppository gently through anus, past internal sphincter, and against rectal wall, 10 cm (4 inches) in adults or 5 cm (2 inches) in infants and children. ____ ____ ____ _____

23. Option: Gave suppository through a colostomy (not ileostomy) if ordered. Positioned patient supine. Used small amount of water-soluble lubricant for insertion. ____ ____ ____ _____

24. Withdrew finger and wiped patient's anal area. ____ ____ ____ _____

	S	U	NP	Comments

25. Asked patient to remain flat or on side for 5 minutes. ___ ___ ___ _____

26. Discarded gloves by turning them inside out and disposed of them and used supplies in an appropriate receptacle. Performed hand hygiene. Used appropriate disposal receptable if patient was on hazardous drugs (ONS, 2018, 2022). ___ ___ ___ _____

27. If suppository contained laxative or fecal softener, placed call light within reach so that patient could obtain help to reach bedpan or toilet. ___ ___ ___ _____

28. If suppository was given for constipation, reminded patient not to flush commode after bowel movement. ___ ___ ___ _____

29. Returned to bedside within 5 minutes to determine if suppository was expelled. ___ ___ ___ _____

30. Helped patient to a comfortable position. ___ ___ ___ _____

31. Raised side rails (as appropriate) and lowered bed to lowest position, locking into position. ___ ___ ___ _____

32. Placed nurse call system in accessible location within patient's reach. ___ ___ ___ _____

33. Evaluated character of stool if passed. ___ ___ ___ _____

34. Used Teach-Back: Revised instruction if patient/family caregiver was not able to teach back correctly. ___ ___ ___ _____

35. Documented the drug, dosage, route, and actual time and date of administration on MAR immediately after administration, not before. Documented patient response to medication. Documented evaluation of patient learning. ___ ___ ___ _____

36. Reported adverse effects/patient response and/or withheld drugs to nurse in charge or health care provider. ___ ___ ___ _____

Student _____ Date _____

Instructor _____ Date _____

PERFORMANCE CHECKLIST SKILL 22.1   **PREPARING INJECTIONS: AMPULES AND VIALS**

	S	U	NP	Comments
ASSESSMENT				
1. Checked accuracy and completeness of each MAR or computer printout with health care provider's written medication order. Checked patient's name, medication name and dosage, route of administration, and time of administration. Clarified incomplete or unclear orders with health care provider before administration.	___	___	___	_____
2. Reviewed medication reference pertinent information related to medication, including action, purpose, normal dose and route, side effects, time of onset and peak action, indication, and nursing implications.	___	___	___	_____
3. Assessed patient's medical and medication history and history of allergies. Listed medication allergies on each page of the MAR and prominently displayed them on the patient's electronic health record (EHR). When allergies were present, ensured patient wore an allergy bracelet.	___	___	___	_____
4. Performed hand hygiene. Assessed patient's body build, muscle size, and weight/BMI when giving subcutaneous or IM medication.	___	___	___	_____
PLANNING				
1. Determined expected outcomes following completion of procedure.	___	___	___	_____
2. Performed hand hygiene.	___	___	___	_____
3. Planned preparation to avoid interruptions. Created a quiet environment. Did not take phone calls or talk with others. Followed agency "No-Interruption Zone" policy. Kept all pages of MARs or computer printouts for one patient together or looked at only one patient's electronic MAR at a time.	___	___	___	_____
IMPLEMENTATION				
1. Prepared medications.	___	___	___	_____
a. If using a medication cart, moved it outside patient's room.	___	___	___	_____
b. Unlocked medication drawer or cart or logged on to automated dispensing machine (ADM).	___	___	___	_____
c. Selected correct medication from stock supply or unit-dose drawer. Compared label of medication with MAR computer printout or computer screen.	___	___	___	_____

S   U   NP   Comments

d. Checked expiration date on each medication, one at a time.

    —— —— —— ——————————

e. Calculated medication dose as necessary. Double-checked calculations. In the case of high-risk medications, asked another nurse to perform an independent double check of dosage (per agency policy).

    —— —— —— ——————————

f. If preparing a controlled substance, checked record for previous medication count and compared it with supply available.

    —— —— —— ——————————

g. Did not leave medications unattended.

    —— —— —— ——————————

h. If in a perioperative or procedural area, labeled the syringe with the name of the medication and dose.

    —— —— —— ——————————

2. Prepared ampule.

    —— —— —— ——————————

a. Tapped top of ampule lightly and quickly with finger until fluid moved from its neck.

    —— —— —— ——————————

b. Placed small gauze pad around neck of ampule.

    —— —— —— ——————————

c. Snapped neck of ampule quickly and firmly away from hands.

    —— —— —— ——————————

d. Held ampule upside down or set it on a flat surface. Inserted filter needle into center of ampule opening. Did not allow needle tip or shaft to touch rim of ampule.

    —— —— —— ——————————

e. Used a filter needle long enough so tip was at bottom of ampule. Drew up medication quickly.

    —— —— —— ——————————

f. Aspirated medication into syringe by gently pulling back on plunger

    —— —— —— ——————————

g. Kept needle tip under surface of liquid. Tipped ampule to bring all fluid within reach of needle.

    —— —— —— ——————————

h. If air bubbles were aspirated, did not expel air into ampule.

    —— —— —— ——————————

i. To expel excess air bubbles, removed needle from ampule. Held syringe vertically with needle pointing up. Tapped side of syringe to cause bubbles to rise toward needle. Drew back slightly on plunger and pushed plunger upward to eject air. Did not eject fluid.

    —— —— —— ——————————

j. If syringe contained excess fluid, used sink for disposal. Held syringe vertically with needle tip up and slanted slightly toward sink. Slowly ejected excess fluid into sink. Rechecked fluid level in syringe by holding it vertically.

    —— —— —— ——————————

k. Covered needle with its safety sheath or cap. Replaced filter needle with regular SESIP needle.

    —— —— —— ——————————

	S	U	NP	Comments

3. Prepared vial containing a solution.   ___ ___ ___ _____

  a. Removed cap covering top of unused vial to expose sterile rubber seal. Firmly and briskly wiped surface of rubber seal with antiseptic swab and allowed it to dry.   ___ ___ ___ _____

  b. Picked up syringe and removed needle cap or cap covering needleless access device. Pulled back on plunger to draw amount of air into syringe equivalent to volume of medication to be aspirated from vial.   ___ ___ ___ _____

  c. With vial on flat surface, inserted tip of needle, needleless device, or blunt filled needle through center of rubber seal. Applied pressure to tip of needle during insertion.   ___ ___ ___ _____

  d. Injected air into air space of vial, holding on to plunger. Held plunger firmly.   ___ ___ ___ _____

  e. Inverted vial while keeping firm hold on syringe and plunger. Held vial between thumb and middle fingers of nondominant hand. Grasped end of syringe barrel and plunger with thumb and forefinger of dominant hand to counteract pressure in vial.   ___ ___ ___ _____

  f. Kept tip of needle or needleless device below fluid level.   ___ ___ ___ _____

  g. Allowed air pressure from vial to fill syringe gradually with medication. If necessary, pulled back slightly on plunger to obtain correct amount of medication.   ___ ___ ___ _____

  h. When desired volume was obtained, positioned needle or needleless device into air space of vial; tapped side of syringe barrel gently to dislodge any air bubbles. Ejected any air remaining at top of syringe into vial.   ___ ___ ___ _____

  i. Removed needle or needleless access device from vial by pulling back on barrel of syringe.   ___ ___ ___ _____

  j. Held syringe at eye level at a 90-degree angle to ensure correct volume and absence of air bubbles. Removed any remaining air by tapping barrel to dislodge any air bubbles. Drew back slightly on plunger; then pushed it upward to eject air. Did not eject fluid. Rechecked volume of medication.   ___ ___ ___ _____

  k. Before injecting medication into patient's tissue, changed needle with regular SESIP to appropriate gauge and length according to a route of medication administration.   ___ ___ ___ _____

  l. Covered needle with its safety sheath or cap following agency safety guidelines.   ___ ___ ___ _____

	S	U	NP	Comments

m. For a multi-dose vial, made a label that included date of opening, concentration of drug per milliliter, and your initials.

___ ___ ___ _____

4. Prepared vial containing powder (reconstituting medications).

___ ___ ___ _____

  a. Removed cap covering vial of powdered medication and cap covering vial of proper diluent. Firmly swabbed both rubber seals with an antiseptic swab and allowed to dry.

___ ___ ___ _____

  b. Drew up manufacturer's suggestion for volume and type of diluent into syringe following Steps 3b through 3j.

___ ___ ___ _____

  c. Inserted tip of needle or needleless device through center of rubber seal of vial of powdered medication. Injected diluent into vial. Removed needle.

___ ___ ___ _____

  d. Mixed medication thoroughly. Rolled in palms. Did not shake.

___ ___ ___ _____

  e. Read label carefully to determine dose after reconstitution.

___ ___ ___ _____

  f. Drew up reconstituted medication into syringe. Inserted needleless device/needle into vial. Did not add air. Then followed Steps 3e through 3j.

___ ___ ___ _____

5. Compared label of medication with MAR, computer screen, or computer printout.

___ ___ ___ _____

6. Vials and/or ampules and the syringe may be barcoded. Both went to the bedside and were barcoded at the bedside prior to administration. If medication prepared in syringe was not given immediately, labeled syringe.

___ ___ ___ _____

7. Disposed of soiled supplies. Placed broken ampule and/or used vials and used needle or needleless device in puncture- and leak-proof container. Cleaned work area and performed hand hygiene.

___ ___ ___ _____

EVALUATION

1. Just before administering drug to patient, compared MAR with label of prepared drug and compared dose in syringe with desired dose.

___ ___ ___ _____

PERFORMANCE CHECKLIST PROCEDURAL GUIDELINE 22.1   **MIXING PARENTERAL MEDICATIONS IN ONE SYRINGE**

	S	U	NP	Comments

PROCEDURAL STEPS

1. Checked accuracy and completeness of MAR or computer printout with health care provider's written medication order. Checked patient's name, medication name and dosage, route of administration, and time of administration. Clarified incomplete or unclear orders with health care provider before administration.

2. Reviewed pertinent information related to medication, including action, purpose, side effects, and nursing implications.

3. Performed hand hygiene. Assessed patient body build, muscle size, and weight/BMI if giving subcutaneous or IM medication.

4. Considered compatibility of medications to be mixed and type of injection.

5. Checked expiration date of medication printed on vial or ampule.

6. Performed hand hygiene.

7. Prepared medication for one patient at a time following the seven rights of medication administration. Selected an ampule or vial from the unit-dose drawer or automated dispensing system. Compared the label of each medication with the MAR or computer printout. In the case of insulin, ensured that correct type(s) of insulin were prepared.

8. Mixed medications from two vials:

   a. Took syringe with needleless device or filter needle and aspirated volume of air equivalent to first medication dose (vial A).

   b. Injected air into vial A and made sure that needle or needleless device did not touch solution.

   c. Holding plunger, withdrew needle or needleless device and syringe from vial A. Aspirated air equivalent to second medication dose (vial B) into syringe.

	S	U	NP	Comments

d. Inserted needle or needleless device into vial B, injected volume of air into vial B, and withdrew medication from vial B into syringe.

___ ___ ___ _____

e. Withdrew needle or needleless device and syringe from vial B. Ensured that proper volume had been obtained.

___ ___ ___ _____

f. Determined by viewing syringe scale the appropriate combined volume of medications.

___ ___ ___ _____

g. Inserted needle or needleless device into vial A, being careful not to push plunger and expel medication within syringe into vial. Inverted vial and carefully withdrew the desired amount of medication from vial A into syringe.

___ ___ ___ _____

h. Withdrew needle or needleless device and expelled any excess air from syringe. Checked fluid level in syringe for proper dose. Medications were now mixed.

___ ___ ___ _____

i. Changed needle or needleless device for appropriate-size needle if medication was being injected. Kept needle or needleless device capped until administration time.

___ ___ ___ _____

9. Mixed insulin:

___ ___ ___ _____

a. If cloudy insulin was being administered, rolled bottle of insulin between hands to resuspend insulin preparation.

___ ___ ___ _____

b. Wiped off tops of both insulin vials with an antiseptic swab.

___ ___ ___ _____

c. Verified insulin dose against MAR.

___ ___ ___ _____

d. If mixing rapid- or short-acting insulin with intermediate- or long-acting insulin, took insulin syringe and aspirated volume of air equivalent to dose to be withdrawn from intermediate- or long-acting insulin first. If two intermediate- or long-acting insulins were mixed, either vial was prepared first.

___ ___ ___ _____

e. Inserted needle and injected air into vial of intermediate- or long-acting insulin. Did not let tip of needle touch solution.

___ ___ ___ _____

f. Removed syringe from vial of insulin without aspirating medication.

___ ___ ___ _____

g. With the same syringe, injected air equal to the dose of rapid- or short-acting insulin into vial and withdrew correct dose into syringe.

___ ___ ___ _____

376

h. Removed syringe from rapid- or short-acting insulin and removed any air bubbles to ensure accurate dose.

    — — — _____

i. Verified short-acting insulin dosage with MAR and verified insulin prepared in syringe with another nurse to ensure that correct dosage of insulin was prepared. Determined which point on syringe scale the combined units of insulin should measure by adding the number of units of both insulins together. Verified combined dosage. A second nurse confirmed.

    — — — _____

j. Placed needle of syringe back into vial of intermediate- or long-acting insulin. Was careful not to push plunger and inject insulin in syringe into vial.

    — — — _____

k. Inverted vial and carefully withdrew desired amount of insulin into syringe.

    — — — _____

l. Withdrew needle and checked fluid level in syringe. Verified with another nurse that correct total dose was prepared. Kept needle of prepared syringe sheathed or capped until ready to administer medication.

    — — — _____

10. Mixed medications from a vial and an ampule:

    — — — _____

a. Prepared medication from vial first, following Skill 22.1, Step 3.

    — — — _____

b. Determined on syringe scale the combined volume of medications that should be measured.

    — — — _____

c. Next, using the same syringe, prepared second medication from ampule, following Step 2 in Skill 22.1.

    — — — _____

d. Withdrew filter needle from ampule and verified fluid level in syringe. Changed filter needle to appropriate SESIP needle. Kept device or needle sheathed or capped until administering medication.

    — — — _____

e. Checked syringe carefully for total combined dose of medications.

    — — — _____

11. Compared MAR, computer screen, or computer printout with prepared medication and labels on vials/ampules.

    — — — _____

12. The vial and/or ampules and syringes were saved if barcoding was required. The labeled syringe (when indicated) was placed next to the vial and both were barcoded at the bedside.

    — — — _____

	S	U	NP	Comments

13. Disposed of soiled supplies. Placed used ampules and/or vials and needle or needleless device in puncture- and leak-proof container. ___ ___ ___ _____

14. Cleaned work area and performed hand hygiene. ___ ___ ___ _____

15. Checked syringe again carefully for total combined dose of medications. ___ ___ ___ _____

16. The third check for accuracy occurred at patient's bedside. ___ ___ ___ _____

Student _____   Date _____

Instructor _____   Date _____

PERFORMANCE CHECKLIST SKILL 22.2   **ADMINISTERING INTRADERMAL INJECTIONS**

	S	U	NP	Comments

ASSESSMENT

1. Checked accuracy and completeness of MAR or computer printout with health care provider's original medication order. Checked patient's name, medication name and dosage, route of administration, and time of administration. Clarified incomplete or unclear orders with health care provider before administration.

2. Reviewed medication reference information about expected reaction/anticipated effects when testing skin with specific allergen and appropriate time to interpret injection site results.

3. Assessed patient's/family caregiver's health literacy.

4. Asked patient to describe history of allergies: known type of allergies and normal allergic reaction. Compared information with health history. Placed allergy band on patient's wrist if allergy was identified.

5. Performed hand hygiene. Inspected skin to assess for contraindication to ID injections. Assessed for history of severe adverse reactions or necrosis that happened after previous ID injection.

6. Checked date of expiration for medication.

7. Assessed patient's knowledge, prior experience with ID injections, test being conducted, and feelings about procedure.

PLANNING

1. Determined expected outcomes following completion of procedure.

2. Determined that the patient could identify signs of skin reaction and their significance.

3. Provided privacy and explained test and procedure to patient. Discussed signs and symptoms of ID reaction. If applicable, taught patient how to report any side effects from injection.

4. Planned preparation to avoid interruptions. Created a quiet environment. Did not accept phone calls or talk with others. Followed agency "No-Interruption Zone" policy. Kept all pages of MARs or computer printouts for one patient together or looked at only one patient's electronic MAR at a time.

	S	U	NP	Comments

5. Obtained and organized equipment for ID injection at bedside. ___ ___ ___ _____

IMPLEMENTATION

1. Performed hand hygiene. Prepared medications for one patient at a time using aseptic technique and avoiding distractions. Checked label of medication carefully with MAR or computer printout when removing medication from storage and after preparing medication. ___ ___ ___ _____

2. Took medication(s) to patient at correct time per agency policy. Gave non-time-critical scheduled medications within a range of 1 or 2 hours of scheduled dose. During administration, applied seven rights of medication administration. ___ ___ ___ _____

3. Identified patient using at least two identifiers according to agency policy. Compared identifiers with information on patient's MAR or EHR. ___ ___ ___ _____

4. At patient's bedside, again compared MAR or computer printout with names of medications on medication labels and patient name. Asked patient about any allergies. ___ ___ ___ _____

5. Performed hand hygiene and applied clean gloves. Kept sheet or gown draped over body parts not requiring exposure. ___ ___ ___ _____

6. Helped patient to a comfortable position. Had patient extend elbow, and support ted elbow and forearm on a flat surface. ___ ___ ___ _____

7. Selected appropriate injection site on inner aspect of forearm. Noted lesions or discolorations of skin. If possible, selected site three to four finger widths below antecubital space and one hand width above wrist. If forearm could not be used, inspected upper back. If necessary, use sites appropriate for subcutaneous injections. ___ ___ ___ _____

8. Instructed patient to keep forearm stable. Cleaned site with antiseptic swab. Applied swab at center of site and rotated outward in a circular direction for about 5 cm (2 inches). *Option:* Used a vapocoolant spray before injection. ___ ___ ___ _____

9. Held swab or gauze between third and fourth fingers of nondominant hand. ___ ___ ___ _____

10. Removed needle cap from needle by pulling it straight off. ___ ___ ___ _____

11. Held syringe between thumb and forefinger of dominant hand with bevel of needle pointing up. ___ ___ ___ _____

12. Administered injection. ___ ___ ___ _____

	S	U	NP	Comments

a. With nondominant hand, stretched skin over site with forefinger or thumb.   ___ ___ ___ _____

b. With needle almost against patient's skin, inserted it slowly at a 5- to 15-degree angle until resistance was felt. Advanced needle through epidermis to approximately 3 mm (1/8 inch) below skin surface. The bulge of the needle tip was visible through skin.   ___ ___ ___ _____

c. Injected medication slowly. If resistance was not felt, removed and began again.   ___ ___ ___ _____

d. While injecting medication, noted that small wheal resembling mosquito bite appeared on skin surface.   ___ ___ ___ _____

   (1) If no wheal formed or if the wheal was less than 6 mm of induration, repeated the test immediately, approximately 5 cm (2 inches) from original site or on the other arm.   ___ ___ ___ _____

e. After withdrawing needle, applied antiseptic swab or gauze gently over site.   ___ ___ ___ _____

13. Discarded uncapped needle or needle enclosed in safety shield and attached syringe in puncture- and leak-proof receptacle.   ___ ___ ___ _____

14. Helped patient to a comfortable position.   ___ ___ ___ _____

15. Placed nurse call system in an accessible location within patient's reach.   ___ ___ ___ _____

16. Raised side rails (as appropriate) and lowered bed to lowest position, locking into position.   ___ ___ ___ _____

17. Disposed of all contaminated supplies in appropriate receptacle, removed and disposed of gloves, and performed hand hygiene.   ___ ___ ___ _____

18. Stayed with patient for several minutes and observed for any allergic reactions.   ___ ___ ___ _____

EVALUATION

1. Returned to room in 15 to 30 minutes and asked if patient felt any acute pain, burning, numbness, or tingling at injection site.   ___ ___ ___ _____

2. Asked patient to discuss implications of skin testing and signs of hypersensitivity.   ___ ___ ___ _____

3. Inspected bleb. *Option:* Used skin pencil and drew a circle around perimeter of injection site. Read TB test site between 48 and 72 hours after injection; looked for induration of skin around injection site of: ___ ___ ___ _____

• 15 mm or more in patients with no known risk factors for TB.   ___ ___ ___ _____

- 10 mm or more in patients who have recently immigrated from countries with high infection rates; injection drug users; residents and employees of high-risk settings; patients with certain chronic illnesses; children younger than 4 years; and infants, children, and adolescents exposed to high-risk adults.

    ____ ____ ____ _____

- 5 mm or more in patients who are human immunodeficiency virus (HIV) positive, have fibrotic changes on chest x-ray film consistent with previous TB infection, have had organ transplants, or are immunosuppressed.

    ____ ____ ____ _____

4. Used Teach-Back: Revised instruction if patient or family caregiver was not able to teach back correctly.

    ____ ____ ____ _____

RECORDING

1. Documented drug, dose, route, site, time, and date on MAR immediately after administration. Correctly signed MAR according to agency policy.

    ____ ____ ____ _____

2. Documented area of ID injection and appearance of skin.

    ____ ____ ____ _____

3. Documented patient teaching, validation of understanding, and patient's response to medication (including adverse effects).

    ____ ____ ____ _____

HAND-OFF REPORTING

1. Reported any undesirable effects from medication to patient's health care provider.

    ____ ____ ____ _____

2. Reported the location, time, and date on which a final reading for a reaction was required.

    ____ ____ ____ _____

Student _____ Date _____

Instructor _____ Date _____

PERFORMANCE CHECKLIST SKILL 22.3 **ADMINISTERING SUBCUTANEOUS INJECTIONS**

	S	U	NP	Comments

ASSESSMENT

1. Checked accuracy and completeness of each MAR or computer printout with health care provider's written medication order. Checked patient's name, medication name and dosage, route of administration, and time of administration. Clarified incomplete or unclear orders with health care provider before administration.   ___ ___ ___ _____

2. Reviewed EHR to assess patient's medical and medication history. If patient was in circulatory shock, withheld subcutaneous injection and chose a different route.   ___ ___ ___ _____

3. Reviewed medication reference information for medication action, purpose, normal dose, side effects, time and peak of onset, and nursing implications.   ___ ___ ___ _____

4. Assessed relevant laboratory results.   ___ ___ ___ _____

5. Assessed patient's/family caregiver's health literacy.   ___ ___ ___ _____

6. Asked patient to describe history of allergies: known allergies and normal allergic reaction. Compared information with health history. Placed allergy band on patient's wrist if allergy was identified.   ___ ___ ___ _____

7. Checked date of expiration for medication on vial/pen.   ___ ___ ___ _____

8. Observed patient's previous verbal and nonverbal responses toward injection.   ___ ___ ___ _____

9. Performed hand hygiene. Assessed condition of skin at potential sites for contraindication to subcutaneous injections.   ___ ___ ___ _____

10. Assessed patient's symptoms before initiating medication therapy.   ___ ___ ___ _____

11. Assessed condition (amount) of patient's adipose tissue. Performed hand hygiene.   ___ ___ ___ _____

12. Assessed patient's knowledge, prior experience with subcutaneous injections, medication to receive, and feelings about procedure.   ___ ___ ___ _____

PLANNING

1. Determined expected outcomes following completion of procedure.   ___ ___ ___ _____

	S	U	NP	Comments

2. Provided privacy and explained medication and procedure to patient. Discussed rationale and expected sensations related to the subcutaneous injection. If applicable, taught patient how to report any side effects.

3. Planned preparation to avoid interruptions. Created a quiet environment. Did not accept phone calls or talk with others. Followed agency "no-interruption-zone" policy. Kept all pages of MARs or computer printouts for one patient together or looked at only one patient's electronic MAR at a time.

4. Obtained and organized equipment for subcutaneous injection at bedside

IMPLEMENTATION

1. Performed hand hygiene. Prepared medications for one patient at a time using aseptic technique and avoiding distractions. Checked label of medication carefully with MAR or computer printout when removing medication from storage and after preparation.

2. Took medication(s) to patient at correct time, per agency policy. Gave non-time-critical scheduled medications within a range of 1 or 2 hours of scheduled dose. During administration, applied seven rights of medication administration.

3. Identified patient using at least two identifiers according to agency policy. Compared identifiers with information on patient's MAR or EHR.

4. At patient's bedside, again compared MAR or computer printout with names of medications on medication labels and patient name. Asked patient about any allergies.

5. Performed hand hygiene and applied clean gloves. Kept sheet or gown draped over body parts not requiring exposure.

6. Positioned patient comfortably for site assessment. Selected appropriate injection site. Inspected skin surface over sites for bruises, inflammation, or edema. Did not use an area that was bruised or had signs associated with infection.

7. Palpated sites and avoided those with masses or tenderness. Ensured that needle was correct size by grasping skinfold at site with thumb and forefinger. Measured fold from top to bottom. Made sure that needle was one-half length of fold.

   a. When administering insulin or heparin, used abdominal injection sites first, followed by thigh injection site.

384

	S	U	NP	Comments

b. When administering LMWH subcutaneously, chose site on right or left side of abdomen, at least 5 cm (2 inches) away from umbilicus. _____ _____ _____ _____

c. Rotated insulin site within an anatomical area and systematically rotated sites within that area. _____ _____ _____ _____

8. Kept patient in a comfortable position. Had patient relax arm, leg, or abdomen, depending on site selection. _____ _____ _____ _____

9. Relocated site using anatomical landmarks. _____ _____ _____ _____

10. Cleaned site with antiseptic swab. Applied swab at center of site and rotated outward in circular direction for about 5 cm (2 inches). _____ _____ _____ _____

11. Held swab or gauze between third and fourth fingers of nondominant hand. _____ _____ _____ _____

12. Removed needle cap or protective sheath by pulling it straight off. _____ _____ _____ _____

13. Held syringe between thumb and forefinger of dominant hand; held as a dart. _____ _____ _____ _____

14. Administered injection (via syringe): _____ _____ _____ _____

a. For average-size patient, held skin across injection site or pinched skin with nondominant hand. _____ _____ _____ _____

b. Injected needle quickly and firmly at a 45- to a 90-degree angle. Released skin if pinched. Option: If using an injection pen or giving heparin, continued to pinch skin while injecting medicine. _____ _____ _____ _____

c. For obese patient, pinched skin at site and injected needle at a 90-degree angle below tissue fold. _____ _____ _____ _____

d. After needle entered site, grasped lower end of syringe barrel with nondominant hand to stabilize it. Moved dominant hand to end of plunger and slowly injected medication over several seconds. If giving heparin, injected over 30 seconds. Avoided moving syringe. _____ _____ _____ _____

e. Withdrew needle quickly while placing antiseptic swab or gauze gently over site. _____ _____ _____ _____

f. Option: When administering heparin, applied a moist ice pack over injection site and left in place for 3 to 5 minutes. _____ _____ _____ _____

15. Administered injection (via injection pen) _____ _____ _____ _____

a. Primed the insulin pen. _____ _____ _____ _____

b. To prime the insulin pen, turned the dosage knob to the 2-units indicator. With the pen pointing upward, pushed the knob all the way. Watched for one drop of insulin to appear. Repeated this step until a drop appeared. _____ _____ _____ _____

	S	U	NP	Comments

c. Selected the dose of insulin that had been prescribed by turning the dosage knob.   ___ ___ ___ _____

d. Removed the pen cap. Inserted the needle with a quick motion into the skin at a 90-degree angle. The needle went all the way into the skin.   ___ ___ ___ _____

e. Slowly pushed the knob of the pen all the way in to deliver the full dose. Held the pen at the site for 6–10 seconds and then pulled the needle out. Placed antiseptic swab or gauze gently over site.   ___ ___ ___ _____

f. Replaced the pen cap and stored at room temperature.   ___ ___ ___ _____

16. Applied gentle pressure to site. Did not massage site. (If heparin was given, or if patient was on an anticoagulant, held alcohol swab or gauze to site for 30–60 seconds and applied ice pack.)   ___ ___ ___ _____

17. Discarded uncapped needle or needle enclosed in safety shield and attached syringe in a puncture- and leak-proof receptacle.   ___ ___ ___ _____

18. Helped patient to a comfortable position.   ___ ___ ___ _____

19. Placed nurse call system in an accessible location within patient's reach.   ___ ___ ___ _____

20. Raised side rails (as appropriate) and lowered bed to lowest position, locking into position.   ___ ___ ___ _____

21. Disposed of all contaminated supplies in appropriate receptacle, removed and disposed of gloves, and performed hand hygiene.   ___ ___ ___ _____

22. Stayed with patient for several minutes and observed for any allergic reactions.   ___ ___ ___ _____

EVALUATION

1. Returned to room in 15 to 30 minutes and asked if patient felt any acute pain, burning, numbness, or tingling at injection site.   ___ ___ ___ _____

2. Inspected site, noting bruising or induration. Provided warm compress to the site.   ___ ___ ___ _____

3. Observed patient's response to medication at times that correlated with onset, peak, and duration of medication. Reviewed laboratory results as appropriate.   ___ ___ ___ _____

4. Used Teach-Back: Revised instruction if patient or family caregiver was not able to teach back correctly.   ___ ___ ___ _____

RECORDING

1. Immediately after administration, documented medication, dose, route, site, time, and date given. Signed MAR according to agency policy.   ___ ___ ___ _____

	S	U	NP	Comments

2. Documented any undesirable effects from the injection.   ___ ___ ___ _____

3. Documented patient teaching, validation of understanding, and patient's response to medication.   ___ ___ ___ _____

HAND-OFF REPORTING

1. Reported any undesirable effects from medication to patient's health care provider.   ___ ___ ___ _____

Student _____ Date _____

Instructor _____ Date _____

PERFORMANCE CHECKLIST SKILL 22.4 **ADMINISTERING INTRAMUSCULAR INJECTIONS**

	S	U	NP	Comments

ASSESSMENT

1. Checked accuracy and completeness of each MAR or computer printout with health care provider's written medication order. Checked patient's name, medication name and dosage, route of administration, and time of administration. Clarified incomplete or unclear orders with health care provider before administration.

2. Reviewed EHR to assess patient's medical and medication history. If patient was in circulatory shock, withheld subcutaneous injection and chose a different route.

3. Reviewed medication reference information for medication action, purpose, normal dose, side effects, time and peak of onset, and nursing implications.

4. Assessed patient's/family caregiver's health literacy.

5. Asked patient to describe history of allergies: known type of allergies and normal allergic reaction. Compared information with health history. Placed allergy band on patient's wrist if allergy was identified.

6. Checked date of expiration for medication.

7. Observed patient's previous verbal and nonverbal responses regarding injection.

8. Performed hand hygiene. Assessed condition of skin at potential sites for contraindication to IM injections. Assessed adequacy of adipose tissue.

9. Assessed patient's symptoms before initiating medication therapy.

10. Assessed patient's knowledge, prior experience with IM injections, type of medicine to receive, and feelings about procedure.

PLANNING

1. Determined expected outcomes following completion of procedure.

2. Provided privacy and explained medication and procedure to patient. Discussed need for and experience of receiving an IM injection. If applicable, taught patient how to report side effects.

388

	S	U	NP	Comments

3. Planned preparation to avoid interruptions. Created a quiet environment. Did not accept phone calls or talk with others. Followed agency "No-Interruption Zone" policy. Kept all pages of MARs or computer printouts for one patient together or looked at only one patient's electronic MAR at a time. ___ ___ ___ _____

4. Obtained and organized equipment for IM at bedside ___ ___ ___ _____

IMPLEMENTATION

1. Performed hand hygiene. Prepared medications for one patient at a time using aseptic technique and avoiding distractions. Checked label of medication carefully with MAR or computer printout when removing drug from storage and after preparation. ___ ___ ___ _____

2. Took medication(s) to patient at correct time per agency policy. Gave non-time-critical scheduled medications within a range of 1 to 2 hours of scheduled dose. During administration, applied seven rights of medication administration. ___ ___ ___ _____

3. Identified patient using at least two identifiers according to agency policy. Compared identifiers with information on patient's MAR or EHR. ___ ___ ___ _____

4. At patient's bedside, again compared MAR or computer printout with names of medications on medication labels and patient's name. Asked patient about allergies. ___ ___ ___ _____

5. Performed hand hygiene and applied clean gloves. Kept sheet or gown draped over body parts not requiring exposure. ___ ___ ___ _____

6. Positioned patient comfortably to access site. Selected an appropriate site. Noted integrity and size of muscle. Palpated for tenderness or hardness. Avoided these areas. If patient received frequent injections, rotated sites. Used ventrogluteal if possible. ___ ___ ___ _____

7. Had patient maintain a comfortable position depending on chosen site. ___ ___ ___ _____

8. Relocated site using anatomical landmarks. ___ ___ ___ _____

9. Cleaned site with antiseptic swab. Applied swab at center of site and rotate outward in a circular direction for about 5 cm (2 inches). ___ ___ ___ _____

   a. Option: Applied 5% topical lidocaine-prilocaine emulsion on injection site at least 1 hour before IM injection or used a vapocoolant spray just before injection. ___ ___ ___ _____

10. Held swab or gauze between third and fourth fingers of nondominant hand. ___ ___ ___ _____

	S	U	NP	Comments

11. Removed needle cap or sheath by pulling it straight off.   ___ ___ ___ _____

12. Held syringe between thumb and forefinger of dominant hand; held as a dart, palm down.   ___ ___ ___ _____

13. Administered injection using Z-track method: ___ ___ ___ _____

    a. Positioned ulnar side of nondominant hand just below site and pulled skin laterally approximately 2.5 to 3.5 cm (1 to 1 ½ inches). Held position until medication was injected. With dominant hand, injected needle quickly at a 90-degree angle into muscle.   ___ ___ ___ _____

    b. Option: If patient's muscle mass was small, grasped body of muscle between thumb and forefingers.   ___ ___ ___ _____

    c. After needle pierced skin, and while still pulling on skin with nondominant hand, grasped lower end of syringe barrel with fingers of nondominant hand to stabilize it. Moved dominant hand to end of plunger. Avoided moving syringe.   ___ ___ ___ _____

    d. Pulled back on plunger 5 to 10 seconds. Exception: Aspiration not required with administration of immunizations). If no blood appeared, injected medication slowly at a rate of 10 sec/mL.   ___ ___ ___ _____

    e. Once medication was injected, waited 10 seconds, then smoothly and steadily withdrew needle, released skin, and applied gauze with gentle pressure over site. If patient was taking anticoagulants, held antiseptic swab or gauze to site for 30 to 60 seconds. Did not massage site.   ___ ___ ___ _____

14. Helped patient to a comfortable position.   ___ ___ ___ _____

15. Discarded uncapped needle or needle enclosed in safety shield and attached syringe into a puncture- and leak-proof receptacle.   ___ ___ ___ _____

16. Placed nurse call system in an accessible location within patient's reach.   ___ ___ ___ _____

17. Raised side rails (as appropriate) and lowered bed to lowest position, locking into place.   ___ ___ ___ _____

18. Disposed of all contaminated supplies in appropriate receptacle, removed and disposed of gloves, and performed hand hygiene.   ___ ___ ___ _____

19. Stayed with patient for several minutes and observed for any allergic reactions.   ___ ___ ___ _____

EVALUATION

1. Returned to room in 15 to 30 minutes and asked if patient felt any acute pain, burning, numbness, or tingling at injection site.   ___ ___ ___ _____

	S	U	NP	Comments

2. Inspected site; noted any bruising or induration. Option: Applied warm compress to site. ___ ___ ___ _____

3. Observed patient's response to medication at times that correlated with onset, peak, and duration of medication. ___ ___ ___ _____

4. Used Teach-Back: Revised instruction if patient or family caregiver was not able to teach back correctly. ___ ___ ___ _____

RECORDING

1. Immediately after administration, documented medication, dose, route, site, time, date given, and any adverse effects. ___ ___ ___ _____

2. Documented any undesirable effects from the injection. ___ ___ ___ _____

3. Documented patient teaching, validation of understanding, and patient's response to medication. ___ ___ ___ _____

HAND-OFF REPORTING

1. Reported any undesirable effects from medication to patient's health care provider. ___ ___ ___ _____

Student _____ Date _____

Instructor _____ Date _____

PERFORMANCE CHECKLIST SKILL 22.5 **ADMINISTERING MEDICATIONS BY INTRAVENOUS PUSH**

	S	U	NP	Comments

ASSESSMENT

1. Checked accuracy and completeness of each MAR or computer printout with health care provider's written medication order. Checked patient's name, medication name and dosage, route of administration, and time of administration. Clarified incomplete or unclear orders with health care provider before administration. ___ ___ ___ _____

2. Reviewed EHR to assess patient's medical and medication history. ___ ___ ___ _____

3. Assessed relevant laboratory results. ___ ___ ___ _____

4. Reviewed medication reference information for medication action, purpose, normal dose, side effects, time and peak of onset, how slowly to give medication, and nursing implications. ___ ___ ___ _____

5. If giving medication through an existing IV line, determined compatibility of medication with IV fluids and any additives within IV solution. ___ ___ ___ _____

6. Performed hand hygiene. Assessed condition of IV needle insertion site for signs of infiltration or phlebitis. ___ ___ ___ _____

7. Assessed patency of patient's existing IV infusion line or saline lock. Performed hand hygiene. ___ ___ ___ _____

8. Assessed patient's/family caregiver's health literacy. ___ ___ ___ _____

9. Asked patient to describe history of allergies: known type of allergens and normal allergic reaction. Compared information with health history. Placed allergy band on patient's wrist if allergy was identified. ___ ___ ___ _____

10. Assessed patient's symptoms before initiating medication therapy. ___ ___ ___ _____

11. Assessed patient's knowledge, prior experience with IV push administration, the medication to be received, and feelings about procedure. ___ ___ ___ _____

PLANNING

1. Determined expected outcomes following completion of procedure. ___ ___ ___ _____

2. Provided privacy and explained medication and procedure to patient. Discussed need for and sensations expected with IV push. If applicable, taught patient how to report any side effects. ___ ___ ___ _____

392

	S	U	NP	Comments

3. Planned preparation to avoid interruptions. Created a quiet environment. Did not accept phone calls or talk with others. Followed agency "No-Interruption Zone" policy. Kept all pages of MARs or computer printouts for one patient together or looked at only one patient's electronic MAR at a time. ⎯ ⎯ ⎯ ⎯⎯⎯⎯⎯

4. Closed room door and bedside curtain. ⎯ ⎯ ⎯ ⎯⎯⎯⎯⎯

5. Obtained and organized equipment for IV push infusion at bedside. ⎯ ⎯ ⎯ ⎯⎯⎯⎯⎯

IMPLEMENTATION

1. Performed hand hygiene. Prepared medications for one patient at a time using aseptic technique and avoiding distractions. Checked label of medication carefully with MAR or computer printout when removing medication from storage and after preparation. ⎯ ⎯ ⎯ ⎯⎯⎯⎯⎯

2. Took medication(s) to patient at correct time per agency policy. Gave non-time-critical scheduled medications within a range of 1 to 2 hours of scheduled dose. During administration, applied seven rights of medication administration. ⎯ ⎯ ⎯ ⎯⎯⎯⎯⎯

3. Identified patient using at least two identifiers according to agency policy. Compared identifiers with information on patient's MAR or EHR. ⎯ ⎯ ⎯ ⎯⎯⎯⎯⎯

4. At patient's bedside, again compared MAR or computer printout with names of medications on medication labels and patient name. Asked patient about allergies. ⎯ ⎯ ⎯ ⎯⎯⎯⎯⎯

5. Performed hand hygiene and applied clean gloves. ⎯ ⎯ ⎯ ⎯⎯⎯⎯⎯

6. Administered IV push (existing IV line): ⎯ ⎯ ⎯ ⎯⎯⎯⎯⎯

   a. Selected injection port of IV tubing closest to patient. Used needleless injection port. ⎯ ⎯ ⎯ ⎯⎯⎯⎯⎯

   b. Cleaned injection port with antiseptic swab. Allowed to dry. ⎯ ⎯ ⎯ ⎯⎯⎯⎯⎯

   c. Connected syringe to IV line: Inserted needleless tip of syringe containing drug through center of port. ⎯ ⎯ ⎯ ⎯⎯⎯⎯⎯

   d. Occluded IV line by pinching tubing just above injection port. Pulled back gently on plunger of syringe to aspirate for blood return. ⎯ ⎯ ⎯ ⎯⎯⎯⎯⎯

   e. Released tubing and injected medication within amount of time recommended by agency policy, pharmacist, or medication reference manual. Used watch to time administrations. Pinched IV line while pushing medication and released it when not pushing medication. Allowed IV fluids to infuse when not pushing medication. ⎯ ⎯ ⎯ ⎯⎯⎯⎯⎯

		S	U	NP	Comments

f. After injecting medication, withdrew syringe and rechecked IV fluid infusion rate.

   ____ ____ ____ _____

g. If IV medication was incompatible with IV fluids, stopped IV fluids, clamped IV line, and flushed with 10 mL of normal saline or sterile water per agency policy. Then gave IV push medication over appropriate amount of time and flushed with another 10 mL of normal saline or sterile water at same rate as medication was administered.

   ____ ____ ____ _____

h. If IV line that currently was hanging was infusing a medication, disconnected it and administered IV push medication, only as outlined in Step 7. Verified agency policy for stopping IV fluids or continuous IV medications. If unable to stop IV infusion, started new IV site and administered medication using IV push (IV lock) method.

   ____ ____ ____ _____

7. Administered IV push (IV lock):

   ____ ____ ____ _____

a. Prepared flush solutions according to agency policy.

   ____ ____ ____ _____

(1) Saline flush method (preferred method): If agency did not provide prefilled normal saline syringes for flushing IV lines, prepared two syringes filled with 2 to 3 mL of normal saline (0.9%). Labeled syringe to distinguish it from the syringe containing the medication that was being administered.

   ____ ____ ____ _____

(2) Heparin flush method (refer to agency policy).

   ____ ____ ____ _____

b. Administered medication:

   ____ ____ ____ _____

(1) Cleaned injection port with antiseptic swab.

   ____ ____ ____ _____

(2) Inserted needleless tip of syringe containing normal saline 0.9% (or heparin if required by agency) through center of injection port of IV lock.

   ____ ____ ____ _____

(3) Pulled back gently on syringe plunger and checked for blood return.

   ____ ____ ____ _____

(4) Flushed IV site by pushing slowly on plunger.

   ____ ____ ____ _____

(5) Removed saline-filled syringe.

   ____ ____ ____ _____

(6) Cleaned injection port with antiseptic swab. Allowed to dry.

   ____ ____ ____ _____

(7) Inserted needleless tip of syringe containing prepared medication through injection port of IV lock.

   ____ ____ ____ _____

(8) Injected medication within amount of time recommended by agency policy, pharmacist, or medication reference manual. Used watch to time administration.

   ____ ____ ____ _____

394

	S	U	NP	Comments

(9) After administering IV push, withdrew syringe. ___ ___ ___ _____

(10) Cleaned injection port with antiseptic swab. Allowed to dry. ___ ___ ___ _____

(11) Flushed injection port. ___ ___ ___ _____

    (a) Attached syringe with normal saline and injected flush at same rate that medication was delivered. ___ ___ ___ _____

8. Ensured that IV continued to run at a proper hourly rate after administering medication. ___ ___ ___ _____

9. Disposed of SESIP-covered needles and syringes in puncture- and leak-proof container. ___ ___ ___ _____

10. Helped patient to a comfortable position. ___ ___ ___ _____

11. Placed nurse call system in an accessible location within patient's reach. ___ ___ ___ _____

12. Raised side rails (as appropriate) and lowered bed to lowest position, locking into position. ___ ___ ___ _____

13. Disposed of all contaminated supplies in appropriate receptacle, removed and disposed of gloves, and performed hand hygiene. ___ ___ ___ _____

14. Stayed with patient for several minutes and observed for any allergic reactions. ___ ___ ___ _____

EVALUATION

1. Observed patient closely for adverse reactions during administration and for several minutes thereafter. ___ ___ ___ _____

2. Observed IV site during injection for sudden swelling and for 48 hours after IV push. ___ ___ ___ _____

3. Assessed patient's status, including relevant lab test results, after giving medication to evaluate effectiveness of the medication. ___ ___ ___ _____

4. Used Teach-Back: Revised instruction if patient or family caregiver was not able to teach back correctly. ___ ___ ___ _____

RECORDING

1. Immediately documented medication administration, including drug, dose, route, time instilled, and date and time administered on MAR. ___ ___ ___ _____

2. Documented patient teaching, validation of understanding, and patient's response to medication. ___ ___ ___ _____

HAND-OFF REPORTING

1. Reported any adverse reactions to patient's health care provider. ___ ___ ___ _____

Student _____ Date _____

Instructor _____ Date _____

PERFORMANCE CHECKLIST SKILL 22.6 **ADMINISTERING INTRAVENOUS MEDICATIONS BY PIGGYBACK AND SYRINGE PUMPS**

	S	U	NP	Comments

ASSESSMENT

1. Checked accuracy and completeness of each MAR or computer printout with health care provider's written medication order. Checked patient's name, medication name and dosage, route of administration, and time of administration. Clarified incomplete or unclear orders with health care provider before administration.   ___ ___ ___ _____

2. Reviewed EHR to assess patient's medical and medication history.   ___ ___ ___ _____

3. Assessed relevant laboratory results.   ___ ___ ___ _____

4. Reviewed medication reference information for medication action, purpose, normal dose, side effects, time and peak of onset, how slowly to give medication, and nursing implications.   ___ ___ ___ _____

5. Assessed patient's/family caregiver's health literacy.   ___ ___ ___ _____

6. Assessed patient's history of allergies: known type of allergens and normal allergic reaction. Applied allergy band to patient's wrist if allergy identified.   ___ ___ ___ _____

7. If giving medication through an existing IV line, determined compatibility of medication with IV fluids and any additives within IV solution.   ___ ___ ___ _____

8. To reduce the risks for administration set misconnections: ___ ___ ___ _____

   a. Performed hand hygiene. Traced all catheters/administration sets/add-on devices between the patient and container.   ___ ___ ___ _____

9. Assessed patency and placement of patient's existing IV infusion line or saline lock.   ___ ___ ___ _____

10. Assessed patient's symptoms before initiating medication therapy.   ___ ___ ___ _____

11. Assessed patient's knowledge of medication, prior experience with IV piggyback or syringe pump medication, and feelings about the procedure.   ___ ___ ___ _____

PLANNING

1. Determined expected outcomes following completion of procedure.   ___ ___ ___ _____

396

	S	U	NP	Comments

2. Provided privacy and explained medication and procedure to patient. Discussed purpose and side effects of IV piggyback or syringe pump medications. If applicable, taught patient how to report any side effects. ___ ___ ___ _____

3. Planned preparation to avoid interruptions. Created a quiet environment. Did not accept phone calls or talk with others. Followed agency "No-Interruption Zone" policy. Kept all pages of MARs or computer printouts for one patient together or looked at only one patient's electronic MAR at a time. ___ ___ ___ _____

4. Closed room door and bedside curtain. ___ ___ ___ _____

5. Obtained and organized equipment for IV piggyback or syringe pump medications at bedside. ___ ___ ___ _____

IMPLEMENTATION

1. Performed hand hygiene. Prepared medications for one patient at a time using aseptic technique and avoiding distractions. Checked label of medication carefully with MAR or computer printout at time medication was removed from storage and after preparation. ___ ___ ___ _____

2. Took medication(s) to patient at correct time per agency policy. Gave non-time-critical scheduled medications within a range of 1 to 2 hours of scheduled dose. During administration, applied seven rights of medication administration. ___ ___ ___ _____

3. Identified patient using at least two identifiers according to agency policy. Compared identifiers with information on patient's MAR or EHR. ___ ___ ___ _____

4. At patient's bedside, again compared MAR or computer printout with names of medications on medication labels and patient name. Asked patient if they had allergies. ___ ___ ___ _____

5. Administered infusion. Performed hand hygiene. Applied clean gloves. ___ ___ ___ _____

   a. Piggyback infusion:

     (1) Connected infusion tubing to piggyback medication bag. Filled tubing by opening regulator flow clamp. Once tubing was full, closed clamp and capped end of tubing. ___ ___ ___ _____

     (2) Hung piggyback medication bag above level of primary fluid bag. (Option: Used hook to lower main bag.) ___ ___ ___ _____

     (3) Connected tubing of piggyback infusion to appropriate connector on upper Y-port of primary infusion line: ___ ___ ___ _____

	S	U	NP	Comments

(a) Continuous Infusion: Wiped off needleless port of main IV line with antiseptic swab and allowed to dry. Then inserted needleless cannula tip of piggyback infusion tubing into port.

    ___ ___ ___ _____

(b) Option: Connected tubing of piggyback infusion to normal saline lock: Followed Steps 7a(1) through 7b(6) in Skill 22.5 to flush and prepare lock. Wiped off port with antiseptic swab, let dry, and inserted tip of piggyback infusion tubing into port via needleless access.

    ___ ___ ___ _____

(4) Regulated flow rate of medication solution by adjusting regulator clamp or IV pump infusion rate. Referred to medication reference or agency policy for safe flow rate.

    ___ ___ ___ _____

(5) Labeled all tubing and IV bags with your initials, patient initials, date, time the drug was hung, and when it was due to be infused.

    ___ ___ ___ _____

(6) Once medication had infused:

    ___ ___ ___ _____

(a) Checked flow rate of primary infusion. Primary infusion automatically began after piggyback solution was empty.

    ___ ___ ___ _____

(b) Checked normal saline lock: Disconnected piggyback tubing, cleaned port of lock with antiseptic swab, and flushed IV line with 2 to 3 mL of sterile 0.9% sodium chloride. Maintained sterility of IV tubing between intermittent infusions.

    ___ ___ ___ _____

(7) Regulated continuous main infusion line to ordered rate.

    ___ ___ ___ _____

(8) Left IV piggyback and tubing in place for future drug administration (per agency policy) or discarded in puncture- and leak-proof container.

    ___ ___ ___ _____

b. Volume-control administration set (e.g., Volutrol):

(1) Filled Volutrol with desired amount of IV fluid (50–100 mL) by opening clamp between Volutrol and main IV bag.

    ___ ___ ___ _____

(2) Closed clamp and checked to be sure that clamp on air vent Volutrol chamber was open.

    ___ ___ ___ _____

(3) Cleaned injection port on top of Volutrol with antiseptic swab.

    ___ ___ ___ _____

	S	U	NP	Comments

(4) Removed needle cap or sheath and inserted needleless tip or syringe needle of medication through port and injected medication. Gently rotated Volutrol between hands. ___ ___ ___ _____

(5) Regulated IV infusion rate to allow medication to infuse in time recommended by agency policy, pharmacist, or medication reference manual. ___ ___ ___ _____

(6) Labeled Volutrol with name of medication; dosage and total volume, including diluent; and time of administration following ISMP (2019) safe-medication label format. ___ ___ ___ _____

(7) If patient was receiving continuous IV infusion, checked infusion rate after Volutrol infusion was complete. ___ ___ ___ _____

(8) Disposed of uncapped needle or needle enclosed in safety shield and syringe in puncture- and leak-proof container. ___ ___ ___ _____

c. Syringe pump administration:

(1) Connected prefilled syringe to mini-infusion tubing; removed end cap of tubing. ___ ___ ___ _____

(2) Carefully applied pressure to syringe plunger, allowing tubing to fill with medication. ___ ___ ___ _____

(3) Placed syringe into a mini-infusion pump (following product directions) and hung it on IV pole. Ensured that syringe was secured. ___ ___ ___ _____

(4) Connected end of mini-infusion tubing to main IV line or saline lock: ___ ___ ___ _____

(a) Existing IV line: Wiped off needleless port on main IV line with antiseptic swab, allowed to dry, and inserted tip of mini-infusion tubing through center of port. ___ ___ ___ _____

(b) Normal saline lock: Followed Steps 7a(1) through 7b(6) in Skill 22.5 to flush and prepare lock. Wiped off port with antiseptic swab, allowed to dry, and inserted tip of mini-infusion tubing. ___ ___ ___ _____

(5) Set pump to deliver medication within time recommended by agency policy, pharmacist, or medication reference manual. Pressed button on pump to begin infusion. ___ ___ ___ _____

(6) Once medication had infused: ___ ___ ___ _____

(a) Main IV infusion: Checked flow rate. Infusion automatically began to flow once pump stopped. Regulated infusion to desired rate as needed. ___ ___ ___ _____

	S	U	NP	Comments

(b) Normal saline lock: Disconnected tubing, cleaned port with antiseptic swab and flushed IV line with 2 to 3 mL of sterile 0.9% sodium chloride. Maintained sterility of IV tubing between intermittent infusions. ___ ___ ___ _____

6. Helped patient to a comfortable position. ___ ___ ___ _____

7. Placed nurse call system in an accessible location within patient's reach. ___ ___ ___ _____

8. Raised side rails (as appropriate) and lowered bed to lowest position, locking into position. ___ ___ ___ _____

9. Disposed of all contaminated supplies in appropriate receptacle, removed and disposed of gloves, and performed hand hygiene. ___ ___ ___ _____

10. Stayed with patient for several minutes and observed for any allergic reactions. ___ ___ ___ _____

EVALUATION

1. Observed patient for signs or symptoms of adverse reaction. ___ ___ ___ _____

2. During infusion, periodically checked infusion rate and condition of IV site. ___ ___ ___ _____

3. Asked patient to explain purpose and side effects of medication. ___ ___ ___ _____

4. Used Teach-Back: Revised instruction if patient or family caregiver was not able to teach back correctly. ___ ___ ___ _____

RECORDING

1. Immediately documented medication, dose, route, infusion rate, and date and time administered in MAR. ___ ___ ___ _____

2. Documented volume of fluid in medication bag or Volutrol on intake and output (I&O) form. ___ ___ ___ _____

3. Documented patient teaching, validation of understanding, and patient's response to medication. ___ ___ ___ _____

HAND-OFF REPORTING

1. Reported any adverse reactions to patient's health care provider. ___ ___ ___ _____

Student _____   Date _____

Instructor _____   Date _____

PERFORMANCE CHECKLIST SKILL 22.7 **ADMINISTERING MEDICATIONS BY CONTINUOUS SUBCUTANEOUS INFUSION**

	S	U	NP	Comments
ASSESSMENT				
1. Checked accuracy and completeness of each MAR or computer printout with health care provider's written medication order. Checked patient's name, medication name and dosage, route of administration, and time of administration. Clarified incomplete or unclear orders with health care provider before administration.	___	___	___	_____
2. Reviewed EHR to assess patient's medical and medication history.	___	___	___	_____
3. Assessed for contraindications to CSQI.	___	___	___	_____
4. Reviewed EHR for the following factors: neonates and older adults; dry skin; dehydration; malnutrition; certain medications; dermatological conditions; and underlying medical conditions that affect the skin.	___	___	___	_____
5. Collected drug reference information necessary to administer drug safely, including action, purpose, side effects, normal dose, time of peak onset, rate setting for pump, and nursing implications.	___	___	___	_____
6. Assessed patient's/family caregiver's health literacy.	___	___	___	_____
7. Assessed patient's history of allergies: known type of allergens and normal allergic reaction. Applied allergy band to patient's wrist if allergy identified.	___	___	___	_____
8. Assessed patient's previous verbal and nonverbal response to needle insertion.	___	___	___	_____
9. If an analgesic was being administered, assessed character of patient's pain and rated severity using a scale from 0 to 10.	___	___	___	_____
10. Performed hand hygiene. Assessed adequacy of patient's adipose tissue to determine appropriate infusion site. If previous insertion site existed, assessed for redness, maceration, or skin tear.	___	___	___	_____
11. Assessed patient's knowledge of medication, prior experience with CSQI, and feelings about procedure.	___	___	___	_____
PLANNING				
1. Determined expected outcomes following completion of procedure.	___	___	___	_____

401

	S	U	NP	Comments

2. Provided privacy and explained procedure to patient. Discussed need for and what to anticipate with the initiation of CSQI. If applicable, taught patient how to perform cannula insertion.   ___ ___ ___ _____

3. Planned preparation to avoid interruptions. Created a quiet environment. Did not accept phone calls or talk with others. Followed agency "No-Interruption Zone" policy. Kept all pages of MARs or computer printouts for one patient together or looked at only one patient's electronic MAR at a time.   ___ ___ ___ _____

4. Reviewed manufacturer directions for how to use pump.   ___ ___ ___ _____

5. Obtained and organized equipment for CSQI at bedside.   ___ ___ ___ _____

IMPLEMENTATION

1. Reviewed manufacturer directions for how to use pump and infusion set.   ___ ___ ___ _____

2. Performed hand hygiene. Checked label of medication carefully with MAR or computer printout when removing medication from storage and after preparation.   ___ ___ ___ _____

3. At bedside, identified patient using at least two identifiers according to agency policy. Compared identifiers with information on patient's MAR or EHR.   ___ ___ ___ _____

4. At patient's bedside, again compared MAR or computer printout with name of medication on medication label on syringe and patient's name. Asked patient again about allergies.   ___ ___ ___ _____

5. Positioned patient comfortably, supine or sitting. Draped extremities.   ___ ___ ___ _____

6. Performed hand hygiene. Programmed infusion pump. If not using a commercial infusion set device, prepared infusion tubing of needle by priming with syringe filled with medication.   ___ ___ ___ _____

7. Prepared commercial infusion set: ___ ___ ___ _____

   a. For a commercial device such as a Quik Set™, used the transfer device and reservoir that comes with the set. Filled reservoir with the prescribed medication per device directions.   ___ ___ ___ _____

   b. Once reservoir was full, removed the transfer device used to fill the reservoir. Discarded in appropriate receptacle.   ___ ___ ___ _____

   c. Connected reservoir to the tubing of the infusion pump. Turned on pump and filled tubing following manufacturer's guidelines or directions shown on pump screen.   ___ ___ ___ _____

	S	U	NP	Comments

d. Prepared cannula/needle insertion device per manufacturer's directions. ___ ___ ___ _____

8. Initiated CSQI: ___ ___ ___ _____

   a. Performed hand hygiene and applied clean gloves. Selected appropriate injection site free of irritation and away from bony prominences and waistline. Chose site that patient could access. Noted condition of skin around proposed insertion site. ___ ___ ___ _____

   b. Cleaned injection site with antiseptic swab. Applied swab at center of site and rotated outward in a circular direction for about 5 cm (2 inches). Allowed to dry. ___ ___ ___ _____

   c. Commercial device:

      (1) Removed guard to expose cannula/needle in insertion device. ___ ___ ___ _____

      (2) Held insertion device against the prepared site on patient's skin. ___ ___ ___ _____

      (3) Followed manufacturer's directions and pushed down on device, inserting cannula/needle into the skin. ___ ___ ___ _____

      (4) Once cannula/needle was in place, pulled inserter away from the body and pressed adhesive disk surrounding the cannula/needle against the skin. ___ ___ ___ _____

   d. Winged needle:

      (1) If using a winged needle attached to prepared pump and tubing, pinched skin at insertion site. Then gently and firmly inserted needle at a 45- to 90-degree angle. Referred to manufacturer's directions. ___ ___ ___ _____

      (2) Released skinfold and applied gentle pressure around adhesive disk. Option: Covered with transparent semipermeable membrane (TSM). ___ ___ ___ _____

9. Initiated medication infusion: ___ ___ ___ _____

   a. Commercial device: Ensured cannula/needle was secure. Turned on pump and checked infusion rate. ___ ___ ___ _____

   b. Winged needle: Attached tubing from needle to tubing from infusion pump and turned on pump. Checked infusion rate. ___ ___ ___ _____

10. Inspected site before leaving patient, and instructed patient to inform you if site became red or swollen or began to leak. ___ ___ ___ _____

11. Helped patient to a comfortable position. ___ ___ ___ _____

	S	U	NP	Comments

12. Placed nurse call system in an accessible location within patient's reach.

13. Raised side rails (as appropriate) and lowered bed to lowest position, locking into position.

14. Disposed of all contaminated supplies in appropriate receptacle, removed and disposed of gloves, and performed hand hygiene.

15. Discontinued CSQI:

   a. Verified order and established alternative method for medication administration if applicable.

   b. Stopped infusion pump.

   c. Performed hand hygiene and applied clean gloves.

   d. Removed disk: Gently loosened a corner of the dressing. Lifted off disk while removing needle from skin at same angle it was inserted.

   e. Removed tape from wings of needle or removed transparent dressing without dislodging or removing needle and without pulling skin. Option: Removed nonbordered transparent membrane dressing by loosening a corner of the dressing and stretching it horizontally in the opposite direction of the wound. Walked fingers under the dressing to continue stretching it, with one hand continuously supporting the skin adhered to the dressing. Repeated the process around the dressing as necessary. Discarded tape/dressing in appropriate receptacle. Pulled needle out at the same angle at which it was inserted.

   f. Applied gentle pressure at site until no fluid leaked out of skin.

   g. Applied small sterile gauze dressing or adhesive bandage to site.

   h. Helped patient to a comfortable position.

   i. Placed nurse call system in an accessible location within patient's reach.

   j. Raised side rails (as appropriate) and lowered bed to lowest position, locking into position.

   k. Disposed of all contaminated supplies in appropriate receptacle, removed and disposed of gloves, and performed hand hygiene.

EVALUATION

1. Evaluated patient's response to medication.

2. Assessed site at least every 4 hours for redness, pain, drainage, or swelling.

	S	U	NP	Comments

3. Used Teach-Back: Revised instruction if patient or family caregiver was not able to teach back correctly. ___ ___ ___ _____

RECORDING

1. After initiating CSQI, immediately documented medication, dose, route, site, time, date, and type of medication pump. ___ ___ ___ _____

2. If medication was an opioid, followed agency policy to document waste. ___ ___ ___ _____

3. Documented patient's response to medication and appearance of site every 4 hours or according to agency policy. ___ ___ ___ _____

4. Documented patient teaching, validation of understanding, and patient's response to medication. ___ ___ ___ _____

HAND-OFF REPORTING

1. Reported any adverse effects from medication or infection or MARSI at insertion site to patient's health care provider and documented according to agency policy. ___ ___ ___ _____

Student _____ Date _____

Instructor _____ Date _____

PERFORMANCE CHECKLIST SKILL 23.1 **APPLYING AN OXYGEN-DELIVERY DEVICE**

	S	U	NP	Comments

ASSESSMENT

1. Identified patient using at least two identifiers according to agency policy. ___ ___ ___ _____

2. Reviewed patient's electronic health record (EHR), including health care provider's order and nurses' notes. ___ ___ ___ _____

3. Reviewed patient's EHR order for oxygen, noting delivery method, flow rate, duration of oxygen therapy, and parameters for titration of oxygen settings. ___ ___ ___ _____

4. Assessed patient's/family caregiver's health literacy. ___ ___ ___ _____

5. Performed hand hygiene and applied clean gloves. ___ ___ ___ _____

6. Performed respiratory assessment and checked for signs and symptoms associated with hypoxia. ___ ___ ___ _____

7. Inspected condition of skin around nose and ears. Noted if patient had any risk factors for MARSI and/or MDRPI. ___ ___ ___ _____

8. Observed for cognitive and behavioral changes. ___ ___ ___ _____

9. Assessed airway patency and removed airway secretions by having patient cough and expectorate mucus, or by suctioning. Auscultated lung sounds. Note: Removed and disposed of gloves and performed hand hygiene. Reapplied gloves if further contact with mucus was likely. ___ ___ ___ _____

10. Assessed patient's/family caregiver's knowledge and prior experience with oxygen administration and feelings about procedure. ___ ___ ___ _____

PLANNING

1. Determined expected outcomes following completion of procedure. ___ ___ ___ _____

2. Provided privacy and explained procedure. ___ ___ ___ _____

3. Organized and set up any equipment needed to perform procedure. ___ ___ ___ _____

4. Instructed patient and/or family caregiver about need for oxygen. If the oxygen was for home use, educated patient about oxygen safety in the home and the equipment that would be used. ___ ___ ___ _____

406

	S	U	NP	Comments

IMPLEMENTATION

1. Performed hand hygiene. Applied face shield if risk of exposure to splashing mucus existed. Applied gloves if patient had oral or nasal secretions. Applied gown if agency protocol dictated the need for one or if there was a risk of splash or excessive secretions..

2. Adjusted bed to appropriate height and lowered side rail on side nearest you. Positioned patient comfortably in semi-Fowler position.

3. Attached oxygen-delivery device to oxygen tubing and attached end of tubing to humidified oxygen source (if needed) adjusted to prescribed flow rate. Checked functioning.

4. Applied oxygen device:

   a. Nasal cannula: Placed tips of the nasal cannula into patient's nares. If tips were curved, they should have pointed downward inside nostrils. Then looped cannula tubing up and over patient's ears. Adjusted lanyard so cannula fit snugly but not too tightly, without pressure to patient nares and ears.

   b. Mask: Applied any type of oxygen mask by placing it over patient's mouth and nose. Then brought straps over patient's head and adjusted to form a comfortable but tight seal.

5. Maintained sufficient slack on oxygen tubing.

6. Observed for proper function of oxygen-delivery device:

   a. Nasal cannula: Cannula was positioned properly in nares; oxygen flowed through tips.

   b. Oxygen-conserving cannula: Fitted as for nasal.

   c. Nonrebreather mask: Applied as regular mask.

   d. Simple face mask: Selected appropriate flow rate.

   e. Venturi mask: Selected appropriate flow rate.

   f. HFNC: Fitted as for nasal cannula.

7. Verified setting on flowmeter and oxygen source for proper setup and prescribed flow rate.

8. Checked cannula/mask and humidity device (if used) every 8 hours or as agency policy indicated. Ensured that humidity container was filled at all times.

9. Posted "Oxygen in use" signs on wall behind bed and at entrance to room (per agency policy).

10. Removed and disposed of gloves.

11. Helped patient to comfortable position.

	S	U	NP	Comments

12. Raised side rails (as appropriate) and lowered bed to lowest position, locking into position. ___ ___ ___ _____

13. Placed nurse call system in an accessible location within the patient's reach. ___ ___ ___ _____

14. Properly disposed of used equipment and performed hand hygiene. ___ ___ ___ _____

EVALUATION

1. Monitored patient's response to changes in oxygen flow rate with SpO2. Note: Monitored ABGs when ordered. ___ ___ ___ _____

2. Performed respiratory assessment. Obtained vital signs. ___ ___ ___ _____

3. Assessed adequacy of oxygen flow each shift or per agency policy. ___ ___ ___ _____

4. Observed patient's external ears, bridge of nose, nares, and nasal mucous membranes for evidence of skin breakdown. ___ ___ ___ _____

5. Used Teach-Back: Revised instruction if patient or family caregiver was not able to teach back correctly. ___ ___ ___ _____

DOCUMENTATION

1. Documented the respiratory assessment findings, method of oxygen delivery, oxygen flow rate, patient's response to intervention, any adverse reactions or side effects, and documented status of patient's skin integrity. ___ ___ ___ _____

2. Documented evaluation of patient and family caregiver learning. ___ ___ ___ _____

HAND-OFF REPORTING

1. Reported patient status, including recent assessment findings, vital signs, SpO2, and skin integrity before and after oxygen administration. ___ ___ ___ _____

2. Reported the type of oxygen-delivery device initiated and used, the initial flow rates, and whether any adjustments to the flow rate were made during the shift. Included the patient response to the flow rate adjustments and what interventions were successful. ___ ___ ___ _____

3. Reported any unexpected outcome to health care provider or nurse in charge. ___ ___ ___ _____

Student _____ Date _____

Instructor _____ Date _____

PERFORMANCE CHECKLIST SKILL 23.2 **ADMINISTERING OXYGEN THERAPY TO A PATIENT WITH AN ARTIFICIAL AIRWAY**

	S	U	NP	Comments

ASSESSMENT

1. Identified patient using at least two identifiers according to agency policy. ___ ___ ___ _____

2. Reviewed patient's electronic health record (EHR), including health care provider's order and nurses' notes. Noted patient's normal and most recent pulse oximetry and $EtCO_2$ values, baseline and trends in respiratory rate and effort of breathing, past medical history, past oxygen requirements, and most recent ABG. Also reviewed for medical order for oxygen, flow rate, and duration of oxygen therapy. ___ ___ ___ _____

3. Assessed patient's/family caregiver's health literacy. ___ ___ ___ _____

4. Performed hand hygiene. Applied mask if there was risk of mucus splash. Assessed patient's respiratory status. Assessed for signs and symptoms associated with hypoxia. ___ ___ ___ _____

5. Observed condition of tissues surrounding ET tube or tracheostomy tube (TT) for impaired skin integrity on nares, lips, cheeks, corner of mouth, or neck; excess nasal or oral secretions; patient moving tube with tongue or biting tube or tongue; or foul-smelling mouth. ___ ___ ___ _____

6. Observed patency of airway. ___ ___ ___ _____

7. Observed for cognitive and behavioral changes. ___ ___ ___ _____

8. Monitored pulse oximetry (SpO2) and, if available, noted patient's most recent ABG results. Removed gloves and other PPE and performed hand hygiene. ___ ___ ___ _____

9. Assessed patient's/family caregiver's knowledge, prior experience with oxygen administration through an artificial airway, and feelings about procedure. ___ ___ ___ _____

PLANNING

1. Determined expected outcomes following completion of procedure. ___ ___ ___ _____

2. Provided privacy and explained procedure. ___ ___ ___ _____

3. Organized and set up any equipment needed to perform procedure. ___ ___ ___ _____

4. Instructed patient and/or family caregiver about need for oxygen. If the oxygen was for home use, educated patient about oxygen safety in the home and the equipment that would be used.

      ___ ___ ___ _____

IMPLEMENTATION

1. Performed hand hygiene, applied clean gloves and PPE as needed (per agency policy).

      ___ ___ ___ _____

2. Adjusted bed to appropriate height and lowered side rail on side nearest you. Positioned patient comfortably in semi-Fowler position.

      ___ ___ ___ _____

3. Attached T tube or tracheostomy mask to large-bore oxygen tubing and to humidified room air or oxygen source as indicated. Ensured that humidity container was filled at all times.

      ___ ___ ___ _____

4. If health care provider ordered oxygen, adjusted flow rate to 10 L/min or as ordered. Adjusted nebulizer to proper oxygen concentration (FiO2) setting. Attached T tube to artificial airway. Placed tracheostomy collar over TT and adjusted straps so it fit snugly.

      ___ ___ ___ _____

5. Observed that T tube did not pull on artificial airway or cause pressure on adjacent skin and tissue. Observed for secretions within T tube or tracheostomy collar and suctioned as necessary.

      ___ ___ ___ _____

6. Observed oxygen tubing frequently for accumulation of fluid caused by condensation. If fluid was present, drained tube away from patient, disconnected from collar or T tube, and discarded fluid in proper receptacle.

      ___ ___ ___ _____

7. Set up suction equipment at patient's bedside.

      ___ ___ ___ _____

8. Ensured patient remained in a comfortable position.

      ___ ___ ___ _____

9. Raised side rails (as appropriate) and lowered bed to lowest position, locking into position.

      ___ ___ ___ _____

10. Placed nurse call system in an accessible location within the patient's reach.

      ___ ___ ___ _____

11. Removed and disposed of PPE; performed hand hygiene.

      ___ ___ ___ _____

EVALUATION

1. Monitored patient's vital signs and SpO2.

      ___ ___ ___ _____

2. Performed respiratory assessment and observed for any cognitive and behavioral changes indicative of hypoxia.

      ___ ___ ___ _____

3. Observed position of oxygen-delivery device and condition of adjacent tissues to ensure that there was no pulling on artificial airway or pressure injuries.

      ___ ___ ___ _____

	S	U	NP	Comments

4. Used Teach-Back: Revised instruction if patient or family caregiver was not able to teach back correctly. ___ ___ ___ _____

DOCUMENTATION

1. Documented the respiratory assessment findings; method of oxygen delivery; flow rate; condition of tracheal stoma, peristomal area, or lips; patient's response; and any adverse reactions. ___ ___ ___ _____

2. Documented evaluation of patient and family caregiver learning. ___ ___ ___ _____

HAND-OFF REPORTING

1. Reported patient status, including recent assessment findings, vital signs, and SpO2 before and after oxygen administration. ___ ___ ___ _____

2. Reported the type of oxygen-delivery device initiated and used, the initial flow rates, and whether any ordered adjustments to the flow rate were made during the shift. Included the patient response to the flow rate adjustments and what interventions were successful. ___ ___ ___ _____

3. Reported any unexpected outcome to health care provider or nurse in charge. ___ ___ ___ _____

Student_____ Date_____

Instructor_____ Date_____

PERFORMANCE CHECKLIST SKILL 23.3 **USING INCENTIVE SPIROMETRY**

	S	U	NP	Comments

ASSESSMENT

1. Identified patient using at least two identifiers according to agency policy. ____ ____ ____ _____

2. Reviewed patient's electronic health record (EHR), including health care provider's order and nurses' notes. Reviewed if patient would benefit from IS. ____ ____ ____ _____

3. Assessed patient's/family caregiver's health literacy. ____ ____ ____ _____

4. Assessed patient for confusion, cognitive impairment, ability to follow directions, age, developmental level, level of consciousness, and decrease in necessary motor skills. ____ ____ ____ _____

5. Performed hand hygiene. Assessed patient's respiratory status. Also obtained a pulse oximetry reading. ____ ____ ____ _____

6. Assessed character of patient's pain and rated acuity on a pain scale of 0 to 10. ____ ____ ____ _____

7. Assessed knowledge, prior experience of patient/family caregiver with the use of the IS, and feelings about procedure. ____ ____ ____ _____

8. Assessed patient's goals or preferences for how incentive spirometry should be performed. ____ ____ ____ _____

PLANNING

1. Determined expected outcomes following completion of procedure. ____ ____ ____ _____

2. Provided privacy and explained procedure. ____ ____ ____ _____

3. Organized and set up any equipment needed to perform procedure. ____ ____ ____ _____

4. Instructed patient about need for IS. Indicated to patient where target volume is on IS. NOTE: If possible, demonstrated to patient how to use IS. ____ ____ ____ _____

IMPLEMENTATION

1. Performed hand hygiene. Appled clean gloves if there was risk of exposure to mucus. ____ ____ ____ _____

2. Adjusted bed to appropriate height and lowered side rail on side nearest you. Positioned patient in most erect position in bed or chair. ____ ____ ____ _____

	S	U	NP	Comments

3. Instructed patient to hold IS upright, exhale normally and completely through mouth, and place lips tightly around mouthpiece ⎯⎯ ⎯⎯ ⎯⎯ ⎯⎯⎯⎯⎯⎯⎯⎯⎯⎯⎯

4. Instructed patient to take a slow, deep breath and maintain constant flow, like pulling through a straw. Removed mouthpiece at point of maximal inhalation; then had patient hold his or her breath for 3 seconds and exhale normally. ⎯⎯ ⎯⎯ ⎯⎯ ⎯⎯⎯⎯⎯⎯⎯⎯⎯⎯⎯

5. Had patient repeat maneuver; encouraged patient to reach prescribed goal. ⎯⎯ ⎯⎯ ⎯⎯ ⎯⎯⎯⎯⎯⎯⎯⎯⎯⎯⎯

6. Encouraged patient to independently use IS at prescribed frequency. ⎯⎯ ⎯⎯ ⎯⎯ ⎯⎯⎯⎯⎯⎯⎯⎯⎯⎯⎯

7. Encouraged patient to cough after cycle of IS breaths. ⎯⎯ ⎯⎯ ⎯⎯ ⎯⎯⎯⎯⎯⎯⎯⎯⎯⎯⎯

8. Helped patient to comfortable position. ⎯⎯ ⎯⎯ ⎯⎯ ⎯⎯⎯⎯⎯⎯⎯⎯⎯⎯⎯

9. Raised side rails (as appropriate) and lowered bed to lowest position, locking into position. ⎯⎯ ⎯⎯ ⎯⎯ ⎯⎯⎯⎯⎯⎯⎯⎯⎯⎯⎯

10. Placed nurse call system in an accessible location within the patient's reach. ⎯⎯ ⎯⎯ ⎯⎯ ⎯⎯⎯⎯⎯⎯⎯⎯⎯⎯⎯

11. Removed and properly disposed of gloves, if used, and performed hand hygiene. ⎯⎯ ⎯⎯ ⎯⎯ ⎯⎯⎯⎯⎯⎯⎯⎯⎯⎯⎯

EVALUATION

1. Observed patient's ability to use incentive spirometry by return demonstration. ⎯⎯ ⎯⎯ ⎯⎯ ⎯⎯⎯⎯⎯⎯⎯⎯⎯⎯⎯

2. Assessed if patient was able to achieve target volume or frequency. ⎯⎯ ⎯⎯ ⎯⎯ ⎯⎯⎯⎯⎯⎯⎯⎯⎯⎯⎯

3. Auscultated chest during respiratory cycle and obtained pulse oximeter reading. ⎯⎯ ⎯⎯ ⎯⎯ ⎯⎯⎯⎯⎯⎯⎯⎯⎯⎯⎯

4. Used Teach-Back: Revised instruction if patient or family caregiver was not able to teach back correctly. ⎯⎯ ⎯⎯ ⎯⎯ ⎯⎯⎯⎯⎯⎯⎯⎯⎯⎯⎯

DOCUMENTATION

1. Documented lung sounds, respiratory rate, and pulse oximetry readings before and after incentive spirometry; frequency of use; volumes achieved; and any adverse effects. ⎯⎯ ⎯⎯ ⎯⎯ ⎯⎯⎯⎯⎯⎯⎯⎯⎯⎯⎯

2. Documented evaluation of patient and/or family caregiver learning. ⎯⎯ ⎯⎯ ⎯⎯ ⎯⎯⎯⎯⎯⎯⎯⎯⎯⎯⎯

HAND-OFF REPORTING

1. Reported patient status, including recent lung sounds, vital signs, and SpO2 before and after the use of the IS. ⎯⎯ ⎯⎯ ⎯⎯ ⎯⎯⎯⎯⎯⎯⎯⎯⎯⎯⎯

2. Reported the frequency of use of the IS, the desired volume/level the patient should reach, the actual volume/level attained, and patient tolerance of the procedure. ⎯⎯ ⎯⎯ ⎯⎯ ⎯⎯⎯⎯⎯⎯⎯⎯⎯⎯⎯

3. Reported the need for any analgesic medication prior to the use of the IS. ⎯⎯ ⎯⎯ ⎯⎯ ⎯⎯⎯⎯⎯⎯⎯⎯⎯⎯⎯

4. Reported any unexpected outcome to health care provider or nurse in charge. ⎯⎯ ⎯⎯ ⎯⎯ ⎯⎯⎯⎯⎯⎯⎯⎯⎯⎯⎯

Student _____ Date _____

Instructor _____ Date _____

PERFORMANCE CHECKLIST SKILL 23.4 **CARE OF A PATIENT RECEIVING NONINVASIVE POSITIVE PRESSURE VENTILATION**

	S	U	NP	Comments

ASSESSMENT

1. Identified patient using at least two identifiers according to agency policy. ___ ___ ___ _____

2. Reviewed patient's electronic health record (EHR), including health care provider's order and nurses' notes for patient's normal pulse oximetry values, baseline and trends in respiratory rate and effort of breathing, past medical history, past oxygen and NIPPV requirements, and most recent ABG results or SpO_2 value. Also reviewed EHR for prescription for NIPPV, noting pressure settings, desired amount of oxygen, desired facial appliance, and duration of therapy. ___ ___ ___ _____

3. Assessed patient's/family caregiver's health literacy. ___ ___ ___ _____

4. Performed hand hygiene and applied clean gloves. ___ ___ ___ _____

5. Assessed patient's respiratory status, including symmetry of chest wall expansion, respiratory rate and depth, oxygen saturation, sputum production, and lung sounds. If possible, asked patient about dyspnea and observed for signs and symptoms associated with hypoxia. ___ ___ ___ _____

6. Observed patient's skin over bridge of nose, around external ears, back of head. ___ ___ ___ _____

7. Observed patient's ability to clear and remove airway secretions by coughing. ___ ___ ___ _____

8. Assessed patient's level of consciousness, cognition and behaviors, and ability to maintain and protect airway. ___ ___ ___ _____

9. Removed and discarded gloves; performed hand hygiene. ___ ___ ___ _____

10. Assessed patient's/family caregiver's knowledge and prior experience with NIPPV and feelings about procedure. ___ ___ ___ _____

PLANNING

1. Determined expected outcomes following completion of procedure. ___ ___ ___ _____

2. Provided privacy and explained procedure. ___ ___ ___ _____

414

	S	U	NP	Comments

3. Collaborated with the respiratory therapist to gather and organize equipment/supplies to perform procedure at patient's bedside. ___ ___ ___ _____

4. Instructed patient and/or family caregiver about need for NIPPV. If NIPPV was for home use, educated patient about oxygen safety, use of equipment, and appropriate vendor and community resources. ___ ___ ___ _____

IMPLEMENTATION

1. Performed hand hygiene; applied clean gloves. Applied mask, gown, and goggles if secretions were projectile or if patient was in isolation. ___ ___ ___ _____

2. Determined correct mask size. Used masking chart to determine correct size (S, M, L, XL). Ensured masks had quick-release straps. ___ ___ ___ _____

3. Adjusted bed to appropriate height and lowered side rail on side nearest you. Checked locks on bed wheels. Placed patient in position of comfort with the head of the bed raised. ___ ___ ___ _____

4. Connected CPAP/BiPAP device-delivery tubing to pressure generator. ___ ___ ___ _____

5. Connected patient to pulse oximetry, if not already being monitored. ___ ___ ___ _____

6. Set CPAP/BiPAP initial settings per health care provider order: ___ ___ ___ _____

   a. CPAP: Initially, pressure was set at 3 to 5 cm H_2O or less, and then changes were guided by ABG and patient tolerance. ___ ___ ___ _____

   b. BiPAP: Inspiratory pressure was set at 5 to 15 cm H_2O initially and was titrated up to 20 to 30 cm H_2O as patient condition dictated; expiratory pressure was set at 3 to 4 cm H_2O initially and was titrated up as patient condition warranted. ___ ___ ___ _____

7. Selected FiO2 level as indicated and per prescriber order. ___ ___ ___ _____

8. Ensured that humidification and heating appliances were connected and on. ___ ___ ___ _____

9. Ensured that mask was tight fitting, no air leak was present, and there were no excessive pressure points. ___ ___ ___ _____

10. If patient was to use CPAP at home, had patient or family caregiver demonstrate mask placement and adjustment of settings. ___ ___ ___ _____

11. Returned patient to comfortable position. ___ ___ ___ _____

12. Raised side rails (as appropriate) and lowered bed to lowest position, locking into position. ___ ___ ___ _____

	S	U	NP	Comments

13. Placed nurse call system in an accessible location within the patient's reach.
_____ _____ _____ _____

14. Removed and disposed of gloves and other PPE, and performed hand hygiene.
_____ _____ _____ _____

15. Continuous care of patient:

   a. Ensured that all ventilator alarms were on and active and that ventilator circuit was intact and properly functioning.
_____ _____ _____ _____

   b. Ensured that emergency resuscitation equipment was at bedside.
_____ _____ _____ _____

   c. Investigated any and all alarms from ventilator/CPAP machine and/or patient monitor.
_____ _____ _____ _____

   d. Changed patient's position every 2 hours or encouraged patient to change position every 2 hours.
_____ _____ _____ _____

EVALUATION

1. Observed for decreased anxiety, improved level of consciousness and cognitive abilities, decreased fatigue, and absence of dizziness.
_____ _____ _____ _____

2. Measured vital signs, performed respiratory assessment, and asked patient to describe sense of dyspnea.
_____ _____ _____ _____

3. Assessed skin under mask every 1 to 2 hours for signs of skin breakdown/pressure injuries. Applied protective dressing/barrier if indicated.
_____ _____ _____ _____

4. Monitored pulse oximetry. Obtained ABG values per health care provider.
_____ _____ _____ _____

5. If NIPPV was planned for use in the home, observed and monitored the patient's and family caregiver's ability to use the NIPPV ventilator and manipulate the mask to have a good fit.
_____ _____ _____ _____

6. Used Teach-Back: Revised instruction if patient or family caregiver was not able to teach back correctly.
_____ _____ _____ _____

DOCUMENTATION

1. Documented type of NIPPV, including pressure settings, oxygen flow rates, assistance needed with positioning, coughing effectiveness, and respiratory assessment findings.
_____ _____ _____ _____

2. Documented patient tolerance of and adherence to NIPPV, mask fit, skin assessment findings, and patient subjective reports of comfort and daytime fatigue.
_____ _____ _____ _____

3. Documented evaluation of patient and family caregiver learning.
_____ _____ _____ _____

HAND-OFF REPORTING

1. Reported patient status, including recent assessment findings, vital signs, and SpO2 before initiation of NIPPV.
_____ _____ _____ _____

416

	S	U	NP	Comments

2. Reported the type of NIPPV device initiated and used, the initial pressure settings and oxygen flow rates, and if any adjustments to the pressure settings and flow rate were made during the shift. Included the patient response to the flow rate adjustments and what interventions were successful. ___ ___ ___ _____

3. Reported any unexpected outcome to health care provider or nurse in charge. ___ ___ ___ _____

PERFORMANCE CHECKLIST PROCEDURAL GUIDELINE 23.1   **USE OF A PEAK FLOWMETER**

	S	U	NP	Comments

PROCEDURAL STEPS

1. Identified patient using at least two identifiers according to agency policy.

2. Reviewed electronic health record (EHR) for patient's baseline PEFR readings (if available).

3. Reviewed the target set by patient's health care provider.

4. Assessed patient's/family caregiver's health literacy.

5. Performed hand hygiene and completed a respiratory assessment.

6. Assessed if patient had the manual dexterity to correctly measure PEFR by having patient manipulate device.

7. Assessed patient/family caregiver's knowledge and prior experience with the peak flowmeter.

8. Assessed patient's goals or preferences for how peak flow rate measurement should be performed.

9. Gathered peak flowmeter and diary at bedside.

10. Performed hand hygiene. Donned clean gloves if exposure to mucus was likely.

11. Closed room door or curtains around bed.

12. Instructed the patient and/or family caregiver about the need for the peak flowmeter.

13. Helped patient to stand or to assume a high-Fowler position or any other position that promoted optimum lung expansion. Removed any gum or food from mouth.

14. Slid the marker on the peak flow meter to the bottom of the scale.

15. Slid clean mouthpiece into base of the numbered scale. Instructed patient on how to place mouthpiece in mouth and close lips, making a firm seal. Instructed patient to keep tongue away from mouthpiece.

	S	U	NP	Comments

16. Instructed patient to take a deep breath and blow out. Then had patient take another deep breath and hold. Had patient quickly place meter mouthpiece in mouth, close lips firmly, and blow out as hard and fast as possible through mouth only. Noted the number on scale and documented on a piece of paper. ___ ___ ___ _____

17. Repeated two more times or as ordered by health care provider. ___ ___ ___ _____

18. Documented the highest number. ___ ___ ___ _____

19. Informed patient of the individualized acceptable range and marked on meter. ___ ___ ___ _____

20. If patient was to record PEFR at home, had the patient or family caregiver demonstrate how to record it accurately on chart using "traffic light" pattern. ___ ___ ___ _____

21. Instructed patient to measure peak flow rate every day, as close as possible to the same time every day. ___ ___ ___ _____

22. Instructed patient to keep a chart of daily peak flow values that could be shared with the health care provider. ___ ___ ___ _____

23. Instructed patient to clean unit weekly, following manufacturer instructions. ___ ___ ___ _____

24. Helped patient to comfortable position. ___ ___ ___ _____

25. Raised side rails (as appropriate) and lowered bed to lowest position, locking into position. ___ ___ ___ _____

26. Placed nurse call system in an accessible location within patient's reach. ___ ___ ___ _____

27. Removed and disposed of gloves and other PPE (if used) and performed hand hygiene. ___ ___ ___ _____

28. Used Teach-Back: Revised instruction if patient or family caregiver was not able to teach back correctly ___ ___ ___ _____

29. Compared patient's PEFR with the patient's personal best. ___ ___ ___ _____

30. Documented PEFR measurement before and after therapy and patient's ability and effort to perform PEFR. ___ ___ ___ _____

31. Reported to health care provider if patient was in yellow or red zone. ___ ___ ___ _____

32. Reported to nurses/respiratory therapists the patient's PEFR values and tolerance of performance of peak flow measurements. ___ ___ ___ _____

PERFORMANCE CHECKLIST SKILL 23.5 **CARE OF A PATIENT ON A MECHANICAL VENTILATOR**

	S	U	NP	Comments

ASSESSMENT

1. Identified patient using at least two identifiers according to agency policy.

2. Reviewed patient's EHR, including health care provider's order and nurses' notes.

3. Reviewed patient's EHR for prescription for oxygen requirements and ventilator settings. Noted any titration parameters.

4. Reviewed EHR to determine patient's age and history of dehydration, malnutrition, exposure to radiation therapy, underlying chronic conditions, and edema of the skin.

5. Assessed patient's/family caregiver's health literacy. Determined method for communication with patient. If possible, reviewed previous communication techniques with patient and family. Used simple language to gather assessment.

6. Assessed patient's level of consciousness (LOC) and ability to cooperate with mechanical ventilation and tolerate need for special positioning.

7. Assessed patient's need for sedation (per agency policy).

8. Performed hand hygiene. Applied gloves and other PPE as patient status indicated.

9. Assessed patient's respiratory status and assessed for signs and symptoms associated with hypoxia.

10. Assessed patient's cardiovascular condition.

11. Assessed for signs and symptoms of inadvertent extubation.

12. Checked ventilator, EtCO2 (if available), SpO2, and cardiac alarms at beginning of each shift and periodically throughout care and compared with health care provider's orders.

13. Verified placement of artificial airway through auscultation of lung sounds, verification of distal tip marking on ET tube, and/or EtCO2 value. Determined that tube was secure and stable.

	S	U	NP	Comments

a. Auscultated over trachea for presence of air leak. Assessed and compared inhaled and exhaled tidal volumes as measured by ventilator. ___ ___ ___ _____

b. Used cuff pressure monitoring device. ___ ___ ___ _____

14. Ensured suctioning system was functioning properly. ___ ___ ___ _____

15. Observed for patent airway and, if necessary, removed airway secretions by suctioning. Removed and disposed of gloves and performed hand hygiene. ___ ___ ___ _____

16. Applied clean gloves. Inspected integrity of patient's oral mucous membrane and skin around tube stabilization device or adhesives. ___ ___ ___ _____

17. If available, noted patient's most recent ABG results or SpO2. Determined if any factors had changed during mechanical ventilation. Removed and disposed of gloves and performed hand hygiene. ___ ___ ___ _____

18. Assessed patient's/family caregiver's knowledge and prior experience with mechanical ventilation and feelings about procedure. ___ ___ ___ _____

PLANNING

1. Determined expected outcomes following completion of procedure. ___ ___ ___ _____

2. Provided privacy and explained procedure. ___ ___ ___ _____

3. Organized and set up any equipment needed to perform procedure. ___ ___ ___ _____

4. Explained ventilator system to patient and family caregiver and included purpose of and reasons for initiation of mechanical ventilation. ___ ___ ___ _____

5. Arranged for extra personnel to help as necessary. ___ ___ ___ _____

IMPLEMENTATION

1. Performed hand hygiene; applied clean gloves. Applied PPE: mask, gown, and goggles if secretions were projectile or if isolation precautions secondary to infectious status were indicated. ___ ___ ___ _____

2. Ensured that suction equipment was set up and functioning, including oral suctioning. ___ ___ ___ _____

3. Ensured that subglottic suctioning equipment (if tube was equipped for such type of suction) was functioning appropriately. ___ ___ ___ _____

4. Checked need for airway suctioning, then positioned patient with HOB elevated 30 to 45 degrees (unless contraindicated). ___ ___ ___ _____

5. Ensured there was proper connection of ET or TT to ventilator with mechanical ventilator functioning. ___ ___ ___ _____

	S	U	NP	Comments

6. Observed patient for synchronization with mechanical ventilation and response to therapy. ___ ___ ___ _____

7. Monitored heart rate, blood pressure, respiratory rate, temperature, and cardiac rhythm routinely during care (per agency policy). ___ ___ ___ _____

8. Reassessed and marked level of ET tube at patient's teeth. Ensured that ET tube continued to be secured. ___ ___ ___ _____

9. Repositioned patient regularly (minimum of every 2 hours), maintaining HOB elevation of 30 to 45 degrees, or, in some cases, prone position. Monitored SpO_2 levels during and after positioning. Assessed ET tube markings at teeth to ensure tube placement had not changed. ___ ___ ___ _____

10. Collaborated with health care provider frequently about status of patient, response to therapy, and ongoing monitoring. ___ ___ ___ _____

    a. Monitored SpO_2 continuously. ___ ___ ___ _____

    b. Monitored $EtCO_2$ continually (if available and indicated). ___ ___ ___ _____

    c. Obtained serial ABG levels with changes in patient's condition or ventilator changes per provider order. ___ ___ ___ _____

11. Performed safety checks on patient and ventilator system: ___ ___ ___ _____

    a. Placed nurse call system in an accessible location within patient's reach. ___ ___ ___ _____

    b. Checked security of all ventilator connections; made sure that alarms were all turned on. ___ ___ ___ _____

    c. Collaborated with RT and verified that all ventilator settings were correct and corresponded to health care provider's orders. ___ ___ ___ _____

    d. Checked and refilled humidifier as needed. Checked corrugated tubing for condensation; drained away from patient but not into humidifier and appropriately discarded liquid. ___ ___ ___ _____

    e. When present, observed temperature gauges on panel of mechanical ventilator, making sure that gas was delivered at correct temperature. Conferred with RT if settings needed adjusting. ___ ___ ___ _____

12. Performed mouth care at least 4 times per 24 hours. Used 0.12% chlorhexidine to brush teeth, gums, and tongue with soft toothbrush at least twice a day. Applied water-based moisturizer every 2 to 4 hours. ___ ___ ___ _____

13. Monitored for the development of oral or lip ulcers or facial skin tears. ___ ___ ___ _____

	S	U	NP	Comments

14. Inserted bite block if patient bit ET tube. ___ ___ ___ _____

15. Administered sedating drugs as indicated. ___ ___ ___ _____

16. Performed daily interruption in sedation; assessed readiness to extubate. ___ ___ ___ _____

17. Instituted deep vein thrombosis (DVT) prophylaxis as ordered per health care provider. ___ ___ ___ _____

18. Performed nursing activities to prevent hazards of immobility. ___ ___ ___ _____

19. Ensured that communication method was in place for patient after administering care. ___ ___ ___ _____

20. Kept patient and family informed about progress and plan for weaning from mechanical ventilator. ___ ___ ___ _____

21. Removed and disposed of PPE; performed hand hygiene. ___ ___ ___ _____

22. Helped patient to a comfortable position with HOB elevated 30 to 45 degrees. ___ ___ ___ _____

23. Raised side rails (as appropriate) and lowered bed to lowest position, locking into position. ___ ___ ___ _____

24. Placed nurse call system in an accessible location within the patient's reach. ___ ___ ___ _____

25. Performed hand hygiene. ___ ___ ___ _____

EVALUATION

1. Monitored and evaluated patient's response to mechanical ventilation every 1 to 4 hours. ___ ___ ___ _____

   a. Neurological assessment: LOC, orientation, sleepiness. changes in anxiety, sedation levels ___ ___ ___ _____

   b. Pulmonary assessment: Lung sounds, airway clearance, work of breathing, breathing pattern, rate of respirations, SpO_2, $EtCO_2$ ___ ___ ___ _____

   c. Cardiovascular assessment: Vital signs, heart rhythm, heart sounds, lower extremity edema, pulse quality ___ ___ ___ _____

2. Observed integrity of patient ventilator system. ___ ___ ___ _____

3. Observed and evaluated effectiveness of communication methods: ___ ___ ___ _____

   a. Asked patient if needs and concerns were addressed. ___ ___ ___ _____

   b. Observed for signs of frustration. ___ ___ ___ _____

   c. Observed patient/family caregiver and health care personnel using communication methods. ___ ___ ___ _____

4. Used Teach-Back: Revised instruction if patient or family caregiver was not able to teach back correctly. ___ ___ ___ _____

	S	U	NP	Comments

DOCUMENTATION

1. Documented the following: respiratory assessment findings, mode of mechanical ventilation, oxygen level, actual patient tidal volume, actual patient respiratory rate, peak inspiratory pressure, vital signs, size and level of the ET tube, ABG results (if performed as a point-of-care test), patient level of comfort, sedation level scores (if sedation was used), and degree of bed elevation.

2. Documented nursing interventions that were performed, including oral care, repositioning, range-of-motion exercises, medications that were administered, and suctioning.

3. Documented evaluation of patient and caregiver learning.

HAND-OFF REPORTING

1. Reported patient status, including recent assessment findings, vital signs, and SpO2 before and after initiation of mechanical ventilation.

2. Reported the type of ventilator used and mode of ventilation. Included the patient response to any ventilator adjustments and what interventions were successful.

3. Reported patient tolerance to nursing interventions.

4. Reported any unexpected outcomes to health care provider or nurse in charge.

424

Student _____ Date _____

Instructor _____ Date _____

PERFORMANCE CHECKLIST SKILL 24.1 **PERFORMING OROPHARYNGEAL SUCTIONING**

	S	U	NP	Comments
ASSESSMENT				
1. Identified patient using at least two identifiers.	—	—	—	_____
2. Reviewed patient's electronic health record (EHR), including health care provider's order and nurses' notes for patient's normal pulse oximeter values, baseline and trends in respiratory rate and effort of breathing, frequency of suctioning, and response to suctioning.	—	—	—	_____
3. Reviewed patient's medical history and identified risk factors for airway obstruction.	—	—	—	_____
4. Reviewed EHR for conditions including recent head and neck surgery or mouth trauma.	—	—	—	_____
5. Assessed patient's/family caregiver's health literacy.	—	—	—	_____
6. Performed hand hygiene. Applied gloves and any other PPE equipment as patient condition dictated.	—	—	—	_____
7. Assessed patient's level of consciousness and obtained vital signs (VS), noted signs and symptoms of hypoxia.	—	—	—	_____
8. Obtained patient's oxygen saturation level via SpO_2. Did not remove probe until after the oropharynx was suctioned.	—	—	—	_____
9. Assessed for signs and symptoms of upper airway obstruction.	—	—	—	_____
10. Auscultated for presence of adventitious sounds.	—	—	—	_____
11. Assessed patient's knowledge, prior experience with oropharyngeal suctioning, and feelings about procedure.	—	—	—	_____
PLANNING				
1. Determined expected outcomes following completion of procedure.	—	—	—	_____
2. Performed hand hygiene. Gathered equipment/supplies at patient's bedside. Checked the suction machine to ensure it was working properly.	—	—	—	_____

425

	S	U	NP	Comments

3. Closed the room door or the curtain. Lowered side rails and assisted patient to comfortable position, typically semi-Fowler or high Fowler. ___ ___ ___ _____

4. Explained to patient how procedure helped clear airway secretions and relieve some breathing problems. Explained that coughing, gagging, or (less commonly) sneezing was normal and lasts only a few seconds. Encouraged patient to cough out secretions and showed how to splint painful areas during procedure. Practiced coughing if able. ___ ___ ___ _____

IMPLEMENTATION

1. Performed hand hygiene. Applied clean gloves. Applied mask or face shield if splashing was likely. Wore gown if isolation precautions were indicated. ___ ___ ___ _____

2. Placed towel, cloth, or paper drape across patient's neck and chest. Placed pulse oximeter on finger, if not already in place. ___ ___ ___ _____

3. Filled cup or basin with approximately 100 mL of water or normal saline. ___ ___ ___ _____

4. Connected one end of connecting tubing to suction machine and other to Yankauer suction catheter. Turned on suction machine; set vacuum regulator to appropriate suction, typically between 80 and 120 mm Hg. ___ ___ ___ _____

5. Checked that suction machine was functioning properly by placing tip of catheter in water or normal saline and suctioning small amount from cup or basin. ___ ___ ___ _____

6. Removed patient's oxygen mask if present. Left nasal cannula in place if present. Kept oxygen mask near patient's face. ___ ___ ___ _____

7. Inserted catheter into mouth along gum line to pharynx. Moved catheter around mouth until secretions were cleared. Encouraged patient to cough. Replaced oxygen mask. ___ ___ ___ _____

8. Rinsed catheter with water or normal saline in cup or basin until connecting tubing was cleared of secretions. Turned off suction. Placed catheter in clean, dry area. Removed and disposed of gloves (and any other PPE). Performed hand hygiene. ___ ___ ___ _____

9. Observed respiratory status. Repeated procedure if indicated. Used standard suction catheter to reach trachea if respiratory status was not improved (as needed). ___ ___ ___ _____

426

	S	U	NP	Comments

10. Removed towel, cloth, or disposable drape and placed in trash or laundry if soiled. Repositioned patient; preferably in lateral recumbent or side-lying position if patient had decreased level of consciousness. ____ ____ ____ _____

11. Discarded remainder of water or normal saline into appropriate receptacle. Rinsed basin in warm, soapy water and dried with paper towels or discarded (per agency policy). Discarded disposable cup into appropriate receptacle. Performed hand hygiene. ____ ____ ____ _____

12. Applied clean gloves to provide personal care. ____ ____ ____ _____

13. Helped patient to a comfortable position. ____ ____ ____ _____

14. Placed nurse call system in an accessible location within the patient's reach. ____ ____ ____ _____

15. Raised side rails (as appropriate) and lowered and locked the bed into the lowest position. ____ ____ ____ _____

16. Removed and disposed of gloves. Performed hand hygiene. ____ ____ ____ _____

EVALUATION

1. Compared assessment findings before and after procedure. ____ ____ ____ _____

2. Auscultated chest and airways for adventitious sounds. ____ ____ ____ _____

3. Inspected mouth for any vomitus or remaining secretions. ____ ____ ____ _____

4. Obtained and documented postsuction SpO_2 value. Compared with presuction level. ____ ____ ____ _____

5. Used Teach-Back. Revised or developed a plan for revised patient/family caregiver teaching if patient or family caregiver was not able to teach back correctly. ____ ____ ____ _____

DOCUMENTATION

1. Documented the amount, consistency, color, and odor of secretions; number of times suctioned; patient's response to suctioning; and presuction and postsuction cardiopulmonary assessment findings. ____ ____ ____ _____

2. Documented evaluation of patient learning. ____ ____ ____ _____

HAND-OFF REPORTING

1. Reported any unresolved outcomes such as worsening respiratory distress to the health care provider. ____ ____ ____ _____

2. Reported frequency of suctioning and patient response to suction, as well as presuction and postsuction assessments. ____ ____ ____ _____

Student _____ Date _____

Instructor _____ Date _____

PERFORMANCE CHECKLIST SKILL 24.2 **SUCTIONING: OPEN FOR NASOTRACHEAL / PHARYNGEAL AND ARTIFICIAL AIRWAYS**

	S	U	NP	Comments

ASSESSMENT

1. Identified patient using at least two identifiers. ____ ____ ____ _____

2. Obtained necessary information from patient's electronic health record (EHR) including history of abnormal anatomy or head and neck surgery / trauma, tumors involving lower airway, pneumonia, chronic obstructive pulmonary disease and neurological abnormalities. ____ ____ ____ _____

3. Reviewed EHR for patient's normal pulse oximeter and end-tidal CO_2 values, vital signs (VS), previous response and tolerance to suctioning procedure, and color and quantity of sputum. ____ ____ ____ _____

4. Reviewed sputum microbiology data in laboratory report. ____ ____ ____ _____

5. Assessed patient's / family caregiver's health literacy. ____ ____ ____ _____

6. Performed hand hygiene and applied clean gloves or other personal protective equipment (PPE) if risk of exposing self to secretions or if patient condition indicates. ____ ____ ____ _____

7. Auscultated lungs and assessed for: ____ ____ ____ _____

   a. Signs and symptoms of upper and lower airway obstruction requiring suctioning. ____ ____ ____ _____

   b. VS and oximetry signs and symptoms associated with respiratory distress or hypoxia and hypercapnia. Kept pulse oximetry on patient for continuous assessment of SpO_2. ____ ____ ____ _____

8. Assessed for risk factors for upper and lower airway obstruction, including chronic obstructive pulmonary disease, impaired mobility, decreased level of consciousness, nasal feeding tube, decreased cough or gag reflex, and decreased swallowing ability. ____ ____ ____ _____

428

	S	U	NP	Comments

9. Assessed for excessive amounts of secretions visible in the artificial airway, signs of respiratory distress from obstructed airway, presence of rhonchi on auscultation, excessive coughing, increased peak inspiratory pressures (if on mechanical ventilator), sawtooth pattern on ventilator monitor, or changes in capnography waveform (if patient on mechanical ventilator) or decrease in patient pulse oximeter. ____ ____ ____ _____

10. Assessed patency of ET with capnography/end-tidal carbon dioxide (CO_2) detector. ____ ____ ____ _____

11. Assessed factors that may affect volume and consistency of secretions. ____ ____ ____ _____

   a. Fluid balance ____ ____ ____ _____

   b. Lack of humidity ____ ____ ____ _____

   c. Infection ____ ____ ____ _____

12. For endotracheal suctioning, assessed patient's peak inspiratory pressure when on volume-controlled ventilation or tidal volume during pressure-controlled ventilation. ____ ____ ____ _____

13. Identified contraindications to nasotracheal suctioning. ____ ____ ____ _____

14. Removed and disposed of gloves. Performed hand hygiene. Kept other PPE on for actual suctioning. ____ ____ ____ _____

15. Determined presence of apprehension, anxiety, decreased ability to concentrate, lethargy, decreased level of consciousness (especially acute), increased fatigue, dizziness, and/or behavioral changes (especially irritability). ____ ____ ____ _____

16. Assessed knowledge and experience of patient and family caregiver with suctioning procedure. ____ ____ ____ _____

PLANNING

1. Determined expected outcomes following completion of procedure. ____ ____ ____ _____

2. Performed hand hygiene. Arranged supplies at patient's bedside. Closed room door or curtain. ____ ____ ____ _____

3. Explained to patient procedure and how procedure will help clear airway and relieve breathing difficulty. Explained that temporary coughing, sneezing, gagging, or shortness of breath was normal during procedure. ____ ____ ____ _____

	S	U	NP	Comments

IMPLEMENTATION

1. Performed hand hygiene and applied appropriate PPE, if not already applied during assessment (mask with face shield or goggles; gown if necessary).   ___ ___ ___ _____

2. If not already present, placed pulse oximeter on patient's finger. Took reading and left oximeter in place.   ___ ___ ___ _____

3. Adjusted bed to appropriate height (if not already done) and lowered side rail on side nearest self. Checked locks on bed wheels. Assisted patient to comfortable position, typically semi-Fowler or high Fowler.   ___ ___ ___ _____

4. Connected one end of connecting tubing to suction device and placed other end in convenient location near patient. Turned suction device on and set suction pressure to as low a level as possible and yet able to effectively clear secretions, typically between 80 and 120 mm Hg. Occluded end of suction tubing to check pressure.   ___ ___ ___ _____

5. Prepared suction catheter for all types of open suctioning.   ___ ___ ___ _____

   a. Using aseptic technique, opened suction kit or catheter package. If sterile drape was available, placed it across patient's chest or on bedside table. Did not allow suction catheter to touch any nonsterile surfaces.   ___ ___ ___ _____

   b. Unwrapped or opened sterile basin and placed on bedside table. Was careful not to touch inside of basin. Filled with about 100 mL sterile normal saline solution or water.   ___ ___ ___ _____

   c. If performing nasotracheal suctioning, opened packet of water-soluble lubricant and applied small amount to sterile field. NOTE: Lubricant was not necessary for artificial airway suctioning.   ___ ___ ___ _____

6. Applied sterile gloves to each hand or clean glove to nondominant hand and sterile glove to dominant hand.   ___ ___ ___ _____

7. Picked up suction catheter with dominant hand without touching nonsterile surfaces. Picked up connecting tubing with nondominant hand. Secured catheter to tubing.   ___ ___ ___ _____

8. Placed tip of catheter into sterile basin and suctioned small amount of normal saline solution from basin by occluding suction vent.   ___ ___ ___ _____

9. Suctioned airway.   ___ ___ ___ _____

	S	U	NP	Comments

a. Nasopharyngeal and nasotracheal:

(1) Asked patient to extend neck back slightly. Had patient take deep breaths, if able, or increased oxygen flow rate with delivery device through cannula or mask (if ordered).

         ___ ___ ___ _____

(2) Lightly coated distal 6 to 8 centimeters (2 to 3 inches) of catheter with water-soluble lubricant.

         ___ ___ ___ _____

(3) Removed oxygen-delivery device, if applicable, with nondominant hand.

         ___ ___ ___ _____

(4) Introduced catheter and applied suction.

         ___ ___ ___ _____

   (a) Nasopharyngeal: As patient took deep breath, inserted catheter (without applying suction) following natural course of naris; slightly slanted catheter downward and advanced to back pharynx. Did not force through naris. In adults, inserted catheter approximately 16 centimeters (6.5 inches); in older children, 8 to 12 centimeters (3 to 5 inches); in infants and young children, 4 to 7.5 centimeters (1.5 to 3 inches).

         ___ ___ ___ _____

     (i) Applied intermittent suction for no more than 10 to 15 seconds by placing and releasing nondominant thumb over catheter vent. Slowly withdrew catheter while rotating it back and forth between thumb and forefinger.

         ___ ___ ___ _____

   (b) Nasotracheal: With head slighting extended, had patient take deep breaths, then advanced catheter (without applying suction) following natural course of naris. Advanced catheter slightly slanted and downward to just above larynx. While patient took deep breath, quickly inserted catheter into larynx. Patient began to cough; then pulled back catheter 1 to 2 centimeters (1/2 inch) before applying suction.

         ___ ___ ___ _____

	S	U	NP	Comments

(i) Positioning option: Turned patient's head to improve suctioning. If resistance was felt after insertion of catheter, pulled catheter back 1 centimeter (0.4 inches) before applying suction.   ___ ___ ___ _____

(ii) Applied intermittent suction for no more than 10 to 15 seconds by placing and releasing nondominant thumb over catheter vent. Slowly withdrew catheter while rotating it back and forth between thumb and forefinger.   ___ ___ ___ _____

(iii) If there were pharyngeal secretions preset, suctioned just before removing catheter from naris. Did not suction nasally again after suctioned mouth.   ___ ___ ___ _____

(5) Reapplied oxygen-delivery device and encouraged patient to take some deep breaths, if able.   ___ ___ ___ _____

(6) Rinsed catheter and connecting tubing with normal saline or water until cleared.   ___ ___ ___ _____

(7) Assessed for need to repeat suctioning. Did not perform more than two passes with catheter. Allowed patient to rest at least 1 minute. Asked patient to deep breathe and cough.   ___ ___ ___ _____

b. Artificial airway:

(1) With assistance from respiratory therapy when patient has an artificial airway, hyperoxygenated, when appropriate, with 100% oxygen for at least 30 to 60 seconds before suctioning by having (1) pressed suction hyperoxygenation button on ventilator, OR (2) increased baseline fraction of inspired oxygen (FiO_2) level on mechanical ventilator, OR (3) disconnected ventilator, attached self-inflating resuscitation bag-valve device to tube with nondominant hand (or had assistant do this), and administered 5 to 6 breaths over 30 seconds (or had assistant do this). NOTE: Some mechanical ventilators had button that, when pushed, delivered 100% oxygen for a few minutes and then reset to previous setting.   ___ ___ ___ _____

432

	S	U	NP	Comments

(2) If patient was receiving mechanical ventilation, opened swivel adapter or, if necessary, removed oxygen- or humidity-delivery device with nondominant hand.

——— ——— ——— ————————————

(3) Advised patient that nurse was about to begin suctioning. Without applying suction, gently but quickly inserted catheter into tracheostomy or artificial airway using dominant thumb and forefinger, timing insertion with airway inspiration. Advanced catheter until patient coughed (usually 0.5 to 1 centimeter below level of the tube). Then pulled back 1 centimeter (0.4 inch) before applying suction.

——— ——— ——— ————————————

(4) Applied intermittent suction for 10 seconds by placing and releasing nondominant thumb over valve of catheter. Slowly withdrew catheter while rotating it back and forth between dominant thumb and forefinger. Did not use suction for greater than 15 seconds. Encouraged patient to cough. Watched for respiratory distress.

——— ——— ——— ————————————

(5) If patient was receiving mechanical ventilation, closed swivel adapter or replaced oxygen-delivery device. Hyperoxygenated patient for 30 to 60 seconds.

——— ——— ——— ————————————

(6) Rinsed catheter and connecting tubing with normal saline until clear. Used continuous suction.

——— ——— ——— ————————————

(7) Assessed patient's vital signs (VS), cardiopulmonary status, and ventilator measures for secretion clearance. Repeated Steps 9b(1) through 9b(6) once or twice more to clear secretions. Allowed adequate time (at least 1 full minute) between suction passes.

——— ——— ——— ————————————

c. When trachea or artificial airways were sufficiently cleared of secretions, performed oropharyngeal suctioning to clear mouth of secretions. Did not suction nose with catheter after suctioning mouth.

——— ——— ——— ————————————

	S	U	NP	Comments

10. When suctioning was complete, disconnected catheter from connecting tubing. Rolled catheter around fingers of dominant hand. Pulled glove off inside out so that catheter remains coiled in glove. Pulled off other glove over first glove in same way. Discarded in appropriate receptacle. Turned off suction device.

_____ _____ _____ _____

11. Removed towel, place in laundry or appropriate receptacle, and repositioned patient. (Applied clean gloves to continue personal care.)

_____ _____ _____ _____

12. If oxygen level was changed during procedure, readjusted oxygen to original ordered level; patient's blood oxygen level should have returned to baseline.

_____ _____ _____ _____

13. Discarded remainder of normal saline. If basin was disposable, discarded into appropriate receptacle. If basin was reusable, rinsed it out and placed it in soiled utility room.

_____ _____ _____ _____

14. Helped patient to comfortable position and provided oral hygiene as needed.

_____ _____ _____ _____

15. Removed and disposed of gloves and other PPE, if used, and performed hand hygiene.

_____ _____ _____ _____

16. Placed unopened suction kit on suction machine table or at head of bed.

_____ _____ _____ _____

17. Raised side rails (as appropriate) and lowered and locked bed into lowest position.

_____ _____ _____ _____

18. Placed nurse call system in an accessible location within the patient's reach.

_____ _____ _____ _____

EVALUATION

1. Compared patient's VS, cardiopulmonary assessments, and EtCO2 and SpO2 values before and after suctioning. If on ventilator, compared FiO2 and tidal volumes and peak inspiratory pressures.

_____ _____ _____ _____

2. Asked patient if breathing was easier and if congestion was decreased.

_____ _____ _____ _____

3. Observed character of airway secretions.

_____ _____ _____ _____

4. Used Teach-Back. Revised instruction or developed a plan for revised patient/family caregiver learning if patient or family caregiver was not able to teach back correctly.

_____ _____ _____ _____

DOCUMENTATION

1. Documented the amount, consistency, color, and odor of secretions; size of catheter; route of suctioning; and patient's response to suctioning.

_____ _____ _____ _____

434

	S	U	NP	Comments

2. Documented patient's presuctioning and postsuctioning VS, cardiopulmonary status, and ventilation measures. ___ ___ ___ _____

3. Documented need for hyperoxygenation, type of hyperoxygenation, and FiO_2 used. ___ ___ ___ _____

4. Documented evaluation of patient and family learning. ___ ___ ___ _____

HAND-OFF REPORTING

1. Reported patient's tolerance of and response to procedure, need for hyperoxygenation, frequency of suctioning, and the quantity and quality of the secretions. ___ ___ ___ _____

2. Reported unexpected physiological changes to health care provider. ___ ___ ___ _____

Student _____ Date _____

Instructor _____ Date _____

PERFORMANCE CHECKLIST PROCEDURAL GUIDELINE 24.1   **CLOSED (IN-LINE) SUCTION**

	S	U	NP	Comments

PROCEDURAL STEPS

1. Identified patient using at least two identifiers. _____ _____ _____ _____

2. Performed assessment as in Skill 24.2. _____ _____ _____ _____

3. Performed hand hygiene. Gathered equipment/supplies at bedside. _____ _____ _____ _____

4. Closed room door or curtains around bed. _____ _____ _____ _____

5. Explained procedure to patient and caregiver and the importance of coughing during the suctioning procedure. _____ _____ _____ _____

6. Performed hand hygiene; donned personal protective equipment (PPE) as patient status indicated. _____ _____ _____ _____

7. If not already placed during assessment, positioned pulse oximeter on patient's finger. Took reading and left oximeter in place. _____ _____ _____ _____

8. Adjusted the bed to appropriate height and lowered side rail on the side nearest nurse. Checked locks on the bed. _____ _____ _____ _____

9. Helped patient assume a position of comfort, usually semi- or high-Fowler position. Placed towel across patient's chest. _____ _____ _____ _____

10. Turned suction device on, set vacuum regulator to appropriate negative pressure (usually 80 to 120 mm Hg), and checked pressure. Consulted manufacturer guidelines for recommended pressure to use with the agency's brand of catheter. _____ _____ _____ _____

11. Attached suction: _____ _____ _____ _____

  a. If catheter was not already in place, opened suction catheter package using aseptic technique and attached closed-system suction catheter to ventilator circuit by removing swivel adapter and placing closed-system suction catheter apparatus on endotracheal tube (ET) or tracheostomy tube (TT). Connected Y on mechanical ventilator circuit to closed system suction catheter with flex tubing. _____ _____ _____ _____

436

	S	U	NP	Comments

b. Connected one end of connecting tubing to suction machine; connected other end to the end of the closed system or in-line suction catheter.

    —— —— —— ————————

12. If ordered, hyperoxygenated patient (usually 100% oxygen) for at least 30 seconds by adjusting the fraction of inspired oxygen (FiO2) setting on the ventilator or by using a temporary oxygen-enrichment program available on microprocessor ventilators according to agency policy or protocol.

    —— —— —— ————————

13. Unlocked suction control mechanism, if required by manufacturer. Opened saline port and attached saline syringe or vial.

    —— —— —— ————————

14. Picked up suction catheter enclosed in plastic sleeve with dominant hand.

    —— —— —— ————————

15. Suctioned patient:

    —— —— —— ————————

a. Waited until patient inhaled to insert catheter. Then inserted catheter using a repeating maneuver of pushing catheter and sliding plastic sleeve back between thumb and forefinger until resistance was felt or patient coughed.

    —— —— —— ————————

b. Pulled back 1 centimeter (0.4 inches) before applying suction to avoid tissue damage to carina. NOTE: If patient had a history of bleeding during previous suction procedures, avoided hitting the carina with the suction catheter.

    —— —— —— ————————

c. Encouraged patient to cough and apply suction by squeezing on suction control mechanism while withdrawing catheter.

    —— —— —— ————————

d. Applied continuous suction for 10 to 15 seconds as nurse removed the suction catheter. Withdrew the catheter completely into the plastic sheath and past the tip of the airway so that it did not obstruct airflow.

    —— —— —— ————————

16. Reassessed cardiopulmonary status, including pulse oximetry (SpO$_2$) and ventilator measures, to determine need for subsequent suctioning or complications. Repeated Steps 15a-d one more time to clear secretions if patient condition indicated. Allowed adequate time (at least 1 full minute) between suction passes for ventilation and reoxygenation.

    —— —— —— ————————

17. When airway was clear, withdrew catheter completely into sheath. Ensured that colored indicator line on catheter was visible in the sheath. Attached sterile solution lavage container or sterile saline or water syringe to side port of suction catheter. Squeezed vial or pushed syringe while applying suction to rinse inner lumen of catheter. NOTE: Did not let the saline go down the ETT or TT. Used at least 5 to 10 mL of saline to rinse the catheter until it was clear of retained secretions. Locked suction mechanism if applicable and turned off suction.

_____ _____ _____ _____

18. Hyperoxygenated for at least 30 seconds.

_____ _____ _____ _____

19. If patient required oral or nasal suctioning, performed Skill 24.1 or 24.2 with separate standard suction catheter.

_____ _____ _____ _____

20. Placed the Yankauer catheter on a clean, dry area for reuse with suction turned off or within patient's reach with suction on if patient was capable of suctioning own mouth.

_____ _____ _____ _____

21. Helped patient to comfortable position.

_____ _____ _____ _____

22. Placed nurse call system in an accessible location within patient's reach.

_____ _____ _____ _____

23. Raised side rails as appropriate and lowered and locked bed into lowest position.

_____ _____ _____ _____

24. Compared patient's vital signs and SpO2 before and after suctioning.

_____ _____ _____ _____

25. Auscultated lung fields and compared with baseline.

_____ _____ _____ _____

26. Observed airway secretions.

_____ _____ _____ _____

27. Asked patient if breathing was easier and congestion was decreased.

_____ _____ _____ _____

28. Removed gloves, face shield, and other PPE; discarded into appropriate receptacle; and performed hand hygiene.

_____ _____ _____ _____

29. Used Teach-Back. Revised instruction or developed plan for revised patient/family caregiver teaching if patient or family caregiver was not able to teach back correctly.

_____ _____ _____ _____

438

Student _____ Date _____

Instructor _____ Date _____

PERFORMANCE CHECKLIST SKILL 24.3 **PERFORMING ENDOTRACHEAL TUBE CARE**

	S	U	NP	Comments

ASSESSMENT

1. Identified patient using at least two identifiers.

2. Reviewed patient's electronic health record (EHR) for depth of endotracheal tube (ETT) insertion, previous ET cuff pressures, last time ETT was repositioned, and patient tolerance of care.

3. Assessed patient's/family caregiver's health literacy. Used communication board with patient.

4. Identified if patient was at risk for medical adhesive-related skin injury (MARSI) from adhesive tape: age, dehydration, malnutrition, exposure to radiation therapy, underlying chronic conditions, and edema of skin.

5. Asked patient to describe history of allergies: known type of allergies and normal allergic reaction. Checked patient's allergy wristband. Focus on adhesive or latex.

6. Performed hand hygiene, applied gloves and other personal protective equipment (PPE) as determined by patient condition and agency policy.

7. Assessed patient's cardiopulmonary status, including lung sounds, pulse oximetry, EtCO2, vital signs (VS), and level of consciousness. Kept pulse oximeter in place.

8. Observed for factors that increase risk for complications from ETT: type and size of tube, movement of tube up and down trachea, duration of tube placement, presence of facial trauma.

9. Observed conditions of tissues surrounding ETT for impaired skin integrity on nares, lips, cheeks, or corner of mouth and for excess nasal or oral secretions. Noted if patient moved tube with tongue, bit tube or tongue, and / or had foul-smelling mouth.

	S	U	NP	Comments

10. Observed patency of airway: excess secretions, diminished airflow, and signs and symptoms of airway obstruction. ___ ___ ___ _____

11. Observe for gurgling on expiration, decreased exhale tidal volume (mechanically ventilated patient), signs and symptoms of inadequate ventilation (rising end-tidal carbon dioxide concentration [EtCO2], patient-ventilator dyssynchrony or dyspnea), spasmodic coughing, tense test balloon on tube, flaccid test balloon on tube, and ability to speak or vocalize. ___ ___ ___ _____

12. Determine current ET depth as noted by centimeters at incisors or gum line. Ensured a line was marked on tube and documented in patent's EHR at time of intubation and every shift. ___ ___ ___ _____

13. Removed and disposed of gloves. Performed hand hygiene. Remaining PPE stayed in place. ___ ___ ___ _____

14. Reviewed EHR and determined when oral and airway care were last performed. Knew the health care agency protocols and procedures, but was aware of patient-specific needs for more frequent care. ___ ___ ___ _____

15. Assessed patient's knowledge, prior experience with ETT care, and feelings about procedure. Used communication board. ___ ___ ___ _____

PLANNING

1. Determined expected outcomes following completion of procedure. ___ ___ ___ _____

2. Performed hand hygiene. Gathered equipment/supplies and arrange at bedside. ___ ___ ___ _____

3. Obtained assistance from available staff for this procedure. ___ ___ ___ _____

4. Closed room door or curtains around bed. ___ ___ ___ _____

5. Explained procedure and patient's need to participant, including not biting or moving ETT with tongue, trying not to cough when tape/holder device was off ETT, keeping hands down, and not pulling on tubing. ___ ___ ___ _____

IMPLEMENTATION

1. Performed hand hygiene. Applied clean gloves. Kept remaining PPE on. Had assistant apply PPE as well. ___ ___ ___ _____

2. Assisted patient in assuming comfortable position. Elevated patient's head of bed at least 30 degrees, unless contraindicated. ___ ___ ___ _____

440

	S	U	NP	Comments

3. Adjusted bed to appropriate height and lowered side rail on side nearest nurse. Checked locks on bed wheel.

4. Placed clean towel across patient's chest.

5. Performed endotracheal or oropharyngeal suction if indicated.

6. Connected Yankauer suction catheter to suction source and had it ready to use. Ensured that suction source/machine for oral suctioning was on and functioning properly.

7. Removed oral airway or bite block, if present, and placed on towel.

8. Brushed teeth with soft toothbrush using toothpaste with fluoride. Suctioned oropharyngeal secretions as needed.

9. Used 0.12% chlorhexidine solution, 1.5% hydrogen peroxide, or 0.05% antiseptic solution and oral swabs to clean mouth. Had assistant suction oropharyngeal secretions as needed. Applied mouth moisturizer to oral mucosa and lips after each cleaning. This was completed every 2 to 4 hours (per agency policy).

10. Performed subglottic secretion drainage (SSD), if not being continuously performed.

11. Prepared to secure the ETT.

    a. Opened commercially available ETT holder package per manufacturer instructions. Set device aside with head guard in place and Velcro strips open.

    b. Removed Velcro strips from ETT and removed ETT holder from patient while assistant held ETT securely in place.

    c. Removed excess secretions or adhesive from patient's face. Cleaned facial skin with mild soap and water and dried thoroughly.

    d. Noted level of ETT by looking at mark or noting centimeter value on tube itself. Moved oral ETT to other side of mouth and ensured that tube marking at incisors or gum line was unchanged. Performed oral care as needed on side where tube was initially positioned. Cleaned oral airway or bite block (if patient was not biting) with warm soapy water and rinsed well. Reinserted as needed.

	S	U	NP	Comments

12. Secured tube. (NOTE: Assistant continued to hold ETT in place.) ___ ___ ___ _____

   a. Threaded ET through opening in holder designed to secure it. Ensured that pilot balloon was accessible. ___ ___ ___ _____

   b. Placed strips of ET holder under patient at occipital region of head. ___ ___ ___ _____

   c. Verified that ET was at established depth using incisors or gum line marker as guide. ___ ___ ___ _____

   d. Attached Velcro strips at base of patient's head. Left 1 centimeter (0.4 inch) slack in strips. ___ ___ ___ _____

   e. Verified that tube was secure, it did not move forward from patient's mouth or backward down into patient's throat, and there were no pressure areas on oral mucosa or occipital region of head. ___ ___ ___ _____

13. For unconscious patient, reinserted oral airway without pushing tongue into oropharynx and secured with tape. ___ ___ ___ _____

14. Ensured proper cuff inflation by using the pressure manometer to keep the pressure between 20 and 25mm Hg. ___ ___ ___ _____

15. Cleaned rest of face and neck with soapy washcloth, rinsed, and dried. Shaved male patient as needed. ___ ___ ___ _____

16. Removed gloves and mask, goggles, or face shield or gown; discarded in receptacle; and performed hand hygiene. (Assistant performed same steps.) Placed clean items in place of storage in patient room. ___ ___ ___ _____

17. Helped patient to a comfortable position. ___ ___ ___ _____

18. Raised side rails (as appropriate) and lowered and locked bed into lowest position. ___ ___ ___ _____

19. Ensured the nurse call system was in an accessible location within the patient's reach. ___ ___ ___ _____

EVALUATION

1. Compared respiratory assessments before and after ETT care. ___ ___ ___ _____

2. Observed depth and position of ETT according to health care provider recommendation. ___ ___ ___ _____

3. Assessed security of holder device or tape by gently tugging at tube. ___ ___ ___ _____

442

	S	U	NP	Comments

4. Assessed skin around mouth and oral mucous membranes for intactness and MDRPI. Checked for MARSI if used adhesive securement. ___ ___ ___ _____

5. Compared EtCO2 and SpO2 values from before and after ETT care. ___ ___ ___ _____

6. Observed for excessive phonation, presence of gastric secretions in airway secretions, or tracheoesophageal fistula. ___ ___ ___ _____

7. Used Teach-Back. Revised or developed a plan for revised patient/family caregiver teaching if patient or family caregiver was not able to teach back correctly. ___ ___ ___ _____

DOCUMENTATION

1. Documented time of care, respiratory assessments (including pulse oximetry and EtCO2) before and after care, cuff pressure after care, patient's tolerance of procedure, frequency and extent of ETT care, integrity of oral and nasal mucosa, and pressure injury care (if performed). ___ ___ ___ _____

2. Documented evaluation of patient/family learning. ___ ___ ___ _____

3. Documented repositioning of ET, side on which it was placed, depth it was placed, and the securement technique used. ___ ___ ___ _____

HAND-OFF REPORTING

1. Reported signs of infection immediately. ___ ___ ___ _____

2. Reported unequal breath sounds, accidental extubation or displacement, cuff leak, or respiratory distress immediately to the health care provider. ___ ___ ___ _____

3. Reported tolerance of procedure, as well as Assessment findings to the next shift nurse and the respiratory therapist (if they did not assist during the procedure). ___ ___ ___ _____

Student _____ Date _____

Instructor _____ Date _____

PERFORMANCE CHECKLIST SKILL 24.4 **PERFORMING TRACHEOSTOMY CARE**

	S	U	NP	Comments
ASSESSMENT				
1. Identified patient using two identifiers.	___	___	___	_____
2. Gathered the following information from the patient's electronic health record (EHR): time care was last performed; tolerance to procedure; type and size of tracheostomy tube (TT) and inner cannula, if present; any specific provider orders regarding the TT care; amount of air or fluid in TT cuff; and trends in patient vital signs (VS) and respiratory assessments.	___	___	___	_____
3. Assessed patient's/family caregiver's health literacy.	___	___	___	_____
4. Performed hand hygiene and applied clean gloves and other PPE as patient condition dictated.	___	___	___	_____
5. Observed for tube dislodgement/decannulation and tube obstruction.	___	___	___	_____
6. Observed for excess peristomal and intratracheal secretions, soiled or damp tracheostomy ties, soiled or damp tracheostomy dressing, or diminished airflow through tracheostomy tube, or signs and symptoms of airway obstruction requiring suctioning.	___	___	___	_____
7. Observed skin around tracheal stoma, under TT flange, and under tracheal ties for pressure injury: blistering, erythema, drainage, or other discoloration.	___	___	___	_____
8. Assessed patient's hydration status, humidity delivered to airway, status of any existing infection, patient's nutritional status, and ability to cough.	___	___	___	_____

444

	S	U	NP	Comments

9. Assessed patient's cardiopulmonary status, including pulse oximetry (SpO2), EtCO2, VS, respiratory effort, lung sounds, and level of consciousness. Kept pulse oximeter in place. ____ ____ ____ _____

10. Removed and disposed of gloves. Performed hand hygiene. Kept on remaining PPE. ____ ____ ____ _____

11. Assessed patient's knowledge, prior experience with performing tracheostomy care, and feelings about procedure. ____ ____ ____ _____

PLANNING

1. Determined expected outcomes following completion of procedure. ____ ____ ____ _____

2. Had another nurse or respiratory therapist (RT) help in this procedure. Ensured this employee performed hand hygiene, applied clean gloves, and donned appropriate PPE as patient condition dictated. Kept all PPE in place until end of procedures. ____ ____ ____ _____

3. Gathered supplies and arranged at bedside. Closed room door or curtain. ____ ____ ____ _____

4. Raised head of bed at least 30 degrees, unless contraindicated. Ensured patient was comfortable. Adjusted bed to appropriate height and lowered side rail on side nearest nurse. Checked locks on bed wheel. ____ ____ ____ _____

5. Explained procedure and patient's need to participate, including trying not to cough when tape or holder is off TT, keeping hands down, and not pulling on staff or tubing. ____ ____ ____ _____

IMPLEMENTATION

1. Performed hand hygiene. Applied clean/sterile gloves for suctioning and other PPE if not already completed. ____ ____ ____ _____

	S	U	NP	Comments

2. Hyperoxygenated patient for 30 seconds or ask patient to take 5 to 6 deep breaths. Then suctioned tracheostomy. Before removing gloves, removed soiled gauze or polyurethane foam tracheostomy dressing and discarded in glove with coiled catheter. Left hydrocolloid or polyurethane foam dressings in place depending on amount of tracheal secretions and manufacturer's directions.

    ____   ____   ____   _____

3. Performed hand hygiene. Prepared equipment on bedside table:

    ____   ____   ____   _____

  a. Opened sterile tracheostomy kit. Opened two 4 x 4–inch gauze packages using aseptic technique and poured normal saline on gauze in one package. Left gauze in second package dry. Opened two cotton-tipped swab packages and poured normal saline on swab tip in one package. Did not recap normal saline.

    ____   ____   ____   _____

  b. Opened sterile tracheostomy dressing package for hydrocolloid, polyurethane foam or precut gauze.

    ____   ____   ____   _____

  c. Unwrapped sterile basin and poured about 0.5 to 2 centimeters (0.2 to 1 inch) of normal saline into it.

    ____   ____   ____   _____

  d. Opened small sterile brush package and placed aseptically into sterile basin.

    ____   ____   ____   _____

  e. Prepared TT fixation device.

    ____   ____   ____   _____

    (1) If using commercially available TT holder, opened package accordingly to manufacturer directions.

    ____   ____   ____   _____

    (2) If using twill tape: Prepared length of twill tape long enough to go around patient's neck 2 times, around 60 to 75 centimeters (24 to 30 inches) for an adult. Cut ends on diagonal. Laid aside in dry area..

    ____   ____   ____   _____

  f. Opened inner cannula package (if new one was to be inserted).

    ____   ____   ____   _____

	S	U	NP	Comments

4. Applied sterile gloves. Kept dominant hand sterile throughout procedure. ____ ____ ____ _____

5. Removed oxygen source if present and if patient could tolerate. ____ ____ ____ _____

6. Care of tracheostomy with reusable inner cannula: ____ ____ ____ _____

   a. While touching only outer aspect of tube, unlocked and removed inner cannula with nondominant hand following line of tracheostomy. Dropped inner cannula into normal saline basin. ____ ____ ____ _____

   b. Placed tracheostomy collar, T tube, or ventilator oxygen source over outer cannula. (NOTE: Understood it may not be possible to attach T tube and ventilator oxygen devices to all outer cannulas when inner cannula is removed.) ____ ____ ____ _____

   c. To prevent oxygen desaturation in affected patients, quickly picked up inner cannula and used small brush to remove secretions inside and outside inner cannula. ____ ____ ____ _____

   d. Held inner cannula over basin and rinsed with sterile normal saline, using nondominant (clean) hand to pour normal saline. ____ ____ ____ _____

   e. Removed oxygen source, replaced inner cannula, and secured "locking" mechanism. Reapplied ventilator, tracheostomy collar, or T tube. Hyperoxygenated patient if needed. ____ ____ ____ _____

7. Tracheostomy with disposable inner cannula: ____ ____ ____ _____

   a. Removed new cannula from manufacturer packaging. ____ ____ ____ _____

   b. While touching only outer aspect of tube, withdrew inner cannula and replaced with new cannula. Locked into position. ____ ____ ____ _____

   c. Disposed of contaminated cannula in appropriate receptacle and reconnected TT to ventilator or oxygen supply. ____ ____ ____ _____

	S	U	NP	Comments

8. Using normal saline-saturated cotton-tipped swabs and 4x4–inch gauze, cleaned exposed outer cannula surfaces and tracheal stoma under faceplate extending 5 to 10 centimeters (2 to 4 inches) in all directions from stoma. Cleaned in circular motion from stoma site outward with dominant hand to handle sterile supplies. Did not go over previously cleaned area.   ____ ____ ____ _____

9. Using dry 4x4–inch gauze, patted lightly at skin and exposed outer cannula surfaces. Inspected condition of skin under tracheostomy flange.   ____ ____ ____ _____

10. Secured tracheostomy.   ____ ____ ____ _____

　a. Used the tracheostomy tube holder method: ____ ____ ____ _____

　　(1) Instructed assistant to continue to hold TT in place. If assistant was not available, left old TT holder in place until new device was secure.   ____ ____ ____ _____

　　(2) Aligned strap under patient's neck. Was sure that Velcro attachments were on either side of TT.   ____ ____ ____ _____

　　(3) Placed narrow end ties under and through faceplate eyelets. Pulled ends even and secured with Velcro closures.   ____ ____ ____ _____

　　(4) Verified that there was space for only one loose or two snug finger widths to be inserted under neck strap.   ____ ____ ____ _____

　　(5) Inserted new hydrocolloid, foam, or 4 x 4-inch gauze precut tracheostomy dressing under clean neck plate. Option: if used gauze dressing, applied barrier cream around stoma, if ordered.   ____ ____ ____ _____

　b. Tracheostomy tie / twill tape method: ____ ____ ____ _____

	S	U	NP	Comments

(1) Instructed assistant to continue holding TT in place while nurse cut old tracheostomy ties. Ensured to not cut pilot balloon of cuff.

(2) Took prepared twill tape, inserted one end of tie through faceplate eyelet, and pulled ends even.

(3) Slid both ends of tie behind head and around neck to other eyelet and inserted one tie through second eyelet.

(4) Pulled snuggly.

(5) Tied ends securely in double square knot, allowing space for insertion of one loose or two snug finger widths between tie and neck.

(6) Inserted new hydrocolloid, foam, or 4 x 4-inch gauze precut tracheostomy dressing under clean neck plate. Option: If used gauze dressing, applied barrier cream around stoma, if ordered.

11. Ensured the tracheostomy tube was midline and secured and that no excess traction was Assistant released TT at this time.

12. Performed oral care with toothbrush or oral swabs and chlorhexidine rinse. Suctioned orally if needed. Performed subglottic suctioning if TT equipped with that capability.

13. Measured cuff pressure with the manometer; added or removed air/saline/water from cuff to maintain pressure between 20 and 25 mm Hg.

14. Helped patient to a more comfortable position with head of bed remaining elevated at least 30 degrees (unless contraindicated) and assessed respiratory status.

15. Ensured that oxygen- or humidification-delivery sources were in place and set at correct levels.

	S	U	NP	Comments

16. Raised side rails (as appropriate) and lowered and locked bed into lowest position.

_____ _____ _____ _____

17. Removed and properly disposed of gloves and other PPE, if used. Performed hand hygiene.

_____ _____ _____ _____

18. Ensured nurse call system was in an accessible location within the patient's reach.

_____ _____ _____ _____

19. Replaced cap on reusable normal saline bottles. Stored reusable liquids, dated container, and stored unused supplies in appropriate place.

_____ _____ _____ _____

EVALUATION

1. Compared respiratory assessments before and after tracheostomy care.

_____ _____ _____ _____

2. Assessed fit of new tracheostomy securement device and asked patient if tube felt comfortable. Palpated tube for pulsation for air under the skin.

_____ _____ _____ _____

3. Inspected inner and outer cannulas for secretions.

_____ _____ _____ _____

4. Assessed stoma, surrounding skin, and skin under ties for MDRPI: inflammation, edema, bleeding or discolored secretions.

_____ _____ _____ _____

5. Observed for excessive phonation, presence of gastric secretions in airway secretions, or tracheoesophageal fistula.

_____ _____ _____ _____

6. Used Teach-Back. Revised instruction or developed a plan for revised patient/family caregiver teaching if patient or family caregiver was not able to teach back correctly.

_____ _____ _____ _____

DOCUMENTATION

1. Documented respiratory, stoma, and skin assessments before and after care; type and size of tracheostomy tube and inner cannula; frequency and extent of care, including inner cannula, dressing, and securement device changes; type, color, and amount of secretions; patient tolerance and understanding of procedure; and any interventions performed in event of unexpected outcomes.

_____ _____ _____ _____

450

	S	U	NP	Comments
2. Documented evaluation of patient/family learning.	___	___	___	_____

HAND-OFF REPORTING

1. Reported patient status, frequency of care, tolerance and response to care, TT size and type of securement device, and last time care was performed.

| | ___ | ___ | ___ | _____ |

2. Reported accidental decannulation, respiratory distress, or other unexpected outcomes to nurse in charge and health care provider.

| | ___ | ___ | ___ | _____ |

Student _____ Date _____

Instructor _____ Date _____

PERFORMANCE CHECKLIST SKILL 25.1   **OBTAINING A 12-LEAD ELECTROCARDIOGRAM**

	S	U	NP	Comments
ASSESSMENT				
1. Identified patient using at least two identifiers.	___	___	___	_____
2. Reviewed electronic health record (EHR) to determine indications for obtaining electrocardiogram (ECG). Assessed patient's history and cardiopulmonary status.	___	___	___	_____
3. Reviewed EHR to determine patient's age and history of dehydration, malnutrition, exposure to radiation therapy, underlying chronic conditions, and edema of the skin.	___	___	___	_____
4. Assessed patient's/family caregiver's health literacy.	___	___	___	_____
5. Assessed for chest pain; asked patient to rate pain on a scale from 0 to 10.	___	___	___	_____
6. Asked patient if there was a history of irritant contact dermatitis from use of adhesives.	___	___	___	_____
7. Assessed patient's ability to follow directions and remain still in supine position.	___	___	___	_____
8. Assessed patient's knowledge, prior experience with ECG, and feelings about procedure.	___	___	___	_____
PLANNING				
1. Determined expected outcomes following completion of procedure.	___	___	___	_____
2. Provided privacy and explained procedure to patient. Discussed the ECG and what the patient might experience.	___	___	___	_____
3. Closed room door and bedside curtain.	___	___	___	_____
4. Obtained and organized equipment for ECG at bedside.	___	___	___	_____
IMPLEMENTATION				
1. Performed hand hygiene, applied clean gloves, and prepared patient for procedure:	___	___	___	_____
a. Removed or repositioned patient's clothing to expose only patient's chest and arms. Kept abdomen and thighs covered.	___	___	___	_____
b. Placed patient in supine position with head of bed no higher than 30 degrees.	___	___	___	_____

	S	U	NP	Comments

c. Instructed patient to lie still without talking and to not cross legs. ___ ___ ___ _____

2. Turned on machine; entered required demographic information. ___ ___ ___ _____

3. Cleaned and prepared skin for isolated electrode placement with soap and water. Wiped area with rough washcloth or gauze, or used edge of electrode to gently scrape skin. Clipped excessive hair from electrode area. Where possible, avoided the use of products that dry the skin, such as alcohol-based skin preps. ___ ___ ___ _____

4. Applied electrodes in correct positions. ___ ___ ___ _____

a. Applied chest (precordial) leads:
- V1—Fourth intercostal space (ICS) at right sternal border
- V2—Fourth ICS at left sternal border
- V3—Midway between V2 and V4
- V4—Fifth ICS at midclavicular line
- V5—Left anterior axillary line at level of V4 horizontally
- V6—Left midaxillary line at level of V4 horizontally ___ ___ ___ _____

b. Extremities: One lead on each extremity; right wrist, left wrist, left ankle, right ankle ___ ___ ___ _____

5. Checked 12-lead machine for messages to correct electrode or lead issues. If no messages occurred, pressed button to obtain 12-lead ECG. ___ ___ ___ _____

6. If obtained ECG tracing without artifact, disconnected leads and gently removed from patient's skin. ___ ___ ___ _____

7. If STAT, immediately delivered ECG tracing (if not computerized) to appropriate health care provider for interpretation. ___ ___ ___ _____

8. Helped patient to a comfortable position. ___ ___ ___ _____

9. Raised side rails (as appropriate) and lowered and locked bed into lowest position. ___ ___ ___ _____

10. Placed nurse call system in an accessible location within patient's reach. ___ ___ ___ _____

11. Disposed of all contaminated supplies in appropriate receptacle, removed and disposed of gloves, and performed hand hygiene. ___ ___ ___ _____

EVALUATION
1. Noted and documented if patient experienced any chest discomfort during procedure. ___ ___ ___ _____

	S	U	NP	Comments

2. Discussed findings and results of 12-lead ECG with health care provider to determine next steps in patient's treatment plan.

   ___ ___ ___   _____

3. Inspected condition of skin after electrode removal for signs of MARSI.

   ___ ___ ___   _____

4. Used Teach-Back technique. Revised instruction or developed a plan for revised patient / family caregiver learning if patient or family caregiver were not able to teach back correctly.

   ___ ___ ___   _____

DOCUMENTATION

1. Documented date and time ECG was obtained, reason for obtaining ECG, and to whom ECG was given for interpretation.

   ___ ___ ___   _____

2. Documented evaluation of patient learning.

   ___ ___ ___   _____

HAND-OFF REPORTING

1. Reported any chest pain or unexpected outcomes immediately.

   ___ ___ ___   _____

454

Student _____ Date _____

Instructor _____ Date _____

PERFORMANCE CHECKLIST SKILL 25.2 **APPLYING A CARDIAC MONITOR**

	S	U	NP	Comments

ASSESSMENT

1. Identified patient using at least two identifiers. ___ ___ ___ _____

2. Reviewed electronic health record (EHR) to determine clinical indication for continuous cardiac monitoring. Assessed patient's history, cardiopulmonary status, and history of chest pain. ___ ___ ___ _____

3. Reviewed EHR to determine patient's age and history of dehydration, malnutrition, exposure to radiation therapy, underlying chronic conditions, edema of the skin, and allergic dermatitis, erythema, blistering, or excoriation of the skin under or around monitor leaders. ___ ___ ___ _____

4. Performed hand hygiene. Checked skin for fragility, presence of oil or excess moisture, and local signs of irritation or damage at the site where the adhesive would be applied. If oil or moisture was present, wiped chest or limbs with clean, dry towel. ___ ___ ___ _____

5. Assessed patient's/family caregiver's health literacy. ___ ___ ___ _____

6. Assessed patient's knowledge, prior experience with ECG monitoring, and feelings about procedure. ___ ___ ___ _____

PLANNING

1. Determined expected outcomes following completion of procedure. ___ ___ ___ _____

2. Provided privacy and explained procedure to patient. Discussed need for ECG. If applicable, taught patient how to report chest pain. ___ ___ ___ _____

3. Closed room door and bedside curtain. ___ ___ ___ _____

4. Obtained and organized equipment for ECG monitoring at bedside. ___ ___ ___ _____

IMPLEMENTATION

1. Performed hand hygiene, applied clean gloves, and prepared patient for procedure: ___ ___ ___ _____

   a. Removed or repositioned patient's gown to expose only patient's chest. Kept abdomen and thighs covered. ___ ___ ___ _____

   b. Placed patient in supine position. ___ ___ ___ _____

S U NP   Comments

2. Cleaned and prepared chest area for electrode placement with soap and water. Wiped area with rough washcloth or gauze, or used edge of electrode to gently scrape area. Where possible, avoided the use of products that dry the skin, such as alcohol-based skin preps. Clipped excessive hair from electrode area rather than shaving.

 ___ ___ ___ _____

3. Applied electrodes in correct positions for either a three- or five-electrode system.

 ___ ___ ___ _____

 a. For females, placed the precordial leads (V3-V6) under the left breast.

 ___ ___ ___ _____

4. Attached monitor leads to electrodes. For two additional leads on five-lead system, placed green lead (positive or negative) and a brown lead (positive) at a V lead location on precordial chest.

 ___ ___ ___ _____

5. Checked bedside monitor or telemetry station for any messages indicating electrode or lead issues. Performed troubleshooting as needed.

 ___ ___ ___ _____

6. Checked that the ECG rhythm could be visualized on bedside monitor, central station, or remote viewing station.

 ___ ___ ___ _____

7. Changed ECG electrodes daily or more often if electrode contact to skin was loose. Inspected skin for allergic dermatitis, erythema, blistering, or excoriation.

 ___ ___ ___ _____

8. Customized alarm limits within 1 hour of assuming care of patient and on condition changes. Made changes in accordance with agency policies and health care provider's orders.

 ___ ___ ___ _____

9. Helped patient to comfortable position.

 ___ ___ ___ _____

10. Ensured that nurse call system was in an accessible location within patient's reach.

 ___ ___ ___ _____

11. Raised side rails (as appropriate) and lowered and locked bed into lowest position.

 ___ ___ ___ _____

12. Disposed of all contaminated supplies in appropriate receptacle, removed and disposed of gloves, and performed hand hygiene.

 ___ ___ ___ _____

EVALUATION

1. Ensured that all appropriate alarms were ON.

 ___ ___ ___ _____

2. Inspected condition of skin after electrode removal for signs of MARSI.

 ___ ___ ___ _____

3. Used Teach-Back technique. Revised instruction or developed a plan for revised patient/family caregiver teaching if patient or family caregiver were not able to teach back correctly.

 ___ ___ ___ _____

	S	U	NP	Comments

DOCUMENTATION

1. Documented alarm trends and waveforms at least once a shift and on report of an alarm. ___ ___ ___ _____

2. Documented at least one rhythm strip per shift per agency policy. ___ ___ ___ _____

3. Documented evaluation of patient and family caregiver learning. ___ ___ ___ _____

HAND-OFF REPORTING

1. Reported any unexpected ECG outcomes immediately to the health care provider. ___ ___ ___ _____

Student _____ Date _____

Instructor _____ Date _____

PERFORMANCE CHECKLIST SKILL 26.1 **MANAGING CLOSED CHEST DRAINAGE SYSTEMS**

	S	U	NP	Comments

ASSESSMENT

1. Identified patient using at least two identifiers according to agency policy. ___ ___ ___ _____

2. Reviewed patient's electronic health record (EHR), including health care provider's order and nurses' notes. Assessed significant medical history or injury. ___ ___ ___ _____

3. Verified that informed consent was obtained before administering any pain medication, per agency policy. ___ ___ ___ _____

4. Reviewed patient's medication record for anticoagulant therapy. ___ ___ ___ _____

5. Assessed patient for known allergies. Asked patient any history of problems with medications, latex, or anything applied to skin. If allergy identified, placed allergy band on patient's wrist. ___ ___ ___ _____

6. Reviewed EHR to determine patient's age and history of dehydration, malnutrition, exposure to radiation therapy, underlying chronic conditions, and edema of the skin. ___ ___ ___ _____

7. If nonemergent, assessed patient's/family caregiver's health literacy. ___ ___ ___ _____

8. Assessed character of patient's pain and rated pain severity on a scale of 0 to 10. ___ ___ ___ _____

9. Performed hand hygiene and inspected condition of skin around chest. If adhesive had been in place, noted any redness, irritation, or blistering. Noted if patient was diaphoretic or had history of impaired poor perfusion, altered tissue tolerance, poor nutrition, or edema. ___ ___ ___ _____

10. Performed a complete respiratory assessment, baseline vital signs, and pulse oximetry (SpO_2). ___ ___ ___ _____

    a. Assessed for signs and symptoms of increased respiratory distress and hypoxia. ___ ___ ___ _____

    b. Assessed for sharp, stabbing chest pain or chest pain on inspiration, hypotension, and tachycardia. If possible, asked patient to again rate level of pain severity on a scale of 0 to 10. ___ ___ ___ _____

458

	S	U	NP	Comments

11. For patients who had chest tubes in place:

    a. Performed hand hygiene and applied gloves. Inspected skin around chest tube dressing and site surrounding tube insertion. Kept box of sterile 4-×-4-inch gauze pads and petroleum gauze at bedside.

    b. Inspected the amount and type of drainage by marking the drainage level on the outside of the drainage-collection chamber in hourly or shift increments or in increments established by the health care provider or per the agency's policy.

    c. Observed tubing for kinks, dependent loops, or clots.

    d. Verified that chest drainage system was kept upright and below level of tube insertion. Removed gloves and performed hand hygiene.

12. Assessed patient's knowledge, prior experience with chest tubes, and feelings about procedure.

PLANNING

1. Determined expected outcomes following completion of procedure.

2. Provided privacy and explained procedure to patient. Discussed chest tube systems and the patient's role. If applicable, taught patient how to move with chest tube in place.

3. Organized and set up any equipment needed for chest tube management at bedside.

IMPLEMENTATION

1. Confirmed informed consent was obtained (if needed). Completed time-out procedure; verified procedure with patient.

2. Reviewed health care provider's order for chest tube placement.

3. Performed hand hygiene and donned appropriate PPE.

4. Set up water-seal or dry suction system; consulted manufacturer guidelines.

    a. Prepared chest drainage system. Removed wrappers and prepared to set up two- or three-chamber system.

    b. While maintaining sterility of drainage tubing, stood system upright and added sterile water or NS to appropriate compartments.

(1) Two-chamber system (without suction): Added sterile solution to water-seal chamber (second chamber), bringing fluid to required level as indicated or ordered by health care provider.

(2) Three-chamber system (with suction): Added sterile solution to water-seal chamber (second chamber). Added amount of sterile solution prescribed by health care provider to suction-control chamber (third chamber), usually 20 cm H_2O pressure. Connected tubing from suction-control chamber to suction source. Note: Ensured that suction-control chamber vent was not occluded when suction was used.

(3) Dry suction system: Filled water-seal chamber with sterile solution. Adjusted suction-control dial to prescribed level of suction; suction ranges from −10 to −40 cm of water pressure. Ensured that suction-control chamber vent was never occluded when suction was used. Did not obstruct positive-pressure relief valve.

5. Set up waterless system per manufacturer guidelines.

6. Secured all tubing connections with tape in double-spiral fashion using 2.5-cm (1-inch) adhesive tape or zip ties with a clamp. Checked system for patency by:

a. Clamping drainage tubing that would connect to patient's chest tube.

b. Connecting tubing from float ball chamber to suction source.

c. Turning on suction to prescribed level.

7. Turned off suction source and unclamped drainage tubing before connecting patient to system. Turned suction source on again after patient was connected. Removed and disposed of gloves.

8. If not already completed, administered premedication such as sedatives or analgesics as ordered.

9. Provided psychological support to patient:

a. Reinforced preprocedure explanation.

b. Coached and supported patient throughout procedure.

10. Performed hand hygiene and applied clean gloves. Positioned patient for tube insertion so side in which tube was to be inserted was accessible to health care provider.

	S	U	NP	Comments

11. Assisted health care provider with chest tube insertion by providing needed equipment and local analgesic. Health care provider anesthetized skin over insertion site, made small skin incision, inserted clamped tube, sutured it in place, and applied occlusive dressing. ___ ___ ___ _____

12. Helped health care provider attach drainage tube to chest tube; removed any existing clamp. Turned on suction to prescribed level. ___ ___ ___ _____

13. Taped or zip-tied all connections between chest tube and drainage tube, as needed. ___ ___ ___ _____

14. Checked systems for proper functioning. Health care provider ordered chest x-ray film. ___ ___ ___ _____

15. After tube placement, positioned patient:

    a. Semi-Fowler or high-Fowler position to evacuate air (pneumothorax). ___ ___ ___ _____

    b. High-Fowler position to drain fluid (hemothorax). ___ ___ ___ _____

16. Checked patency of air vents in system. ___ ___ ___ _____

    a. Water-seal vent had no occlusion. ___ ___ ___ _____

    b. Suction-control chamber vent was not occluded when suction was used. ___ ___ ___ _____

    c. Waterless systems had relief valves without caps. ___ ___ ___ _____

17. Positioned excess tubing horizontally on mattress next to patient. Secured with clamp that attached to bottom sheet so it did not obstruct tubing. ___ ___ ___ _____

18. Adjusted tubing to hang in straight line from chest tube to drainage chamber. ___ ___ ___ _____

19. Placed two rubber-tipped hemostats (for each chest tube) in easily accessible position. Kept these with patient when ambulating. ___ ___ ___ _____

20. Disposed of all contaminated supplies in appropriate receptacle, removed and disposed of gloves, and performed hand hygiene. ___ ___ ___ _____

21. Care of patient after chest tube insertion:

    a. Performed hand hygiene and applied clean gloves. Assessed vital signs; oxygen saturation; pain; skin color; breath sounds; rate, depth, and ease of respirations; and insertion site every 15 min for first 2 hours and then at least every shift (per agency policy). ___ ___ ___ _____

    b. For severe pain, medicated with ordered analgesics and used complementary pain relief methods as needed. ___ ___ ___ _____

	S	U	NP	Comments

c. Monitored color, consistency, and amount of chest tube drainage every 15 minutes for first 2 hours. Indicated level of drainage fluid, date, and time on write-on surface of chamber.

d. Observed chest dressing for drainage and determined whether it was still occlusive.

e. Inspected condition of skin around adhesive tape for redness, blistering, and edema.

f. Palpated around tube for swelling and crepitus as indicated by crackling.

g. Checked tubing to ensure that it was free of kinks and dependent loops.

h. Observed for fluctuation of drainage in tubing and water-seal chamber during inspiration and expiration. Observed for clots or debris in tubing.

i. Kept drainage system upright and below level of patient's chest.

j. Checked for air leaks by monitoring bubbling in water-seal chamber.

22. Instructed patient on how to regularly take deep breaths and to reposition as often as possible.

23. Assisted patient to semi- or high-Fowler position. Verified that patient was comfortable.

24. Raised side rails (as appropriate) and lowered bed to lowest position, locking into position.

25. Placed nurse call system in an accessible location within patient's reach.

26. Disposed of all contaminated supplies in appropriate receptacle, removed and disposed of gloves, and performed hand hygiene.

EVALUATION

1. Evaluated patient for decreased respiratory distress and chest pain. Auscultated patient's lungs and observed chest expansion.

2. Monitor vital signs and SpO_2.

3. Reassessed patient's character of pain and level of severity on a scale of 0 to 10, comparing level with comfort before chest tube insertion.

4. Evaluated patient's ability to use deep-breathing exercises while maintaining comfort.

5. Monitored functioning of chest tube system.

6. Used Teach-Back: Revised instruction if patient or family caregiver was not able to teach back correctly.

462

	S	U	NP	Comments

RECORDING

1. Documented respiratory assessment, type of chest tube and drainage device, amount of suction if used, amount and appearance of drainage in chamber, and presence or absence of an air leak. ____ ____ ____ _____

2. Documented the integrity of the dressing, color and type of drainage, and condition of skin around tape for comparison between shifts. ____ ____ ____ _____

3. Documented level of patient comfort and baseline vital signs, including oxygen saturation. ____ ____ ____ _____

4. Documented patient teaching and validation of patient understanding. ____ ____ ____ _____

HAND-OFF REPORTING

1. Reported patient tolerance of chest tube insertion, comfort level and any analgesia, and respiratory assessment before and after chest tube insertion. ____ ____ ____ _____

2. Reported the quantity and quality of the chest tube drainage. ____ ____ ____ _____

Student _____   Date _____

Instructor _____   Date _____

PERFORMANCE CHECKLIST SKILL 26.2 **ASSISTING WITH REMOVAL OF CHEST TUBES**

	S	U	NP	Comments

ASSESSMENT

1. Identified patient using at least two identifiers according to agency policy. _____ _____ _____ _____

2. Reviewed patient's electronic health record (EHR) regarding health care order, patient response to chest tube, and status of tube functioning. _____ _____ _____ _____

3. Reviewed EHR to determine patient's age and history of dehydration, malnutrition, exposure to radiation therapy, underlying chronic conditions, and edema of the skin. _____ _____ _____ _____

4. Assessed patient's/family caregiver's health literacy. _____ _____ _____ _____

5. Performed hand hygiene. Performed respiratory assessment and gathered measures for indication of lung reexpansion. _____ _____ _____ _____

   a. Provided health care provider with results of most recent chest x-ray study. _____ _____ _____ _____

   b. Noted trend in water-seal fluctuation over last 24 hours. Determined if bubbling was present. _____ _____ _____ _____

   c. Confirmed that drainage had decreased to less than 50 to 100 mL/day. _____ _____ _____ _____

   d. Percussed lung for resonance. _____ _____ _____ _____

   e. Auscultated lung sounds. _____ _____ _____ _____

6. Assessed patient's skin around and under chest tube insertion site for skin injury. _____ _____ _____ _____

7. Assessed patient's character of pain and rated severity on a scale of 0 to 10 and determined when last analgesic medication was given. _____ _____ _____ _____

8. Assessed patient's knowledge, prior experience with chest tube removal, and feelings about procedure. _____ _____ _____ _____

PLANNING

1. Determined expected outcomes following completion of procedure. _____ _____ _____ _____

2. Planned to administer prescribed medication for pain relief approximately 30 minutes before procedure. _____ _____ _____ _____

464

	S	U	NP	Comments

3. Provided privacy and explained procedure to patient.

4. Organized and set up equipment for chest tube removal at bedside.

IMPLEMENTATION

1. Performed hand hygiene and applied clean gloves and face shield and other personal protective equipment (PPE) as needed.

2. Performed time-out procedure with health care provider to verify patient identification, planned procedure, correct tube(s), and that chest tube was visible and patient position was correct.

3. Helped patient to sitting position on edge of bed, lying supine or on side without chest tubes. Placed pad under chest tube site.

4. Assisted health care provider with preparation and procedure.

   a. Assisted with discontinuing suction from chest-drainage system and checked for leaks while patient coughed.

   b. Assisted with gently removing existing tape and cleaned areas around tubes with antiseptic wipe.

   c. Assisted with clamping each tube to be removed with two Kelly clamps or clamp associated with chest-drainage setup.

5. Assisted health care provider in preparing an occlusive dressing of petrolatum-impregnated gauze on pressure dressing. Set it aside on sterile field while provider applied sterile gloves.

6. Supported patient physically and emotionally while health care provider removed dressing and clipped sutures.

7. Health care provider asked patient to exhale completely and hold it while bearing down.

8. Health care provider quickly pulled out chest tube. *Option:* tightened and tied purse-string suture, if present, after which patient was instructed to breathe normally.

9. Health care provider applied sterile occlusive dressing over wound and firmly secured it in position with wide tape. Assisted as needed.

10. Health care provider inspected end of chest tube(s) before disposal to ensure entire removal.

11. Helped patient to upright position supported by pillows or in comfortable position.

	S	U	NP	Comments

12. Assessed the patient's condition immediately after the procedure and compared with preprocedure findings.

13. Raised side rails (as appropriate) and lowered bed to lowest position, locking into position.

14. Placed nurse call system in an accessible location within patient's reach.

15. Disposed of all contaminated supplies in appropriate receptacle, removed and disposed of gloves, and performed hand hygiene.

EVALUATION

1. Auscultated lung sounds.

2. Palpated skin over area where tube was inserted for subcutaneous emphysema and inspected for redness, inflammation, and blistering.

3. Evaluated vital signs, oxygen saturation, and ventilatory movement to detect signs of respiratory distress after tube removal and during first few hours after removal.

4. Evaluated patient's psychological status.

5. Reviewed chest x-ray film, if ordered.

6. Evaluated character of patient's pain and level of severity on a scale of 0 to 10. Observed for nonverbal cues of pain.

7. Checked chest dressing for drainage per agency policy. When changing dressing, noted wound for signs of healing.

8. Used Teach-Back: Revised instruction if patient or family caregiver was not able to teach back correctly.

RECORDING

1. Documented removal of tube, amount and appearance of drainage in the collection bottle, appearance of wound, surrounding skin, and dressing, and patient's response/tolerance and understanding of the procedure.

2. Documented vital signs and respiratory assessment.

3. Documented the results of chest radiograph, and any unexpected outcomes.

4. Documented patient learning.

HAND-OFF REPORTING

1. Reported patient tolerance of chest tube removal, comfort level and any analgesia, and respiratory assessment before and after chest tube removal.

466

	S	U	NP	Comments
2. Reported any persistent bleeding, crepitus, purulent drainage, tenderness, or warmth at the site.	___	___	___	_____
3. Reported any continued or severe pain despite pain interventions.	___	___	___	_____
4. Reported chest radiograph results.	___	___	___	_____
5. Reported unexpected outcomes to nurse in charge or health care provider.	___	___	___	_____

Student _____   Date _____

Instructor _____   Date _____

PERFORMANCE CHECKLIST SKILL 26.3   **AUTOTRANSFUSION OF CHEST TUBE DRAINAGE**

	S	U	NP	Comments
ASSESSMENT				
1. Identified patient using at least two identifiers according to agency policy. Compared identifiers with information on patient's medication administration record (MAR) or electronic health record (EHR).	___	___	___	_____
2. Reviewed patient's EHR regarding history of coagulation disorders, cancer, active infection, and kidney or liver disease, including health care provider's order and nurses' notes.	___	___	___	_____
3. Assessed patient's/family caregiver's health literacy.	___	___	___	_____
4. Performed assessment per Skill 26.1.	___	___	___	_____
5. Determined presence of active bleeding (at least 100 mL/h) through an existing chest tube or collection of more than 300 mL in a collection system.	___	___	___	_____
6. Performed hand hygiene. Assessed IV site. Noted size of IV catheter (18-gauge angiocatheter preferred).	___	___	___	_____
7. Obtained baseline laboratory data.	___	___	___	_____
8. Assessed patient's knowledge, prior experience with autotransfusion, and feelings about procedure.	___	___	___	_____
PLANNING				
1. Determined expected outcomes following completion of procedure.	___	___	___	_____
2. Provided privacy and explained procedure to patient.	___	___	___	_____
3. Organized and set up equipment for autotransfusion at bedside.	___	___	___	_____
IMPLEMENTATION				
1. Performed hand hygiene and applied clean gloves and and mask and/or face shield and other PPE as needed.	___	___	___	_____
2. Prepared AT System:				
a. Followed manufacturer's guidelines and agency policy.	___	___	___	_____
b. Made certain that all connections were tight and all clamps were open.	___	___	___	_____

468

	S	U	NP	Comments

c. Noted that 200-μm double-sided mesh filter was located in AT bag to filter drainage. Checked manufacturer's instructions. ___ ___ ___ _____

d. Noted AT system collection bag had capacity of 1000 mL marked in increments of 25 mL and an area for marking times and amounts. ___ ___ ___ _____

3. Prepared chest drainage for reinfusion. ___ ___ ___ _____

   a. Following manufacturer directions, opened replacement bag and closed two white clamps. ___ ___ ___ _____

   b. Used high-negativity relief valve to reduce excessive negativity. ___ ___ ___ _____

   c. Bag transfer:

     (1) Closed clamps on chest drainage tubing. ___ ___ ___ _____

     (2) Closed clamps on top of initial AT system collection bag. ___ ___ ___ _____

     (3) Connected chest drainage tube to new AT system bag. ___ ___ ___ _____

     (4) Made certain that all connections were tight. ___ ___ ___ _____

     (5) Opened all clamps on chest drainage tube and replacement bag. ___ ___ ___ _____

   d. Connected connectors on top of initial collection bag and removed bag by lifting it from side hook and then from foot hook. ___ ___ ___ _____

   e. Secured replacement bag by connecting foot hook, replacing metal frame into side hook of chest drainage unit (CDU), and pushing down to secure frame onto hook. ___ ___ ___ _____

   f. Placed thumbs on top of metal frame and pushed up with fingers to slide bag out; removed replacement bag. ___ ___ ___ _____

4. Reinfused chest drainage. ___ ___ ___ _____

   a. Used new microaggregate filter to reinfuse each autotransfusion bag. ___ ___ ___ _____

   b. Accessed bag by inverting it, wiping off port with antiseptic swab, and spiking through port with microaggregate filter by twisting. ___ ___ ___ _____

   c. With bag upside down, gently squeezed it to remove air and primed filter with blood. ___ ___ ___ _____

   d. Hung bag on IV pole and continued to prime tubing until all air was gone. Clamped tubing, attached it to patient's IV access, and adjusted clamp to deliver reinfusion at appropriate rate. ___ ___ ___ _____

	S	U	NP	Comments

e. If ordered, anticoagulants were added to reinfusion through self-sealing port in autotransfusion connector.
      —   —   —   _____

f. Monitored patient's vital signs and SpO_2 according to patient condition and agency policy.
      —   —   —   _____

5. Helped patient to comfortable position.
      —   —   —   _____

6. Raised side rails (as appropriate) and lowered bed to lowest position, locking into position.
      —   —   —   _____

7. Placed nurse call system in an accessible location within patient's reach.
      —   —   —   _____

8. Disposed of all contaminated supplies in appropriate receptacle, removed and disposed of gloves and other PPE, and performed hand hygiene.
      —   —   —   _____

EVALUATION

1. Monitored vital signs every 15 minutes for the first hour and then according to agency policy, hematocrit, and hemoglobin.
      —   —   —   _____

2. Monitored chest drainage system and patient's lung sounds.
      —   —   —   _____

3. Evaluated IV infusion site for infiltration and phlebitis.
      —   —   —   _____

4. Used Teach-Back: Revised instruction if patient or family caregiver was not able to teach back correctly.
      —   —   —   _____

RECORDING

1. Documented drainage and reinfusion with times and amounts of each; included patient's response to reinfusion.
      —   —   —   _____

2. Documented condition of IV infusion site.
      —   —   —   _____

3. Documented patient teaching and validation of understanding.
      —   —   —   _____

HAND-OFF REPORTING

1. Reported to health care provider any drainage > 200 mL/h, new-onset clots, absence of drainage, or any unexpected outcomes.
      —   —   —   _____

Student _____ Date _____

Instructor _____ Date _____

PERFORMANCE CHECKLIST SKILL 27.1   **INSERTING AN OROPHARYNGEAL AIRWAY**

	S	U	NP	Comments

ASSESSMENT

1. Identified need to insert an oropharyngeal airway (OPA). ___ ___ ___ _____

2. Assessed for factors that might have contributed to upper airway obstruction. NOTE: Once established that airway obstruction was developing, proceeded immediately to implementation. ___ ___ ___ _____

3. Performed hand hygiene. ___ ___ ___ _____

4. Measured the OPA size for the patient. Held the flange of the OPA parallel to the front teeth. The end of the OPA reached the angle of the jaw. ___ ___ ___ _____

PLANNING

1. Determined expected outcomes following completion of procedure. ___ ___ ___ _____

2. Closed room door and bedside curtain. ___ ___ ___ _____

3. Obtained and organized equipment for airway insertion at bedside. ___ ___ ___ _____

4. Positioned unconscious patient in semi-Fowler position if possible. ___ ___ ___ _____

IMPLEMENTATION

1. Performed hand hygiene and applied clean gloves and face shield (when possible). ___ ___ ___ _____

2. Ensured that the patient did not have dentures in place before attempting an OPA insertion. Removed dentures that were in place. ___ ___ ___ _____

3. If difficult to open mouth, used a padded tongue blade or used thumb and forefinger of nondominant hand to open jaws and teeth. ___ ___ ___ _____

4. Suctioned out the oral cavity to rid it of excess secretions. ___ ___ ___ _____

5. Inserted OPA. ___ ___ ___ _____

	S	U	NP	Comments

a. Held oral airway with curved end toward the hard palate. As the OPA was inserted and it approached the posterior pharynx, rotated the OPA 180 degrees into the correct position. Option: Held airway sideways, inserted halfway, and rotated 90 degrees while gliding it over natural curvature of tongue. Made sure that outer flange was just outside patient's lips.

   ____ ____ ____ _____

6. Suctioned secretions as needed.

   ____ ____ ____ _____

7. Reassessed patient's respiratory status.

   ____ ____ ____ _____

8. Cleaned patient's face with soft tissue or washcloth.

   ____ ____ ____ _____

9. Helped patient to comfortable, preferably side-lying position.

   ____ ____ ____ _____

10. Once airway was established, determined family caregiver's health literacy and knowledge of purpose of airway. Explained how airway functions and the reasons that the patient required one.

   ____ ____ ____ _____

11. Placed nurse call system in an accessible location within patient's reach so it could be used if patient regained consciousness.

   ____ ____ ____ _____

12. Raised side rails (as appropriate) and lowered bed to lowest position, locking into position.

   ____ ____ ____ _____

13. Disposed of all contaminated supplies in appropriate receptacle, removed and disposed of gloves and face mask, and performed hand hygiene.

   ____ ____ ____ _____

14. Administered mouth care frequently.

   ____ ____ ____ _____

EVALUATION

1. Observed patient's respiratory status and compared respiratory assessments before and after insertion of OPA.

   ____ ____ ____ _____

2. Evaluated that airway was patent and that patient's tongue did not obstruct it.

   ____ ____ ____ _____

3. Observed adjacent and underlying tissue for signs of redness, abrasion, or bruising.

   ____ ____ ____ _____

4. Observed patient for signs of improved mental status.

   ____ ____ ____ _____

5. Used Teach-Back technique: Revised instruction if patient or family caregiver were not able to teach back correctly.

   ____ ____ ____ _____

	S	U	NP	Comments

DOCUMENTATION

1. Documented assessment findings; patient's status prior to and after airway insertion; size of OPA; other interventions performed at same time, especially positioning and suctioning; and patient's response to procedure.

2. Documented evaluation of patient and family caregiver learning.

HAND-OFF REPORTING

1. Reported any airway obstruction, changes in secretions, or changes in patient's tolerance of airway. If patient attempted to push out the OPA, did not reinsert.

Student _____ Date _____

Instructor _____ Date _____

PERFORMANCE CHECKLIST SKILL 27.2   **USING AN AUTOMATED EXTERNAL DEFIBRILLATOR**

	S	U	NP	Comments

ASSESSMENT

1. Established person's unresponsiveness and called for help. (In community settings, had someone call 9-1-1.)

2. Established absence of respirations and lack of circulation within 10 seconds: no pulse, no respirations, no movement.

PLANNING

1. Determined expected outcomes following completion of procedure.

IMPLEMENTATION

1. Assessed patient for unresponsiveness, not breathing and pulselessness, and no movement within 10 seconds.

2. Activated code team in accordance with agency policy and procedure.

3. Started chest compressions and continued until AED was attached to patient and verbal prompt of device advised you "Do not touch the patient."

4. Placed AED next to patient near chest or head.

5. Turned on power.

6. Attached device. Placed first AED pad on upper right sternal border directly below clavicle. Placed second AED pad lateral to left nipple with top of pad a few inches below axilla. Ensured that cables were connected to AED.

7. Did NOT touch patient when AED prompted. Directed rescuers and bystanders to avoid touching patient by announcing "Clear!" Allowed AED to analyze the rhythm. Pressed analysis button if required.

8. Before pressing the shock button, announced loudly to clear the victim and performed a visual check to ensure that no one was in contact with the patient.

474

	S	U	NP	Comments

9. Immediately began chest compression after the shock and continued for 2 minutes with a ratio of 30:2 (30 compressions and two breaths). Did NOT remove pads.   ____   ____   ____   _____

10. Delivered two breaths using mouth-to-mouth with barrier device, mouth-to-mask device, or bag-valve mask device. Watched for chest rise and fall. If second rescuer was available, delivered 10 to 12 breaths/min or 1 breath every 5 to 6 seconds while continuing chest compressions.   ____   ____   ____   _____

11. After 2 minutes of CPR, AED prompted not to touch patient and analysis of patient's rhythm resumed. Cycle continued until patient regained pulse or health care provider determined death.   ____   ____   ____   _____

12. Removed and disposed of gloves and other PPE. Performed hand hygiene.   ____   ____   ____   _____

EVALUATION

1. Inspected pad adhesion to chest wall. If pads were not in good contact with chest wall, removed them and applied a new set.   ____   ____   ____   _____

2. Checked for palpable pulse and responsiveness. Continued resuscitative efforts until patient regained pulse or health care provider determined death.   ____   ____   ____   _____

3. Provided updates to family on patient's status.   ____   ____   ____   _____

DOCUMENTATION

1. Cardiopulmonary arrest requires immediate and accurate documentation. Immediately documented arrest using the form designed specifically for in-agency arrests.   ____   ____   ____   _____

2. Documented onset of arrest, time and number of AED shocks (will not know the exact energy level used by the AED), and additional resuscitation activities.   ____   ____   ____   _____

HAND-OFF REPORTING

1. Immediately reported arrest via the agency-wide communication system, indicating exact location of victim.   ____   ____   ____   _____

2. Shared all documented information regarding patient status prearrest and postarrest to the postarrest team.   ____   ____   ____   _____

Student _____ Date _____

Instructor _____ Date _____

PERFORMANCE CHECKLIST SKILL 27.3 **RESUSCITATION MANAGEMENT**

	S	U	NP	Comments
ASSESSMENT				
1. Determined if patient was unconscious by shaking them and shouting, "Are you OK?" Assessed patient unresponsiveness.	____	____	____	_____
PLANNING				
1. Determined expected outcomes following completion of procedure.	____	____	____	_____
2. Immediately activated the agency's code team or emergency medical services (EMS). Told coworkers to bring AED (if available) and crash cart to bedside.	____	____	____	_____
IMPLEMENTATION				
PRIMARY SURVEY: C (CIRCULATION) AND D (DEFIBRILLATION, AS SOON AS AVAILABLE)				
1. Applied clean gloves and face shield, if needed.	____	____	____	_____
2. Checked carotid pulse on adult or child; used brachial or femoral pulse in infant. Palpated for no more than 10 seconds.	____	____	____	_____
3. If pulse was absent and an AED was unavailable, immediately initiated chest compressions.	____	____	____	_____
a. Placed victim on hard surface. Ensured that victim was flat. Logrolled victim to flat, supine position using spine precautions if trauma was suspected.	____	____	____	_____
b. Assumed correct hand position and compression ratio for patient.	____	____	____	_____
4. If pulse was absent and AED was available, applied AED immediately as appropriate.	____	____	____	_____
a. After one shock, resumed CPR for five cycles (30:2, adult compressions: breath ratio) and began rhythm analysis and shock sequence again.	____	____	____	_____
PRIMARY SURVEY: A (AIRWAY):				
Performed after first 2 minutes of chest compression and AED use.				
5. Opened airway.	____	____	____	_____
a. Head tilt-chin lift (no trauma) or	____	____	____	_____
b. Jaw thrust (used if cervical trauma suspected)	____	____	____	_____

476

	S	U	NP	Comments

6. Determined if patient had spontaneous respirations. ____ ____ ____ _____

PRIMARY SURVEY: B (BREATHING)

7. Attempted to ventilate patient with slow breaths using one of these methods:

   a. Mouth-to-mouth using barrier device ____ ____ ____ _____

   b. Mouth-to-mask using pocket mask ____ ____ ____ _____

   c. Bag-mask device ____ ____ ____ _____

8. If ventilation was difficult, inserted an oral airway. ____ ____ ____ _____

9. Suctioned secretions if necessary or turned victim's head to one side unless trauma was suspected. ____ ____ ____ _____

SECONDARY SURVEY: IMPLEMENTATION

1. Gave code leader brief verbal report on events performed before code team's arrival. Reported immediate prearrest events, medical diagnosis, and any prearrival code intervention. ____ ____ ____ _____

2. On arrival of sufficient personnel, delegated tasks as appropriate while the primary group continued with resuscitation efforts. ____ ____ ____ _____

   a. Helped victim's roommate and visitors away from code scene. Assigned pastoral care or other nurses to communicate with patient's family. Considered allowing family to witness resuscitation (per agency policy). ____ ____ ____ _____

   b. Delegated someone to remove excess furniture or equipment from room. ____ ____ ____ _____

   c. Had someone bring patient's chart to bedside or had access to patient's electronic health record (EHR). ____ ____ ____ _____

   d. Assigned nurses to one of three major roles:

      (1) Bedside nurse ____ ____ ____ _____

      (2) Crash cart nurse ____ ____ ____ _____

      (3) Recorder nurse ____ ____ ____ _____

SECONDARY SURVEY: C (ANALYSIS OF CARDIAC RHYTHM)

3. Attached manual defibrillator/monitor to patient or switched over from the AED to the manual defibrillator using "hands-off" defibrillation electrode to visualize cardiac rhythm. ____ ____ ____ _____

	S	U	NP	Comments

4. If cardiac rhythm was "shockable," continued CPR and helped code team with manual defibrillation.

   a. Turned on defibrillator and selected proper energy level following agency policy and equipment directions.

   b. Applied conductive gel or gel pads to patient's chest where defibrillator paddles were to be placed.

   c. Placed paddles or pads on patient's chest wall.

   d. Verified that no one was in physical contact with patient, bed, or any item contacting patient during defibrillation. Called out warning before initiating charge.

5. Established IV access with large-bore IV needle (14- to 22-gauge) and began infusion of 0.9% NS or lactated Ringer solution.

   a. If peripheral IV access could not be obtained, health care provider may have pursued central venous or intraosseous access.

6. Helped with procedures as needed.

7. Continued CPR until relieved. Rotated chest compressors every 2 minutes to maintain high-quality CPR.

SECONDARY SURVEY: A (INTUBATE AIRWAY)

8. If respirations were absent, helped code team with endotracheal intubation.

   a. Had available laryngoscope handle, laryngoscope blades, curved and straight blades, ET tubes, stylet, suction, and tape or ET tube holder. Ensured that light source on laryngoscope was functional. Note: During the COVID-19 pandemic, the AHA recommended using video laryngoscopy to reduce exposure to aerosolized particles during intubation.

SECONDARY SURVEY: B (CONFIRMATION OF AIRWAY AND VENTILATION)

9. Helped in confirmation of ET tube placement or advanced airway support by auscultating lungs for bilateral breath sounds and monitoring the carbon dioxide (CO_2) detector to confirm correct airway placement

10. Ventilated using bag device on intubation. Avoided hyperventilation.

478

	S	U	NP	Comments

SECONDARY SURVEY: D (DIFFERENTIAL DIAGNOSIS)

11. Obtained ordered laboratory and diagnostic studies.   ____ ____ ____ _____

EVALUATION

1. Reassessed primary and secondary surveys throughout code event.   ____ ____ ____ _____

2. Palpated carotid or femoral pulse at five cycles or 2 minutes of CPR.   ____ ____ ____ _____

3. Observed for spontaneous return of respirations or heart rate every 2 minutes, usually performed during chest compressors rotation. Performed check in less than 10 seconds.   ____ ____ ____ _____

4. Ensured that interruptions in CPR were minimized.   ____ ____ ____ _____

5. Used Teach-Back with family caregiver: Revised instruction if family caregiver was not able to teach back correctly.   ____ ____ ____ _____

DOCUMENTATION

1. Documented the onset of arrest, time, and number of AED shocks (will not know the exact energy level used by the AED), time and energy level of manual defibrillations, medications given (including time), procedures performed, cardiac rhythm, use of CPR, patient's response, education, and support provided to family.   ____ ____ ____ _____

HAND-OFF REPORTING

1. Immediately reported arrest, indicating exact location of victim. In agency setting, followed agency policy. In community setting, activated the emergency response system.   ____ ____ ____ _____

2. Used the CPR worksheet as reference during a hand-off to accepting nurse. Reported the prearrest assessment and major interventions during the arrest.   ____ ____ ____ _____

Student _____ Date _____

Instructor _____ Date _____

PERFORMANCE CHECKLIST SKILL 28.1   **INSERTION OF A PERIPHERAL INTRAVENOUS DEVICE**

	S	U	NP	Comments

ASSESSMENT

1. Reviewed patient's electronic health record (EHR) for accuracy of health care provider's order: date and time, IV solution, route of administration, volume, rate, duration, and signature of ordering health care provider. Followed the seven rights of medication administration.

   a. Used approved online database or drug reference book or consulted pharmacist for information about IV solution composition, purpose, potential incompatibilities, adverse reactions, and side effects.

2. Assessed patient's/family caregiver's health literacy.

3. Performed hand hygiene following Aseptic Non-Touch Technique (ANTT). Obtained data from patient's EHR for clinical factors/conditions that would respond to or be affected by administration of IV solutions, or performed physical examination of the following:

   a. Body weight

   b. Clinical markers of vascular volume

   c. Clinical markers of interstitial volume

   d. Thirst

   e. Behavior and level of consciousness

4. After completing any physical examination, performed hand hygiene.

5. Reviewed EHR to determine patient's risk for developing a MARSI with use of adhesive devices or tape.

6. Reviewed EHR and asked patient about allergy to iodine, adhesive, latex, or chlorhexidine (CHG). If allergy identified, applied allergy ID band to patient's wrist.

7. Determined whether patient was to undergo any planned surgeries or procedures.

8. Assessed available laboratory data.

	S	U	NP	Comments

9. Assessed patient's knowledge, prior experience with infusion therapy, and feelings about procedure.   ___ ___ ___ _____

PLANNING

1. Determined expected outcomes following completion of procedure.   ___ ___ ___ _____

2. Provided privacy and explained the rationale for infusion, including solution and medications ordered, procedure for initiating an IV line, and signs and symptoms of complications.   ___ ___ ___ _____

3. Collected and organized equipment on clean, clutter-free bedside stand or overbed table. Ensured that you had the correct infusion set for the EID that was to be used. Selected integrated securement device or proper adhesive tape to reduce risk of MARSI. Option: Had vein visualization device at hand.   ___ ___ ___ _____

4. Helped patient to comfortable sitting or supine position. Changed patient's gown to one more easily removed with snaps at shoulder if available. Provided adequate lighting.   ___ ___ ___ _____

IMPLEMENTATION

1. Identified patient using at least two identifiers according to agency policy. Compared identifiers with information on patient's medication administration record (MAR) or EHR.   ___ ___ ___ _____

2. Performed hand hygiene following ANTT. Selected appropriate-size catheter based on assessment; opened and prepared sterile packages using sterile aseptic technique.   ___ ___ ___ _____

3. Option: Prepared short extension tubing with fused needleless connector or separate needleless connector (injection cap) to attach to catheter hub.   ___ ___ ___ _____

   a. Removed protective cap from needleless connector and attached syringe with 1 to 3 mL 0.9% sodium chloride (NS), maintaining sterility. Slowly injected enough saline to prime (fill) short extension tubing and connector, removing all air. Left syringe attached to end of tubing.   ___ ___ ___ _____

   b. Maintained sterility of end of connector by reapplying end caps, and set aside for attaching to catheter hub after successful venipuncture.   ___ ___ ___ _____

4. Prepared IV tubing and solution for continuous infusion.   ___ ___ ___ _____

a. Checked IV solution using seven rights of medication administration and reviewed label for name and concentration of solution, type and concentration of any additives, volume, beyond-use and expiration dates, and sterility state. If using bar code system, scanned code on patient's wristband and then on IV fluid container. Ensured prescribed additives had been added. Checked solution for color and clarity. Checked bag for leaks.   ___   ___   ___   _____

b. Opened IV infusion set, maintaining sterility. Note: If EID had dedicated administration set, followed manufacturer's instructions.   ___   ___   ___   _____

c. Placed roller clamp about 2 to 5 cm (1–2 inches) below drip chamber and moved roller clamp to "off" position.   ___   ___   ___   _____

d. Removed protective sheath over IV tubing port on plastic IV solution bag or top of IV solution bottle while maintaining sterility.   ___   ___   ___   _____

e. Inserted spike into port of IV bag using a twisting motion.   ___   ___   ___   _____

f. Compressed drip chamber and released, allowing it to fill one-third to one-half full.   ___   ___   ___   _____

g. Primed air out of IV tubing by filling with IV solution: Removed protective cover on end of IV tubing (or primed without removing protective cover if using that type of tubing) and slowly opened roller clamp to allow fluid to flow from drip chamber to distal end of IV tubing. Returned roller clamp to "off" position after priming tubing (filled with IV fluid). Replaced protective cover on distal end of tubing. Labeled IV tubing with date according to agency policy and procedure.   ___   ___   ___   _____

h. Ensured IV tubing was clear of air and air bubbles. To remove small air bubbles, firmly tapped tubing where they were located. Checked entire length of tubing to ensure that all air bubbles were removed.   ___   ___   ___   _____

i. If using optional long extension tubing (not short tubing mentioned in Step 3), removed protective cover and attached it to distal end of IV tubing, maintaining sterility. Then primed long extension tubing. Inserted tubing into EID with power off.   ___   ___   ___   _____

5. Performed hand hygiene and applied clean gloves following ANTT.   ___   ___   ___   _____

	S	U	NP	Comments

6. Applied tourniquet around upper arm about 10 to 15 cm (4–6 inches) above proposed insertion site. Did not apply tourniquet too tightly. Checked for presence of pulse distal to tourniquet.   ___ ___ ___ _____

(Option A: Applied tourniquet on top of thin layer of clothing, such as gown sleeve, to protect fragile or hairy skin.)   ___ ___ ___ _____

(Option B: Used blood pressure cuff in place of tourniquet: activated cuff and held at approximately 50 mm Hg. Avoided performing venipuncture too close to the blood pressure cuff.)   ___ ___ ___ _____

(Option C: Instead of applying a tourniquet, used a vein visualization device.)   ___ ___ ___ _____

7. Selected vein for VAD insertion.   ___ ___ ___ _____

   a. Used most distal site in nondominant arm if possible.   ___ ___ ___ _____

   b. Following ANTT, with your fingertip, palpated vein at intended insertion site by pressing downward. Noted resilient, soft, bouncy feeling while releasing pressure.   ___ ___ ___ _____

   c. Selected well-dilated vein.   ___ ___ ___ _____

   d. Improved vascular distention: ___ ___ ___ _____

      (1) Positioned extremity lower than heart, had patient open and close fist slowly, and lightly stroked vein downward.   ___ ___ ___ _____

      (2) Used controlled warming to extremity for several minutes.   ___ ___ ___ _____

8. When selecting a vein, avoided selection in:

   a. Dominant hand. Chose site that would not interfere with patient's activities of daily living (ADLs), use of assistive devices, or planned procedures.   ___ ___ ___ _____

   b. Areas with pain on palpation, compromised areas, sites distal to compromised areas.   ___ ___ ___ _____

   c. Upper extremity on side of breast surgery with axillary node dissection or lymphedema or after radiation; arteriovenous (AV) fistulas/grafts; or affected extremity from cerebrovascular accident (CVA).   ___ ___ ___ _____

   d. Site distal to previous venipuncture site, sclerosed or hardened veins, previous infiltrations or extravasations, areas of venous valves, or phlebitic vessels.   ___ ___ ___ _____

   e. Fragile dorsal hand veins in older adults. Veins of lower extremities should not be used for routine IV therapy in adults because of risk of tissue damage and thrombophlebitis.   ___ ___ ___ _____

	S	U	NP	Comments

f. Areas of flexion such as wrist or antecubital area. ____ ____ ____ _____

g. Ventral surface of wrist (10 to 12.5 cm [4-5 inches]). ____ ____ ____ _____

9. Released tourniquet temporarily. Removed gloves and disposed of in appropriate container. ____ ____ ____ _____

10. Performed hand hygiene and applied clean gloves following ANTT. Wore eye protection and mask (per agency policy) if splash or spray of blood was possible. ____ ____ ____ _____

11. Placed adapter end of short extension set (prepared in Step 3) or needless connector (injection cap) for saline lock nearby in sterile package. ____ ____ ____ _____

12. If area of insertion was visibly soiled, cleaned site with antiseptic soap and water first and dried. Performed skin antisepsis with alcoholic CHG solution in back-and-forth motion and allowed to dry completely, following manufacturer's recommendations. If using alcohol or povidone-iodine, cleaned in concentric circle, moving from insertion site outward with swab. Allowed drying time between agents if agents were used in combination (alcohol and povidone-iodine). ____ ____ ____ _____

13. Used visualization device or reapplied tourniquet 10 to 15 cm (4–6 inches) above anticipated insertion site. Checked for presence of pulse distal to tourniquet. ____ ____ ____ _____

14. Performed venipuncture. Anchored vein below anticipated insertion site by placing thumb over vein 4 to 5 cm (1 1/2 to 2 inches) distal to site and gently stretching skin against direction of insertion. Instructed patient to relax hand. ____ ____ ____ _____

a. Warned patient of a sharp stick. Held ONC or metal stylet with needle bevel up. Aligned catheter on top of vein at 10- to 30-degree angle. Punctured skin and anterior vein wall. ____ ____ ____ _____

15. Observed for blood return in catheter or flashback chamber of catheter, indicating that bevel of needle has entered vein. Advanced ONC approximately 0.6 cm (1/4 inch) into vein and loosened stylet (needle) of ONC. Continued to hold skin taut while stabilizing ONC and, with index finger on push-off tab of ONC, advanced catheter off needle into vein until hub rested at venipuncture site. Did not reinsert stylet into catheter once catheter had been advanced into vein. Advanced catheter while safety device automatically retracted stylet. Placed stylet directly into sharps container. ____ ____ ____ _____

16. Stabilized ONC with nondominant hand and re-leased tourniquet or blood pressure cuff with other. Applied gentle but firm pressure with middle finger of nondominant hand 3 cm (1 1/4 inches) above in-sertion site. Kept catheter stable with index finger. ___ ___ ___ _____

17. Quickly connected Luer-Lok end of short extension tubing with needleless connector to end of catheter hub. Secured connection. Avoided touching sterile connection ends. ___ ___ ___ _____

    Option: attached main IV tubing directly to cath-eter hub in place of short extension tubing with needleless connector. ___ ___ ___ _____

18. Took the prefilled flush syringe of 0.9% sodium chloride already attached to short extension set and aspirated to assess blood return. Did not rein-ject air. After blood return, slowly injected NS from prefilled syringe into ONC. Removed syringe and discarded. ___ ___ ___ _____

    Option: To begin primary infusion, swabbed needle-less connector of short extension set with antiseptic swab and attached Luer-Lok end of IV tubing. Opened roller clamp of IV tubing, turned on EID, and programed it. Began infusion at correct rate. If using gravity flow instead of EID, began infusion by slowly opening roller clamp to regulate rate. ___ ___ ___ _____

19. Observed insertion site for swelling. ___ ___ ___ _____

20. Applied protective skin barrier. Allowed to dry completely. ___ ___ ___ _____

21. Applied sterile dressing over site. ___ ___ ___ _____

    a. Integrated securement device:

       (1) Continued to secure catheter with nondomi-nant hand. Took first securement strip and placed over catheter hub; secured to skin. ___ ___ ___ _____

       (2) Peeled paper from paper-framed dressing. Using dressing handles and, using ANNT technique, placed dressing over catheter so that transparent film covered insertion site. ___ ___ ___ _____

       (3) Removed paper border and pressed down on dressing edges. ___ ___ ___ _____

       (4) Smoothed over the soft cloth sections under the catheter hub. ___ ___ ___ _____

       (5) Used second securement strip and placed under catheter hub and across soft cloth sec-tion of dressing. ___ ___ ___ _____

   b. TSM dressing:

     (1) Continued to secure catheter with nondominant hand. Removed adherent backing of dressing. Applied one edge of dressing and gently smoothed over IV insertion site. Did not apply with tension or stretching. Left the Luer-Lok connection between tubing and catheter hub uncovered. Applied in the correct orientation to allow for stretching of body part if movement or swelling anticipated. Smoothed into place without gaps or wrinkles. Removed outer covering and smoothed dressing gently over site.

     (2) Placed 2.5 cm (2-inch) piece of tape over Luer-Lok connector. Did not cover connection between connector and catheter hub. Did not apply tape on top of TSM dressing.

   c. Sterile gauze dressing:

     (1) Ensured skin was dry, and then placed a 5-cm (2-inch) piece of sterile tape over catheter hub.

     (2) Placed 2- × 2–inch gauze pad over insertion site and edge of catheter hub. Secured all edges with tape. Did not place tape over insertion site. Did not cover connection between IV tubing and catheter hub.

     (3) Folded 2- × 2–inch gauze in half and covered with 2.5-cm-wide (1 inch) tape so that about 1 inch would extend on each side of dressing. Placed under Luer-Lok connection.

22. Secured Luer-Lok connector and tubing.

   a. Secured using engineered stabilization device (followed manufacturer directions and agency policy).

     (1) Applied skin protectant to area of skin where stabilization device was to be placed and allowed to dry completely.

     (2) Aligned anchoring pads with directional arrow pointing to insertion site. Pressed device retainer over top of Luer-Lok connection while supporting underneath connection.

     (3) Stabilized catheter and peeled off one side of liner and pressed to adhere to skin. Repeated on other side.

	S	U	NP	Comments

b. Secured using tape. Applied 2.5-cm (1-inch) piece of tape over the folded gauze that was placed under Luer-Lok connector. Avoided applying tape or gauze around arm. Did not used rolled bandages with or without elastic to secure ONC. Did not tape Luer-Lok connection if engineered stabilization device was to be used. ___ ___ ___ _____

23. Option: Applied site protection device. ___ ___ ___ _____

24. Looped extension or IV tubing alongside dressing on arm and secured with second piece of tape directly over tubing. ___ ___ ___ _____

25. For continuous infusion, verified ordered rate of infusion and ensured EID was programmed correctly. If infusing by gravity drip, adjusted flow rate to correct drops per minute. ___ ___ ___ _____

26. Labeled dressing per agency policy. Included date and time of IV insertion, VAD gauge size and length, and initials. ___ ___ ___ _____

27. Disposed of all contaminated supplies in appropriate receptacle; removed and disposed of gloves and any other PPE. ___ ___ ___ _____

28. Assisted patient to a comfortable position and instructed how to move and turn without dislodging VAD. ___ ___ ___ _____

29. Raised bed rails (as appropriate) and lowered bed to lowest position, locking into position. ___ ___ ___ _____

30. Placed nurse call system in an accessible location within patient's reach. Instructed patient in its use. ___ ___ ___ _____

31. Performed hand hygiene. ___ ___ ___ _____

EVALUATION

1. Observed patient every 1 to 2 hours or at established intervals per agency policy and procedure for function, intactness, and patency of IV system and for correct infusion rate and accurate type/amount of IV solution infused by observing level in IV container. ___ ___ ___ _____

2. Evaluated patient to determine response to therapy. ___ ___ ___ _____

3. Evaluated patient at established intervals per agency policy and procedure for signs and symptoms of phlebitis and infiltration by inspecting and gently palpating skin around and above IV site over the dressing. ___ ___ ___ _____

4. Monitored IV dressing site for MARSI. ___ ___ ___ _____

5. Used Teach-Back. Revised instruction if patient or family caregiver was not able to teach back correctly. ___ ___ ___ _____

	S	U	NP	Comments

DOCUMENTATION

1. Documented number of attempts at insertion, both successful and unsuccessful; precise description of insertion site by location and vessel (if possible); brand, length, and gauge of IV device; type of solution and additives infusing; rate and method of infusion; and patient's response to insertion.

    ___ ___ ___ _____

2. Documented patient's status, purpose of infusion, when infusion was started, IV fluid, amount infused, and integrity and patency of system according to agency policy. Used an infusion therapy flow sheet when available.

    ___ ___ ___ _____

3. If using an EID, documented type and rate of infusion and device identification number.

    ___ ___ ___ _____

4. Documented patient's and family caregiver's level of understanding following instruction.

    ___ ___ ___ _____

HAND-OFF REPORTING

1. Reported placement of ONC with reason for insertion with signs or symptoms of observed or patient-reported IV site-related complications, type of fluid, flow rate, status of ONC, amount of fluid remaining in present solution, expected time to hang subsequent IV container, and patient condition.

    ___ ___ ___ _____

2. Reported to health care provider any adverse events occurring upon ONC placement.

    ___ ___ ___ _____

Student _____ Date _____

Instructor _____ Date _____

PERFORMANCE CHECKLIST SKILL 28.2 **REGULATING INTRAVENOUS FLOW RATES**

	S	U	NP	Comments

ASSESSMENT

1. Reviewed patient's electronic health record (EHR), including accuracy and completeness of health care provider's order for patient name, type and volume of IV fluid, additives, infusion rate, and duration of IV therapy. Followed seven rights of medication administration. ___ ___ ___ _____

2. Reviewed EHR to identify patient's risk for fluid and electrolyte imbalance given type of IV solution ordered. ___ ___ ___ _____

3. Performed hand hygiene and applied clean gloves following Aseptic Non-Touch Technique (ANTT). ___ ___ ___ _____

4. Checked infusion system from solution container down to VAD insertion site for integrity. ___ ___ ___ _____

   a. Assessed IV container for discoloration, cloudiness, leakage, and expiration date. ___ ___ ___ _____

   b. Assessed IV tubing for puncture, contamination, or occlusion. ___ ___ ___ _____

5. Assessed the integrity, patency, and functioning of the existing VAD. Assessed the VAD catheter-skin junction site and surrounding area by visually inspecting and palpating through the intact dressing for redness, tenderness, swelling, and drainage. ___ ___ ___ _____

6. Removed and disposed of gloves and performed hand hygiene. ___ ___ ___ _____

7. Assessed patient's/family caregiver's health literacy regarding positioning of IV site. ___ ___ ___ _____

8. Assessed patient's knowledge, prior experience with IV flow rates, and feelings about procedure. ___ ___ ___ _____

PLANNING

1. Determined expected outcomes following completion of procedure. ___ ___ ___ _____

2. Prepared and organized equipment at patient's bedside: ___ ___ ___ _____

   a. Had paper and pencil or calculator to calculate flow rate. ___ ___ ___ _____

	S	U	NP	Comments

b. Checked order to see how long each liter of fluid should infuse. If hourly rate (mL/h) was not provided in health care provider order, calculated it by dividing total volume in infusion by hours of infusion.

c. If a keep-vein-open (KVO) rate was ordered, checked agency policy regarding flow rate of KVO.

d. Used hourly rate to program EID or, if gravity-flow infusion, used the hourly rate to calculate minute flow rate (gtt/mL).

e. Knew calibration (drop factor), in drops per milliliter (gtt/mL), of infusion set used by agency:

(1) Microdrip: 60 gtt/mL

(2) Macrodrip: 10 to 15 gtt/mL

f. Selected correct formula to calculate minute flow rate (drops per minute) based on drop factor of infusion set.

3. Provided privacy and explained procedure, its purpose, and what was expected of the patient.

IMPLEMENTATION

1. Identified patient using at least two identifiers according to agency policy. Compared identifiers with information on patient's medical administration record (MAR) or EHR.

2. Regulated gravity infusion.

a. Ensured that IV container was at least 76.2 cm (30 inches) above IV site for adults, and increased height for more viscous fluids.

b. Slowly opened roller clamp on tubing until drops in drip chamber were visible. Held a watch with second hand at same level as drip chamber and counted drip rate for 1 minute. Adjusted roller clamp to increase or decrease rate of infusion.

c. Monitored drip rate at least hourly.

3. Regulated EID (infusion pump or smart pump): Followed manufacturer guidelines for setup of EID. Ensured infusion tubing was compatible with EID.

a. Closed roller clamp on primed IV infusion tubing.

b. Inserted infusion tubing into chamber of control mechanism, per manufacturer's directions. Ensured roller clamp on IV tubing went between EID and patient.

490

	S	U	NP	Comments

c. Secured part of IV tubing through "air in line" alarm system. Closed door and turned on power button, selected required drops per minute or volume per hour, closed door to control chamber, and pressed start button. If infusing medication, accessed the EID library of medications and set appropriate rate and dose limits. ___ ___ ___ _____

d. Opened infusion tubing drip regulator completely while EID was in use. ___ ___ ___ _____

e. Monitored infusion rate and IV site for complications according to agency policy. Used watch to verify rate of infusion, even when using EID. ___ ___ ___ _____

f. Assessed IV system from container to VAD insertion site if alarm signaled. ___ ___ ___ _____

4. Attached label to IV solution container with date and time container changed, per agency policy. ___ ___ ___ _____

5. Taught patient to avoid touching control clamp, lying on tubing, or raising hand or arm in a way that affects flow rate. If infusion therapy was delivered by EID, explained purpose of alarms and taught patient to avoid trying to adjust settings. ___ ___ ___ _____

6. Disposed of all contaminated supplies in appropriate receptacle. ___ ___ ___ _____

7. Assisted patient to a comfortable position and instructed how to move and turn without dislodging VAD. ___ ___ ___ _____

8. Raised bed rails (as appropriate) and lowered bed to lowest position, locking into position. ___ ___ ___ _____

9. Placed nurse call system in an accessible location within patient's reach. Instructed patient in its use. ___ ___ ___ _____

10. Performed hand hygiene. ___ ___ ___ _____

EVALUATION

1. Observed patient every 1 to 2 hours (per agency policy), noting volume of IV fluid infused and rate of infusion. ___ ___ ___ _____

2. Evaluated patient's response to therapy. ___ ___ ___ _____

3. Evaluated condition of IV site at established intervals per agency policy and procedure for signs and symptoms of IV site-related complications. ___ ___ ___ _____

4. Used Teach-Back. Revised instruction if patient or family caregiver was not able to teach back correctly. ___ ___ ___ _____

	S	U	NP	Comments

DOCUMENTATION

1. Documented IV solution and volume in container, rate of infusion in drops per minute (gtt/min) or milliliters per hour (mL/h), and integrity and patency of system.

2. If an EID was used, documented type and rate of infusion and device identification number.

3. Documented patient response to therapy and unexpected outcomes.

4. Documented patient's and family caregiver's level of understanding following instruction.

HAND-OFF REPORTING

1. Reported rate of infusing and remaining volume.

2. Reported to health care provider any infusion-related complications, interventions, and response to treatment.

492

PERFORMANCE CHECKLIST SKILL 28.3 **CHANGING INTRAVENOUS SOLUTIONS**

	S	U	NP	Comments

ASSESSMENT

1. Reviewed patient's electronic health record (EHR), including accuracy and completeness of health care provider's order for patient name and correct solution: type, volume, additives, infusion rate, and duration of IV therapy. Followed the seven rights of medication administration.

2. Noted date and time when IV tubing and solution were last changed.

3. Assessed patient's/family caregiver's health literacy.

4. Performed hand hygiene and applied clean gloves, following Aseptic Non-Touch Technique (ANTT); inspected and gently palpated skin around and above IV site over dressing. Assessed VAD for patency and signs and symptoms of IV site-related complications.

5. Checked infusion system from solution container down to VAD insertion site for integrity, including, but not limited to, discoloration, cloudiness, leakage, and expiration date. Determined compatibility of all IV solutions and additives by consulting approved online database, drug reference, or pharmacist. Removed and disposed of gloves and performed hand hygiene.

6. Checked pertinent laboratory data.

7. Assessed patient's/family caregiver's knowledge and understanding of need for continued IV therapy and feelings about procedure.

PLANNING

1. Determined expected outcomes following completion of procedure.

2. Provided privacy and explained procedure, its purpose, and what was expected of patient.

3. Organized and set up any equipment needed to perform procedure.

	S	U	NP	Comments

4. Performed hand hygiene following ANTT. Collected equipment. Had next solution prepared at least 1 hour before needed. If solution was prepared in pharmacy, ensured that it had been delivered to patient care unit. Allowed solution to warm to room temperature if it had been refrigerated. Checked that solution was correct and properly labeled. Checked solution expiration date. Ensured that any light sensitivity restrictions were followed.

    _____ _____ _____ _____

IMPLEMENTATION

1. Identified patient using at least two identifiers according to agency policy. Compared identifiers with information on patient's medical administration record (MAR) or EHR.

    _____ _____ _____ _____

2. Changed solution when fluid remained only in neck of container (about 50 mL), when new type of solution had been ordered, or when existing solution hang time had expired.

    _____ _____ _____ _____

3. Prepared new solution for changing. If using plastic bag, hung on IV pole and removed protective cover from IV tubing port. If using glass bottle, removed metal cap and metal and rubber disks.

    _____ _____ _____ _____

4. Applied clean gloves. Closed roller clamp on existing solution to stop flow rate. Removed IV tubing from EID (if used). Then removed old IV solution container from IV pole. Held container with tubing port pointing upward.

    _____ _____ _____ _____

5. Quickly removed spike from old solution container and, without touching tip, inserted spike into new container

    _____ _____ _____ _____

6. Hung new container of solution on IV pole.

    _____ _____ _____ _____

7. Checked for air in IV tubing. If air bubbles had formed, removed them by closing roller clamp, stretching tubing downward, and tapping tubing with finger (bubbles rose in fluid to drip chamber).

    _____ _____ _____ _____

8. Made sure that drip chamber was one-third to one-half full. If drip chamber was too full, decreased level by removing bag from IV pole, pinching off IV tubing below drip chamber, inverting container, squeezing drip chamber, releasing, turning solution container upright, and releasing pinch on tubing.

    _____ _____ _____ _____

9. Regulated flow to ordered rate by opening and adjusting roller clamp on IV tubing or by opening roller clamp and programming and turning on EID.

    _____ _____ _____ _____

494

	S	U	NP	Comments

10. Placed time label on side of container and labeled with time hung, time of completion, and appropriate hourly intervals. If using plastic bags, marked only on label and not container. ___ ___ ___ _____

11. Instructed patient on purpose of new IV solution, additives, flow rate, potential side effects, how to avoid occluding tubing, and what to report. ___ ___ ___ _____

12. Disposed of all contaminated supplies in appropriate receptacle; removed and disposed of gloves. ___ ___ ___ _____

13. Assisted patient to a comfortable position and instructed how to move and turn without dislodging VAD. ___ ___ ___ _____

14. Raised bed rails (as appropriate) and lowered bed to lowest position, locking into position. ___ ___ ___ _____

15. Placed nurse call system in an accessible location within patient's reach. Instructed patient in its use. ___ ___ ___ _____

16. Performed hand hygiene. ___ ___ ___ _____

EVALUATION

1. Observed patient every 1 to 2 hours or at established intervals per agency policy and procedure for function, intactness, and patency of IV system; correct infusion rate; and type/amount of IV solution infused. ___ ___ ___ _____

2. Evaluated patient to determine response to therapy. ___ ___ ___ _____

   a. Monitored patient for signs of fluid volume excess (FVE), fluid volume deficit (FVD), or signs and symptoms of electrolyte imbalances. ___ ___ ___ _____

3. Evaluated IV site at established intervals per agency policy and procedure for signs and symptoms of phlebitis or infiltration. ___ ___ ___ _____

4. Used Teach-Back. Revised instruction if patient or family caregiver was not able to teach back correctly. ___ ___ ___ _____

DOCUMENTATION

1. Documented solution changes, type of infusion solution including any additives, volume of container, time of change, rate of infusion, and integrity and patency of system. ___ ___ ___ _____

2. Documented use of any EID or control device and identification number on that device. ___ ___ ___ _____

3. Documented patient response to therapy and unexpected outcomes. ___ ___ ___ _____

HAND-OFF REPORTING

1. Reported time and reason for IV solution change, new solution, rate of and volume left in infusion, and any significant information about IV site or system.

___ ___ ___ _____

Student _____ Date _____

Instructor _____ Date _____

PERFORMANCE CHECKLIST SKILL 28.4   **CHANGING INFUSION TUBING**

	S	U	NP	Comments

ASSESSMENT

1. Noted date and time when IV tubing was last changed.

2. Performed hand hygiene, following Aseptic Non-Touch Technique (ANTT). Assessed IV tubing for puncture, contamination, or occlusion that required immediate change.

3. Assessed patient's/family caregiver's health literacy.

4. Assessed patient's knowledge, prior experience with need for IV tubing change, and feelings about procedure.

PLANNING

1. Determined expected outcomes following completion of procedure.

2. Provided privacy and explained procedure, its purpose, and what was expected of patient.

3. Coordinated IV tubing changes with solution changes when possible.

4. Obtained and organized equipment for tubing change at bedside.

5. Assisted patient to comfortable position with easy access to IV site.

IMPLEMENTATION

1. Identified patient using at least two identifiers according to agency policy. Compared identifiers with information on patient's medication administration record (MAR) or EHR.

2. Performed hand hygiene following ANTT. Opened new infusion set and connected add-on pieces using aseptic technique. Kept protective coverings over infusion spike and distal adapter. Placed roller clamp about 2 to 2.5 cm (1–2 inches) below drip chamber and moved roller clamp to "off" position. Secured all connections.

3. Applied clean gloves. If patient's IV cannula hub was not visible, removed IV dressing. Did not remove tape or securement device securing cannula to skin.

		S	U	NP	Comments

4. Prepared IV tubing with new IV container. _____ _____ _____ _____

5. Prepared IV tubing with existing continuous IV infusion bag. _____ _____ _____ _____

   a. Ensured roller clamp on new IV tubing was still in the "off" position. _____ _____ _____ _____

   b. Slowed rate of infusion through old tubing to keep-vein-open (KVO) rate using EID or roller clamp. _____ _____ _____ _____

   c. Compressed and filled drip chamber of old tubing. _____ _____ _____ _____

   d. Inverted container and removed old tubing. Disposed of container. Held old tubing upright or hung on IV pole until end of change was over. Kept spike of tubing sterile and upright. _____ _____ _____ _____

   e. Inserted spike of new infusion tubing into solution container. Hung solution bag on IV pole, compressed drip chamber on new tubing, and released, allowing it to fill one-third to one-half full. _____ _____ _____ _____

   f. Primed air out of IV tubing by filling with IV solution: Removed protective cover on end of tubing and slowly opened roller clamp to allow solution to flow from drip chamber to distal end of IV tubing. If tubing had Y connector, inverted Y connector when solution reached it to displace air. Returned roller clamp to "off" position after priming tubing. Replaced protective cover on end of IV tubing. Placed end of adapter near patient's IV site. _____ _____ _____ _____

   g. Stopped EID or turned roller clamp on old tubing to "off" position. _____ _____ _____ _____

6. Prepared tubing with extension set or saline lock. _____ _____ _____ _____

   a. If short extension tubing was needed, used sterile technique to connect new injection cap to new extension set or IV tubing. _____ _____ _____ _____

   b. Scrubbed injection cap with antiseptic swab for at least 15 seconds and allowed to dry completely. Attached syringe with 3 to 5 mL of NS flush solution and injected through injection cap into extension set. _____ _____ _____ _____

7. Reestablished infusion. _____ _____ _____ _____

   a. Gently disconnected old tubing from extension tubing (or from IV catheter hub). Quickly inserted Luer-Lok end of new tubing or saline lock into extension tubing connection (or IV catheter hub). _____ _____ _____ _____

   b. For continuous infusion, opened roller clamp on new tubing and regulated drip rate using roller clamp, or inserted tubing into EID, programmed to desired rate, and pushed "on." _____ _____ _____ _____

498

		S	U	NP	Comments

c. Attached piece of tape or preprinted label with date and time of IV tubing change onto tubing below drip chamber.

d. Formed loop of tubing and secured it to patient's arm with strip of tape.

8. Removed and discarded old IV tubing. If necessary, applied new dressing.

9. Taught patient how to move and turn properly with IV tubing.

10. Disposed of all contaminated supplies in appropriate receptacle; removed and disposed of gloves.

11. Assisted patient to a comfortable position.

12. Raised bed rails (as appropriate) and lowered bed to lowest position, locking into position.

13. Placed nurse call system in an accessible location within patient's reach. Instructed patient in its use.

14. Performed hand hygiene.

EVALUATION

1. Observed patient every 1 to 2 hours or at established intervals per agency policy and procedure for function, intactness, and patency of IV system and leaking at connection sites.

2. Evaluated patient at established intervals per agency policy and procedure for signs and symptoms of IV site-related complications.

3. Used Teach-Back. Revised instruction if patient or family caregiver was not able to teach back correctly.

DOCUMENTATION

1. Documented tubing change, type of solution, volume, and rate of infusion. Used an infusion therapy flow sheet for parenteral solutions per agency policy.

2. If using an EID, documented type and rate of infusion and device identification number.

3. Documented patient's and family caregiver's level of understanding following instruction, including what problems to report.

HAND-OFF REPORTING

1. Reported any significant information about IV site or system, and time IV tubing was changed.

Student _____ Date _____

Instructor _____ Date _____

PERFORMANCE CHECKLIST SKILL 28.5 **CHANGING A PERIPHERAL INTRAVENOUS DRESSING**

	S	U	NP	Comments

ASSESSMENT

1. Referred to electronic health record (EHR) to determine when dressing was last changed.

2. Reviewed EHR to determine patient's risk for developing a MARSI with use of adhesive devices or tape.

3. Assessed patient's/family caregiver's health literacy.

4. Performed hand hygiene and applied clean gloves, following Aseptic Non-Touch Technique (ANTT). Observed present dressing for moisture and intactness. Determined if moisture was from site leakage or external source.

5. Inspected and gently palpated skin around and above IV site over dressing and asked if patient felt tenderness or discomfort. Assessed area for swelling.

   a. Assessed VAD for patency and checked site for signs and symptoms of IV site–related complications.

   b. Assessed skin around dressing: temperature, color, moisture level, turgor, fragility, and integrity. Observed for local signs of irritation or skin damage at the site where any adhesive had been or would be applied.

6. Removed and disposed of gloves in appropriate receptacle and performed hand hygiene.

7. Assessed patient for allergy to iodine, adhesive, latex, or chlorhexidine (CHG). If allergy identified, placed allergy band on patient's wrist.

8. Assessed patient's knowledge, prior experience with the need for IV dressing change, and feelings about the procedure.

PLANNING

1. Determined expected outcomes following completion of procedure.

500

	S	U	NP	Comments

2. Provided privacy and explained procedure and purpose to patient and family caregiver. Explained that patient would need to hold affected extremity still. Explained how long procedure would take.

3. Assisted patient to comfortable position with IV site easily accessible.

4. Collected equipment and organized on clean, clutter-free bedside stand or overbed table.

IMPLEMENTATION

1. Identified patient using at least two identifiers according to agency policy. Compared identifiers with information on patient's medication administration record (MAR) or EHR.

2. Performed hand hygiene, following ANTT, and applied clean gloves. Removed existing dressing:

   a. For integrated securement device/TSM dressing:

      (1) Stabilized catheter with nondominant hand.

      (2) Loosened edges of the dressing with the fingers of the nondominant hand by pushing the skin down and away from integrated securement device/TSM dressing. (For integrated securement device, gently lifted edges of two strips of tape covering dressing.)

      (3) With fingers of the dominant hand, loosened a corner of the dressing and stretched it horizontally in the opposite direction of the wound. Walked fingers under the dressing to continue stretching it. One hand continuously supported the skin adhered to the dressing.

      (4) Repeated process around dressing. Used medical adhesive remover if needed. Followed the manufacturer's instructions for use.

   b. For gauze dressing:

      (1) Stabilized catheter hub.

      (2) Removed tape strips by slowly lifting and removing each side toward the center of dressing. When both sides were completely loosened, lifted the strip up from the center of dressing.

	S	U	NP	Comments

(3) Removed old dressing one layer at a time by pulling toward the insertion site. Used caution if tubing became tangled between two layers of dressing. Used medical adhesive remover if needed.

    ____ ____ ____ _____

3. Assessed VAD insertion site for signs and symptoms of IV site-related complications. If complication existed, determined if VAD required removal. Removed catheter if ordered by health care provider.

    ____ ____ ____ _____

4. If catheter was to remain in place, assessed integrity of engineered stabilization device. Continued to stabilize catheter and removed as recommended by manufacturer directions for use. Inspected for signs of MARSI from adhesive-based engineered stabilization devices.

    ____ ____ ____ _____

5. NOTE: Understood that some stabilization devices are designed to remain in place for length of time VAD is in as long as adequate stabilization was evident.

    ____ ____ ____ _____

6. While stabilizing IV line, performed skin antisepsis to insertion site with CHG solution using friction in back-and-forth motion following manufacturer's guidelines. If using alcohol or povidone-iodine, cleaned in concentric circle, moving from insertion site outward with the swab. Allowed any antiseptic solution to dry completely.

    ____ ____ ____ _____

7. Optional: Applied skin protectant to area where tape, dressing, or engineered stabilization device would be applied. Allowed to dry.

    ____ ____ ____ _____

8. While stabilizing catheter, applied sterile dressing over site per agency policy. Ensured skin surface was dry.

    ____ ____ ____ _____

   a. Integrated securement device/TSM dressing: Applied dressings as directed in Skill 28.1, Step 21a, 21b.

    ____ ____ ____ _____

   b. Sterile gauze dressing: Applied sterile gauze dressing as directed in Skill 28.1, Step 21c.

    ____ ____ ____ _____

9. Option: Secured with new engineered catheter stabilization device. Applied device as directed in Skill 28.1, Step 22.

    ____ ____ ____ _____

10. Optional: Applied site protection device.

    ____ ____ ____ _____

11. Anchored extension tubing or IV tubing alongside dressing on arm and secured with tape directly over tubing. When using integrated securement device/TSM dressing, avoided placing tape over dressing.

    ____ ____ ____ _____

502

	S	U	NP	Comments

12. Labeled dressing per agency policy.

13. Disposed of all contaminated supplies in appropriate receptacle. Removed and disposed of gloves.

14. Assisted patient to a comfortable position and instructed how to move and turn without dislodging VAD.

15. Raised bed rails (as appropriate) and lowered bed to lowest position, locking into position.

16. Placed nurse call system in an accessible location within patient's reach. Instructed patient in its use.

17. Performed hand hygiene.

EVALUATION

1. Evaluated function, patency of IV system, and flow rate after changing dressing.

2. Evaluated patient at established intervals per agency policy and procedure for signs and symptoms of IV site–related complications.

3. Used Teach-Back. Revised instruction if patient or family caregiver was not able to teach back correctly.

DOCUMENTATION

1. Documented the time peripheral dressing was changed, reason for change, type of dressing material used, patency of system, description of VAD site, and any complications, interventions, and response to treatment.

2. Documented patient's and family caregiver's understanding of what IV problems to report.

HAND-OFF REPORTING

1. Reported dressing was changed and any significant information about integrity of system.

2. Reported to health care provider any IV-related complications, interventions, and response to treatment.

Student _____ Date _____

Instructor _____ Date _____

PERFORMANCE CHECKLIST PROCEDURAL GUIDELINE 28.1 **DISCONTINUING A PERIPHERAL INTRAVENOUS DEVICE**

	S	U	NP	Comments

PROCEDURAL STEPS

1. Reviewed accuracy and completeness of health care provider's order for discontinuation of vascular access device (VAD).

2. Performed hand hygiene, following Aseptic Non-Touch Technique (ANTT), and collected equipment.

3. Identified patient using at least two identifiers according to agency policy. Compared identifiers with information on patient's electronic health record (EHR).

4. Applied clean gloves. Observed existing IV site for signs and symptoms of IV-related complications. Palpated catheter site through intact dressing.

5. Assessed if patient was receiving an anticoagulant or had a history of a coagulopathy.

6. Assessed patient's/family caregiver's health literacy and understanding of the reason for IV infusion to be discontinued.

7. Provided privacy and explained procedure to patient before removing catheter. Explained that patient needed to hold affected extremity still.

8. Turned IV tubing roller clamp to "off" position or turned electronic infusion device (EID) off and roller clamp to "off" position.

9. Carefully removed VAD dressing and engineered stabilization device following guidelines in Skill 28.5 for preventing medical adhesive-related skin injury (MARSI).

10. Stabilized IV catheter hub with middle finger of nondominant hand.

11. Placed clean sterile gauze above insertion site and, using dominant hand, withdrew catheter using a slow, steady motion and kept the hub parallel to skin. Did not raise or lift catheter before it was completely out of the vein to avoid trauma or hematoma formation.

504

	S	U	NP	Comments

12. Applied pressure to site for a minimum of 30 seconds until bleeding had stopped. Applied pressure for at least 5 to 10 minutes if patient was on anticoagulants.

13. Inspected catheter for intactness after removal; noted tip integrity and length.

14. Observed IV site for evidence of redness, pain, tenderness, swelling, bleeding, or drainage. Monitored for 24 to 48 hours after removal for postinfusion phlebitis.

15. Applied clean, folded gauze dressing over insertion site and secured firmly with plastic tape.

16. Discarded of used supplies, removed and disposed of gloves, and performed hand hygiene.

17. Used Teach-Back. Revised instruction if patient/family caregiver was not able to teach back correctly.

18. Documented removal of peripheral IV device and patient's tolerance of procedure.

19. Provided hand-off reporting to oncoming nursing staff: time and reason for removal of peripheral IV device. Reported to health care provider and documented any complications.

Student _____ Date _____

Instructor _____ Date _____

PERFORMANCE CHECKLIST SKILL 28.6 **MANAGING CENTRAL VASCULAR ACCESS DEVICES**

	S	U	NP	Comments

ASSESSMENT

1. Reviewed patient's electronic health record (EHR), including accuracy and completeness of health care provider's order for insertion of CVAD for size and type. Assessed treatment schedule. Followed seven rights of medication administration. Confirmed that informed consent had been obtained and witnessed by health care provider who would perform procedure. ___ ___ ___ _____

2. Reviewed EHR to determine patient's risk for developing a medical adhesive-related skin injury (MARSI) with use of adhesive devices or tape. ___ ___ ___ _____

3. Assessed patient's/family caregiver's health literacy. ___ ___ ___ _____

4. Performed hand hygiene following ANTT. Applied gloves if risk of contacting blood. Assessed patient's hydration status. ___ ___ ___ _____

5. Prior to a new insertion, assessed patient for any surgical procedures of upper chest or anatomical irregularities of proposed insertion site. ___ ___ ___ _____

6. Assessed existing or potential CVAD placement site for skin integrity and signs of infection. Also assessed skin temperature, color, moisture level, fragility, and overall integrity, including presence of irritation around potential IV site. Applied gloves if drainage was present. ___ ___ ___ _____

7. Assessed patient for allergy to iodine, lidocaine, adhesive, latex, or chlorhexidine (CHG). If allergy identified, placed allergy band on patient's wrist. ___ ___ ___ _____

8. Assessed type of CVAD intended for placement. Reviewed manufacturer directions concerning catheter and maintenance. ___ ___ ___ _____

9. Assessed for proper function of existing CVAD before therapy. Removed and disposed of gloves (if worn). Performed hand hygiene. ___ ___ ___ _____

10. Assessed if any existing catheter lumens required flushing or if CVAD site needed dressing change by referring to EHR, nurses' notes, agency policies, and manufacturer-recommended guidelines for use. ___ ___ ___ _____

506

	S	U	NP	Comments

11. Assessed patient's knowledge and prior experience with CVAD, including purpose, care, and maintenance, and feelings about procedure. For long-term use, asked patient or family caregiver to discuss steps in care and perform procedure. ____ ____ ____ _____

PLANNING

1. Determined expected outcomes following completion of procedure. ____ ____ ____ _____

2. Provided privacy and explained procedure and purpose to patient and family caregiver. Explained to patient that patient must not move during procedure. Offered opportunity at this time to toilet and offered pain medication (if needed). ____ ____ ____ _____

3. Performed hand hygiene. Collected and organized equipment on clean, clutter-free bedside stand or overbed table. ____ ____ ____ _____

IMPLEMENTATION

1. Identified patient using at least two identifiers according to agency policy. Compared identifiers with information on medication administration record (MAR) or EHR. ____ ____ ____ _____

2. Catheter insertion: nontunneled device:

   a. Health care provider, with help from nurse, positioned patient in Trendelenburg or supine position for placement of CVAD in vessels above heart, unless contraindicated. ____ ____ ____ _____

      (1) Nurse placed rolled towel or bath blanket between patient's shoulder blades, rotating them slightly to 10-degree angle. Turned patient's head away from intended insertion site. ____ ____ ____ _____

   b. If necessary, used scissors or electric clippers to remove any hair around insertion site. Explained rationale to patient. ____ ____ ____ _____

   c. Performed hand hygiene, following Surgical ANTT techniques. ____ ____ ____ _____

   d. Health care provider and nurse applied cap, mask, eyewear, surgical gown, and powder-free sterile gloves. Patient applied mask. ____ ____ ____ _____

   e. Nurse or health care provider opened central vascular access kit. Nurse added additional needed sterile equipment to kit for use during insertion. ____ ____ ____ _____

	S	U	NP	Comments

f. Site preparation:

  (1) Performed skin antisepsis over proposed insertion site with CHG solution, using friction in back-and-forth motion according to manufacturer's directions; allowed to dry completely.

    ___ ___ ___ _____

g. After cleaning site, health care provider and nurse removed and disposed of gloves. Health care provider changed into second pair of sterile gloves, and nurse performed hand hygiene. Followed agency policy.

    ___ ___ ___ _____

h. Health care provider used large sterile drape and sterile towels to create sterile field. Health care provider found anatomical landmarks and placed sterile fenestrated drape appropriately over proposed insertion site.

    ___ ___ ___ _____

i. Health care provider arranged equipment in kit in preparation for catheter insertion.

    ___ ___ ___ _____

j. Nurse set up IV bag, primed and filled tubing, and covered end of tubing with sterile cap.

    ___ ___ ___ _____

k. Nurse scrubbed top of 1% lidocaine bottle with antiseptic swab, allowed to dry completely, and held bottle upside down if not in insertion kit. Optional: Applied topical local anesthetic agents before insertion with health care provider's order.

    ___ ___ ___ _____

l. Health care provider injected needle into bottle and withdrew approximately 3 to 4 mL lidocaine. Health care provider injected needle into site for internal jugular puncture and anesthetized venipuncture site, waiting 1 to 2 minutes for effect to take place.

    ___ ___ ___ _____

m. Health care provider used ultrasound imaging with an introducer needle, micropuncture needle, or angiocath cannula to insert CVAD into internal jugular vein. Once vein was entered, health care provider removed needle from cannula, threaded wire into cannula and vein, removed cannula over wire, advanced central vein catheter over wire to appropriate location, and removed the guidewire (Seldinger technique).

    ___ ___ ___ _____

n. Health care provider determined patency of line by withdrawing blood with 5-mL syringe, flushing with 0.9% sodium chloride, and placing needleless connectors on hub of each lumen. Option: VAD flushed with heparin based on type of catheter and agency policy and procedure.

    ___ ___ ___ _____

508

	S	U	NP	Comments

o. Covered insertion site with integrated secure-ment device/TSM dressing. Health care provid-er applied catheter securement device to secure central vascular catheter in place.

____ ____ ____ _____

p. Health care provider removed sterile drapes and completed procedure. Patient removed mask once dressing was applied. External cath-eter length was measured and documented by nurse.

____ ____ ____ _____

q. Nurse initiated and regulated IV infusion to pre-scribed rate and connected to EID after receiv-ing confirmation of appropriate tip placement.

____ ____ ____ _____

3. Insertion site care and dressing change:

a. Positioned patient in comfortable position with head slightly elevated. Had arm extended for PICC or midline device.

____ ____ ____ _____

b. Prepared dressing materials.
- Integrated securement device/TSM dressing: changed at least every 7 days
- Gauze dressing: changed at least every 2 days
- Gauze under TSM: changed at least every 2 days (not recommended)

____ ____ ____ _____

c. Performed hand hygiene and applied mask, fol-lowing ANTT. Instructed patient to apply mask and turn head away from site during dressing change.

____ ____ ____ _____

d. Applied clean gloves. Carefully removed old dressing.

____ ____ ____ _____

e. Removed catheter stabilization device if used and required changing. Used adhesive remover to remove adhesive stabilization devices.

____ ____ ____ _____

f. Inspected catheter, insertion site, and surround-ing skin. Measured external CVAD length and compared to measurement from insertion if dis-lodgement was suspected. For PICC and mid-lines, measured upper-arm circumference 10 cm above antecubital fossa if clinically indicated and compared with baseline.

____ ____ ____ _____

g. Removed and disposed of clean gloves; per-formed hand hygiene. Opened CVAD dressing kit using sterile technique and applied sterile gloves, following surgical ANTT.

____ ____ ____ _____

h. Cleaned site:

____ ____ ____ _____

(1) Performed skin antisepsis with CHG solu-tion, using friction in back-and-forth motion according to manufacturer's directions, and allowed to dry completely.

____ ____ ____ _____

	S	U	NP	Comments

     (2) If using alcohol or povidone-iodine, cleaned in concentric circle, moving from insertion site outward with swab. Allowed to dry completely.

  i. Applied polymer-based skin protectant to area and allowed to dry completely so that skin was not tacky. Used skin protectant if adhesive stabilization device was to be used.

  j. Option: Used CHG-impregnated dressing for short-term CVADs.

  k. Applied sterile integrated securement device/TSM dressing over insertion site.

  l. Applied new catheter stabilization device according to manufacturer directions for use. Applied new injection caps to lumens of CVAD every 72 hours, per agency policy. Applied disinfecting cap to end of injection caps of catheter.

  m. Applied label to dressing with date, time, and initials.

  n. Had patient remove mask. Disposed of all contaminated supplies in appropriate receptacle, removed and disposed of gloves, and performed hand hygiene.

4. Blood sampling:

  a. Performed hand hygiene. Applied clean gloves and face mask using Surgical ANTT.

  b. Put the EID on hold for at least 1 to 5 minutes before drawing blood. NOTE: If infusion could not be stopped, drew blood from peripheral vein.

  c. Used a dedicated lumen for blood sampling from a multilumen CVAD. When drawing through staggered multilumen catheters, drew from the lumen exiting at the point farthest away from the heart (or one recommended by manufacturer).

  d. Clamped the CVAD lumen using the small slide clamp. Did not clamp valved catheter.

  e. Syringe method:

     (1) Removed disinfection cap from CVAD lumen. Scrubbed catheter injection cap hub with antiseptic swab for at least 15 seconds and allowed to dry completely.

     (2) Attached syringe containing 5 to 10 mL of NS, per agency policy, to end of hub. Unclamped CVAD if necessary. Flushed CVAD slowly with NS. Reclamped CVAD.

510

	S	U	NP	Comments

(3) Cleaned catheter hub with antiseptic swab and allowed to dry completely. Attached empty 5-mL syringe to hub and unclamped catheter (if necessary). To withdraw blood, first aspirated gently, pulling back 1 to 2 mL. Paused and held pressure to allow valve to open. Then continued pulling plunger slowly, staying just ahead of blood flow, until 2 to 25 mL of blood was obtained for discard sample (depending on the internal volume of CVAD and agency policy). ___ ___ ___ _____

(4) Reclamped catheter (if necessary); removed syringe with blood and discarded in appropriate biohazard container. ___ ___ ___ _____

(5) Scrubbed catheter hub with another antiseptic swab for 15 seconds and allowed to dry completely. ___ ___ ___ _____

(6) Attached syringe(s) to obtain required volume of blood needed for specimen(s) ordered. ___ ___ ___ _____

(7) Unclamped catheter (if necessary) to withdraw blood. Obtained necessary blood volume for specimens. ___ ___ ___ _____

(8) Once specimens were obtained, clamped catheter (if necessary) and removed syringe. ___ ___ ___ _____

(9) Scrubbed catheter hub with antiseptic swab for 15 seconds and allowed to dry completely. ___ ___ ___ _____

(10) Attached prefilled syringe with 10-mL 0.9% sodium chloride (NS). Unclamped catheter if necessary. Flushed catheter using the appropriate flush/clamp/disconnect sequence based on the type of needleless connector. Ensured that clamp was engaged (if available). ___ ___ ___ _____

(11) Removed syringe and discarded into appropriate biohazard container. ___ ___ ___ _____

(12) Transferred blood from syringe into blood tubes using transfer vacuum device. ___ ___ ___ _____

(13) Option: Flushed catheter with heparin flush based on type of catheter and agency policy and procedure using appropriate flush/clamp/disconnect sequence. Ensured that clamp was engaged (if available). ___ ___ ___ _____

(14) Scrubbed exposed hub or CVAD with antiseptic swab for 15 seconds and allowed to dry. Attached new injection cap to accessed lumen. Applied disinfection cap to injection cap. Resumed infusion as ordered. ___ ___ ___ _____

f. NOTE: Checked agency policy for use of vacuum tube method for blood sampling with CVADs.

    ___ ___ ___   _____

g. Disposed of all contaminated supplies in appropriate receptacle; removed and disposed of gloves and mask, and performed hand hygiene.

    ___ ___ ___   _____

5. Changing needleless injection cap:

a. Determined if injection caps should be changed.

    ___ ___ ___   _____

b. Prepared new injection cap(s):

(1) Performed hand hygiene. Applied clean gloves and mask, following Surgical ANTT. (Had patient apply mask.) Removed cap from package. Did not contaminate sterile injection port.

    ___ ___ ___   _____

(2) Kept protective cover on tip of injection cap.

    ___ ___ ___   _____

(3) Attached prefilled syringe to end of injection cap by pushing in and then turning clockwise. Primed injection cap by flushing with preservative-free 0.9% sodium chloride (NS) through cap until fluid escaped from tip of cap. Kept syringe attached to cap and kept connection sterile.

    ___ ___ ___   _____

c. Based on catheter type, clamped catheter lumen by using slide or squeeze clamp.

    ___ ___ ___   _____

d. Removed old injection cap by turning counterclockwise. Disposed of old injection cap using aseptic technique. Continued holding catheter lumen.

    ___ ___ ___   _____

e. Scrubbed exposed catheter hub with antiseptic swab, twisting back and forth vigorously for 15 seconds, and allowed to dry completely. Took the new injection cap and attached syringe, removed the protective cover from the tip, and connected new injection cap(s) on catheter hub, turning clockwise just until resistance was felt. Removed and disposed of syringe. Option: Placed disinfecting cap on end of injection cap.

    ___ ___ ___   _____

f. Repeated procedure for additional CVAD lumens.

    ___ ___ ___   _____

g. Disposed of all contaminated supplies in appropriate receptacle, removed and disposed of gloves and mask, removed patient's mask (if worn), and performed hand hygiene.

    ___ ___ ___   _____

	S	U	NP	Comments

6. Discontinuing nontunneled catheters:

a. Verified health care provider's order to discontinue line. Checked agency policy because most require health care providers to discontinue CVAD. ___ ___ ___ _____

b. If IV solutions or medications were to continue, arranged placement of a peripheral or midline before CVAD discontinuation. ___ ___ ___ _____

c. NOTE: Was aware of osmolarity of solution or medication for appropriateness of conversion to peripheral or midline catheter. ___ ___ ___ _____

d. Positioned patient in supine flat or 10-degree Trendelenburg position unless contraindicated. ___ ___ ___ _____

e. Performed hand hygiene, following Surgical ANTT. ___ ___ ___ _____

f. Turned off IV solutions infusing through central line and converted to alternate VAD. ___ ___ ___ _____

g. Placed moisture-proof pad under central line site. ___ ___ ___ _____

h. Applied gown, clean gloves, mask, and goggles. ___ ___ ___ _____

i. Gently removed CVAD dressing by stabilizing catheter with nondominant hand, pulling up one corner, and gently pulling straight out and parallel to skin. Repeated on all sides until dressing had been removed. ___ ___ ___ _____

j. If catheter securement device was present, carefully removed catheter from device and removed device with adhesive remover. ___ ___ ___ _____

k. Removed and disposed of gloves and performed hand hygiene; opened CVAD dressing change kit. Added items to sterile field. Applied sterile gloves. ___ ___ ___ _____

l. Performed skin antisepsis of insertion site with CHG solution, using friction in back-and-forth motion according to manufacturer's guidelines and allowed to dry completely. ___ ___ ___ _____

m. Using nondominant hand, applied sterile 4- × 4–inch gauze to site. Instructed patient to take deep breath and perform Valsalva maneuver as catheter was withdrawn. ___ ___ ___ _____

n. With dominant hand, slowly removed catheter in smooth, continuous motion an inch at a time. Kept fingers near insertion site and immediately applied digital pressure to site and continued until bleeding stopped. Stopped removal procedure if resistance was met while removing catheter. ___ ___ ___ _____

	S	U	NP	Comments

o. Applied gauze to exit site. Applied sterile occlusive dressing to site. Changed dressing every 24 hours until healed. ___ ___ ___ _____

p. Labeled dressing with date, time, and initials. ___ ___ ___ _____

q. Inspected catheter integrity for intactness, especially along tip; checked that length was appropriate for device. Discarded in appropriate biohazard container. ___ ___ ___ _____

r. NOTE: Obtained catheter culture when catheter was removed for suspected catheter-related bloodstream infection (CRBSI), per agency policy. ___ ___ ___ _____

s. Positioned patient in a supine position for 30 minutes after nontunneled CVAD removal. Ensured that peripheral IV line or midline was infusing at correct rate. ___ ___ ___ _____

t. Disposed of all contaminated supplies in appropriate receptacle, removed and disposed of gloves and other PPE. ___ ___ ___ _____

7. Assisted patient to a comfortable position and instructed how to move and turn without dislodging VAD. ___ ___ ___ _____

8. Raised bed rails (as appropriate) and lowered bed to lowest position, locking into position. ___ ___ ___ _____

9. Placed nurse call system was in an accessible location within patient's reach. Instructed patient in its use. ___ ___ ___ _____

10. Performed hand hygiene. ___ ___ ___ _____

EVALUATION

1. Consulted ECG, fluoroscopy, x-ray film, or ultrasound reports for catheter placement. ___ ___ ___ _____

2. Determined daily, in consultation with health care provider, the continued need for the CVAD. ___ ___ ___ _____

3. Evaluated for postinsertion complications: ___ ___ ___ _____

a. Auscultated breath sounds and evaluated for shortness of breath, chest pain, and absent breath sounds. ___ ___ ___ _____

b. Monitored vital signs, including heart rate and rhythm. ___ ___ ___ _____

c. Monitored patient complaints of pain, numbness, tingling, or weakness. ___ ___ ___ _____

4. Evaluated patient to determine response to infusion therapy. ___ ___ ___ _____

514

	S	U	NP	Comments

5. Evaluated patient at established intervals for signs and symptoms of CVAD-related complications according to agency policy and procedure.

      —— —— —— ————————

6. Observed all connection points, ensuring that they were secure as directed by agency policy and procedure.

      —— —— —— ————————

7. Used Teach-Back. Revised instruction if patient or family caregiver was not able to teach back correctly.

      —— —— —— ————————

DOCUMENTATION

1. Documented catheter site insertion/care, including catheter location; size of catheter; number of lumens; condition of catheter insertion site or port site; skin integrity; external catheter length; mid-arm circumference for PICC; condition and type of securement device; date and time of dressing change; change of injection caps; patency of catheter, including presence or absence of blood return or resistance; and patient's tolerance of the procedure.

      —— —— —— ————————

2. Documented catheter flushes to include solution, volume, and concentration.

      —— —— —— ————————

3. Documented catheter removal: patient position, appearance of site, length of catheter removed, integrity of catheter after removal, dressing applied, patient's tolerance of procedure, presence/absence of bleeding from site, and any problems with removal.

      —— —— —— ————————

4. Documented blood draw: date, time, sample drawn and tests ordered, waste volume, and flushes used.

      —— —— —— ————————

5. Documented unexpected outcomes and CVAD complications, interventions, and patient response to treatment.

      —— —— —— ————————

6. Documented patient's and family caregiver's ability to explain instructions.

      —— —— —— ————————

HAND-OFF REPORTING

1. Reported placement of CVAD with reason for insertion, signs or symptoms of observed or patient-reported IV-related complications, status of VAD, and patient condition.

      —— —— —— ————————

2. Reported to health care provider any CVAD-related complications, interventions, and response to treatment.

      —— —— —— ————————

PERFORMANCE CHECKLIST SKILL 29.1 **INITIATING BLOOD THERAPY**

	S	U	NP	Comments

ASSESSMENT

1. Identified patient using at least two identifiers according to agency policy. Compared identifiers with information on patient's medical administration record (MAR) or electronic health record (EHR).

2. Verified health care provider's orders for specific blood or blood product with appropriate date, time to begin transfusion, special instructions, duration, and any pretransfusion or posttransfusion medications to administer.

3. Verified that any pretransfusion laboratory studies were completed and documented in patient's EHR. Reviewed current laboratory values: hematocrit (Hct), coagulation studies, platelet count, and potassium (K).

4. Obtained patient's transfusion history and noted known allergies and previous transfusion reactions. Verified that type and crossmatch had been completed within 72 hours of transfusion.

5. Assessed patient's/family caregiver's health literacy.

6. Performed hand hygiene and applied clean gloves. Verified that intravenous (IV) cannula was patent and without complications such as infiltration or phlebitis.

   • Assessed the vascular access device (VAD) catheter-skin junction site and surrounding area for catheter-related complications by visually inspecting and palpating through the intact dressing for redness, tenderness, swelling, and drainage.

   • Assessed the patency of the VAD by aspiration of a blood return, absence of resistance when flushing, and complaints of patient pain or discomfort when flushing.

   • If necessary, placed a VAD for transfusion purposes:

	S	U	NP	Comments

a. Administered blood or blood components to an adult through short peripheral catheter (18- to 20-gauge catheter for general population).

b. Transfused an adult patient using proper gauge catheter:
Adults: Used a 20- to 24-gauge device. For rapid transfusion, used an 18- to 20-gauge device.
Infants/children: Used umbilical vein for neonates; 22- to 24-gauge device for other children.

c. Used appropriate gauge central vascular access device (CVAD), if indicated.

7. Removed and disposed of gloves. Performed hand hygiene.

8. Checked that patient had completed and signed transfusion consent form properly before retrieving blood. Determined if patient had questions.

9. Reviewed EHR to confirm indications or reasons for transfusion.

10. Obtained and documented pretransfusion baseline vital signs within 30 minutes prior to transfusion. If patient was febrile (temperature greater than 37.8°C [100°F]), notified health care provider before initiating transfusion.

11. Assessed patient's need for IV fluids or medications to be given while transfusion was infusing. Administered blood or blood components only with 0.9% sodium chloride (NS).

12. Assessed patient's knowledge, prior experience with a blood transfusion, and feelings about procedure. Allowed patient to express religious/cultural beliefs about transfusion.

PLANNING

1. Determined expected outcomes following completion of procedure.

2. Closed room doors and prepared environment.

3. Asked patient to void. If patient was unable to void, applied clean gloves and emptied urine drainage collection container.

4. Performed hand hygiene. Collected and then organized equipment on clean, clutter-free bedside stand or overbed table.

	S	U	NP	Comments

5. Explained procedure to patient and family caregiver. Reviewed compatibility testing and vascular access. Explained signs and symptoms associated with complications of transfusion. ___ ___ ___ _____

IMPLEMENTATION

1. Preadministration protocol:

a. Obtained blood component from blood bank, following agency protocol. ___ ___ ___ _____

b. Observed and checked blood bag for any signs of contamination at the time it was released from blood bank. Did not use if container was not intact or if abnormal color, clots, excessive air/bubbles, or unusual odor was present. ___ ___ ___ _____

c. At bedside, identified patient using at least two identifiers according to agency policy. Compared identifiers with information on patient's MAR or EHR. ___ ___ ___ _____

d. With another RN at patient's bedside, verified information on blood unit and in EHR: ___ ___ ___ _____

- Checked that transfusion record number and patient's identification number matched. ___ ___ ___ _____

- Checked that patient's name was correct on all documents. ___ ___ ___ _____

- Checked unit number on blood bag with blood bank form to ensure they matched. ___ ___ ___ _____

- Checked blood type matches on transfusion record and blood bag. Verified that component received from blood bank was the same component that health care provider ordered. ___ ___ ___ _____

- Checked that patient's blood type and Rh type were compatible with donor blood type and Rh type. ___ ___ ___ _____

- Checked special transfusion requirements. ___ ___ ___ _____

- Checked expiration date/time on blood unit and date/time released from blood bank. ___ ___ ___ _____

e. Just before initiating transfusion, checked patient identification information one more time with blood unit label information. Ensured patient's name was on the label. Did not administer blood to patient without identification bracelet or blood identification bracelet (per agency policy). Checked one more time that patient's blood type and Rh type were compatible with donor blood type and Rh type. ___ ___ ___ _____

f. Both nurses verified patient and unit identification record process as directed by agency policy. ___ ___ ___ _____

518

g. Reviewed purpose of transfusion and asked patient to report any changes noticed during the transfusion.

    ___ ___ ___ _____

2. Administration:

a. Performed hand hygiene. Applied clean gloves. Reinspected blood product for signs of leakage or unusual appearance.

    ___ ___ ___ _____

b. Opened standard Y-tubing blood administration set with filter for single unit. Used multiset if multiple units were to be transfused.

    ___ ___ ___ _____

c. Set all clamp(s) to "off" position.

    ___ ___ ___ _____

d. Used aseptic technique and spiked 0.9% sodium chloride NS IV bag with one set of Y-tubing spikes. Hung bag on IV pole and primed tubing. Opened upper clamp on NS side of tubing and squeezed drip chamber until fluid covered filter and one-third to one-half of drip chamber.

    ___ ___ ___ _____

e. Maintained clamp on blood product side of Y-tubing in "off" position. Opened common tubing clamp to finish priming tubing to distal end of tubing connector with NS. Closed tubing clamp when tubing was filled with saline. Ensured that all three tubing clamps were closed. Maintained protective sterile cap on tubing connector.

    ___ ___ ___ _____

f. Prepared blood component for administration. Gently inverted bag 2 or 3 times, turning back and forth. Removed protective covering from access port. Spiked blood component unit with other Y-connection. Closed NS clamp above filter, opened clamp above filter to blood unit, and primed tubing with blood. Tapped filter chamber to remove residual air. Closed clamp when tubing was filled. Applied cap to end of tubing.

    ___ ___ ___ _____

g. *Option:* Infused with electronic infusion device (EID). Maintaining asepsis, inserted infusion tubing into chamber of control mechanism of EID. Ensured EID being used was indicated for blood administration (followed manufacturer's directions). Ensured roller clamp on IV tubing was between EID and patient. Secured tubing through "air in line" alarm system. Closed door and turned on power button. Selected required administration rate.

    ___ ___ ___ _____

h. Removed cap and attached primed tubing to patient's VAD by first cleansing the catheter hub with an antiseptic swab. Then connected NS-primed blood administration tubing directly to patient's VAD.

    ___ ___ ___ _____

i. Opened common tubing clamp and the clamp to blood bag. Regulated blood infusion to allow only 2 mL/min to infuse in initial 15 minutes. Remained with patient during first 15 minutes of transfusion. Initial flow rate during this time should be 1–2 mL/min or 10–20 gtt/min (using macrodrip of 10 gtt/mL).

_____ _____ _____ _____

j. Monitored patient's vital signs within 15 minutes of initiating transfusion, upon completion of transfusion, and 1 hour after transfusion completed or more often if patient condition is warranted.

_____ _____ _____ _____

k. Assessed the patient for any adverse reactions at least every 30 minutes during transfusion.

l. If there was no transfusion reaction, regulated rate of transfusion according to health care provider's orders based on drop factor for blood administration tubing.

_____ _____ _____ _____

m. After blood had infused, turned off EID and turned off clamp to blood bag. Removed tubing from EID. Cleared IV line with 0.9% sodium chloride (NS) by opening clamp to NS bag and infusing slowly. Discarded blood bag according to agency policy. If consecutive units were ordered, maintained line patency with 0.9% sodium chloride (NS) at keep vein open (KVO) rate as ordered by health care provider, and then retrieved subsequent unit for administration.

_____ _____ _____ _____

3. Helped patient to comfortable position.

_____ _____ _____ _____

4. Placed nurse call system in an accessible location within patient's reach.

_____ _____ _____ _____

5. Raised side rails (as appropriate) and lowered bed to lowest position, locking into position.

_____ _____ _____ _____

6. Disposed of all contaminated supplies in appropriate receptacle, removed and disposed of gloves, and performed hand hygiene.

_____ _____ _____ _____

EVALUATION

1. Observed IV site and status of infusion each time vital signs were taken.

_____ _____ _____ _____

2. Observed for any signs of transfusion reactions for at least 4 to 6 hours to detect febrile or pulmonary reactions.

_____ _____ _____ _____

3. Observed patient and assessed laboratory values to determine response to administration of blood component.

_____ _____ _____ _____

4. Monitored urine output.

_____ _____ _____ _____

520

	S	U	NP	Comments

5. Used Teach-Back. Revised instruction if patient or family caregiver were not able to teach back correctly. ___ ___ ___ _____

DOCUMENTATION

1. Before transfusion, documented pretransfusion medications, vital signs, location and condition of IV site, and patient/family caregiver education. ___ ___ ___ _____

2. Documented the type and volume of blood component, blood unit/donor/recipient identification, compatibility, and expiration date according to agency policy, along with patient's response to therapy. ___ ___ ___ _____

3. Documented volume of NS and blood component infused. ___ ___ ___ _____

4. Documented amount of blood received by autotransfusion and patient's response to therapy. ___ ___ ___ _____

5. Documented vital signs 15 minutes after iinitiating transfusion, on completion of transfusion and 1 hour after completion. ___ ___ ___ _____

6. Documented evaluation of patient and family caregiver learning. ___ ___ ___ _____

HAND-OFF REPORTING

1. Reported signs and symptoms of a transfusion reaction immediately to the health care provider. ___ ___ ___ _____

2. Reported to health care provider any intratransfusion or posttransfusion deterioration in cardiac, pulmonary, and/or renal status. ___ ___ ___ _____

Student _____ Date _____

Instructor _____ Date _____

PERFORMANCE CHECKLIST SKILL 29.2   **MONITORING FOR ADVERSE TRANSFUSION REACTIONS**

	S	U	NP	Comments

ASSESSMENT

1. Identified patient using at least two identifiers according to agency policy. ___ ___ ___ _____

2. Assessed patient's/family caregiver's health literacy. ___ ___ ___ _____

3. Performed hand hygiene and applied clean gloves (as needed). Monitored vital signs and pulse oximetry continuously every 15 minutes or per agency policy. Specifically noted the following: ___ ___ ___ _____

   a. With initiation of a transfusion, observed patient for fever with or without chills. ___ ___ ___ _____

   b. Assessed patient for tachycardia and/or tachypnea and dyspnea. ___ ___ ___ _____

   c. Assessed patient for drop in blood pressure. ___ ___ ___ _____

   d. Auscultated lungs before and during the procedure and observed patient for wheezing, chest pain, and possible cardiac arrest. ___ ___ ___ _____

4. Observed patient for urticaria or skin rash and itching, including assessment of trunk and back. ___ ___ ___ _____

5. Observed patient for flushing. ___ ___ ___ _____

6. Observed patient for gastrointestinal symptoms. ___ ___ ___ _____

7. Was alert to patient complaints of headache or muscle pain in presence of fever. ___ ___ ___ _____

8. Monitored patient for disseminated intravascular coagulation (DIC), renal failure, anemia, and hemoglobinemia/hemoglobinuria by reviewing laboratory test results. ___ ___ ___ _____

9. Monitored pulse oximetry and central venous pressure (CVP) if possible. ___ ___ ___ _____

10. Observed patient for jaundice and laboratory values for increased liver enzyme levels, indicating liver damage, and for decreased RBCs, white blood cells (WBCs), and platelets, indicating bone marrow suppression. ___ ___ ___ _____

	S	U	NP	Comments

11. In patients receiving massive transfusions, observed for mild hypothermia, cardiac dysrhythmias, hypotension, hypocalcemia, and hemochromatosis (iron overload). ___ ___ ___ _____

12. Ensured that patient understood what was occurring during your response. ___ ___ ___ _____

13. Assessed patient's knowledge of and prior experience with transfusion reaction, and feelings about outcome. ___ ___ ___ _____

PLANNING

1. Determined expected outcomes following completion of procedure. ___ ___ ___ _____

2. Explained need for monitoring to patient. Discussed signs and symptoms of transfusion reaction. ___ ___ ___ _____

3. Closed room door and bedside curtain. Performed hand hygiene. ___ ___ ___ _____

IMPLEMENTATION

1. When a transfusion reaction was suspected:

   a. Immediately stopped transfusion. ___ ___ ___ _____

   b. Removed blood component and tubing containing blood product. Replaced them with new bag of 0.9% sodium chloride (normal saline [NS]) and tubing. Connected tubing directly to hub of VAD. Exception: If patient symptoms suggested mild allergic reaction, stopped transfusion, administered antihistamine, and later restarted or discontinued transfusion per health care provider's order. ___ ___ ___ _____

   c. Maintained patent VAD by opening 0.9% sodium chloride (NS) infusion and regulated at a keep vein open (KVO) rate until you contacted health care provider for order. ___ ___ ___ _____

   d. Notified health care provider. ___ ___ ___ _____

   e. Notified blood bank. ___ ___ ___ _____

   f. Remained with patient for continuous monitoring and assessment. Did not leave patient alone. ___ ___ ___ _____

   g. Obtained blood samples (if needed) from extremity opposite extremity receiving transfusion. Checked agency policy regarding number and type of tubes to be used. ___ ___ ___ _____

   h. Returned remainder of blood component and attached blood tubing to blood bank according to agency policy. ___ ___ ___ _____

	S	U	NP	Comments

i. Administered prescribed medications according to type and severity of transfusion reaction.

j. In event of cardiac arrest, initiated cardiopulmonary resuscitation (CPR).

k. Obtained first voided urine sample following reaction and sent to laboratory. Inserted Foley catheter to obtain urine if indicated.

2. Helped patient to comfortable position.

3. Placed nurse call system in an accessible location within patient's reach.

4. Raised side rails (as appropriate) and lowered bed to lowest position, locking into position.

5. Disposed of all contaminated supplies in appropriate receptacle, removed and disposed of gloves, and performed hand hygiene.

EVALUATION

1. Continued monitoring patient for signs and symptoms of transfusion reactions.

2. Used Teach-Back. Revised instruction if patient or family caregiver was not able to teach back correctly.

DOCUMENTATION

1. Documented the exact time transfusion reaction was first noted, all vital signs and other physiological assessments, treatments instituted, and patient response. Completed transfusion reaction report (per agency policy).

2. Documented evaluation of patient and family caregiver learning.

HAND-OFF REPORTING

1. Immediately reported presence of transfusion reaction and patient's physical assessment findings to nurse in charge and health care provider.

Student _____   Date _____

Instructor _____   Date _____

PERFORMANCE CHECKLIST SKILL 30.1   **PERFORMING A NUTRITION SCREENING**

	S	U	NP	Comments
ASSESSMENT				
1. Identified patient using at least two identifiers, according to agency policy.	___	___	___	_____
2. Assessed patient's/family caregiver's health literacy.	___	___	___	_____
3. Asked patient to report usual body weight (UBW), noting recent changes in weight. Asked if weight loss was intentional or unintentional.	___	___	___	_____
4. Performed hand hygiene. Measured actual body weight (ABW).	___	___	___	_____
a. Had patient void. Ensured that patient was wearing underwear or hospital gown. Weighed patient barefoot or with same shoes. Weighed at same time of day.	___	___	___	_____
b. Made sure that beam scale had been calibrated. If patient was ambulatory, had patient stand as straight as possible, without shoes or a hat. Ensured weight was evenly distributed on both feet with heels together.	___	___	___	_____
c. If patient was unable to stand, used wheelchair or bed scale.	___	___	___	_____
d. Documented weight to nearest 0.1 kg (1/4 lb).	___	___	___	_____
5. Measured actual height.	___	___	___	_____
a. Helped patient to standing position, standing erect with weight equally distributed on both feet and heels together.	___	___	___	_____
b. Instructed patient to let arms hang freely at sides with palms facing thighs.	___	___	___	_____
c. Had patient look straight ahead, take a deep breath, and hold position while nurse brought horizontal bar firmly on top of head. Measured to nearest 0.1 cm (1/8 inch). Ensured that the nurse's eyes were level with bar to read measurement.	___	___	___	_____
6. Knew the formula for calculating ideal body weight (IBW).	___	___	___	_____
a. Calculated via standard height and weight chart.	___	___	___	_____
b. Used the following formulas: Male: 48.1 kg (106 lb) for first 5 ft; add 2.7 kg (6 lb) per additional 2.5 cm (inch). Female: 45.4 kg (100 lb) for first 5 ft; add 2.25 kg (5 lb) per additional 2.5 cm (inch).	___	___	___	_____

	S	U	NP	Comments
7. Calculated body mass index (BMI).	___	___	___	_____
a. Divided ABW in pounds by 2.2.	___	___	___	_____
b. Converted height to inches. Multiplied inches by 2.54.	___	___	___	_____
c. Divided height in centimeters by 100.	___	___	___	_____
d. Divided weight in kilograms by the square of height in meters (m^2).	___	___	___	_____
e. Used optional formula for BMI: weight (lb)/ height (inches)^2 ×703.	___	___	___	_____
8. Assessed patient's knowledge, prior experience with nutrition screening and physical examination, and feelings about procedure.	___	___	___	_____

PLANNING

	S	U	NP	Comments
1. Determined expected outcomes following completion of procedure.	___	___	___	_____
2. Explained to patient and/or family caregiver intent of assessment and how the information will allow the health care team to develop a diet plan.	___	___	___	_____
3. Closed room door and bedside curtain.	___	___	___	_____

IMPLEMENTATION

	S	U	NP	Comments
1. Reviewed information collected from nursing history:	___	___	___	_____
a. Assessed patients dietary history, including current diet, food choices and preferences, appetite, food allergies, and food intolerances. Note: In outpatient setting, had patient bring 7-day food diary report.	___	___	___	_____
b. Assessed for any cultural, social, and religious preferences and/or restrictions in diet.	___	___	___	_____
c. Determined medications and other dietary/herbal supplements that patient was taking. Was aware of common drug-drug and drug-nutrient interactions. Consulted pharmacist.	___	___	___	_____
2. Synthesized information gathered during physical assessment.	___	___	___	_____
3. Reviewed results of relevant laboratory tests. Compared with known standards.	___	___	___	_____
4. During first meal, determined patient's ability to manipulate eating utensils and self-feed.	___	___	___	_____
5. Completed a nutrition screening tool within 24 hours of patient admission, per agency policy.	___	___	___	_____
6. While critically analyzing findings, conducted education sessions with patient and family caregiver about the *Dietary Guidelines for Americans* and healthy food choices. Used MyPlate as a guide. Adapted to patient's food preferences when possible.	___	___	___	_____

	S	U	NP	Comments

7. Provided patient help with feeding based on assessment findings. ___ ___ ___ _____

8. Instituted aspiration precautions if needed. ___ ___ ___ _____

9. Helped patient to a comfortable position. ___ ___ ___ _____

10. Raised side rails (as appropriate) and lowered bed to lowest position, locking into position. ___ ___ ___ _____

11. Placed nurse call system in an accessible location within patient's reach. ___ ___ ___ _____

EVALUATION

1. Reviewed history and physical findings. Noted abnormal findings or areas of concern. ___ ___ ___ _____

2. Compared patient's actual weight for height with IBW. Compared BMI with recommended BMI for height/weight. ___ ___ ___ _____

3. Compared normal laboratory test levels with patient's levels. ___ ___ ___ _____

4. Computed and reviewed score on nutritional screening tool. ___ ___ ___ _____

5. Used Teach-Back. Revised instruction if patient or family caregiver was not able to teach back correctly. ___ ___ ___ _____

RECORDING

1. Documented assessment results. ___ ___ ___ _____

2. Documented evaluation of patient and family caregiver learning. ___ ___ ___ _____

HAND-OFF REPORTING

1. Notified health care provider and RDN of abnormal findings. ___ ___ ___ _____

PERFORMANCE CHECKLIST SKILL 30.2   **ASSISTING AN ADULT PATIENT WITH ORAL NUTRITION**

	S	U	NP	Comments

ASSESSMENT

1. Identified patient using at least two identifiers, according to agency policy.

2. Reviewed electronic health record (EHR) for patient's most recent weight and laboratory values.

3. Reviewed EHR for history of conditions that might have impaired patient's ability to eat normally.

4. Assessed patient's/family caregiver's health literacy.

5. Performed hand hygiene. Assessed presence and condition of teeth. (Applied clean gloves if there was risk of exposure to saliva.) Determined if dentures were poorly fitted. If patient had mouth discomfort, measured pain severity on a pain scale of 0 to 10.

6. Had patient speak and swallow. Watched for laryngeal movement. Asked patient to say "Ah" while using tongue blade and penlight. Checked for midline uvula and symmetrical rise of uvula and soft palate. Used tongue blade to elicit gag reflex.

7. Assessed physical motor skills and strength of grasp.

8. Assessed patient's cognitive status, level of consciousness, and ability to attend to feeding.

9. Assessed patient's visual acuity and peripheral vision.

10. Assessed patient's appetite, recent food and fluid intake, cultural and religious preferences for participating in mealtime, and food likes and dislikes.

11. Assessed for presence of generalized fatigue, pain, or shortness of breath.

12. Asked if patient felt nauseated. Also assessed recent bowel pattern. Auscultated for bowel sounds.

13. Assessed need for toileting, handwashing, and oral care (including dentures) before feeding.

14. Assessed patient's/family caregiver's knowledge, prior experience regarding eating limitations, and need for assistance with nutritional intake.

	S	U	NP	Comments

PLANNING

1. Determined expected outcomes following completion of procedure. ⎯⎯ ⎯⎯ ⎯⎯ ⎯⎯⎯⎯⎯⎯

2. After assessment, allowed patient to rest 30 minutes before mealtime. ⎯⎯ ⎯⎯ ⎯⎯ ⎯⎯⎯⎯⎯⎯

3. Administered ordered analgesic 30 minutes before meal if patient had discomfort. ⎯⎯ ⎯⎯ ⎯⎯ ⎯⎯⎯⎯⎯⎯

4. Explained to patient how the nurse planned to set up and help with meal. Allowed time for questions. ⎯⎯ ⎯⎯ ⎯⎯ ⎯⎯⎯⎯⎯⎯

5. Prepared patient's room for mealtime. ⎯⎯ ⎯⎯ ⎯⎯ ⎯⎯⎯⎯⎯⎯

   a. Performed hand hygiene. Cleared over-bed table and arranged any needed supplies. ⎯⎯ ⎯⎯ ⎯⎯ ⎯⎯⎯⎯⎯⎯

   b. Helped patient with elimination needs and hand hygiene. ⎯⎯ ⎯⎯ ⎯⎯ ⎯⎯⎯⎯⎯⎯

   c. Helped patient to comfortable sitting position in chair or placed bed in high-Fowler position. If patient was unable to sit, turned patient on side with head of bed elevated and chin in downward position. ⎯⎯ ⎯⎯ ⎯⎯ ⎯⎯⎯⎯⎯⎯

IMPLEMENTATION

1. Prepared patient for meal. ⎯⎯ ⎯⎯ ⎯⎯ ⎯⎯⎯⎯⎯⎯

   a. Applied clean gloves and offered oral hygiene. If patient had dentures, removed and rinsed them thoroughly, then reinserted. Removed and disposed of gloves and performed hand hygiene. ⎯⎯ ⎯⎯ ⎯⎯ ⎯⎯⎯⎯⎯⎯

   b. Consulted with health care provider to determine best therapy for patients with oral mucositis. ⎯⎯ ⎯⎯ ⎯⎯ ⎯⎯⎯⎯⎯⎯

   c. Helped patient put on eyeglasses or insert contact lenses if used. ⎯⎯ ⎯⎯ ⎯⎯ ⎯⎯⎯⎯⎯⎯

2. Checked environment for distractions. Reduced noise level from care activities if possible. Option: If patient enjoys music, played a soothing, low-volume selection. ⎯⎯ ⎯⎯ ⎯⎯ ⎯⎯⎯⎯⎯⎯

3. Obtained special assistive devices as needed and instructed on use. ⎯⎯ ⎯⎯ ⎯⎯ ⎯⎯⎯⎯⎯⎯

4. Assessed meal tray for completeness and correct diet. Used this time (and during actual feeding) to instruct patient about diet, rationale for diet, food options, and dysphagia risks. Focused on principles that were easily applied at home. ⎯⎯ ⎯⎯ ⎯⎯ ⎯⎯⎯⎯⎯⎯

5. Began feeding. Asked in which order patient would like to eat the meal. Helped to set up meal tray if patient was unable to do so. ⎯⎯ ⎯⎯ ⎯⎯ ⎯⎯⎯⎯⎯⎯

6. Watched patient successfully swallow first bites of food and drink. If patient was able to eat independently, stopped there. Reinforced positive results. Returned after 15 or 20 minutes or stayed at side for communication and additional teaching. ⎯⎯ ⎯⎯ ⎯⎯ ⎯⎯⎯⎯⎯⎯

	S	U	NP	Comments

7. Helped patient who could not eat independently. ___ ___ ___ _____

   a. Assumed comfortable position. ___ ___ ___ _____

   b. If patient was visually impaired, identified food location on plate as if it were a clock. ___ ___ ___ _____

   c. Asked in which order patient preferred to eat, and cut food into bite-sized pieces. ___ ___ ___ _____

   d. Provided fluids as requested. Discouraged patient from drinking all fluids at beginning of meal. ___ ___ ___ _____

   e. Paced feeding to avoid patient fatigue. Interacted with patient during mealtime. Verbally encouraged self-feeding attempts. ___ ___ ___ _____

   f. Used mealtime as opportunity to communicate with and educate patient about nutrition topics and discharge plan. ___ ___ ___ _____

   g. Fed patient in manner that facilitated chewing and swallowing. Positioned patient's chin down and placed food in stronger side of the mouth. ___ ___ ___ _____

8. Used appropriate feeding techniques for patients with special needs: ___ ___ ___ _____

   a. Older adult: Fed small amounts at a time, observing biting, chewing, ability to manipulate tongue to form bolus of food, swallowing, and fatigue between bites. Ensured that patient had swallowed food. Offered variety of foods and frequent rest periods. If aspiration was suspected, stopped feeding immediately and suctioned airway. ___ ___ ___ _____

   b. Neurologically impaired patient: Fed small amounts at a time and observed ability to chew, manipulate tongue to form bolus, and swallow. Had patient open mouth and checked for food left inside cheeks (pocketing). Gave small amount of thin liquid between bites. ___ ___ ___ _____

   c. Patients with cancer: Checked for food aversions before and during meal. Monitored for fatigue. ___ ___ ___ _____

9. Helped patient with hand hygiene and mouth care after meal was completed. (Applied gloves as needed.) ___ ___ ___ _____

10. Helped patient to comfortable resting position; left head of bed elevated at least 45 degrees for 30 to 60 min after meal. ___ ___ ___ _____

11. Placed nurse call system in an accessible location within patient's reach. ___ ___ ___ _____

12. Raised side rails (as appropriate) and lowered bed to lowest position, locking into position. ___ ___ ___ _____

13. Returned patient's tray to appropriate place, removed and disposed of gloves, and performed hand hygiene. ___ ___ ___ _____

EVALUATION

1. Monitored body weight daily or weekly. ___ ___ ___ _____

	S	U	NP	Comments
2. Monitored laboratory values as indicated.	——	——	——	———————
3. Monitored intake and output (I&O) and completed intake measurement.	——	——	——	———————
4. Observed patient's ability to self-feed, including ability to feed certain items and part or all of meal.	——	——	——	———————
5. Observed patient for choking, coughing, gagging, or food left in mouth during eating.	——	——	——	———————
6. Used Teach-Back. Revised instruction if patient or family caregiver was not able to teach back correctly.	——	——	——	———————

RECORDING

	S	U	NP	Comments
1. Documented the patient's type of diet, amount of feeding assistance needed, tolerance of diet, amount or percentage of the meal eaten, and calorie count (if ordered).	——	——	——	———————
2. If measuring I&O, documented fluid intake.	——	——	——	———————
3. If patient was receiving oral nutritional supplements, documented the amount taken, as well as patient's tolerance and likes and dislikes in EHR or chart.	——	——	——	———————
4. Documented evaluation of patient/family caregiver learning.	——	——	——	———————

HAND-OFF REPORTING

	S	U	NP	Comments
1. Reported any swallowing difficulties, food dislikes or intolerances, or refusal to eat to health care provider and RDN.	——	——	——	———————
2. Reported to registered nurse (RN) on upcoming shift any new approaches needed that would promote patient's ability to eat.	——	——	——	———————

Student _____ Date _____

Instructor _____ Date _____

PERFORMANCE CHECKLIST SKILL 30.3 **ASPIRATION PRECAUTIONS**

	S	U	NP	Comments

ASSESSMENT

1. Identified patient using at least two identifiers, according to agency policy.

2. Reviewed patient's medical history, nutritional risks, and results of nutrition screening in electronic health record (EHR). Assessed for presence of conditions that cause dysphagia. Noted patient's weight.

3. Assessed patient's current medications for use of sedatives, hypnotics, or other agents that may impair cough or swallowing reflex, and for any medications that dry oral secretions.

4. Assessed patient's/family caregiver's health literacy.

5. Performed hand hygiene. Assessed patient for signs and symptoms of dysphagia. Used a screening tool if recommended by agency.

6. Assessed patient's mental status.

7. Applied gloves. Assessed patient's oral cavity, level of dental hygiene, missing teeth, or poorly fitting dentures. Removed and disposed of gloves and performed hand hygiene.

8. Option: Obtained baseline assessment oxygen saturation. Performed hand hygiene.

9. Indicated in patient's health record that dysphagia/aspiration risks were present. Note: some agencies use different-colored food trays to signify patient at risk for aspiration.

10. Assessed patient's/family caregiver's knowledge of and experience with dysphagia risk and diet options.

PLANNING

1. Determined expected outcomes following completion of procedure.

2. Provided patient 30 minutes of rest.

3. Explained to patient the purpose of mealtime observation.

	S	U	NP	Comments

4. Explained to patient and family caregiver about aspiration precautions and specifically what the nurse was going to do and why.

5. Closed room door and bedside curtain.

6. Obtained and organized equipment for aspiration precautions at bedside.

IMPLEMENTATION

1. Performed hand hygiene and had patient or family caregiver (if going to help with feeding) perform hand hygiene.

2. Applied clean gloves. Provided thorough oral hygiene, including brushing tongue, before meal.

3. Positioned patient upright (90 degrees) in chair or elevated head of patient's bed to a 90-degree angle or highest position allowed by medical condition.

4. Option: If not previously applied, placed pulse oximeter on patient's finger; monitored during feeding.

5. Using penlight and tongue blade, gently inspected mouth for pockets of food.

6. Provided appropriate thickness of liquids per SLP and type of liquids per RDN. Encouraged patient to feed self.

7. Had patient assume chin-down position. Reminded patient to not tilt head backward when eating or while drinking. Option: Had patient assume head-turn-plus-chin-down position.

8. Adjusted the rate of feeding and size of bites to match the patient's tolerance. If patient was unable to feed self, placed 1/2 to 1 teaspoon of food in unaffected side of mouth, allowing utensil to touch mouth or tongue.

9. Observed patient during eating for signs of dysphagia. Observed patient attempt to feed self; noted type of food consistencies and liquids able to swallow. Noted during and at end of meal if patient tired.

10. Provided verbal coaching: Reminded patient to chew and think about swallowing.

11. Avoided mixing food of different textures in same mouthful. Alternated liquids and bites of food. Referred to SLP for next meal if patient had difficulty with a particular consistency.

12. During the meal, explained to patient and family caregiver the techniques being used to promote swallowing. Allowed family caregiver to coach patient.

   ___ ___ ___ _____

13. Monitored swallowing and observed for any respiratory difficulty. Suctioned airway as needed.

   ___ ___ ___ _____

14. Minimized distractions, did not talk (except for explanations being provided), and did not rush patient. Allowed time for adequate chewing and swallowing. Provided rest periods as needed during meal.

   ___ ___ ___ _____

15. Used sauces, condiments, and gravies (if part of dysphagia diet) to facilitate cohesive food bolus formation.

   ___ ___ ___ _____

16. Asked patient to remain sitting upright for at least 30 to 60 minutes after a meal. Provided access to nurse call system to patient and instructed patient to use if needed.

   ___ ___ ___ _____

17. Applied clean gloves. Provided thorough oral hygiene after meal.

   ___ ___ ___ _____

18. Ensured that patient was comfortable in upright position.

   ___ ___ ___ _____

19. Placed nurse call system in an accessible location within patient's reach.

   ___ ___ ___ _____

20. Returned patient's tray to appropriate place. Removed and disposed of gloves, if worn.

   ___ ___ ___ _____

21. Raised side rails (as appropriate) and lowered bed to lowest position, locking into position. Performed hand hygiene.

   ___ ___ ___ _____

EVALUATION

1. Observed patient's ability to swallow food and fluids of various textures and thickness without choking.

   ___ ___ ___ _____

2. Monitored pulse oximetry readings (if ordered) for high-risk patients during eating.

   ___ ___ ___ _____

3. Monitored patient's intake and output (I&O), calorie count, and food intake.

   ___ ___ ___ _____

4. Weighed patient daily or weekly.

   ___ ___ ___ _____

5. Observed patient's oral cavity after meal.

   ___ ___ ___ _____

6. Used Teach-Back. Revised instruction if patient or family caregiver was not able to teach back correctly.

   ___ ___ ___ _____

	S	U	NP	Comments

RECORDING

1. Documented positioning for eating, assessment findings, type of patient's diet, tolerance of liquids and food textures, amount of assistance required, response to instruction, absence or presence of any symptoms of dysphagia, fluid intake, and amount of food eaten. ___ ___ ___ _____

2. Documented evaluation of patient/family caregiver learning. ___ ___ ___ _____

HAND-OFF REPORTING

1. Described patient's tolerance to diet and degree of assistance required during hand-off reporting. ___ ___ ___ _____

2. Reported any coughing, gagging, choking, or other swallowing difficulties to health care provider. ___ ___ ___ _____

PERFORMANCE CHECKLIST SKILL 31.1   **INSERTION AND REMOVAL OF A SMALL-BORE FEEDING TUBE**

	S	U	NP	Comments

ASSESSMENT

1. Identified patient using at least two identifiers, according to agency policy.

2. Verified health care provider's orders for type of tube and enteric feeding schedule. Also checked order to determine if health care provider wanted prokinetic agent given before tube placement.

3. Reviewed patient's electronic health record (EHR) medical history.

4. Reviewed EHR to determine patient's risk for developing a MARSI with use of adhesive devices or tape.

5. Assessed patient's height, weight, hydration status, electrolyte balance, caloric needs, and intake and output (I&O).

6. Asked patient to describe history of allergies; known type of allergies and normal allergic reaction. Focused on foods and adhesives. Checked patient's allergy wristband.

7. Performed hand hygiene. Had patient close each nostril alternately and breathe. Examined each naris for patency and skin breakdown (applied clean gloves if drainage present).

8. Assessed patient's/family caregiver's health literacy.

9. Assessed patient's mental status (ability to cooperate with procedure, sedation), presence of cough and gag reflex, ability to swallow, critical illness, and presence of artificial airway.

10. Performed physical assessment of abdomen. Removed and disposed of gloves (if worn). Performed hand hygiene.

11. Assessed patient's knowledge of and prior experience with small-bore feeding tube insertion, and feelings about procedure.

PLANNING

1. Determined expected outcomes following completion of procedure.

	S	U	NP	Comments

2. Explained procedure to patient, including sensations that would be felt during insertion.

    —— —— —— ————————————

3. Provided privacy and explained to patient how to communicate during intubation by raising index finger to indicate gagging or discomfort.

    —— —— —— ————————————

4. Organized and set up equipment for small-bore feeding tube insertion at bedside.

    —— —— —— ————————————

IMPLEMENTATION

1. Performed hand hygiene. Stood on same side of bed as naris chosen for insertion and positioned patient upright in high-Fowler position (unless contraindicated). If patient was comatose, raised head of bed as tolerated in semi-Fowler position with head tipped forward, using a pillow chin to chest. If necessary, had the AP help with positioning of confused or comatose patients. If patient was forced to lie supine, placed in reverse Trendelenburg position.

    —— —— —— ————————————

2. Applied pulse oximeter/capnograph and measured vital signs. Maintained oximetry or capnography continuously.

    —— —— —— ————————————

3. Placed bath towel over patient's chest. Kept facial tissues within reach.

    —— —— —— ————————————

4. Determined length of tube to be inserted and marked location with tape or indelible ink.

    —— —— —— ————————————

    a. Option, adult: Measured distance from tip of nose to earlobe to xiphoid process (NEX) of sternum. Marked this distance on tube with tape.

    —— —— —— ————————————

    b. Option, adult: Measured distance from tip of nose to earlobe to mid-umbilicus (NEMU) to estimate appropriate NG tube placement.

    —— —— —— ————————————

    c. Option, adult: Measured distance from xiphoid process to earlobe to nose (XEN), + 4 inches (10 cm).

    —— —— —— ————————————

    d. Option, child: Used the NEMU option.

    —— —— —— ————————————

    e. Added 8 to 12 inches (20-30 cm) for postpyloric tubes.

    —— —— —— ————————————

5. Prepared tube for intubation. Did not ice tubes.

    —— —— —— ————————————

    a. Obtained order for stylet tube and checked agency policy for trained clinician to insert tube.

    —— —— —— ————————————

    b. If tube had guidewire or stylet, injected 10 mL of water from ENFit syringe into tube

    —— —— —— ————————————

    c. If using stylet, made certain that it was positioned securely within tube. Injected 10 mL of water from ENFit syringe into tube.

    —— —— —— ————————————

	S	U	NP	Comments

6. Prepared tube fixation materials. Cut hypoallergenic tape 4 inches (10 cm) long or prepared membrane dressing or other tube fixation device. ___ ___ ___ _____

7. Performed hand hygiene and applied clean gloves. ___ ___ ___ _____

8. Option: Dipped tube with surface lubricant into glass of room-temperature water or applied water-soluble lubricant, per manufacturer's directions. ___ ___ ___ _____

9. Offered alert patient a cup of water with straw (if able to safely swallow). ___ ___ ___ _____

10. Explained next steps and gently inserted tube through nostril to back of throat (posterior nasopharynx). Aimed back and down toward ear. ___ ___ ___ _____

11. Had patient take deep breath, relax, and flex head toward chest after tube had passed through nasopharynx. ___ ___ ___ _____

12. Encouraged patient to swallow small sips of water. Advanced tube as patient swallowed. Rotated tube gently 180 degrees while inserting. ___ ___ ___ _____

13. Emphasized need to mouth breathe and swallow during insertion. ___ ___ ___ _____

14. Did not advance tube during inspiration or coughing. Monitored oximetry and capnography at that time. ___ ___ ___ _____

15. Advanced tube each time patient swallowed until desired length was reached. ___ ___ ___ _____

16. Checked for position of tube in back of throat using penlight and tongue blade. ___ ___ ___ _____

17. Temporarily anchored tube to nose with small piece of tape. ___ ___ ___ _____

18. Kept tube secure and checked its placement by aspirating stomach contents to measure gastric pH. Also measured amount, color, and quality of return. ___ ___ ___ _____

19. Anchored tube to patient's nose, avoiding pressure on nares. Marked exit site on tube with indelible ink. Made sure skin over nose was clean and dry. Applied liquid barrier spray or wipe on bridge of patient's nose and allowed it to dry completely. Selected one of the following options for anchoring: ___ ___ ___ _____

   a. Applied membrane dressing or tube fixation device: ___ ___ ___ _____

     (1) Membrane dressing: ___ ___ ___ _____

       (a) Applied tincture of benzoin or other skin protector to patient's cheek and area of tube to be secured. ___ ___ ___ _____

	S	U	NP	Comments

(b) Placed tube against patient's cheek and secured tube with membrane dressing, out of patient's line of vision. ___ ___ ___ _____

(2) Tube fixation device: ___ ___ ___ _____

(a) Applied wide end of patch to bridge of nose. ___ ___ ___ _____

(b) Slipped connector around feeding tube as it exited nose. ___ ___ ___ _____

b. Applied tape: ___ ___ ___ _____

(1) Applied tincture of benzoin or other skin adhesive on tip of patient's nose and allowed it to become "tacky." ___ ___ ___ _____

(2) Removed gloves and tore two horizontal slits on each side of tape at one-third and two-thirds length. Did not split tape. Folded middle sections forward. ___ ___ ___ _____

(3) Tore vertical strip at bottom of tape. Printed date and time on nasal part of tape. ___ ___ ___ _____

(4) Placed intact end of tape over bridge of patient's nose. Wrapped each strip around tube as it exited. ___ ___ ___ _____

20. Fastened end of tube to patient's gown using clip or piece of tape. Did not use safety pins to secure tube to gown. ___ ___ ___ _____

21. Helped patient to comfortable position but kept head of the bed elevated at least 30 degrees (preferably 45 degrees) unless contraindicated. For intestinal tube placement, placed patient on right side when possible until radiographic confirmation of correct placement was made. ___ ___ ___ _____

22. Removed and disposed of gloves and performed hand hygiene. ___ ___ ___ _____

23. Contacted radiology department to obtain x-ray film of chest/abdomen. ___ ___ ___ _____

24. Performed hand hygiene and applied clean gloves. Administered oral hygiene. Cleaned tubing at nostril with washcloth dampened in mild soap and water. ___ ___ ___ _____

25. Placed nurse call system in an accessible location within patient's reach. ___ ___ ___ _____

26. Raised side rails (as appropriate) and lowered bed to lowest position, locking into position. ___ ___ ___ _____

27. Disposed of all contaminated supplies in appropriate receptacle, removed and disposed of gloves, and performed hand hygiene. ___ ___ ___ _____

	S	U	NP	Comments
28. Tube removal:	___	___	___	_____
a. Verified health care provider's order for tube removal.	___	___	___	_____
b. Gathered equipment.	___	___	___	_____
c. Provided privacy and explained procedure to patient and that patient would be instructed to take a deep breath and hold it.	___	___	___	_____
d. Performed hand hygiene. Applied clean gloves.	___	___	___	_____
e. Positioned patient in high-Fowler position unless contraindicated.	___	___	___	_____
f. Placed disposable pad or towel over patient's chest.	___	___	___	_____
g. Disconnected tube from feeding administration set (if present) and clamped or capped end.	___	___	___	_____
h. Removed tape or tube fixation device from patient's nose. Unclipped tube from patient's gown.	___	___	___	_____
i. Instructed patient to take deep breath and hold it. Then, as you kinked end of tube securely (folding it over on itself), completely withdrew it by pulling it out steadily and smoothly onto towel or disposable bag. Disposed of it into appropriate receptacle.	___	___	___	_____
j. Offered tissues to patient to blow nose.	___	___	___	_____
k. Provided oral hygiene.	___	___	___	_____
l. Helped patient to a comfortable position.	___	___	___	_____
m. Placed nurse call system in an accessible location within the patient's reach.	___	___	___	_____
n. Raised side rails (as appropriate) and lowered bed to lowest position, locking into position.	___	___	___	_____
o. Disposed of all contaminated supplies in appropriate receptacle, removed and disposed of gloves, and performed hand hygiene.	___	___	___	_____

EVALUATION

	S	U	NP	Comments
1. Observed patient's response to tube placement. Assessed lung sounds; had patient speak; checked vital signs; and noted any coughing, dyspnea, cyanosis, or decrease in oxygen saturation or increase in end-tidal CO_2.	___	___	___	_____
2. Confirmed radiographic film results with health care provider.	___	___	___	_____

	S	U	NP	Comments

3. Removed stylet after radiographic film verification of correct placement. Reviewed agency policy regarding requirement of trained clinician for insertion. ___ ___ ___ _____

4. Routinely observed condition of nares, location of external exit site marking on tube, and color and pH of fluid aspirated from tube. ___ ___ ___ _____

5. After removal, assessed patient's level of comfort. ___ ___ ___ _____

6. Used Teach-Back technique. Revised instruction if patient or family caregiver was not able to teach back correctly. ___ ___ ___ _____

DOCUMENTATION

1. Documented type and size of tube placed, location of distal tip of tube, patient's tolerance of procedure, condition of naris, and confirmation of tube position by radiographic film examination. ___ ___ ___ _____

2. Documented removal of tube, condition of naris, and patient's tolerance. ___ ___ ___ _____

3. Documented evaluation of patient learning.

HAND-OFF REPORTING

1. Reported any type of unexpected outcome and the interventions performed to the health care provider. ___ ___ ___ _____

2. During hand-off, reported tube placement, when confirmation of placement was received, and condition of nares. ___ ___ ___ _____

Student _____ Date _____

Instructor _____ Date _____

PERFORMANCE CHECKLIST SKILL 31.2 **VERIFYING PLACEMENT OF A FEEDING TUBE**

	S	U	NP	Comments

ASSESSMENT

1. Identified patient using at least two identifiers, according to agency policy.

2. Reviewed agency policy and procedures for frequency and method of checking tube placement. Did not insufflate air into tube to check placement.

3. Reviewed patient's medication record for orders for enteral feeding, a gastric acid inhibitor, or a proton pump inhibitor.

4. Reviewed patient's electronic health record (EHR) for history of prior tube displacement.

5. Identified conditions that increase risk for spontaneous tube migration or dislocation: altered level of consciousness, agitation, retching, vomiting, nasotracheal suction.

6. Observed for signs and symptoms of respiratory distress during feeding: coughing, choking, or reduced oxygen saturation.

7. Performed hand hygiene. Assessed bowel sounds and abdomen.

8. Observed external part of tube for movement of ink or tape mark away from mouth or naris.

9. Obtained baseline pulse oximetry reading.

10. Assessed patient's/family caregiver's health literacy.

11. Assessed patient's knowledge of and prior experience with tube placement, and feelings about procedure.

PLANNING

1. Determined expected outcomes following completion of procedure.

2. Explained procedure to patient. Discussed need for procedure prior to tube feeding. If applicable, taught patient or family caregiver how to check tube placement.

3. Closed room door and bedside curtain.

542

	S	U	NP	Comments

4. Obtained and organized equipment for tube feeding at bedside.

IMPLEMENTATION

1. Performed hand hygiene and applied clean gloves. Ensured that pulse oximeter was in place.

2. Verified tube placement at the following times:

   a. For intermittent tube feedings, tested placement immediately before each feeding (usually a period of at least 4 hours would have elapsed since previous feeding) and before medications.

   b. For continuous tube feedings, followed agency policy to test placement of the tube.

   c. Waited to verify placement at least 1 hour after medication administration by tube or mouth.

3. To assess the gastric or small-bore feeding tube when tube feeding was infusing, first turned off or placed tube feeding on hold. Then clamped or kinked feeding tube and disconnected from end of infusion bag tubing. For intermittent feedings, removed plug at end of feeding tube.

4. Drew up 30 mL of air into a 60-mL ENFit syringe. Placed tip of syringe into end of gastric or small-bore tube and flushed with air before attempting to aspirate fluid.

5. Drew back on syringe slowly and obtained 5 to 10 mL of gastric aspirate. Observed appearance of aspirate.

6. Gently mixed aspirate in syringe. Expelled a few drops into clean medicine cup. Noted color of aspirate. Measured pH of aspirated GI contents by dipping pH strip into fluid or applying a few drops of fluid to strip. Compared color of strip with color on chart provided by manufacturer.

7. If after repeated attempts it was not possible to aspirate fluid from tube that was confirmed by x-ray film to be in desired position and if (1) there were no risk factors for tube dislocation, (2) tube had remained in original taped position, and (3) patient was not in respiratory distress, assumed that tube was correctly placed. Continued with irrigation.

8. Irrigated tube.

9. Helped patient to comfortable position.

	S	U	NP	Comments

10. Placed nurse call system in an accessible location within patient's reach. ___ ___ ___ _____

11. Raised side rails (as appropriate) and lowered bed to lowest position, locking into position. ___ ___ ___ _____

12. Disposed of all contaminated supplies in appropriate receptacle, removed and disposed of gloves, and performed hand hygiene. ___ ___ ___ _____

EVALUATION

1. Observed patient for respiratory distress: persistent gagging, paroxysms of coughing, drop in oxygen (O_2) saturation, or respiratory patterns that were inconsistent with baseline measures. ___ ___ ___ _____

2. Verified that external length of tube, pH, and appearance of aspirate was consistent with initial tube placement. ___ ___ ___ _____

3. Used Teach-Back technique. Revised instruction if patient or family caregiver was not able to teach back correctly. ___ ___ ___ _____

DOCUMENTATION

1. Documented pH, appearance of aspirate, and any irrigation. ___ ___ ___ _____

2. Documented evaluation of patient and family caregiver learning. ___ ___ ___ _____

HAND-OFF REPORTING

1. Reported to health care provider if tubing was clogged or there were indications of tube displacement. ___ ___ ___ _____

2. During hand-off report, noted most current gastric pH and status of feeding. ___ ___ ___ _____

PERFORMANCE CHECKLIST SKILL 31.3 **IRRIGATING A FEEDING TUBE**

	S	U	NP	Comments
ASSESSMENT				
1. Identified patient using at least two identifiers, according to agency policy.	___	___	___	_____
2. Performed hand hygiene and applied clean gloves. Inspected volume, color, and character of previous gastric aspirates (if obtainable).	___	___	___	_____
3. Auscultated for bowel sounds.	___	___	___	_____
4. Noted ease with which tube feeding infused through tubing.	___	___	___	_____
5. Monitored volume of continuous enteral formula administered during shift and compared with ordered amount.	___	___	___	_____
6. Referred to agency policies regarding routine irrigation or health care provider's order.	___	___	___	_____
7. Assessed patient's/family caregiver's health literacy.	___	___	___	_____
8. Assessed patient's knowledge of and prior experience with feeding tube irrigation, and feelings about procedure.	___	___	___	_____
PLANNING				
1. Determined expected outcomes following completion of procedure.	___	___	___	_____
2. Explained procedure to patient. Discussed need for and procedure related to feeding tube irrigation. If applicable, taught patient or family caregiver how to perform feeding tube irrigation.	___	___	___	_____
3. Provided privacy and explained procedure to patient.	___	___	___	_____
4. Obtained and organized equipment for feeding tube irrigation at bedside.	___	___	___	_____
5. Positioned patient in high-Fowler (if tolerated) or semi-Fowler position.	___	___	___	_____
IMPLEMENTATION				
1. Performed hand hygiene and applied clean gloves.	___	___	___	_____
2. Verified tube placement if fluid could be aspirated for pH testing.	___	___	___	_____

	S	U	NP	Comments

3. Irrigated routinely before, between, and after final medication (before feedings were reinstituted), as well as before an intermittent feeding was administered.

   ___ ___ ___ _____

4. Drew up 30 mL of water in ENFit syringe. Did not use irrigation fluids from bottles that had been used on other patients. Ensured patient had individual bottle of solution.

   ___ ___ ___ _____

5. Changed irrigation bottle every 24 hours. Ensured that syringe in tray had ENFit adaptor.

   ___ ___ ___ _____

6. Stopped continuous feeding or intermittent feeding. Kinked feeding tube while disconnecting it from administration tubing or while removing plug at end of tube.

   ___ ___ ___ _____

7. Inserted tip of ENFit syringe into end of feeding tube. Released kink and slowly instilled irrigation solution.

   ___ ___ ___ _____

8. If unable to instill fluid, repositioned patient on left side and tried again.

   ___ ___ ___ _____

9. When water had been instilled, removed syringe. Reinstituted tube feeding or administered medication as ordered. Flushed each medication completely through tube.

   ___ ___ ___ _____

10. Helped patient to comfortable position.

   ___ ___ ___ _____

11. Placed nurse call system in an accessible location within patient's reach.

   ___ ___ ___ _____

12. Raised side rails (as appropriate) and lowered bed to lowest position, locking into position.

   ___ ___ ___ _____

13. Disposed of all contaminated supplies in appropriate receptacle, removed and disposed of gloves, and performed hand hygiene.

   ___ ___ ___ _____

EVALUATION

1. Observed ease with which tube feeding instilled through tubing.

   ___ ___ ___ _____

2. Used Teach-Back technique. Revised instruction if patient or family caregiver was not able to teach back correctly.

   ___ ___ ___ _____

DOCUMENTATION

1. Documented time of irrigation and amount, and type of fluid instilled.

   ___ ___ ___ _____

2. Documented evaluation of patient and family caregiver learning.

   ___ ___ ___ _____

HAND-OFF REPORTING

1. Reported to health care provider if tubing had become clogged.

   ___ ___ ___ _____

PERFORMANCE CHECKLIST SKILL 31.4 **ADMINISTERING ENTERAL NUTRITION**

	S	U	NP	Comments

ASSESSMENT

1. Identified patient using at least two identifiers, according to agency policy.

2. Verified health care provider's order for type of formula, rate, route, and frequency.

3. Assessed patient's/family caregiver's health literacy.

4. Assessed patient for food allergies. If allergy present, applied allergy wristband.

5. Assessed patient for aspiration risk factors.

6. Performed hand hygiene. Performed physical assessment of abdomen, including auscultation for bowel sounds, before feeding.

7. Obtained baseline weight and reviewed serum electrolytes and blood glucose measurement. Assessed patient for fluid volume excess or deficit, electrolyte abnormalities, and metabolic abnormalities.

8. Collaborated with RDN to determine patient's caloric and protein requirements. Then set goal for delivery of EN.

9. Assessed patient's knowledge of and prior experience with enteral feedings, and feelings about procedure.

PLANNING

1. Determined expected outcomes following completion of procedure.

2. Provided privacy and explained procedure to patient. Discussed need for and procedure related to EN. If applicable, taught patient or family caregiver how to perform enteral feeding.

3. Obtained and organized equipment for enteral feeding at bedside.

IMPLEMENTATION

1. Performed hand hygiene. Applied clean gloves.

	S	U	NP	Comments

2. Reverified correct formula and checked expiration date; noted integrity of container and appearance of formula.

    ___ ___ ___   _____

3. Prepared formula for administration, following manufacturer guidelines.

    ___ ___ ___   _____

   a. Had formula at room temperature.

    ___ ___ ___   _____

   b. Used aseptic technique to connect tubing to container as needed. Used proper ENFit connecter and avoided handling feeding system or touching can tops, container openings, spike, and spike port.

    ___ ___ ___   _____

   c. Shook formula container well. Cleaned top of canned formula with alcohol swab before opening it.

    ___ ___ ___   _____

   d. Connected administration tubing to formula bag. If using open system, poured formula from brick pack or can into administration bag.

    ___ ___ ___   _____

4. Opened roller clamp and allowed administration tubing to fill. Clamped off tubing with roller clamp. Hung container on intravenous (IV) pole.

    ___ ___ ___   _____

5. Kept patient in high-Fowler position or elevated head of bed at least 30 degrees (45 degrees is recommended). For patient forced to remain supine, placed in reverse Trendelenburg.

    ___ ___ ___   _____

6. Verified tube placement using EnFit 60 mL syringe. Observed appearance of aspirate and noted pH. When checking a jejunostomy tube, checked pH if significant amounts were returned that resemble gastric secretions.

    ___ ___ ___   _____

7. Checked gastric residual volume (GRV) per agency policy. Because routine use is no longer recommended, did not use GRV as a single measure of tolerance.

    ___ ___ ___   _____

   a. Drew up 10 to 30 mL of air into ENFit syringe and connected to end of feeding tube. Injected air slowly into tube. Pulled back slowly and aspirated total amount of gastric contents that could be aspirated.

    ___ ___ ___   _____

   b. Returned aspirated contents to stomach slowly. Referred to agency policy for any cutoff to hold aspirated contents.

    ___ ___ ___   _____

   c. GRVs in range of 200 to 500 mL raised concern and lead to implementation of measures to reduce risk of aspiration. Automatic cessation of feeding did not occur for GRV less than 500 mL in absence of other signs of intolerance.

    ___ ___ ___   _____

	S	U	NP	Comments

d. Flushed feeding tube with 30 mL water.

8. Intermittent feeding (administered at certain times during the day):

   a. Pinched proximal end of feeding tube and removed cap. Attached distal end of administration set tubing to ENFit connection system on feeding tube and released tubing.

   b. Set rate by adjusting roller clamp on tubing or attached tubing to feeding pump. Allowed bag to empty gradually over 30 to 45 minutes (length of time of a comfortable meal). Labeled bag with patient identifiers, formula type, enteral delivery site (route and access), administration method and volume and frequency of water flushes. Also included label with date, time, and initials when hanging a feeding.

   c. Immediately followed feeding with prescribed amount of water (per health care provider's orders or agency policy). Covered end of feeding tube with cap when not in use. Kept bag as clean as possible. Changed administration set every 24 hours.

9. Continuous infusion method:

   a. Removed cap on tubing and connected distal end of administration set tubing to feeding tube using ENFit connector as in Step 8a.

   b. Threaded tubing through feeding pump; set rate on pump and turned on.

   c. Advanced rate of tube feeding (and concentration of feeding) gradually, as ordered.

10. After feeding, flushed tubing with 30 mL water every 4 hours during continuous feeding (per agency policy) or before and after an intermittent feeding. Had RDN recommend total free-water requirement per day and obtained health care provider's orders.

11. Rinsed bag and tubing with warm water whenever feedings were interrupted. Used new administration set every 24 hours.

12. Helped patient to assume and remain in comfortable position with head of bed elevated 30 to 45 degrees.

13. Placed nurse call system in an accessible location within patient's reach.

14. Raised side rails (as appropriate) and lowered bed to lowest position, locking into position.

	S	U	NP	Comments

15. Disposed of all contaminated supplies in appropriate receptacle, removed and disposed of gloves, and performed hand hygiene.

_____ _____ _____ _____

EVALUATION

1. Monitored patient's tolerance to feeding by evaluating for abdominal distention, firmness, feeling of fullness, or nausea. Measured GRV per agency policy.

_____ _____ _____ _____

2. Monitored intake and output (I&O) at least every 8 hours and calculated daily totals every 24 hours.

_____ _____ _____ _____

3. Weighed patient daily until maximum administration rate was reached and maintained for 24 hours, then weighed patient 3 times per week.

_____ _____ _____ _____

4. Monitored patient for appropriate tube feeding placement at least every 4 hours or per agency policy. Monitored visible length of tubing or marking at tube exit site and checked placement when deviation was noted.

_____ _____ _____ _____

5. Monitored laboratory values as ordered by health care provider.

_____ _____ _____ _____

6. Observed patient's respiratory status for coughing, dyspnea, tachypnea, change in oxygen saturation, hoarseness, or crackles in lungs.

_____ _____ _____ _____

7. For gastrostomy and jejunostomy tubes, inspected site for signs of impaired skin integrity and symptoms of infection, injury, or tightness of tube.

_____ _____ _____ _____

8. Observed nasoenteral tube insertion site at least daily (per agency policy). Noted skin integrity and looked for edema under device, excoriation, or presence of injury.

_____ _____ _____ _____

9. Used Teach-Back technique. Revised instruction if patient or family caregiver was not able to teach back correctly.

_____ _____ _____ _____

DOCUMENTATION

1. Documented amount and type of feeding, infusion rate (continuous feeding) or time of infusion (bolus method), GRV measurements, position of feeding tube, patient's response to tube feeding, patency of tube, and condition of skin at tube site.

_____ _____ _____ _____

2. Documented evaluation of patient and family caregiver learning.

_____ _____ _____ _____

3. Documented volume of formula and any additional water.

_____ _____ _____ _____

550

	S	U	NP	Comments

HAND-OFF REPORTING

1. Reported adverse outcomes to the health care provider. ___ ___ ___ _____

2. During hand-off, reported the type of feeding, infusion rate, and patient's tolerance, and traced the administration set tubing to the enteral tube connection point to ensure feeding was being infused enterally. ___ ___ ___ _____

PERFORMANCE CHECKLIST PROCEDURAL GUIDELINE 31.1   **CARE OF GASTROSTOMY OR JEJUNOSTOMY TUBE**

	S	U	NP	Comments

PROCEDURAL STEPS

1. Identified patient using at least two identifiers, according to agency policy. ___ ___ ___ _____

2. Determined whether exit site was left open to air or if a dressing was indicated. Checked health care provider's order or verified agency policy. If dressing was indicated, obtained and organized dressing supplies. ___ ___ ___ _____

3. Provided privacy and explained procedure to patient. Arranged equipment for care of tube at bedside. Performed hand hygiene. ___ ___ ___ _____

4. Positioned patient in comfortable position lying supine or supine with head of bed slightly elevated. ___ ___ ___ _____

5. Assessed patient's/family caregiver's health literacy. Explained procedure to patient. ___ ___ ___ _____

6. Assessed patient's knowledge of and prior experience with PEG or PEJ tube care, and feelings about procedure. ___ ___ ___ _____

7. Performed hand hygiene and applied clean gloves. Removed old dressing. Folded dressing with drainage contained inside and removed gloves inside out over dressing. Discarded in appropriate container. Performed hand hygiene. ___ ___ ___ _____

8. Assessed exit site for evidence of tenderness, leakage, swelling, excoriation, infection, bleeding, or excessive movement (more than 6 mm [1/4 inch]) of the tube in or out of the stomach. ___ ___ ___ _____

9. Applied clean gloves. Cleaned skin around stoma site with warm water and mild soap or saline (according to agency policy) with 4 x 4–inch gauze. Cleaned starting next to the stoma site and worked outward using circular strokes. ___ ___ ___ _____

10. Rinsed and dried site completely. ___ ___ ___ _____

11. Applied thin layer of protective skin barrier to exit site if indicated. ___ ___ ___ _____

	S	U	NP	Comments

12. If dressing was ordered, placed a drain-gauze dressing over external bar or disk. Did not place dressing under external bar. ___ ___ ___ _____

13. Secured dressing with tape. ___ ___ ___ _____

14. Placed date, time, and initials on new dressing. ___ ___ ___ _____

15. Removed gloves and disposed of supplies in appropriate receptacle. Performed hand hygiene. ___ ___ ___ _____

16. Helped patient to comfortable position. Placed nurse call system in an accessible location within patient's reach. Raised side rails (as appropriate) and lowered bed to lowest position, locking into position. ___ ___ ___ _____

17. Evaluated condition of site routinely, per agency policy. ___ ___ ___ _____

18. Used Teach-Back technique. Revised instruction if patient or family caregiver was not able to teach back correctly. ___ ___ ___ _____

19. Documented appearance of exit site, drainage noted, and dressing application. ___ ___ ___ _____

20. Reported to health care provider any exit site complications. ___ ___ ___ _____

21. Provided hand-off report to health care provider of any changes or abnormal findings. ___ ___ ___ _____

Student _____ Date _____

Instructor _____ Date _____

PERFORMANCE CHECKLIST SKILL 32.1   ADMINISTERING CENTRAL PARENTERAL NUTRITION

	S	U	NP	Comments

ASSESSMENT

1. Identified patient using at least two identifiers, according to agency policy.   ___ ___ ___ _____

2. Reviewed electronic health record (EHR) for lab test measurement of levels of electrolytes, serum albumin, total protein, transferrin, prealbumin, and triglycerides.   ___ ___ ___ _____

3. Assessed patient's medical history for factors influenced by CPN administration: electrolyte levels; renal, cardiac, and hepatic function. Assessed for history of allergies, including egg allergy with lipids.   ___ ___ ___ _____

4. Reviewed EHR to determine patient's age and history of dehydration, malnutrition, exposure to radiation therapy, underlying chronic conditions, and edema of the skin.   ___ ___ ___ _____

5. Assessed patient's/family caregiver's health literacy.   ___ ___ ___ _____

6. Assessed indications of and risks for protein/calorie malnutrition: weight loss from baseline or ideal, muscle atrophy/weakness, edema, lethargy, failure to wean from ventilatory support, chronic illness, and nothing by mouth for more than 7 days. Conferred with nutrition support team.   ___ ___ ___ _____

7. Performed hand hygiene and applied clean gloves. Checked blood glucose level by fingerstick. Removed and disposed of gloves and performed hand hygiene.   ___ ___ ___ _____

8. Applied new pair of clean gloves. Inspected condition of central vein access site for presence of inflammation, edema, and tenderness. Inspected tubing of access device for patency and kinking. Note: If necessary to touch site or connections, applied sterile gloves.   ___ ___ ___ _____

9. Assessed vital signs, auscultated patient's lung sounds, inspected for edema of extremities, and measured weight. Removed and disposed of gloves and performed hand hygiene.   ___ ___ ___ _____

10. Consulted with members of nutrition support team on calculation of calorie, protein, and fluid requirements for patient.   ___ ___ ___ _____

11. Verified order for nutrients, minerals, vitamins, trace elements, electrolytes, added medications, and flow rate. Checked for compatibility of added medications.   ___ ___ ___ _____

12. Assessed patient's knowledge, prior experience with CPN, and feelings about procedure.   ___ ___ ___ _____

554

	S	U	NP	Comments

PLANNING

1. Determined expected outcomes following completion of procedure. ___ ___ ___ _____

2. Explained purpose of CPN to patient and family caregiver. ___ ___ ___ _____

3. If CPN solution was refrigerated, removed from refrigeration 1 hour before infusion. ___ ___ ___ _____

4. Performed hand hygiene. Assembled necessary equipment and supplies at bedside. ___ ___ ___ _____

IMPLEMENTATION

1. Performed hand hygiene. ___ ___ ___ _____

2. In medication room, checked label on CPN bag with health care provider's order on MAR or computer printout and patient's name. Also checked any additives and noted solution expiration date. ___ ___ ___ _____

3. Inspected 2:1 CPN solution for particulate matter. ___ ___ ___ _____

4. Before leaving medication room, checked IV solution a second time using seven rights of medication administration. Checked label of CPN bag against MAR or computer printout. ___ ___ ___ _____

5. Took CPN solution to patient before the existing infusion PN solution emptied. Compared names of solution and additives with MAR at bedside. ___ ___ ___ _____

6. Identified patient using at least two identifiers, per agency policy. Compared identifiers with information on patient's MAR or EHR. ___ ___ ___ _____

7. Closed room doors and/or bedside curtain. ___ ___ ___ _____

8. Positioned patient comfortably, either sitting or lying supine with head of bed elevated. ___ ___ ___ _____

9. Performed hand hygiene. Applied clean gloves. Prepared IV tubing for CPN solution: ___ ___ ___ _____

   a. Attached 1.2-μm filter to IV tubing. ___ ___ ___ _____

   b. Positioned filter to be as close to patient as possible. ___ ___ ___ _____

   c. Primed tubing with CPN solution, making sure that no air bubbles remained, and turned off flow with roller clamp. Added sterile-capped needle or placed sterile cap on end of tubing. ___ ___ ___ _____

10. Scrubbed end port of CVAD with chlorhexidine antiseptic swab, allowed to dry, then attached syringe of 0.9% normal saline (NS) solution to needleless port, aspirated for blood return, and flushed saline per agency policy. ___ ___ ___ _____

11. Removed syringe. Removed sterile lock cap and connected sterile Luer-Lok end of CPN IV tubing to dedicated end port of CVAD; for multilumen lines, labeled tubing used for CPN. ___ ___ ___ _____

12. Placed IV tubing in EID. Opened roller clamp. Set and regulated flow rate as ordered. ___ ___ ___ _____

    a. Continuous infusion: Flow rate was immediately set at ordered rate and given over 24-hour period. ___ ___ ___ _____

    b. Cycle infusion: Flow rate was initiated about 40 to 60 mL/h, and the rate was gradually increased until patient's nutrition needs were met. Before completion of infusion, rate was decreased at about the same rate in milliliters per hour until the CPN was completed. ___ ___ ___ _____

13. Did not interrupt CPN infusion, and ensured that rate did not exceed ordered rate. ___ ___ ___ _____

14. A 3-in-1 CPN solution containing the three macronutrients had a hang time that did not exceed 24 hours. Fat emulsions alone did not have a hang time that exceeded 12 hours. ___ ___ ___ _____

15. Changed IV administration sets with each new CPN solution container, which is usually every 24 hours and immediately on suspected contamination. ___ ___ ___ _____

16. Removed and disposed of supplies and gloves. Performed hand hygiene. ___ ___ ___ _____

17. Helped patient to comfortable position. ___ ___ ___ _____

18. Placed nurse call system in an accessible location within patient's reach. ___ ___ ___ _____

19. Raised side rails (as appropriate), and lowered bed to lowest position, locking into position. ___ ___ ___ _____

EVALUATION

1. Monitored flow rate according to agency policy and procedure. If infusion was not running on time, did not attempt to catch up. ___ ___ ___ _____

2. Monitored fluid intake and urine and gastrointestinal (GI) fluid output every 8 hours. ___ ___ ___ _____

3. Measured vital signs every 4 hours. ___ ___ ___ _____

4. Obtained initial weight and then weighed at least 3 times weekly. ___ ___ ___ _____

5. Evaluated for fluid retention; palpated skin of extremities; auscultated lung sounds. ___ ___ ___ _____

6. Monitored patient's glucose levels daily or as ordered and other laboratory parameters daily or as ordered. ___ ___ ___ _____

7. Inspected central venous access site for signs and symptoms of swelling, inflammation, drainage, redness, warmth, tenderness, or edema. ___ ___ ___ _____

8. Monitored for temperature, elevated white blood cell count, and malaise. ___ ___ ___ _____

9. Used Teach-Back. Revised instruction if patient or family caregiver was not able to teach back correctly. ___ ___ ___ _____

556

	S	U	NP	Comments

RECORDING

1. Documented condition of CVAD site, function of CVAD, rate and type of infusion, catheter lumen used for infusion, intake and output (I&O), blood glucose levels, vital signs, and weights.   ___ ___ ___ _____

2. Documented any adverse reactions.   ___ ___ ___ _____

3. Documented evaluation of patient and family caregiver learning.   ___ ___ ___ _____

HAND-OFF REPORTING

1. In a hand-off report, communicated condition of CVAD site, status of infusion, type of CPN solution infusing, and patient response.

2. If signs of infection, occlusion, fluid retention, or infiltration occurred, notified the health care provider.   ___ ___ ___ _____

PERFORMANCE CHECKLIST SKILL 32.2   **ADMINISTERING PERIPHERAL PARENTERAL NUTRITION WITH LIPID (FAT) EMULSION**

	S	U	NP	Comments

ASSESSMENT

1. Identified patient using at least two identifiers, according to agency policy.

2. Reviewed electronic health record (EHR) for history of patient having hypertriglyceridemia. Consulted with health care provider and obtained orders for serum triglyceride level before initiation of PPN and weekly.

3. Assessed patient's/family caregiver's health literacy.

4. Assessed for history of allergies, including egg allergy with lipids.

5. Obtained patient's weight and vital signs.

6. Performed hand hygiene, and applied clean gloves using ANTT®. Note: If necessary to touch site or connections, applied sterile gloves. Selected or initiated appropriate functional IV site to administer PPN and lipid emulsion. Assessed its patency and function.

7. Obtained blood glucose level by fingerstick. Removed and disposed of gloves and performed hand hygiene.

8. Assessed patient for edema in extremities, lung sounds, or fluid intake greater than fluid output.

9. Assessed patient's knowledge, prior experience with PPN, and feelings about procedure.

PLANNING

1. Determined expected outcomes following completion of procedure.

2. Explained purposes of PPN and fat emulsion.

3. If PPN solution was refrigerated, removed from refrigeration 1 hour before infusion.

4. Placed patient in comfortable position for IV line insertion or initiation of infusion.

IMPLEMENTATION

1. Performed hand hygiene.

2. Checked health care provider's order against MAR for volume of fat emulsion, PPN solution, and administration time for PPN solution/fat emulsion. Then checked name of solution on label with MAR.

	S	U	NP	Comments

3. Read label of fat emulsion solution.

4. Compared label of PPN bag/lipid emulsion bottle with MAR or computer printout; checked for correct additives and solution expiration date. Also checked patient's name.

5. Examined lipid solution for separation of emulsion into layers or fat globules or presence of froth.

6. Identified patient again at bedside using at least two identifiers, according to agency policy. Compared identifiers with information on patient's MAR or EHR.

7. Compared identifiers with information on solution bag label and patient's MAR or EHR at the bedside.

8. Took new PPN solution to patient before the existing PPN infusion solution emptied.

9. Closed room doors and/or bedside curtain.

10. Positioned patient comfortably, either sitting or lying supine with head of bed elevated.

11. Performed hand hygiene. Applied clean gloves (surgical gloves if touching key connecting parts).

12. Prepared IV tubing and administered PPN solution:

   a. Applied 1.2-μm filter to PPN solution tubing using ANTT.

   b. Positioned filters to be as close to patient as possible.

   c. Ran solution through PPN tubing to remove excess air. Turned roller clamp to "off" position. Added sterile-capped needle or placed sterile cap on end of tubing.

   d. Wiped end port of PPN IV infusion tubing with antimicrobial swab and allowed to air dry. Removed cap and prepared to connect needleless connector at end of PPN tubing to end port of patient's functional peripheral IV line. Gently disconnected old PPN tubing from IV site and inserted adapter of new PPN infusion tubing. Opened roller clamp on new tubing. Allowed solution to run to ensure that tubing was patent; regulated IV drip rate using EID.

13. Prepared IV tubing and administered lipid emulsion:

   a. Applied the 1.2-μm filter for lipid infusion to infusion tubing using ANTT.

   b. Positioned filters to be as close to patient as possible.

   c. Ran solution through tubing to remove excess air. Turned roller clamp to "off" position. Added sterile-capped needle or placed sterile cap on end of tubing.

	S	U	NP	Comments

d. Cleaned needless peripheral IV line tubing injection cap with antimicrobial swab and allowed to dry. ___ ___ ___ _____

e. Attached end of fat emulsion infusion tubing to injection cap of PPN IV line. Labeled tubing. ___ ___ ___ _____

f. Opened roller clamp completely on fat emulsion infusion and checked flow rate on infusion pump. ___ ___ ___ _____

g. Infused lipids as follows: ___ ___ ___ _____

(1) Infused at 0.1 mL/min for the first 10 to 15 minutes. ___ ___ ___ _____

(2) If no allergic reaction, increased to the ordered hourly rate of IV lipid emulsion. ___ ___ ___ _____

14. Removed and disposed of gloves and used supplies. Performed hand hygiene. ___ ___ ___ _____

15. Helped patient to comfortable position. ___ ___ ___ _____

16. Placed nurse call system in an accessible location within patient's reach. ___ ___ ___ _____

17. Raised side rails (as appropriate), and lowered bed to lowest position, locking into position. ___ ___ ___ _____

EVALUATION

1. Monitored flow rate routinely on an hourly basis or more frequently if necessary, per agency policy. ___ ___ ___ _____

2. Measured vital signs and patient's general comfort level every 10 minutes for first 30 minutes, then vital signs every 4 hours. ___ ___ ___ _____

3. Monitored patient's laboratory values daily and performed blood glucose monitoring as ordered. Measured serum lipids 4 hours after discontinuing infusion. ___ ___ ___ _____

4. Monitored temperature every 4 hours, and regularly inspected venipuncture site for signs of phlebitis or infiltration. ___ ___ ___ _____

5. Evaluated patient's weight, intake and output (I&O), condition of peripheral extremities (for edema), and breath sounds. ___ ___ ___ _____

6. Used Teach-Back. Revised instruction if patient or family caregiver was not able to teach back correctly. ___ ___ ___ _____

RECORDING

1. Documented location and condition of IV site, type of solutions, rate and status of infusion, catheter lumen size used for infusion, I&O, blood glucose levels, vital signs, weights, and other assessment findings. ___ ___ ___ _____

2. Documented any adverse reactions. ___ ___ ___ _____

3. Documented evaluation of patient and family caregiver learning. ___ ___ ___ _____

560

	S	U	NP	Comments

HAND-OFF REPORTING

1. During hand-off, reported type of infusion, rate and status of IV access site, patient's response, and any abnormal assessment findings. ___ ___ ___ _____

2. If signs of fat intolerance, infection, occlusion, fluid retention, or infiltration occurred, notified the health care provider. ___ ___ ___ _____

Student _____ Date _____

Instructor _____ Date _____

PERFORMANCE CHECKLIST PROCEDURAL GUIDELINE 33.1 **ASSISTING WITH USE OF A URINAL**

	S	U	NP	Comments

PROCEDURAL STEPS

1. In determining the need for a urinal, assessed patient's electronic health record (EHR) for conditions that may place patient at risk for falling during ambulation.

2. Assessed patient's normal urinary elimination habits, including normal frequency and any episodes of incontinence.

3. Determined how much help was needed to place and remove the urinal. (Asked the patient or observed previous use.)

4. Reviewed EHR for health care provider orders to determine if a urine specimen needed to be collected.

5. Assessed patient's/family caregiver's health literacy.

6. Provided privacy and explained procedure to patient.

7. Performed hand hygiene and applied clean gloves.

8. Assessed for a distended bladder by inspecting the lower one-third of the abdomen or palpating gently above symphysis pubis.

9. Helped patient into appropriate position:

   • Male patient on side, back, sitting with head of bed elevated, or in standing position.

   • Female patient lying supine.

10. If needed, placed an absorbent pad under patient's buttocks to protect bed linens from accidental spills.

11. If possible, a patient of male gender should have held urinal and positioned penis in it. If needed, helped patient by positioning penis completely in urinal and holding it in place or by helping to hold urinal. Ensured that the urinal was placed dependent of the flow of urine.

	S	U	NP	Comments

12. Helped a patient of female gender by positioning the urinal against the genitalia and stabilizing it to keep it in position and dependent of urine flow. Option: If the female urinal did not fit, had patient void into a bedpan.   ___ ___ ___ _____

13. Covered patient with bed linens and placed the nurse call system within reach. If possible, gave patient further privacy by leaving the bedside after ensuring that they were in a safe and comfortable position. Removed and disposed of gloves and performed hand hygiene.   ___ ___ ___ _____

14. After patient had finished voiding, applied gloves and removed urinal and assessed characteristics of the urine for color, clarity, odor, and amount. Helped patient wash and dry genitalia.   ___ ___ ___ _____

15. Emptied and cleaned urinal. Returned urinal to patient for future use. Removed and disposed of gloves.   ___ ___ ___ _____

16. Helped patient perform hand hygiene as needed.   ___ ___ ___ _____

17. Performed hand hygiene.   ___ ___ ___ _____

18. Helped patient to comfortable position.   ___ ___ ___ _____

19. Placed nurse call system in an accessible location within patient's reach.   ___ ___ ___ _____

20. Raised side rails (as appropriate) and lowered bed to lowest position, locking into position.   ___ ___ ___ _____

21. Used Teach-Back. Revised instruction if patient or family caregiver was not able to teach back correctly.   ___ ___ ___ _____

22. Documented the amount and character of urine on I&O form.   ___ ___ ___ _____

23. Provided hand-off report to health care provider of any changes or abnormal findings.   ___ ___ ___ _____

PERFORMANCE CHECKLIST SKILL 33.1   **INSERTION OF A STRAIGHT OR AN INDWELLING URINARY CATHETER**

	S	U	NP	Comments

ASSESSMENT

1. Identified patient using at least two identifiers, according to agency policy. ___ ___ ___ _____

2. Reviewed patient's EHR for previous catheterization, including catheter size, response of patient, and time of catheterization. ___ ___ ___ _____

3. Reviewed EHR for any pathological or anatomical conditions that may impair passage of catheter. ___ ___ ___ _____

4. Reviewed EHR to determine patient's age and history of dehydration, malnutrition, exposure to radiation therapy, underlying chronic conditions, and edema of the skin.

5. Assessed patient's gender. ___ ___ ___ _____

6. Assessed patient's/family caregiver's health literacy. ___ ___ ___ _____

7. Asked patient and checked EHR for history of allergies. Checked allergy bracelet. ___ ___ ___ _____

8. Performed hand hygiene. Assessed patient's weight, level of consciousness, developmental level, ability to cooperate, and mobility. ___ ___ ___ _____

9. Assessed for pain and bladder fullness. Palpated bladder over symphysis pubis or used bladder scanner (if available). ___ ___ ___ _____

10. Applied clean gloves. Inspected perineal region, observing for perineal anatomical landmarks, erythema, drainage or discharge, and odor. Removed and disposed of gloves and performed hand hygiene. ___ ___ ___ _____

11. Assessed patient's knowledge of and prior experience with catheterization, and feelings about procedure. ___ ___ ___ _____

PLANNING

1. Determined expected outcomes following completion of procedure. ___ ___ ___ _____

2. Provided privacy and explained procedure to patient. ___ ___ ___ _____

564

	S	U	NP	Comments

3. Organized and set up equipment needed to perform procedure at bedside.

4. Arranged for extra personnel to help as necessary. .

IMPLEMENTATION

1. Checked patient's plan of care for size and type of catheter (if this was a reinsertion). Used smallest-size catheter possible.

2. Performed hand hygiene.

3. Raised bed to appropriate working height. If side rails were in use, raised side rail on opposite side of bed and lowered side rail on working side.

4. Had patient log roll or bend knees and raise hips to place a waterproof pad under patient.

5. Positioned patient:

   a. **Female patient:**

   (1) Helped to dorsal recumbent position. Asked patient to relax thighs so hips could be rotated.

   (2) Alternate female position: Positioned side-lying position with upper leg flexed at knee and hip. Supported patient with pillows, if necessary, to maintain position.

   b. **Male patient:**

   (1) Positioned supine with legs extended and thighs slightly abducted.

6. Draped patient:

   a. **Female patient:**

   (1) Draped with bath blanket. Placed blanket diamond fashion over patient, with one corner at patient's midsection, side corners over each thigh and abdomen, and last corner over perineum.

   b. **Male patient:**

   (1) Draped patient by covering upper part of body with small sheet or towel; draped with separate sheet or bath blanket so only perineum was exposed.

7. Positioned portable light to illuminate genitals or had assistant available to hold light.

	S	U	NP	Comments

8. Applied clean gloves. Cleaned perineal area with soap and water, rinsed, and dried. Used fingers to retract tissues for examining patient and identified urinary meatus. Removed and disposed of gloves. Performed hand hygiene.

9. Opened outer wrapping of catheterization kit. Placed inner wrapped catheter kit tray on clean, accessible surface such as bedside table or, if possible, between patient's open legs.

10. Removed the cover of the tray by taking the edge of the outer cover and peeling it away to open the tray while ensuring that hand did not extend over the sterile contents.

   a. Indwelling catheterization opened system: Opened separate package containing drainage bag, checked to make sure that clamp on drainage port was closed, and placed drainage bag and tubing in easily accessible location. Opened outer package of sterile catheter, maintaining sterility of inner wrapper.

   b. Indwelling catheterization closed system: All supplies were in sterile tray and arranged in sequence of use.

   c. Straight catheterization: All needed supplies were in sterile tray that contained supplies and could be used for urine collection.

11. Applied sterile gloves. NOTE: Used special gloves, if needed, if patient was receiving hazardous drugs.

12. *Option:* Applied sterile drape with ungloved hands if drape was packed as first item. Touched only 2.5 cm (1-inch) edges of drape. Then applied sterile gloves.

13. Draped perineum, keeping gloves and working surface of drape sterile.

   a. **Draped female:**

   (1) Picked up square sterile drape touching only edges (2.5 cm [1 inch]).

   (2) Allowed drape to unfold without touching unsterile surfaces. Allowed top edge of drape (2.5 to 5 cm [1 to 2 inches]) to form cuff over both gloved hands.

	S	U	NP	Comments

(3) Placed drape with shiny side down on bed between patient's thighs. Slipped cuffed edge just under buttocks as nurse asked patient to lift hips. Took care not to touch contaminated surfaces or patient's thighs with sterile gloves. If gloves were contaminated, removed and applied new pair.

(4) Picked up fenestrated sterile drape out of tray. Allowed drape to unfold without touching unsterile surfaces. Allowed top edge of drape to form cuff over both gloved hands. Applied drape over perineum so that opening was over exposed labia.

b. **Draped male:**

(1) Used square drape or fenestrated drape.

(2) Picked up edges of square drape and allowed to unfold without touching unsterile surfaces. Placed over thighs, with shiny side down, just below penis. Took care not to touch contaminated surfaces with sterile gloves.

(3) Placed fenestrated drape with opening centered over penis.

14. Placed sterile tray with cleaning solution (premoistened swab sticks or cotton balls, forceps, and solution), lubricant, catheter, and prefilled syringe for inflating balloon (indwelling catheterization only) on sterile drape close to patient. Arranged any remaining sterile supplies on sterilized field, maintaining sterile of gloves.

a. If kit contained sterile cotton balls, opened package of sterile antiseptic solution and poured over cotton balls. Opened end of package of premoistened swab sticks, if using, for easy access.

b. Opened sterile specimen container if specimen was to be obtained.

c. For indwelling catheterization, opened sterile inner wrapper of catheter and left catheter on sterile field or in tray. If part of closed system kit, removed tray with catheter and preattached drainage bag and placed on sterile drape. Made sure that clamp on drainage port of bag was closed. If needed and if part of sterile tray, attached catheter to drainage tubing.

d. Opened packet of lubricant and squeezed out on sterile field. Lubricated catheter tip by dipping it into water-soluble gel 2.5 to 5 cm (1–2 inches) for women and 12.5 to 17.5 cm (5–7 inches) for men.   ___ ___ ___ _____

15. Cleaned urethral meatus: ___ ___ ___ _____

a. **Female patient:**

(1) Separated labia with fingers of nondominant hand (now contaminated) to fully expose urethral meatus.   ___ ___ ___ _____

(2) Maintained position of nondominant hand throughout procedure.   ___ ___ ___ _____

(3) While maintaining sterility, picked up one moistened cotton ball with forceps or picked up one swab stick at a time. Cleaned labia and urinary meatus from clitoris toward anus. Used new cotton ball or swab for each area that you cleaned. Cleaned by wiping far labial fold, near labial fold, and last, directly over center of urethral meatus   ___ ___ ___ _____

b. **Male patient:**

(1) With nondominant hand (now contaminated), retracted foreskin (if uncircumcised) and gently grasped penis at shaft just below glans. Held shaft of penis at right angle to body. This hand remained in this position for remainder of procedure.   ___ ___ ___ _____

(2) Using dominant hand and maintaining sterility, cleaned meatus with cotton balls and forceps/swab sticks, using circular strokes, beginning at meatus and working outward in spiral motion.   ___ ___ ___ _____

(3) Repeated cleaning 3 times using clean cotton ball/swab stick each time.   ___ ___ ___ _____

16. Picked up and held catheter 7.5 to 10 cm (3 to 4 inches) from catheter tip with catheter loosely coiled in palm of hand. If catheter was not attached to drainage bag, made sure to position urine tray so end of catheter could be placed there once insertion began.   ___ ___ ___ _____

17. Inserted catheter. Explained to patient that feeling of discomfort or pressure may be experienced as catheter is inserted into urethra.   ___ ___ ___ _____

a. **Female patient:**

(1) Asked patient to bear down gently and slowly inserted catheter through urethral meatus.   ___ ___ ___ _____

568

	S	U	NP	Comments

(2) Advanced catheter total of 5 to 7.5 cm (2–3 inches) or until urine flowed out of catheter. Stopped advancing with straight catheter. When urine appeared, advanced catheter another 2.5 to 5 cm (1–2 inches) for indwelling catheter. Did not use force to insert catheter.   ___ ___ ___ _____

(3) Released labia and held catheter securely with nondominant hand.   ___ ___ ___ _____

b. **Male patient:**

(1) Lifted penis to position perpendicular (90 degrees) to patient's body and applied gentle upward traction.   ___ ___ ___ _____

(2) Asked patient to bear down as if to void and slowly inserted catheter through urethral meatus.   ___ ___ ___ _____

(3) Advanced catheter 17 to 22.5 cm (7–9 inches) or until urine flowed out end of catheter. Did not use force to advance catheter.   ___ ___ ___ _____

(4) Stopped advancing with straight catheter. When urine appeared in indwelling catheter, advanced it to bifurcation (inflation and deflation ports exposed).   ___ ___ ___ _____

(5) Lowered penis and held catheter securely in nondominant hand.   ___ ___ ___ _____

18. Allowed bladder to empty fully unless agency policy restricted maximum volume of urine drained (consulted agency policy).   ___ ___ ___ _____

19. Collected urine specimen as needed. Filled specimen container to 20 to 30 mL by holding end of catheter over the cup. Set container aside. Kept end of catheter sterile.   ___ ___ ___ _____

20. Option for straight catheterization: When urine stopped flowing, withdrew catheter slowly and smoothly with dominant hand until removed.   ___ ___ ___ _____

21. For indwelling catheter: Inflated catheter balloon with amount of fluid designated by manufacturer.   ___ ___ ___ _____

a. Continued to hold catheter with nondominant hand.   ___ ___ ___ _____

b. With free dominant hand, connected prefilled syringe to injection port at end of catheter.   ___ ___ ___ _____

c. Slowly injected total amount of solution.   ___ ___ ___ _____

	S	U	NP	Comments

d. After inflating catheter balloon, released catheter from nondominant hand. *Gently* pulled catheter until resistance was felt. Then advanced catheter slightly.

    ____   ____   ____   _____

e. Connected drainage tubing to catheter if it was not already preconnected.

    ____   ____   ____   _____

22. Secured indwelling catheter with catheter strap or other securement device. Attached securement device at tubing just above catheter bifurcation.

    ____   ____   ____   _____

    a. **Female patient:**

        (1) Secured catheter tubing to inner thigh, allowing enough slack to allow leg movement and prevent tension.

    ____   ____   ____   _____

    b. **Male patient:**

        (1) Secured catheter tubing to upper thigh or lower abdomen (with penis directed toward chest). Allowed slack in catheter so movement did not create tension on catheter.

        (2) If retracted, replaced foreskin over glans penis.

    ____   ____   ____   _____

23. Clipped drainage tubing to edge of mattress. Positioned drainage bag below level of bladder by attaching to bedframe. Did not attach to side rails of bed and did not rest bag on floor.

    ____   ____   ____   _____

24. Checked to ensure that there was no obstruction to urine flow. Coiled excess tubing on bed and fastened to bottom sheet with clip or other securement device.

    ____   ____   ____   _____

25. Provided perineal hygiene as needed. Helped patient to comfortable position.

    ____   ____   ____   _____

26. Labeled and bagged specimen according to agency policy. Labeled specimen in front of patient. Had specimen sent to laboratory as soon as possible.

    ____   ____   ____   _____

27. Measured urine and documented.

    ____   ____   ____   _____

28. Disposed of supplies in appropriate receptacles.

    ____   ____   ____   _____

29. Removed and disposed of gloves.

    ____   ____   ____   _____

30. Raised side rails (as appropriate) and lowered bed to lowest position, locking into position.

    ____   ____   ____   _____

31. Placed nurse call system in an accessible location within patient's reach.

    ____   ____   ____   _____

32. Performed hand hygiene.

	S	U	NP	Comments

EVALUATION

1. Palpated bladder for distention or used bladder scan as per agency protocol. ___ ___ ___ _____

2. Asked patient to describe level of comfort and if sensation of bladder fullness was relieved. ___ ___ ___ _____

3. Indwelling catheter: Observed character and amount of urine in drainage system. ___ ___ ___ _____

4. Indwelling catheter: Determined that there was no urine leaking from catheter or tubing connections. ___ ___ ___ _____

5. Used Teach-Back. Revised instruction if patient or family caregiver was not able to teach back correctly. ___ ___ ___ _____

DOCUMENTATION

1. Documented reason for catheterization, type and size of catheter inserted, amount of fluid used to inflate balloon, specimen collection (if applicable), characteristics and amount of urine, patient's response to procedure, and evaluation of patient learning. ___ ___ ___ _____

2. Documented I&O. ___ ___ ___ _____

HAND-OFF REPORTING

1. Reported reason for catheterization, type and size of catheter inserted, amount of fluid used to inflate balloon, specimen collection (if applicable), characteristics and amount of urine, patient's response to procedure, and any education. Verified that specimen was sent to the lab (if applicable). ___ ___ ___ _____

2. Reported to health care provider persistent catheter-related pain and discomfort. ___ ___ ___ _____

Student _____ Date _____

Instructor _____ Date _____

PERFORMANCE CHECKLIST SKILL 33.2 **CARE AND REMOVAL OF AN INDWELLING CATHETER**

	S	U	NP	Comments

ASSESSMENT

1. Identified patient using at least two identifiers, according to agency policy.

2. Assessed patient's/family caregiver's health literacy.

3. Performed hand hygiene.

4. Assessed need for catheter care:

   a. Observed urinary output and urine characteristics.

   b. Assessed for recent history or presence of bowel incontinence.

   c. Applied clean gloves. Positioned patient and retracted labial or foreskin to observe for any discharge, redness, bleeding, or presence of tissue trauma around urethral meatus (this may have been deferred until catheter care).

   d. Removed and disposed of gloves and performed hand hygiene.

5. Assessed need for catheter removal:

   a. Reviewed patient's EHR for length of time catheter had been in place.

   b. Assessed urine color, clarity, odor, and amount. Noted any urethral discharge, irritation of genital region, or trauma to urinary meatus (this may have been deferred until just before removal).

   c. Assessed patient for history of dehydration, malnutrition, exposure to radiation therapy, underlying chronic conditions, and edema of the skin.

   d. Determined size of catheter inflation balloon by looking at balloon inflation valve.

	S	U	NP	Comments

e. Assessed patient's knowledge and prior experience with catheter care and/or catheter removal, and feelings about procedure. ___ ___ ___ _____

PLANNING

1. Determined expected outcomes following catheter care. ___ ___ ___ _____

2. Determined expected outcomes following catheter removal. ___ ___ ___ _____

3. Provided privacy and explained procedure to patient. Discussed signs and symptoms of UTI and MARSI. If patient was to be discharged with a catheter, taught patient or family caregiver how to perform catheter hygiene. ___ ___ ___ _____

4. Obtained and organized equipment at bedside. ___ ___ ___ _____

IMPLEMENTATION

1. Performed hand hygiene. ___ ___ ___ _____

2. Raised bed to appropriate working height. If side rails were raised, lowered side rail on working side. ___ ___ ___ _____

3. Positioned patient with waterproof pad under buttocks and covered with bath blanket, exposing only genital area and catheter. ___ ___ ___ _____

   a. Female in dorsal recumbent position. ___ ___ ___ _____

   b. Male in supine position. ___ ___ ___ _____

4. Applied clean gloves. ___ ___ ___ _____

5. Removed catheter securement device while maintaining connection with drainage tubing. ___ ___ ___ _____

6. Catheter care: ___ ___ ___ _____

   a. *Female:* Used nondominant hand to gently separate labia to fully expose urethral meatus and catheter. Maintained position of hand throughout procedure. ___ ___ ___ _____

   b. *Male:* Used nondominant hand to retract foreskin if not circumcised and held penis at shaft just below glans. Maintained hand position throughout procedure. ___ ___ ___ _____

   c. Grasped catheter with two fingers of nondominant hand to stabilize it. ___ ___ ___ _____

   d. If not performed earlier, assessed urethral meatus and surrounding tissues for inflammation, swelling, discharge, or tissue trauma and asked patient if burning or discomfort was present. ___ ___ ___ _____

	S	U	NP	Comments

e. Provided perineal hygiene using mild soap and warm water. *Option:* Used chlorhexidine gluconate (CHG) 2% cloth.

    ___ ___ ___ _____

f. Using clean washcloth or CHG cloth, cleaned along length of catheter.

    ___ ___ ___ _____

  (1) Starting close to urinary meatus, cleaned catheter in circular motion along its length for about 10 cm (4 inches), moving away from body. Removed all traces of soap. *For male patients:* Reduced or repositioned foreskin after care.

    ___ ___ ___ _____

g. Reapplied catheter securement device. Allowed slack in catheter so movement did not create tension on it.

    ___ ___ ___ _____

7. Routinely checked drainage tubing and bag.

    ___ ___ ___ _____

a. Catheter was secured to upper thigh.

    ___ ___ ___ _____

b. Tubing was positioned without loops and secured onto bed linen.

    ___ ___ ___ _____

c. Tubing was not kinked or clamped.

    ___ ___ ___ _____

d. Drainage bag was positioned below level of bladder with urine flowing freely into bag.

    ___ ___ ___ _____

e. Drainage bag was not over full. Emptied drainage bag when half full.

    ___ ___ ___ _____

8. Catheter removal (Performed catheter care [Step 6] before catheter removal.):

    ___ ___ ___ _____

a. With clean gloves still on, moved syringe plunger up and down to loosen and then pulled it back to 0.5 mL. Inserted hub of syringe into inflation valve (balloon port). Allowed balloon fluid to drain into syringe by gravity. Syringe should have filled. Made sure that entire amount of fluid was removed by comparing removed amount with volume needed for inflation.

    ___ ___ ___ _____

b. Pulled catheter out smoothly and slowly. Examined it to ensure that it was whole. Did not use force. If any resistance noted, repeated Step 8a to remove remaining water.

    ___ ___ ___ _____

c. Wrapped contaminated catheter in waterproof pad. Unhooked collection bag and drainage tubing from bed.

    ___ ___ ___ _____

d. Emptied, measured, and documented urine present in drainage bag. Ensured proper gloving if patient was on hazardous drugs.

    ___ ___ ___ _____

e. Encouraged patient to maintain or increase fluid intake (unless contraindicated).

    ___ ___ ___ _____

574

	S	U	NP	Comments

f. Initiated voiding record or bladder diary. Instructed patient to report need to empty bladder, and that all urine needed to be measured. Made sure that patient understood how to use collection container. ___ ___ ___ _____

g. Explained that many patients experience mild burning, discomfort, or small-volume voiding with first voiding, which soon subsides. ___ ___ ___ _____

h. Measured PVR volume (if ordered) within 5 to 15 minutes after helping the patient to void. ___ ___ ___ _____

i. Informed patient to report any signs of UTI. ___ ___ ___ _____

j. Ensured easy access to toilet, commode, bedpan, or urinal. Placed urine "hat" on toilet seat if patient was using toilet. ___ ___ ___ _____

9. Provided patient personal hygiene as needed. ___ ___ ___ _____

10. Helped patient to comfortable position. ___ ___ ___ _____

11. Placed nurse call system in an accessible location within patient's reach. ___ ___ ___ _____

12. Raised side rails (as appropriate) and lowered bed to lowest position, locking into position. ___ ___ ___ _____

13. Disposed of all contaminated supplies in appropriate receptacle, removed and disposed of gloves, and performed hand hygiene. ___ ___ ___ _____

EVALUATION

1. Inspected catheter, securement area, and genital area for soiling, irritation, signs of MARSI, and skin breakdown. Asked patient about discomfort. ___ ___ ___ _____

2. Observed time and measured amount of first voiding after catheter removal. ___ ___ ___ _____

3. Evaluated patient for signs and symptoms of UTI. ___ ___ ___ _____

4. Used Teach-Back. Revised instruction if patient or family caregiver was not able to teach back correctly. ___ ___ ___ _____

DOCUMENTATION

1. Documented time catheter was removed; teaching related to increasing fluid intake and signs and symptoms of UTI; and time, amount, and characteristics of first voiding. ___ ___ ___ _____

2. Documented intake and voiding times and amounts. ___ ___ ___ _____

	S	U	NP	Comments

3. Documented patient symptoms experienced upon and after catheter removal.

    ____ ____ ____ _____

4. Documented evaluation of patient learning.

    ____ ____ ____ _____

HAND-OFF REPORTING

1. Reported time catheter was removed; teaching provided to patient; and time, amount, and characteristics of first voiding..

    ____ ____ ____ _____

2. Reported hematuria, dysuria, inability or difficulty voiding, and any new incontinence after a catheter was removed to health care provider.

    ____ ____ ____ _____

Student _____ Date _____

Instructor _____ Date _____

PERFORMANCE CHECKLIST PROCEDURAL GUIDELINE 33.2   **BLADDER SCAN**

	S	U	NP	Comments

PROCEDURAL STEPS

1. Identified patient using at least two identifiers, according to agency policy. ___ ___ ___ _____

2. Assessed intake and output (I&O) record to determine urine output trends and checked the plan of care to verify correct timing of the bladder scan measurement. ___ ___ ___ _____

3. Assessed patient's/family caregiver's health literacy. ___ ___ ___ _____

4. Assessed patient for inadequate bladder emptying. ___ ___ ___ _____

5. Provided privacy and explained procedure to patient. ___ ___ ___ _____

6. Performed hand hygiene and applied clean gloves. ___ ___ ___ _____

7. Raised bed to working height. If side rails were raised, lowered side rail on working side. ___ ___ ___ _____

8. If measurement was for PVR, asked patient to void and measured voided urine volume. Measured within 5 to 15 minutes of voiding. ___ ___ ___ _____

9. Measured PVR with the bladder scan. ___ ___ ___ _____

   a. Helped patient to supine position with head slightly elevated. ___ ___ ___ _____

   b. Exposed patient's lower abdomen. ___ ___ ___ _____

   c. Turned on scanner per manufacturer's guidelines. ___ ___ ___ _____

   d. Set gender designation per manufacturer guidelines. Designated women who have had a hysterectomy as male. ___ ___ ___ _____

   e. Wiped scanner head with alcohol pad or other cleaner and allowed to air dry. ___ ___ ___ _____

   f. Palpated patient's symphysis pubis. Applied generous amount of ultrasound gel (or if available a bladder scan gel pad) to midline abdomen 2.5 to 4 cm (1–1.5 inches) above symphysis pubis. ___ ___ ___ _____

	S	U	NP	Comments

g. Placed scanner head on gel, ensuring that scanner head was oriented per manufacturer guidelines.

    ___ ___ ___ _____

h. Applied light pressure, kept scanner head steady, and pointed it slightly downward toward bladder. Pressed and released the scan button

    ___ ___ ___ _____

i. Verified accurate aim (referred to manufacturer guidelines). Completed scan and printed image (if needed).

    ___ ___ ___ _____

10. Removed ultrasound gel from patient's abdomen with paper towel or moist cloth.

    ___ ___ ___ _____

11. Removed ultrasound gel from scanner head and wiped with alcohol pad or other cleaner; allowed to air-dry.

    ___ ___ ___ _____

12. Helped patient to comfortable position.

    ___ ___ ___ _____

13. Placed nurse call system in an accessible location within patient's reach.

14. Raised side rails (as appropriate) and lowered bed to lowest position, locking into position.

    ___ ___ ___ _____

15. Measured PVR after voiding or after using straight/intermittent catheterization. Compared results with pre-voiding scan. For patients with expected urinary retention, determined if results revealed residual urine in bladder.

    ___ ___ ___ _____

16. Disposed of all contaminated supplies in appropriate receptacle and removed and disposed of gloves.

    ___ ___ ___ _____

17. Performed hand hygiene.

    ___ ___ ___ _____

18. Used Teach-Back. Revised instruction if patient/family caregiver was not able to teach back correctly.

    ___ ___ ___ _____

19. Reviewed health care provider's order to determine how often to assess residual urine.

    ___ ___ ___ _____

20. Reviewed I&O record to determine urine output trends.

    ___ ___ ___ _____

21. Documented findings of scan, PVR, and patient tolerance of procedure.

    ___ ___ ___ _____

22. Reported to health care provider outcome of bladder scan and need to catheterize for residual volume.

    ___ ___ ___ _____

Student _____   Date _____

Instructor _____   Date _____

PERFORMANCE CHECKLIST SKILL 33.3   **PERFORMING CATHETER IRRIGATION**

	S	U	NP	Comments

ASSESSMENT

1. Identified patient using at least two identifiers, according to agency policy.

2. Verified in electronic health record (EHR):

3. Assessed patient's/family caregiver's health literacy.

   a. Order for irrigation method (continuous or intermittent), type (sterile saline or medicated solution), and amount of irrigant.

   b. Type of catheter in place.

4. Performed hand hygiene. Palpated bladder for distention and tenderness or used bladder scan.

5. Assessed patient for abdominal pain or spasms, sensation of bladder fullness, or leaking around catheter. Wore clean gloves if there was risk of contacting urine.

6. Observed urine for color, amount, clarity, and presence of mucus, clots, or sediment.

7. Monitored I&O. If CBI was being used, amount of fluid draining from bladder should have exceeded amount of fluid infused into bladder.

8. Assessed patient's or family caregiver's knowledge of and prior experience with catheter irrigation, and feelings about procedure.

PLANNING

1. Determined expected outcomes following completion of procedure.

2. Provided privacy and explained procedure to patient. Discussed what was involved in catheter irrigation and what the patient may expect to experience.

3. Obtained and organized equipment at bedside.

		S	U	NP	Comments

IMPLEMENTATION

1. Performed hand hygiene. Raised bed to appropriate working height. If side rails were raised, lowered side rail on working side. ___ ___ ___ _____

2. Positioned patient supine and exposed catheter junctions (catheter and drainage tubing). ___ ___ ___ _____

3. Removed catheter securement device. ___ ___ ___ _____

4. Closed continuous irrigation:

   a. Closed clamp on new irrigation tubing and hung bag of irrigating solution on IV pole. Inserted (spike) tip of sterile irrigation tubing into designated port of irrigation solution bag using aseptic technique. ___ ___ ___ _____

   b. Filled drip chamber half full by squeezing chamber. Removed cap at end of tubing, and then opened clamp and allowed solution to flow (prime) through tubing, keeping end of tubing sterile. Once fluid had filled tubing, closed clamp and recapped end of tubing. ___ ___ ___ _____

   c. Using aseptic technique, cleansed port on catheter with antiseptic swab, removed cap on tubing, and connected end of tubing securely to port for infusing irrigation fluid into double/triple–lumen catheter. ___ ___ ___ _____

   d. Adjusted clamp on irrigation tubing to begin flow of solution into bladder. If set volume rate was ordered, calculated drip rate and adjusted rate at roller clamp. If urine was bright red or had clots, increased irrigation rate until drainage appeared pink (according to ordered rate or agency protocol). ___ ___ ___ _____

   e. Observed for outflow of fluid into drainage bag. Emptied catheter drainage bag as needed. ___ ___ ___ _____

5. Closed intermittent irrigation:

   a. Poured prescribed sterile irrigation solution into sterile container. ___ ___ ___ _____

   b. Drew prescribed volume of irrigant (usually 30–50 mL) into sterile syringe using aseptic technique. Placed sterile cap on tip of needleless syringe. ___ ___ ___ _____

   c. Clamped catheter tubing below soft injection port with screw clamp (or folded catheter tubing onto itself and secured with rubber band). ___ ___ ___ _____

   d. Using circular motion, cleaned catheter port (specimen port) with antiseptic swab. ___ ___ ___ _____

   e. Inserted tip of needleless syringe into port using twisting motion. ___ ___ ___ _____

580

	S	U	NP	Comments
f. Injected solution using slow, even pressure.	___	___	___	_____
g. Removed syringe and clamp (or rubber band), allowing solution to drain into urinary drainage bag.	___	___	___	_____
6. Anchored catheter with catheter securement device.	___	___	___	_____
7. Helped patient to comfortable position.	___	___	___	_____
8. Placed nurse call system in an accessible location within patient's reach.	___	___	___	_____
9. Raised side rails (as appropriate) and lowered bed to lowest position, locking into position.	___	___	___	_____
10. Disposed of all contaminated supplies in appropriate receptacle, removed and disposed of gloves, and performed hand hygiene.	___	___	___	_____

EVALUATION

	S	U	NP	Comments
1. Measured actual urine output by subtracting total amount of irrigation fluid infused from total volume drained into basin.	___	___	___	_____
2. Reviewed I&O flow sheet to verify that hourly output into drainage bag was in appropriate proportion to irrigating solution entering bladder. Expected more output than fluid instilled because of urine production.	___	___	___	_____
3. Inspected urine for blood clots and sediment and ensured that tubing was not kinked or occluded.	___	___	___	_____
4. Evaluated patient's comfort level.	___	___	___	_____
5. Monitored for signs and symptoms of infection.	___	___	___	_____
6. Used Teach-Back. Revised instruction if patient or family caregiver was not able to teach back correctly.	___	___	___	_____

DOCUMENTATION

	S	U	NP	Comments
1. Documented irrigation method, amount of and type of irrigation solution, amount returned as drainage, characteristics of output, and urine output.	___	___	___	_____
2. Documented I&O.	___	___	___	_____
3. Documented evaluation of patient learning.	___	___	___	_____

HAND-OFF REPORTING

	S	U	NP	Comments
1. Reported status of urine output, catheter occlusion, sudden bleeding, infection, or increased pain.	___	___	___	_____

PERFORMANCE CHECKLIST SKILL 33.4   **APPLYING AN INCONTINENCE DEVICE**

	S	U	NP	Comments

ASSESSMENT

1. Identified patient using at least two identifiers, according to agency policy.

2. Reviewed electronic health record (EHR) and assessed urinary pattern, ability to empty bladder effectively, and degree of urinary continence.

3. Reviewed EHR for history of allergy to rubber or latex. Checked patient's allergy wristband and confirmed with patient.

4. Reviewed EHR to determine patient's age and history of dehydration, malnutrition, exposure to radiation therapy, underlying chronic conditions, and edema of the skin.

5. Assessed patient's/family caregiver's health literacy.

6. Performed hand hygiene and applied clean gloves. Assessed skin of penis or genitalia for rashes, erythema, and/or open areas. (This may have been deferred until just before device application.)

7. Verified patient's size and type of male incontinence device from plan of care or used manufacturer measuring guide to measure length and diameter of penis in flaccid state (applied gloves for measurement). Removed and disposed of gloves and performed hand hygiene.

8. Assessed patient's knowledge and prior experience with and feelings about an incontinence device.

PLANNING

1. Determined expected outcomes following completion of procedure.

2. Provided privacy and explained procedure to patient. Discussed the type of device, why it was being placed, and how to manage the device.

3. Obtained and organized equipment at bedside.

	S	U	NP	Comments

IMPLEMENTATION

1. Performed hand hygiene.

2. Raised bed to appropriate working height. Lowered side rail on working side.

3. Condom catheter: Prepared urinary drainage collection bag and tubing (large-volume drainage bag or leg bag). Clamped off drainage bag port. Placed nearby, ready to attach to condom after applied.

4. Helped patient to supine or sitting position. Placed bath blanket over upper torso. Folded sheets so only penis was exposed.

5. Applied clean gloves. Provided perineal care. Dried thoroughly before applying device. In uncircumcised male, ensured that foreskin was replaced to normal position before applying condom catheter. Did not apply barrier cream.

6. Removed and disposed of gloves. Performed hand hygiene. Reapplied clean gloves.

7. Clipped hair at base of penis as needed before application of condom sheath.

8. Applied incontinence device

   a. **Condom catheter.** With nondominant hand, grasped penis along shaft. With dominant hand, held rolled condom sheath at tip of penis with head of penis in cone. Smoothly rolled sheath onto penis. Allowed 2.5 to 5 cm (1–2 inches) of space between tip of glans penis and end of condom catheter.

   b. **Hydrocolloid device.** Placed the device onto the tip of the penis, not the shaft, per manufacturer directions.

9. Applied appropriate securement device as indicated in manufacturer guidelines.

   a. Self-adhesive condom catheters: After application, applied gentle pressure on penile shaft for 10 to 15 seconds.

   b. Outer securing strip-type condom catheters: Spiral wrapped penile shaft with strip of supplied elastic adhesive. Strip should not have overlapped itself. Elastic strip should have been snug, not tight.

   c. Hydrocolloid incontinence device: Removed release papers from adhesive on faceplate of device. Centered faceplate over opening of urinary meatus. Smoothed hydrocolloid adhesive backing strips onto tip of penis. Then covered with hydrocolloid seal.

	S	U	NP	Comments

10. Removed hair guard if used. Connected drainage tubing to end of condom catheter. Ensured that condom was not twisted. If using large drainage bag, placed excess tubing on bed and secured to bottom sheet.   ___ ___ ___ _____

11. Prepared PureWick Urine Collection System: ___ ___ ___ _____

   a. Plugged the power cord into device outlet and into an A/C power outlet. NOTE: Ensured the power switch was in the OFF position.   ___ ___ ___ _____

   b. Inserted the collection canister into the base of device and pressed the lid down firmly, ensuring the lid was sealed.   ___ ___ ___ _____

   c. Attached the short pump tubing to the PureWick Urine Collection System connector port and to the connector port on canister lid.   ___ ___ ___ _____

   d. Attached the elbow connector to the long collector tubing, then attached other end of the elbow connector to the connector port on canister lid.   ___ ___ ___ _____

   e. Connected the PureWick Female External Catheter to the PureWick Urine Collection canister: ___ ___ ___ _____

   (1) Performed hand hygiene and applied clean gloves. Performed perineal care and assessed skin integrity.   ___ ___ ___ _____

   (2) Separated the patient's legs, gluteus muscles, and labia.   ___ ___ ___ _____

   (3) With the soft gauze side of the device facing the patient, aligned the distal end of the PureWick Female External Catheter at the gluteal cleft.   ___ ___ ___ _____

   (4) Gently tucked the soft gauze side between the gluteus and labia. Ensured that the top of the gauze was aligned to the pubic bone.   ___ ___ ___ _____

   (5) Slowly placed the legs back together once the PureWick Female External Catheter was positioned.   ___ ___ ___ _____

12. Helped patient to a comfortable position.   ___ ___ ___ _____

13. Placed nurse call system in an accessible location within patient's reach.   ___ ___ ___ _____

14. Raised side rails (as appropriate) and lowered bed to lowest position, locking into position.   ___ ___ ___ _____

	S	U	NP	Comments

15. Disposed of all contaminated supplies in appropriate receptacle, removed and disposed of gloves, and performed hand hygiene. ___ ___ ___ _____

16. Removed and reapplied condom catheter daily following Steps 8 to 10 unless an extended-wear device was used. To remove condom, washed penis with warm, soapy water and gently rolled sheath and adhesive off penile shaft. ___ ___ ___ _____

17. Removed and replaced PureWick Female External Catheter every 8 to 12 hours or if soiled with feces or blood. Performed perineal care before replacement of system.

EVALUATION

1. Observed urinary drainage. ___ ___ ___ _____

2. Inspected penis with condom catheter in place within 15 to 30 minutes after application. Assessed for swelling and discoloration and asked patient if there was any discomfort. ___ ___ ___ _____

3. Inspected skin on penile shaft or genitalia for signs of erythema, irritation, or skin breakdown at least daily, when performing hygiene, and before reapplying condom or Purewick Female External Catheter. ___ ___ ___ _____

4. Used Teach-Back. Revised instruction if patient or family caregiver was not able to teach back correctly. ___ ___ ___ _____

DOCUMENTATION

1. Documented condom/device application; condition of genitalia or penis, skin, and scrotum; urinary output and voiding pattern; patient response to external catheter application, and patient learning. ___ ___ ___ _____

HAND-OFF REPORTING

1. During hand-off report, communicated condition of skin and incontinence device. ___ ___ ___ _____

2. Reported erythema, rashes, or skin breakdown to health care provider. ___ ___ ___ _____

Student _____ Date _____

Instructor _____ Date _____

PERFORMANCE CHECKLIST SKILL 33.5 **SUPRAPUBIC CATHETER CARE**

	S	U	NP	Comments

ASSESSMENT

1. Identified patient using at least two identifiers, according to agency policy. ___ ___ ___ _____

2. Reviewed electronic health record (EHR) for history of allergies. ___ ___ ___ _____

3. Reviewed EHR to determine patient's age and history of dehydration, malnutrition, exposure to radiation therapy, underlying chronic conditions, and edema of the skin.

4. Assessed patient's/family caregiver's health literacy.

5. Assessed urine in drainage bag for amount, clarity, color, odor, and sediment. ___ ___ ___ _____

6. Performed hand hygiene and applied clean gloves. Observed dressing around catheter insertion site for drainage and intactness. ___ ___ ___ _____

7. Removed outer dressing and disposed of it in proper receptacle. Assessed catheter insertion site (may have been deferred until you cleaned site) for signs of inflammation and for growth of overgranulation tissue. Asked patient if there was any pain at site; if so, had patient rate pain on scale of 0 to 10. Removed and disposed of gloves and performed hand hygiene. ___ ___ ___ _____

8. Assessed for elevated temperature and chills. ___ ___ ___ _____

9. Assessed patient's knowledge of, prior experience with, and feelings about management of a suprapubic catheter. ___ ___ ___ _____

PLANNING

1. Determined expected outcomes following completion of procedure. ___ ___ ___ _____

2. Provided privacy and explained procedure to patient. Discussed signs and symptoms of UTI and MARSI. If applicable, taught patient and family caregiver how to perform suprapubic catheter hygiene. ___ ___ ___ _____

3. Obtained and organized equipment at bedside. ___ ___ ___ _____

IMPLEMENTATION

1. Performed hand hygiene. ___ ___ ___ _____

586

	S	U	NP	Comments

2. Raised bed to appropriate working height. If side rails were raised, lowered side rail on working side. ___ ___ ___ _____

3. Prepared supplies and opened gauze packets in same manner as for applying dry dressing. ___ ___ ___ _____

4. Applied clean gloves. Loosened tape and removed existing dressing. Noted presence and type of drainage. Removed and disposed of gloves and performed hand hygiene. ___ ___ ___ _____

5. Cleaned insertion site using sterile aseptic technique for newly established catheter: *Option*: reviewed agency policy or considered individual patient need. In some agencies, clean gloves are appropriate. ___ ___ ___ _____

   a. Applied sterile gloves, per agency policy. ___ ___ ___ _____

   b. Without creating tension, held catheter up with nondominant hand while cleaning. Used sterile gauze moistened in saline and cleaned skin around insertion site in circular motion, starting near insertion site and continuing in outward widening circles. Used new sterile gauze for each circular swipe out to approximately 5 cm (2 inches). ___ ___ ___ _____

   c. With fresh, moistened gauze, gently cleaned base of catheter, moving up and away from site of insertion (proximal to distal). ___ ___ ___ _____

   d. Once insertion site was dry, used sterile gloved hand to apply drain dressing (split gauze) around catheter. Taped in place. ___ ___ ___ _____

6. Cleaned insertion site using medical aseptic technique for long-term/established catheter: ___ ___ ___ _____

   a. Applied clean gloves. ___ ___ ___ _____

   b. Without creating tension, held catheter erect with nondominant hand while cleaning. Cleaned with soap and water in circular motion, starting near catheter insertion site and continuing in outward widening circles for approximately 5 cm (2 inches). ___ ___ ___ _____

   c. With a fresh washcloth or gauze, gently cleaned base of catheter, moving up and away from site of insertion (proximal to distal). ___ ___ ___ _____

   d. *Option:* Applied drain dressing (split gauze) around catheter and taped in place. ___ ___ ___ _____

7. Secured catheter to lateral abdomen with tape or hook-and-loop fastener multipurpose tube holder. ___ ___ ___ _____

	S	U	NP	Comments

8. Coiled excess tubing on bed. Kept drainage bag below level of bladder at all times.

9. Helped patient to comfortable position.

10. Placed nurse call system in an accessible location within patient's reach.

11. Raised side rails (as appropriate) and lowered bed to lowest position, locking into position.

12. Disposed of all contaminated supplies in appropriate receptacle, removed and disposed of gloves, and performed hand hygiene.

EVALUATION

1. Asked patient to describe discomfort from suprapubic catheter and rate severity on scale of 0 to 10.

2. Monitored for signs of infection and observed urine for clarity, sediment, unusual color, or odor.

3. Observed catheter insertion site for erythema, edema, discharge, or tenderness. Checked dressing at minimum of every 8 hours.

4. If catheter was secured with adhesive device, evaluated for presence of MARSI.

5. Used Teach-Back. Revised instruction if patient or family caregiver was not able to teach back correctly.

DOCUMENTATION

1. Documented condition of insertion site, character of urine, type of dressing change, and patient's comfort level with the catheter and dressing change.

2. Documented urine output on I&O. In a situation in which there was both a suprapubic and a urethral catheter, documented outputs from each catheter separately.

3. Documented evaluation of patient learning.

HAND-OFF REPORTING

1. Reported condition of insertion site, character of urine, type of dressing change, and patient's comfort level with the catheter and dressing change.

2. Reported any complications with catheter to health care provider.

Student _____ Date _____

Instructor _____ Date _____

PERFORMANCE CHECKLIST PROCEDURAL GUIDELINE 34.1 **PROVIDING AND POSITIONING A BEDPAN**

	S	U	NP	Comments
PROCEDURAL STEPS				
1. Assessed patient's normal bowel elimination habits.	___	___	___	_____
2. Determined need for stool specimen prior to bedpan use.	___	___	___	_____
3. Performed hand hygiene.	___	___	___	_____
4. Assessed patient to determine level of mobility.	___	___	___	_____
5. Assessed patient's level of comfort.	___	___	___	_____
6. Provided privacy by closing curtains around bed or door of room.	___	___	___	_____
7. Applied clean gloves. Inspected condition of perianal and perineal skin. Removed gloves and performed hand hygiene.	___	___	___	_____
8. For patient comfort prepared metal bedpan by running warm water over it for a few minutes.	___	___	___	_____
9. Applied clean gloves.	___	___	___	_____
10. Raised side rail on opposite side of bed.	___	___	___	_____
11. Raised bed horizontally according to nurse's height.	___	___	___	_____
12. Assisted patient to the supine position.	___	___	___	_____
13. Placed patient who could assist on bedpan.	___	___	___	_____
a. Raised head of patient's bed 30–60 degrees.	___	___	___	_____
b. Removed upper bed linens so they were out of the way, but did not expose patient.	___	___	___	_____
c. Had patient flex knees and lift hips upward.	___	___	___	_____
d. Placed hand closest to patient's head palm up under patient's sacrum to help lift. Asked patient to bend knees and raise hips. As patient raised hips, used other hand to slip bedpan under patient. Ensured that open rim of bedpan was facing toward foot of bed. Did not force bedpan under patient's knees.	___	___	___	_____

	S	U	NP	Comments

e. Optional: If using fracture pan, slipped it under patient as hips were raised. Ensured that deep, open, lower end of bedpan was facing toward foot of bed. ___ ___ ___ _____

14. Placed patient who was immobile or had mobility restrictions on bedpan. ___ ___ ___ _____

   a. Lowered head of bed flat or raised head slightly (if tolerated by medical condition). ___ ___ ___ _____

   b. Removed top linens as necessary to turn patient while minimizing exposure. ___ ___ ___ _____

   c. Assisted patient to roll onto side with back toward nurse. Placed bedpan firmly against patient's buttocks and down into mattress. Ensured that open rim of bedpan was facing toward foot of bed. ___ ___ ___ _____

   d. Kept one hand against bedpan; placed other hand around far hip of patient. Helped patient to roll back onto bedpan, flat in bed. Did not force pan under patient. ___ ___ ___ _____

   e. Raised patient's head 30 degrees or to a comfortable level (unless contraindicated). ___ ___ ___ _____

   f. Had patient bend knees (unless contraindicated). ___ ___ ___ _____

15. Maintained patient's comfort, privacy, and safety. Covered patient for warmth. Placed small pillow or rolled towel under lumbar curve of back. ___ ___ ___ _____

16. Placed nurse call system in an accessible location within patient's reach. Ensured toilet tissue was within reach for patient. ___ ___ ___ _____

17. Raised side rails (as appropriate) and lowered bed to lowest position, locking into position. ___ ___ ___ _____

18. Removed and disposed of supplies and gloves and performed hand hygiene. ___ ___ ___ _____

19. Left the room. Allowed patient to be alone, but monitored status and responded promptly. ___ ___ ___ _____

20. Removed bedpan: ___ ___ ___ _____

   a. Performed hand hygiene and applied clean gloves. ___ ___ ___ _____

   b. Maintained privacy; determined if patient was able to wipe own perineal area. If nurse cleaned perineal area, used clean gloves and several layers of toilet tissue or disposable washcloths. For female patients, cleaned from mons pubis toward rectal area. ___ ___ ___ _____

590

	S	U	NP	Comments

c. Deposited contaminated tissue in bedpan if no specimen or intake and output (I&O) was needed.
_____ _____ _____ _____

d. For mobile patient: Asked patient to flex knees, placing body weight on lower legs, feet, and upper torso; lifted buttocks up from bedpan. At same time, placed hand farther from patient on side of bedpan to support it (prevent spillage) and placed other hand (closer to patient) under sacrum to help lift. Had patient lift and remove bedpan.
_____ _____ _____ _____

e. For immobile patient: Lowered head of bed. Helped patient roll onto side away from nurse and off bedpan. Held bedpan flat and steady while patient was rolling off. Placed bedpan on draped bedside chair and covered.
_____ _____ _____ _____

f. Assisted patient with hand and perineal hygiene as needed.
_____ _____ _____ _____

g. Changed soiled linens, removed and disposed of gloves, performed hand hygiene, and returned patient to comfortable position.
_____ _____ _____ _____

h. Raised side rails (as appropriate) and lowered bed to lowest position, locking into position.
_____ _____ _____ _____

i. Placed nurse call system in an accessible location within patient's reach.
_____ _____ _____ _____

j. Placed drinking water, and desired personal items within easy access.
_____ _____ _____ _____

21. Option: Obtained stool specimen as ordered. Wore clean gloves when emptying contents of bedpan into toilet or in special receptacle in utility room. Used spray faucet attached to most institution toilets to rinse bedpan thoroughly. Used disinfectant if required by agency; stored pan. Removed and disposed of gloves. Performed hand hygiene.
_____ _____ _____ _____

22. Used Teach-Back. Revised instruction if patient or family caregiver was not able to teach back correctly.
_____ _____ _____ _____

23. Assessed and recorded characteristics of stool. Noted color, odor, consistency, frequency, amount, shape, and constituents.
_____ _____ _____ _____

24. Included in hand-off report if patient voided in bedpan. Reported any skin irritation, discoloration, or break in skin integrity noted when cleansing patient.
_____ _____ _____ _____

PERFORMANCE CHECKLIST PROCEDURAL GUIDELINE 34.2 **REMOVING FECAL IMPACTION DIGITALLY**

	S	U	NP	Comments

PROCEDURAL STEPS

1. Identified patient using at least two identifiers.

2. Assessed patient's/family caregiver's health literacy.

3. Performed hand hygiene, pulled curtains around bed, obtained patient's baseline vital signs and assessed level of comfort, and palpated for abdominal distention before the procedure.

4. Explained the procedure and helped patient lie on left side in the lateral position with knees flexed and back toward the nurse.

5. Applied clean gloves. Draped trunk and lowered extremities with a bath blanket and placed a waterproof pad under buttocks. Kept a bedpan next to patient.

6. Lubricated index finger of dominant hand with water-soluble lubricant.

7. Instructed patient to take slow, deep breaths. Gradually and gently inserted index finger into the rectum and advanced the finger slowly along the rectal wall.

8. Gently loosened the fecal mass by massaging around it. Worked the finger into the hardened mass.

9. Worked the feces downward toward the end of the rectum. Removed small pieces one at a time and discarded into bedpan.

10. Periodically reassessed patient's pulse and looked for signs of fatigue. Stopped the procedure if pulse rate dropped significantly or rhythm changed.

11. Continued to clear rectum of feces and allowed patient to rest at intervals.

12. After completion, washed and dried buttocks and anal area.

	S	U	NP	Comments
13. Removed bedpan; inspected feces for color and consistency. Disposed of feces. Removed gloves by turning them inside out and then discarded.	___	___	___	_____
14. Helped patient to toilet or onto a bedpan if urge to defecate developed.	___	___	___	_____
15. Performed hand hygiene.	___	___	___	_____
16. Followed procedure with enemas or cathartics as ordered by health care provider.	___	___	___	_____
17. Helped patient to a comfortable position. Reassessed patient's vital signs and level of comfort and observed status of abdominal distention.	___	___	___	_____
18. Placed nurse call system in an accessible location within patient's reach.	___	___	___	_____
19. Raised side rails (as appropriate) and lowered bed to lowest position, locking into position.	___	___	___	_____
20. Used Teach-Back. Revised instruction if patient or family caregiver was not able to teach back correctly.	___	___	___	_____
21. Documented patient's tolerance of procedure, fecal characteristics, amount of stool removed, vital signs, and adverse effects.	___	___	___	_____
22. Reported any changes in vital signs and adverse effects to health care provider.	___	___	___	_____

Student _____   Date _____

Instructor _____   Date _____

PERFORMANCE CHECKLIST SKILL 34.1   **ADMINISTERING AN ENEMA**

	S	U	NP	Comments

ASSESSMENT

1. Identified patient using at least two identifiers.

2. Reviewed health care provider's order for enema and clarified reason for administration.

3. Assessed patient's/family caregiver's health literacy.

4. Checked electronic health record (EHR) to assess last bowel movement, normal versus most recent bowel pattern, presence of hemorrhoids, and presence of abdominal pain or cramping.

5. Assessed patient's mobility and ability to turn and position on side.

6. Assessed patient for allergy to any active ingredients of prepackaged enema.

7. Performed hand hygiene.

8. Inspected and palpated abdomen for presence of distention.

9. Assessed patient's knowledge, prior experience with enemas, and feelings about procedure.

PLANNING

1. Determined expected outcomes following completion of procedure.

2. Explained enema administration procedure to patient and/or caregiver. Provided privacy and performed hand hygiene.

3. Arranged supplies at bedside. Placed bedpan or bedside commode in easily accessible position. If patient would be expelling contents in toilet, ensured that toilet was available and placed patient's nonskid slippers and bathrobe in easily accessible position.

	S	U	NP	Comments

IMPLEMENTATION

1. Checked accuracy and completeness of each medication administration record (MAR) with health care provider's written order. Checked patient's name, type of enema, and time for administration. Compared MAR with label of enema solution. ___ ___ ___ _____

2. Performed hand hygiene. Applied clean gloves. ___ ___ ___ _____

3. With side rail raised on patient's right side and bed raised to appropriate working height, helped patient turn onto left side-lying position with right knee flexed. Determined that patient was comfortable and encouraged patient to remain in position until procedure was complete. Placed a child in the dorsal recumbent position. ___ ___ ___ _____

4. Placed waterproof pad, absorbent side up, under hips and buttocks. Covered patient with bath blanket, exposing only rectal area, clearly visualizing anus. ___ ___ ___ _____

5. Separated buttocks and examined perianal region for abnormalities, including hemorrhoids, anal fissure, and rectal prolapse. ___ ___ ___ _____

6. Administered enema. Verbalized to patient when buttocks would be touched and tubing inserted. ___ ___ ___ _____

   a. Administered prepackaged disposable enema: ___ ___ ___ _____

      (1) Removed plastic cap from tip of container. Applied more water-soluble lubricant as needed. ___ ___ ___ _____

      (2) Gently separated buttocks and located anus. Instructed patient to relax by breathing out slowly through mouth. Informed patient when tip was to be inserted. ___ ___ ___ _____

      (3) Held container upright and expelled any air from enema container. ___ ___ ___ _____

      (4) Inserted lubricated tip of container gently into anal canal toward umbilicus. ___ ___ ___ _____

      (5) Squeezed and rolled plastic bottle from bottom to tip until all of solution entered rectum and colon. Instructed patient to retain solution until urge to defecate occurred, usually in 2–5 min. ___ ___ ___ _____

   b. Administered enema in standard enema bag: ___ ___ ___ _____

      (1) Added warmed prescribed type of solution and amount to enema bag. Warmed tap water as it flowed from faucet. Placed saline container in basin of warm water before adding saline to enema bag. Checked temperature of solution by pouring small amount of solution over inner wrist. ___ ___ ___ _____

	S	U	NP	Comments

(2) If soapsuds enema (SSE) was ordered, added castile soap after water.

(3) Raised container, released clamp, and allowed solution to flow long enough to fill tubing.

(4) Reclamped tubing.

(5) Lubricated 6–8 cm (2½–3 inches) of tip of rectal tube with lubricant.

(6) Gently separated buttocks and located anus. Verbalized when enema tip was going to be inserted. Instructed patient to relax by breathing out slowly through mouth. Touched patient's skin next to anus with tip of rectal tube.

(7) Inserted tip of rectal tube slowly by pointing it in direction of patient's umbilicus.

(8) Held tubing in rectum constantly until end of fluid instillation.

(9) Opened regulating clamp and allowed solution to enter slowly with container at patient's hip level.

(10) Raised height of enema container slowly to appropriate level above anus: 30–45 cm (12–18 inches) for high enema; 30 cm (12 inches) for regular enema; 7.5 cm (3 inches) for low enema. May have used an IV pole to hold an enema bag once a slow flow of fluid was established.

(11) Instilled all solution and clamped tubing. Told patient that procedure was completed and that the tubing would be removed.

7. Placed layers of toilet tissue around tube at anus and gently withdrew rectal tube and tip.

8. Explained to patient that some distention and abdominal cramping are normal. Asked the patient to retain solution as long as possible until urge to defecate occured. Stayed at bedside. Had patient lie quietly in bed if possible. (For infant or young child, gently held buttocks together for a few minutes.)

9. Discarded enema container or disposable bag and tubing in proper receptacle. Removed and discarded gloves and performed hand hygiene.

10. Helped patient to bathroom or commode if possible. If using bedpan, applied clean gloves and helped patient to as near a normal position for evacuation as possible.

	S	U	NP	Comments

11. Observed character of stool and solution (instructed patient not to flush toilet before inspection). ___ ___ ___ _____

12. Helped patient as needed to wash anal area with warm soap and water (used gloves for perineal care). ___ ___ ___ _____

13. Removed and disposed of gloves and performed hand hygiene. ___ ___ ___ _____

14. Helped patient to a comfortable position. ___ ___ ___ _____

15. Placed nurse call system in an accessible location within patient's reach. ___ ___ ___ _____

16. Raised side rails (as appropriate) and lowered bed to lowest position, locking into position. ___ ___ ___ _____

EVALUATION

1. Inspected color, consistency, and amount of stool; odor; and fluid passed. ___ ___ ___ _____

2. Palpated for abdominal distention. ___ ___ ___ _____

3. Used Teach-Back. Revised instruction if patient or family caregiver was not able to teach back correctly. ___ ___ ___ _____

DOCUMENTATION

1. Documented the time, type, and volume of enema administered; patient's signs and symptoms; response to enema; and results, including color, amount, and appearance of stool. ___ ___ ___ _____

HAND-OFF REPORTING

1. Reported to health care provider failure of patient to defecate or any adverse reactions. ___ ___ ___ _____

PERFORMANCE CHECKLIST SKILL 34.2   **INSERTION, MAINTENANCE, AND REMOVAL OF A NASOGASTRIC TUBE FOR GASTRIC DECOMPRESSION**

	S	U	NP	Comments

ASSESSMENT

1. Identified patient using at least two identifiers.

2. Verified health care provider order for type of NG tube to be placed and whether tube was to be attached to suction or drainage bag.

3. Assessed patient's level of consciousness and ability to follow instructions.

4. Assessed patient's/family caregiver's health literacy.

5. Asked patient or family caregiver about history of allergies and type of allergic reaction.

6. Performed hand hygiene and applied gloves. Inspected condition of skin integrity around patient's nares and nasal and oral cavity.

7. Asked if patient had history of nasal surgery or congestion and allergies and noted if deviated nasal septum was present.

8. Auscultated for bowel sounds. Palpated patient's abdomen for distention, pain, and rigidity. Removed and disposed of gloves and performed hand hygiene.

9. Determined if patient had previous NG tube and, if so, which naris was used.

10. Assessed patient's knowledge, prior experience with NG tubes, and feelings about procedure.

11. Assessed patient's goals or preferences for how skill was to be performed or what patient expected.

PLANNING

1. Determined expected outcomes following completion of procedure.

2. Explained procedure. Informed patient that procedure might make them gag and that there would be a burning sensation in nasopharynx as tube was passed. Developed hand signal with patient.

3. Provided privacy. Organized and set up any equipment needed to perform procedure.

598

	S	U	NP	Comments

IMPLEMENTATION

1. Performed hand hygiene and applied gloves. Raised the bed to working height. Positioned patient upright in high Fowler position unless contraindicated. If patient was comatose, raised head of bed as tolerated, with patient in semi-Fowler position and head tipped forward, chin to chest.   ___ ___ ___ _____

2. Placed bath towel over patient's chest; gave facial tissues to patient. Allowed to blow nose if necessary. Placed emesis basin within reach.   ___ ___ ___ _____

3. Washed bridge of nose with soap and water or alcohol swab. Dried thoroughly.   ___ ___ ___ _____

4. Stood on patient's right side if right-handed, left side if left-handed. Lowered side rail.   ___ ___ ___ _____

5. Instructed patient to relax and breathe normally while occluding one naris. Then repeated this action for other naris. Selected nostril with greater airflow.   ___ ___ ___ _____

6. Determined length of tube to be inserted and marked location with tape or indelible ink.   ___ ___ ___ _____

   a. Option for Adult: Measured distance from tip of nose to earlobe to xiphoid process (NEX) of sternum. Marked this distance on tube with tape.   ___ ___ ___ _____

   b. Option for Adult: Measured distance from tip of nose to earlobe to mid-umbilicus (NEMU).   ___ ___ ___ _____

   c. Option for Adult: Measured distance from xiphoid process to earlobe to nose (XEN) + 10 cm (4 inches).   ___ ___ ___ _____

   d. Option for Child: Used the NEMU method.   ___ ___ ___ _____

   e. Added 20 to 30 cm (8—12 inches) for postpyloric tube.   ___ ___ ___ _____

7. With small piece of tape placed around tube, marked length that would be inserted.   ___ ___ ___ _____

8. Prepared materials for tube fixation. Tore off a 7.5- to 10-cm (3- to 4-inch) length of hypoallergenic tape, or open membrane dressing or another fixation device.   ___ ___ ___ _____

9. Removed and disposed of gloves. Performed hand hygiene and applied clean gloves.   ___ ___ ___ _____

10. Applied pulse oximetry/capnography device and measured vital signs. Monitored oximetry/capnography during insertion.   ___ ___ ___ _____

11. Option: Dipped tube with surface lubricant into glass of room temperature water or lubricate 7.5–10 cm (3–4 inches) of end of tube with water-soluble lubricant.   ___ ___ ___ _____

12. Handed an alert patient a cup of water if able to hold cup and swallow. Explained that tube was about to be inserted.

   ___ ___ ___ _____

13. Explained next steps. Inserted tube gently and slowly through naris to back of throat (posterior nasopharynx). Aimed back and down toward patient's ear.

   ___ ___ ___ _____

14. Had patient relax and flex head toward chest after tube was passed through nasopharynx.

   ___ ___ ___ _____

15. Encouraged patient to swallow by taking small sips of water when possible. Advanced tube as patient swallowed. Rotated tube gently 180 degrees while inserting.

   ___ ___ ___ _____

16. Emphasized need to mouth breathe during procedure.

   ___ ___ ___ _____

17. Did not advance tube during inspiration or coughing. Monitored oximetry/capnography.

   ___ ___ ___ _____

18. Advanced tube each time patient swallowed until reaching desired length.

   ___ ___ ___ _____

19. Using penlight and tongue blade, checked to be sure that tube was not positioned in back of throat.

   ___ ___ ___ _____

20. Temporarily anchored tube to nose with small piece of tape.

   ___ ___ ___ _____

21. Verified tube placement. Checked agency policy for recommended methods of checking tube placement.

   ___ ___ ___ _____

   a. Followed order for bedside x-ray study and notified radiology department for examination of chest and abdomen.

   ___ ___ ___ _____

   b. While waiting for x-ray film, followed these procedures: Attached Asepto or catheter-tipped syringe to end of tube. Aspirated gently back on syringe to obtain gastric contents, observing amount, color, and quality of return.

   ___ ___ ___ _____

   c. Used pH test paper to measure aspirate for pH with color-coded pH paper. Ensured that paper range of pH is at least 1.0–11.0.

   ___ ___ ___ _____

22. After tube was properly inserted and positioned, either clamped end or connected it to drainage bag or suction source. Anchored tube with a fixation device, avoiding pressure on the nares. Selected one of the following fixation methods.

   ___ ___ ___ _____

   a. Applied tape.

   ___ ___ ___ _____

     (1) Ensured skin on bridge of nose was dry, not oily.

   ___ ___ ___ _____

	S	U	NP	Comments

(2) Removed gloves. Tore two small horizontal slits at one-third and two-thirds length of tape without splitting tape. Folded middle sections toward each other to form a closed strip. ___ ___ ___ _____

(3) Tore vertical strip at bottom of tape. Printed date and time on tape and placed top end of tape over bridge of patient's nose. ___ ___ ___ _____

(4) Placed intact end of tape over bridge of patient's nose. Wrapped bottom end of tape around tube as it exited nose. ___ ___ ___ _____

b. Applied tube fixation device using shaped adhesive patch. Optionally placed a small strip of skin barrier directly on nose; applied patch over it. ___ ___ ___ _____

(1) Applied wide end of patch to bridge of nose. ___ ___ ___ _____

(2) Slipped connector around tube as it exited nose. ___ ___ ___ _____

23. Fastened end of NG tube to patient's gown using clip or piece of tape. Did not use safety pins to fasten tube to gown. ___ ___ ___ _____

24. Kept head of bed elevated 30–45 degrees (preferably 45 degrees) unless contraindicated. ___ ___ ___ _____

25. Assisted radiology staff as needed in obtaining ordered x-ray film of chest and abdomen. ___ ___ ___ _____

26. Removed and disposed of gloves, performed hand hygiene, and helped patient to comfortable position. Cleaned tubing at nostril with washcloth dampened in mild soap and water. Administered oral hygiene. ___ ___ ___ _____

27. Once placement was confirmed, measured amount of tube that was external and marked exit of tube at nares with indelible marker as guide for any tube displacement. Documented this information in electronic health record (EHR). ___ ___ ___ _____

28. Attached NG tube to suction as ordered. Confirmed suction settings any time the patient was disconnected or at the beginning of each nurse's shift. ___ ___ ___ _____

29. NG tube irrigation:

a. Performed hand hygiene and applied clean gloves. ___ ___ ___ _____

b. Verified tube placement in stomach by disconnecting NG tube, connecting irrigating syringe, and aspirating contents. Temporarily clamped NG tube or reconnected to connecting tube and removed syringe. ___ ___ ___ _____

c. Emptied syringe of aspirate and used it to draw up 30 mL of normal saline. ___ ___ ___ _____

	S	U	NP	Comments

d. Disconnected NG from connecting tubing and laid end of connection tubing on towel.

   ___ ___ ___ _____

e. Inserted tip of irrigating syringe into end of NG tube. Removed clamp. Held syringe with tip pointed at floor and injected saline slowly and evenly. Did not force solution.

   ___ ___ ___ _____

f. If resistance occurred, checked for kinks in tubing. Turned patient onto left side. Repeated resistance was reported to health care provider.

   ___ ___ ___ _____

g. After instilling saline, immediately aspirated or pulled back slowly on syringe to withdraw fluid. If amount aspirated was greater than amount instilled, documented difference as output. If amount aspirated was less than amount instilled, documented difference as intake.

   ___ ___ ___ _____

h. Used an Asepto syringe to place 10 mL of air into blue pigtail.

   ___ ___ ___ _____

i. Reconnected NG tube to drainage or suction. (Repeated irrigation if solution did not return.)

   ___ ___ ___ _____

30. Removal of NG tube:

a. Verified health care provider order to remove NG tube.

   ___ ___ ___ _____

b. Per agency policy, stopped suction briefly to auscultate abdomen for presence of bowel sounds or clamped the tube for a short period of time, assessing for nausea or discomfort.

   ___ ___ ___ _____

c. Provided privacy and explained procedure to patient, including that patient would be instructed to take a deep breath and hold it.

   ___ ___ ___ _____

d. Performed hand hygiene and applied clean gloves.

   ___ ___ ___ _____

e. Positioned patient in high-Fowler position unless contraindicated.

   ___ ___ ___ _____

f. Turned off suction and disconnected NG tube from drainage bag or suction. With irrigating syringe, inserted 20 mL of air into lumen of NG tube. Gently removed tape or fixation device from bridge of nose and patient's gown.

   ___ ___ ___ _____

g. Handed patient facial tissue; placed disposable towel across chest. Instructed patient to take and hold breath as tube was removed.

   ___ ___ ___ _____

h. Clamped or kinked tubing securely and pulled tube out steadily and smoothly into towel held in other hand while patient held breath.

   ___ ___ ___ _____

i. Inspected intactness of tube.

   ___ ___ ___ _____

	S	U	NP	Comments

j. Measured amount of drainage and noted character of content. Disposed of tube and drainage equipment into proper container.

k. Cleaned nares and provided oral hygiene.

l. Positioned patient comfortably and explained procedure for drinking fluids if not contraindicated. Instructed patient to notify nurse if nausea occurred.

31. For all procedures, cleaned equipment and returned to proper place. Placed soiled linen in utility room or proper receptacle.

32. Removed and disposed of gloves and performed hand hygiene.

33. Helped patient to a comfortable position

34. Placed nurse call system in an accessible location within patient's reach.

35. Raised side rails (as appropriate) and lowered bed to lowest position, locking into position.

EVALUATION

1. Observed amount and character of contents draining from NG tube. Asked if patient felt nauseated.

2. Auscultated for presence of bowel sounds. Turned off suction while auscultating. Assessed for nausea and patient discomfort if tube was clamped for short trial period.

3. Palpated patient's abdomen periodically. Noted any distention, pain, and rigidity.

4. Inspected condition of nares, nose, and all skin and tissue around NG tubing as per agency policy.

5. Observed position of tubing.

6. Explained that it was normal if patient felt sore throat or irritation in pharynx.

7. Used Teach-Back. Revised instruction if patient or family caregiver was not able to teach back correctly.

DOCUMENTATION

1. Documented length, size, and type of gastric tube inserted, and naris in which tube was introduced. Also documented patient's tolerance of procedure, confirmation of tube placement, character and pH of gastric contents, results of x-ray film, whether the tube was clamped or connected to drainage bag or to suction, and amount of suction supplied.

	S	U	NP	Comments

2. When irrigating NG tube, documented difference between amount of normal saline instilled and amount of gastric aspirate removed. Documented amount and character of contents draining from NG tube every shift. ____ ____ ____ _____

3. Documented removal of tube "intact," patient's tolerance of procedure, and final amount and character of drainage. ____ ____ ____ _____

HAND-OFF REPORTING

1. Set up a schedule to remove the tape and assess the skin and mucosa to avoid MDRPI and MARSI. ____ ____ ____ _____

2. Reported occurrence of abdominal distention, unexpected increase or sudden stoppage in gastric drainage, and patient complaint of gastric distress to health care provider. ____ ____ ____ _____

PERFORMANCE CHECKLIST SKILL 35.1   **POUCHING A COLOSTOMY OR AN ILEOSTOMY**

	S	U	NP	Comments
ASSESSMENT				
1. Identified patient using at least two identifiers.	___	___	___	_____
2. Assessed patient's/family caregiver's health literacy.	___	___	___	_____
3. Reviewed electronic health record (EHR) and assessed if patient was at risk for MARSI.	___	___	___	_____
4. Performed hand hygiene and applied clean gloves.	___	___	___	_____
5. Had patient assume semi-reclining or supine position. Observed existing skin barrier and pouch for leakage and checked EHR for length of time in place. If an opaque pouch was being used, removed it to fully observe stoma. Emptied and measured effluent and disposed of pouch in proper receptacle.	___	___	___	_____
6. Observed amount of effluent in pouch and emptied when it was one-third to one-half full by opening the pouch and draining it into a container for measurement of output. Noted consistency of effluent and documented output.	___	___	___	_____
7. Observed stoma if pouch was transparent for type, location, color, swelling, presence of sutures, trauma, and healing or irritation of peristomal skin.	___	___	___	_____
8. Inspected area for placement of stoma in relation to abdominal contours and presence of scars or incisions. Removed and disposed of gloves; performed hand hygiene.	___	___	___	_____
9. Assessed patient's knowledge, prior experience with stoma and ostomy care, and feelings about procedure.	___	___	___	_____
10. Discussed interest in learning self-care. Identified others who would be helping patient after leaving agency.	___	___	___	_____
PLANNING				
1. Determined expected outcomes following completion of procedure.	___	___	___	_____
2. Explained procedure to patient; encouraged patient's interaction and questions.	___	___	___	_____
3. Performed hand hygiene. Assembled equipment at bedside and closed room curtains or door.	___	___	___	_____

IMPLEMENTATION

S   U   NP   Comments

1. Made patient comfortable, continuing to assume semi-reclining or supine position. If possible, provided patient with mirror for observation. ___ ___ ___ _____

2. Performed hand hygiene and applied clean gloves. ___ ___ ___ _____

3. Placed towel or disposable waterproof barrier under patient and across patient's lower abdomen. ___ ___ ___ _____

4. If not done during assessment, removed used pouch and skin barrier gently by pushing skin away from barrier in direction of hair growth. Loosened and lifted the edge with one hand and pressed down on the skin near the sticky backing with the other hand. Used adhesive releaser to facilitate removal of skin barrier. Emptied pouch and disposed of it in an appropriate receptacle. ___ ___ ___ _____

5. Cleaned peristomal skin gently with warm tap water using washcloth; did not scrub skin. If stoma was touched, understood minor bleeding was normal. Patted skin dry. Had washcloth handy for additional cleaning if there was output from the stoma while preparing pouch. ___ ___ ___ _____

6. Measured stoma. Expected size of stoma to change for first 4–6 weeks after surgery. ___ ___ ___ _____

7. Traced pattern of stoma measurement on pouch backing or skin barrier. ___ ___ ___ _____

8. Cut opening on backing or skin barrier wafer. If using moldable or a shape-to-fit barrier, used fingers to mold shape-to-fit stoma. ___ ___ ___ _____

9. Removed protective backing from adhesive backing or wafer. ___ ___ ___ _____

10. Applied pouch over stoma. Pressed firmly into place around stoma and outside edges. Had patient hold hand over pouch to apply heat to secure seal. ___ ___ ___ _____

11. Closed end of pouch with clip or integrated closure. Removed drape from patient. Helped patient to assume comfortable position. ___ ___ ___ _____

12. Placed disposables in trash. Removed and disposed of gloves. Performed hand hygiene. ___ ___ ___ _____

13. Raised side rails as appropriate and lowered bed to lowest position, locking into position. ___ ___ ___ _____

14. Placed nurse call system in an accessible location within patient's reach. ___ ___ ___ _____

606

	S	U	NP	Comments

EVALUATION

1. Observed condition of skin barrier and adherence of pouch to abdominal surface. ____ ____ ____ _____

2. During pouch change, observed appearance of stoma, peristomal skin, abdominal contours, and suture line. ____ ____ ____ _____

3. Noted if there was presence of any flatus during pouch change. ____ ____ ____ _____

4. Observed patient's and family caregiver's willingness to view stoma and ask questions about procedure. ____ ____ ____ _____

5. Used Teach-Back technique. Revised instruction if patient or family caregiver were not able to teach back correctly. ____ ____ ____ _____

DOCUMENTATION

1. Documented type of pouch and skin barrier applied; time of procedure; amount and appearance of effluent in pouch; location, size and appearance of stoma; and condition of peristomal skin. ____ ____ ____ _____

2. Documented patient's and family caregiver's level of participation, teaching that was done, and response to teaching. ____ ____ ____ _____

HAND-OFF REPORTING

1. Reported any of the following to nurse and/or health care provider: abnormal appearance of stoma, suture line, peristomal skin, or character of output. ____ ____ ____ _____

Student _____ Date _____

Instructor _____ Date _____

PERFORMANCE CHECKLIST SKILL 35.2 **POUCHING A UROSTOMY**

	S	U	NP	Comments

ASSESSMENT

1. Identified patient using at least two identifiers.

2. Assessed patient's/family caregiver's health literacy.

3. Reviewed electronic health record (EHR) and assessed if patient was at risk for MARSI.

4. Performed hand hygiene and applied clean gloves.

5. Had patient assume semi-reclining or supine position. Observed existing skin barrier and pouch for leakage and length of time in place. If urine was leaking under wafer, changed pouch.

6. Observed characteristics of urine in pouch or bedside drainage bag. Emptied pouch before it was one-third to one-half full by opening valve and draining it into container for measurement.

7. Observed stoma for color, swelling, presence of sutures, trauma, and healing of peristomal skin. Assessed type of stoma. Removed and disposed of gloves. Performed hand hygiene.

8. Assessed patient's knowledge, prior experience with urostomy pouching, and feelings about procedure.

9. Explored patient's perceptions, acceptance of change in function, and interest in learning self-care. Identified others who would be helping patient after leaving hospital.

PLANNING

1. Determined expected outcomes following completion of procedure.

2. Explained procedure to patient; encouraged questions and interaction.

3. Performed hand hygiene. Assembled equipment at bedside and closed room curtains or door.

IMPLEMENTATION

1. Made patient comfortable, continuing to assume semi-reclining or supine position. If possible, provided patient with mirror for observation.

2. Performed hand hygiene and applied clean gloves.

608

	S	U	NP	Comments

3. Placed towel or disposable waterproof barrier under patient and across patient's lower abdomen.

4. If not done during assessment, removed used pouch and skin barrier gently by pushing skin away from barrier, away from direction of hair growth. Loosened and lifted the edge with one hand and pressed down on the skin near the sticky backing with the other hand. If stents were present, pulled pouch gently around them and laid towel underneath. Emptied pouch and measured output. Disposed of pouch in appropriate receptacle.

5. If stoma was draining continuously, used rolled gauze placed at stoma opening. Encouraged patient or family caregiver to hold gauze at stoma opening continuously during pouch measurement and change.

6. While keeping rolled gauze in contact with stoma, cleaned peristomal skin gently with warm tap water and washcloth; did not scrub skin. Understood that after touching stoma, minor bleeding was normal. Patted skin completely dry.

7. Measured stoma. Expected size of stoma to change for first 4–6 weeks after surgery.

8. Traced pattern on pouch backing or skin barrier.

9. Cut opening in pouch. If using a moldable or shape-to-fit barrier, used fingers to mold shape to shape-to-fit stoma.

10. Removed protective backing from adhesive backing or wafer surface. Removed rolled gauze from stoma.

11. Applied pouch. Pressed adhesive barrier firmly into place around stoma and outside edges. Had patient hold hand over pouch 1–2 min to secure seal.

12. Used adapter provided with pouches to connect pouch to bedside urinary bag. Kept tubing below level of bag.

13. Removed drape from patient. Helped patient to assume comfortable position.

14. Placed disposables in the trash. Removed and disposed of gloves. Performed hand hygiene.

15. Raised side rails as appropriate and lowered bed to lowest position, locking into position.

16. Placed nurse call system in an accessible location within patient's reach.

	S	U	NP	Comments

EVALUATION

1. Observed appearance of stoma, peristomal skin, and suture line during pouch change.

2. Evaluated character and volume of urinary drainage.

3. Observed patient's and family caregiver's willingness to view stoma and ask questions about procedure.

4. Used Teach-Back technique. Revised instruction if patient or family caregiver were not able to teach back correctly.

DOCUMENTATION

1. Documented type of pouch, time of change, condition and appearance of stoma/stents and peristomal skin, and character of urine.

2. Documented urinary output.

3. Documented patient's and family caregiver's reaction to stoma and level of participation. Documented evaluation of patient and family caregiver learning.

HAND-OFF REPORTING

1. Reported abnormalities in stoma or peristomal skin and absence of urinary output to nurse in charge or health care provider.

610

Student _____   Date _____

Instructor _____   Date _____

PERFORMANCE CHECKLIST SKILL 35.3   **CATHETERIZING A URINARY DIVERSION**

	S	U	NP	Comments

ASSESSMENT

1. Identified patient using at least two identifiers.

2. Reviewed electronic health record (EHR) and observed for signs and symptoms of urinary tract infection (UTI).

3. Obtained health care provider's order for catheterization.

4. Assessed patient's/family caregiver's health literacy.

5. Assessed patient's understanding of need for procedure and how it was done.

6. Assessed patient's knowledge, experience with urinary diversion catheterization, and feelings about procedure.

7. Assessed for allergies to antiseptics and substituted chlorhexidine for another antiseptic if patient showed a skin or allergic reaction to this solution. Had patient describe typical allergic response when allergy was identified.

PLANNING

1. Determined expected outcomes following completion of procedure.

2. Performed hand hygiene. Assembled equipment at bedside and closed room curtain or door.

3. Explained procedure to patient, including sensations that would be felt. If possible, obtained specimen when patient was due to change pouch if using one-piece system.

IMPLEMENTATION

1. If possible, positioned patient sitting and draped towel across lower abdomen.

2. Performed hand hygiene and applied clean gloves.

3. Removed pouch. If patient used two-piece system, removed pouch but left skin barrier attached to skin.

4. Removed and disposed of gloves and performed hand hygiene.

	S	U	NP	Comments

5. Opened sterile catheterization set according to instructions or opened needed equipment and placed on sterile barrier using aseptic technique. If not using catheterization kit, placed gauze pad on sterile field and squeezed small amount of lubricant onto gauze. Applied sterile gloves. ___ ___ ___ _____

6. If needed, had patient hold absorbent gauze wick on stoma while nurse prepared catheterization supplies. ___ ___ ___ _____

7. Cleaned surface of stoma with antiseptic swabs using circular motion from center outward. Used new swab each time; repeated twice. Allowed chlorhexidine antiseptic to dry completely or, or if another antiseptic was used, wiped off excess antiseptic with dry sterile gauze or cotton ball. ___ ___ ___ _____

8. Removed lid from sterile specimen container. ___ ___ ___ _____

9. Lubricated tip of catheter with water-soluble lubricant, keeping catheter sterile. ___ ___ ___ _____

10. With dominant hand, gently inserted catheter tip into stoma. Did not force catheter; redirected course as needed. Placed distal end of catheter into specimen container. Had patient cough; massaged abdomen near stoma or turned patient on side. ___ ___ ___ _____

11. Held container below level of stoma. If needed, waited several minutes to get adequate amount of urine. ___ ___ ___ _____

12. Withdrew catheter slowly; placed absorbent pad over stoma. ___ ___ ___ _____

13. Applied lid to specimen container. ___ ___ ___ _____

14. Reapplied new pouch or reattached pouch if patient used two-piece system. ___ ___ ___ _____

15. Disposed of used pouch and equipment properly. ___ ___ ___ _____

16. Removed and disposed of gloves; performed hand hygiene. Labeled specimen in presence of patient, placed in biohazard bag, and sent to laboratory at once. ___ ___ ___ _____

17. Helped patient to a comfortable position. ___ ___ ___ _____

18. Placed nurse call system in an accessible location within patient's reach. ___ ___ ___ _____

19. Raised side rails if appropriate and lowered bed to lowest position, locking into position. ___ ___ ___ _____

EVALUATION

1. Compared results of culture and sensitivity with expected findings. ___ ___ ___ _____

612

	S	U	NP	Comments

2. Used Teach-Back technique. Revised instruction if patient or family caregiver were not able to teach back correctly. ___ ___ ___ _____

DOCUMENTATION

1. Documented time specimen collected; patient's tolerance of procedure; and appearance of urine, skin, and stoma. ___ ___ ___ _____

2. Documented evaluation of patient and family caregiver learning. ___ ___ ___ _____

HAND-OFF REPORTING

1. Reported results of laboratory test to nurse in charge or health care provider. ___ ___ ___ _____

PERFORMANCE CHECKLIST SKILL 36.1   **PREOPERATIVE ASSESSMENT**

	S	U	NP	Comments

ASSESSMENT

1. Identified patient using at least two identifiers. ___ ___ ___ _____

2. Performed hand hygiene. Prepared equipment and room for assessment. ___ ___ ___ _____

3. Assessed patient's/family caregiver's health literacy. ___ ___ ___ _____

4. Determined if patient had any communication impairment, could read and understand English, and was mentally competent. Obtained a professional interpreter if needed. ___ ___ ___ _____

5. Assessed patient's understanding of the intended surgery and anesthesia. Asked patient to offer description rather than simple yes or no question. Asked about patient's and family caregiver's expectations of surgery and care. ___ ___ ___ _____

6. Asked about advance directives. ___ ___ ___ _____

7. Collected nursing history and identified surgical risk factors, including: ___ ___ ___ _____

   a. Condition requiring surgery ___ ___ ___ _____

   b. Chronic illnesses and risks ___ ___ ___ _____

   c. Presence of obstructive sleep apnea (OSA) ___ ___ ___ _____

   d. Last menstrual period, if appropriate ___ ___ ___ _____

   e. Previous hospitalizations ___ ___ ___ _____

   f. Full medication history, including prescription, over-the-counter (OTC), and herbal remedies, and date/time of last doses ___ ___ ___ _____

   g. Previous experience with surgery and anesthesia ___ ___ ___ _____

   h. Family history of complications from surgery or anesthesia ___ ___ ___ _____

   i. Patient history of chronic pain disorders and home treatments ___ ___ ___ _____

	S	U	NP	Comments
j. Allergies to medications, food, topical solutions or adhesives, and natural rubber latex	___	___	___	_____
k. Physical impairment	___	___	___	_____
l. Prostheses and implants	___	___	___	_____
m. Smoking, alcohol, and illicit drug use	___	___	___	_____
n. Occupation	___	___	___	_____
8. Obtained patient's weight, height, and vital signs.	___	___	___	_____
9. Assessed patient's respiratory status.	___	___	___	_____
10. Auscultated heart sounds and assessed patient's circulatory status, including apical pulse, ECG report, peripheral pulses, and capillary refill.	___	___	___	_____
11. Assessed for patient's risk for postoperative thrombus formation. Asked patient about any leg pain. Observed calves for swelling, warmth, redness, symmetry, and palpated pedal pulses	___	___	___	_____
12. Completed a gastrointestinal assessment; identified time of patient's last intake of food or drink.	___	___	___	_____
13. Completed neurological assessment; determined patient's neurological status, including level of consciousness (LOC), cognitive function, and sensation, and noted neurological deficits.	___	___	___	_____
14. Assessed patient's musculoskeletal system, including range of motion (ROM) of joints.	___	___	___	_____
15. Examined patient's skin; identified any breaks in skin integrity and determined level of hydration. Paid attention to area of body on which patient would be positioned.	___	___	___	_____
16. Determined patient's age and history of dehydration, malnutrition, exposure to radiation therapy, underlying chronic conditions, and edema of the skin.	___	___	___	_____
17. Assessed patient's emotional status, including level of anxiety, coping ability, and family caregiver support. Considered using Hospital Anxiety and Depression Scale (HADS). Assessed potential for abuse from a partner or family member.	___	___	___	_____
18. Reviewed results of laboratory tests.	___	___	___	_____
19. Assessed patient's knowledge, prior experience with preoperative assessment, and feelings about procedure.	___	___	___	_____

	S	U	NP	Comments

PLANNING

1. Determined expected outcomes following completion of procedure.

2. Provided privacy and explained assessment procedure to patient. Encouraged patient to ask questions. If applicable, taught patient how to perform postoperative exercises.

3. Obtained and organized equipment for preoperative assessment at bedside.

IMPLEMENTATION

1. Communicated to preoperative team any risk factors that had the potential for making the patient vulnerable to intraoperative complications.

2. Based on the patient's cognitive status, experience, and nature of planned surgery, presented preoperative instruction to patient and family caregiver.

3. Helped patient to comfortable position.

4. Placed nurse call system in an accessible location within patient's reach.

5. Raised side rails (as appropriate) and lowered bed to lowest position, locking into position.

6. Disposed of all contaminated supplies in appropriate receptacle, removed and disposed of gloves, and performed hand hygiene.

EVALUATION

1. Determined if patient information was complete so that plan of care could be established. Validated unclear information with family caregiver.

2. Used Teach-Back. Revised instruction if patient or family caregiver were not able to teach back correctly.

DOCUMENTATION

1. Documented findings on the preoperative flow sheet or preoperative note in the EHR.

2. Documented evaluation of patient and family caregiver learning.

HAND-OFF REPORTING

1. Reported abnormal laboratory values or other operative risks to the surgeon, anesthesiologist, and OR nurse. If patient had known history of opioid use for pain control or previous history of postoperative nausea and vomiting, communicated to health care provider.

616

Student _____ Date _____

Instructor _____ Date _____

PERFORMANCE CHECKLIST SKILL 36.2 **PREOPERATIVE TEACHING**

	S	U	NP	Comments

ASSESSMENT

1. Identified patient using at least two identifiers. ___ ___ ___ _____

2. Assessed patient's electronic health record (EHR) for type of surgery and approach. ___ ___ ___ _____

3. Assessed patient's/family caregiver's health literacy. ___ ___ ___ _____

4. Asked about patient's previous experiences with surgery and anesthesia. ___ ___ ___ _____

5. Assessed patient's level of alertness and orientation and identified primary language and culture. If patient did not speak English, had a professional interpreter on hand to assist. ___ ___ ___ _____

6. Assessed patient's risk for postoperative respiratory complications. Checked nursing history for patient's height and age. ___ ___ ___ _____

7. Assessed patient's anxiety related to surgery. ___ ___ ___ _____

8. Assessed family caregiver's willingness to learn and support patient following surgery. ___ ___ ___ _____

9. Assessed patient's understanding of the intended surgery and anesthesia. Asked patient to offer description rather than asking simple yes-or-no question. Asked about patient's and family caregiver's expectations of surgery and care. ___ ___ ___ _____

10. Assessed patient's knowledge, prior experience with preoperative teaching, and feelings about procedure. ___ ___ ___ _____

PLANNING

1. Determined expected outcomes following completion of procedure. ___ ___ ___ _____

2. Provided privacy and explained importance of patient participation in performing postoperative exercises. Discussed surgical procedure and expected postoperative experiences and exercises. ___ ___ ___ _____

3. Obtained and organized equipment for preoperative teaching at bedside. ___ ___ ___ _____

IMPLEMENTATION

S   U   NP   Comments

1. Performed hand hygiene. Informed patient and family caregiver of date, time, and location of surgery; anticipated length of surgery; additional time in postanesthesia recovery area; and where to wait.

2. Encouraged and answered questions asked by patient and family caregiver.

3. Instructed patient about preoperative bowel or skin preparations as needed. Checked medical orders and agency policy regarding number of preoperative showers and agent to be used for each shower. Following each preoperative shower, instructed patient to rinse the skin thoroughly and dry with a fresh, clean, dry towel. Patient should have donned clean clothing.

4. Instructed patient about extent and purpose of food and fluid restrictions for period specified before surgery.

5. Described perioperative routines applicable to patient.

6. Described planned effect of preoperative medications.

7. Reviewed which routine medications patient needed to discontinue before surgery and when.

8. Described perioperative sensations to expect.

9. Described pain-control methods to be used after surgery.

10. Described what patient would experience after surgery.

11. Taught turning:

   a. Instructed patient on turning and sitting up:

      (1) Turned onto right side: Had patient assume supine position and moved to side of bed (in this case, left side) if permitted by surgery. Had patient move by bending knees and pressing heels against mattress to raise and move buttocks. Top side rails on both sides of bed should have been in up position.

      (2) Had patient splint incision with right hand or with right hand with pillow over incisional area; keep right leg straight and flex left knee up; grab right side rail with left hand; pull toward right; and roll onto right side. Had patient reverse process to turn to left side.

618

	S	U	NP	Comments

(3) Instructed patient to turn every 2 h from side to side while awake.

(4) Sat up on right side of bed. Elevated head of bed and had patient turn onto right side. While lying on right side, patient pushed on mattress with left arm and swung feet over edge of bed with nurse's help. To sit up on left side of bed, patient reversed this process. Monitored for signs of orthostatic hypotension when patient performed maneuver.

12. Taught coughing and deep breathing:

a. Assisted patient to high-Fowler position in bed with knees flexed, or had patient sit on side of bed or chair in upright position.

b. Instructed patient to place palms of hands across from one another lightly along lower border of rib cage or upper abdomen.

c. Had patient take slow, deep breaths, inhaling through nose. Explained that patient would feel normal downward movement of diaphragm during inspiration. Demonstrated as needed.

d. Had patient avoid using chest and shoulder muscles while inhaling.

e. Had patient take slow, deep breath; hold for count of 3 seconds; and slowly exhale through mouth as if blowing out candle (pursed lips).

f. Had patient repeat breathing exercise three to five times.

g. Had patient take two slow, deep breaths, inhaling through nose and exhaling through pursed lips.

h. Had patient inhale deeply a third time and hold breath to count of three. Had patient cough fully for two to three consecutive coughs without inhaling between those coughs. Cautioned patient against just clearing throat.

i. Had patient practice several times. Instructed patient to perform turning, coughing, and deep breathing every 2 h. Had family caregiver coach patient to exercise.

13. Taught use of an incentive spirometer:

a. Positioned patient in sitting position in chair or in reclining position with head of bed elevated at least 45 degrees in bed.

b. Set targeted tidal volume on the incentive spirometer according to manufacturer directions. Explained that this is the volume level to be reached with each breath.

	S	U	NP	Comments

c. Explained to patient how to place mouthpiece of incentive spirometer so that patient's lips completely covered mouthpiece. Had patient demonstrate until position was correct. _____ _____ _____ _____

d. Instructed patient to exhale completely, then position mouthpiece so that patient's lips completely covered it. Had patient inhale slowly, maintaining constant flow through unit until goal volume was reached. _____ _____ _____ _____

e. Once maximum inspiration was reached, had patient hold breath for 2–3 seconds and exhale slowly. _____ _____ _____ _____

f. Instructed patient to breathe normally for short period between each of the 10 breaths taken on incentive spirometer. Repeated every hour while awake. _____ _____ _____ _____

14. Taught positive expiratory pressure (PEP) therapy and "huff" coughing: _____ _____ _____ _____

a. Set PEP device for setting ordered. _____ _____ _____ _____

b. Instructed patient to assume semi-Fowler or high-Fowler position in bed or to sit in a chair and place nose clip on patient's nose. _____ _____ _____ _____

c. Had patient place lips around mouthpiece. Instructed patient to take full breath and exhale 2 or 3 times longer than inhalation. Repeated pattern for 10–20 breaths. _____ _____ _____ _____

d. Removed device from mouth and had patient take slow, deep breath and hold for 3 seconds. _____ _____ _____ _____

e. Instructed patient to exhale in quick, short, forced "huffs." Repeated exercise every 2 hours while awake. _____ _____ _____ _____

15. Taught controlled coughing: _____ _____ _____ _____

a. Applied clean gloves if expecting patient to cough and expectorate mucus. Explained importance of maintaining upright position. _____ _____ _____ _____

b. Demonstrated coughing. Took two slow, deep breaths, inhaling through nose and exhaling through (pursed lips) mouth. _____ _____ _____ _____

c. To exhale, had patient lean forward, pressing arms against their abdomen. Coughed 2–3 times without inhaling between coughs. Coughed through a slightly open mouth. Coughs should have been short and sharp. Told patient to push all air out of lungs. _____ _____ _____ _____

d. Cautioned patient against just clearing throat instead of coughing deeply. _____ _____ _____ _____

620

	S	U	NP	Comments

e. If surgical incision was either thoracic or abdominal, taught patient to place either hands or pillow over incisional area and placed hands over pillow to splint incision. During breathing and coughing exercises, pressed gently against incisional area for splinting and support. ___ ___ ___ _____

f. Instructed patient to practice coughing exercises, splinting imaginary incision. Instructed patient to cough 2–3 times every 2 hours while awake. ___ ___ ___ _____

g. Instructed patient to examine sputum for consistency, odor, amount, and color changes, and to notify a nurse if any changes were noted. ___ ___ ___ _____

16. Taught leg exercises: ___ ___ ___ _____

a. Instructed and encouraged patient in leg exercises to be performed every 1–2 hours while awake: ankle rotation, dorsiflexion and plantar flexion, leg extension and flexion, and straight leg raises. ___ ___ ___ _____

b. Positioned patient supine. ___ ___ ___ _____

c. Instructed patient to rotate each ankle in complete circle and draw imaginary circles with big toe 5 times. ___ ___ ___ _____

d. Alternated dorsiflexion and plantar flexion while instructing patient to feel calf muscles tighten and relax. Repeated 5 times. ___ ___ ___ _____

e. Performed quadriceps setting by tightening thigh and bringing knee down toward mattress and relaxing. Repeated 5 times. ___ ___ ___ _____

f. Instructed patient to alternate raising knee and leg straight up from bed surface. Kept leg straight and then knee drawn up. Repeated 5 times. ___ ___ ___ _____

17. Had patient continue to practice exercises before surgery at least every 2 hours while awake. Taught patient to coordinate turning and leg exercises with diaphragmatic breathing and use of incentive spirometer. ___ ___ ___ _____

18. Verified that patient's expectations of surgery were realistic. Corrected expectations as needed. ___ ___ ___ _____

19. Reinforced therapeutic coping strategies. If ineffective, encouraged alternatives. ___ ___ ___ _____

20. Helped patient to comfortable position. ___ ___ ___ _____

21. Placed nurse call system in an accessible location within patient's reach. ___ ___ ___ _____

	S	U	NP	Comments

22. Raised side rails (as appropriate) and lowered bed to lowest position, locking into position.

23. Disposed of all contaminated supplies in appropriate receptacle, removed and disposed of gloves, and performed hand hygiene.

EVALUATION

1. Observed patient demonstrating splinting, turning and sitting, deep breathing, use of incentive spirometer, PEP therapy, and leg exercises.

2. Asked family caregiver to identify location of waiting room and validated if correct.

3. Asked family caregiver to explain how to help prepare patient at home before surgery.

4. Observed level of emotional support family caregiver provided to patient.

5. Used Teach-Back. Revised instruction if patient or family caregiver were not able to teach back correctly.

DOCUMENTATION

1. Documented all preoperative patient and family caregiver teaching and their response to teaching.

HAND-OFF REPORTING

1. Reported patient's inability to identify procedure and site of surgery, as well as understanding of postoperative exercise(s) and teaching to health care provider.

Student _____ Date _____

Instructor _____ Date _____

PERFORMANCE CHECKLIST SKILL 36.3 **PATIENT PREPARATION FOR SURGERY**

	S	U	NP	Comments

ASSESSMENT

1. Identified patient using at least two identifiers.   ___ ___ ___ _____

2. Performed hand hygiene. Completed preoperative assessment, including patient health literacy.   ___ ___ ___ _____

3. Assessed and documented patient's heart rate, blood pressure, respiratory rate, oxygen saturation, and temperature. *Option:* Kept oximeter attached to patient.   ___ ___ ___ _____

4. If patient was same-day admit or ambulatory, validated that admission preparations were completed at home as ordered. Ensured that patient followed appropriate fluid and food restrictions per surgeon or anesthesiologist orders.   ___ ___ ___ _____

5. Asked if patient had advance directive. If so, ensured that a copy was in the electronic health record (EHR).   ___ ___ ___ _____

6. Assessed patient's knowledge, prior experience with surgical preparation, and feelings about procedure.   ___ ___ ___ _____

PLANNING

1. Determined expected outcomes following completion of procedure.   ___ ___ ___ _____

2. Provided privacy and explained preoperative preparations to patient.   ___ ___ ___ _____

3. Planned preparation of any preoperative medications to avoid interruptions. Created a quiet environment. Did not take phone calls or talk with others. Followed agency "No Interruption Zone" policy.   ___ ___ ___ _____

4. Obtained and organized equipment for preparing patient at bedside.   ___ ___ ___ _____

IMPLEMENTATION

	S	U	NP	Comments

1. Performed hand hygiene. Helped patient put on hospital gown and removed personal items. Before any procedure, decreased anxiety by explaining how equipment or preparation would feel before touching patient.

    ____ ____ ____ _____

2. Instructed patient to remove makeup, nail polish, hairpins, and jewelry.

    ____ ____ ____ _____

3. Ensured that money and valuables were locked up or given to a family caregiver.

    ____ ____ ____ _____

4. Verified that patient followed appropriate medication, fluid, and food restrictions per surgeon or anesthesiologist order.

    ____ ____ ____ _____

5. Verified presence of allergies and ensured that allergy/sensitivity band was present.

    ____ ____ ____ _____

6. Assessed patient's fall risks; applied fall risk armband if appropriate.

    ____ ____ ____ _____

7. Verified that bowel preparation was completed by patient or family caregiver at home if ordered.

    ____ ____ ____ _____

8. Ensured that medical history and physical examination results were in the EHR.

    ____ ____ ____ _____

9. Verified that surgical consent, anesthesia consent, and consent for blood transfusion were complete. The name of procedure; name of surgeon; date; name of person authorized to obtain surgical consent; signature of surgeon (or authorized person) obtaining consent; anesthesia provider delivering anesthesia and witness (often the nurse); and patient's signature should all have been present.

    ____ ____ ____ _____

10. Ensured that necessary laboratory work, electrocardiogram (ECG), and chest x-ray film studies were completed and results were documented.

    ____ ____ ____ _____

11. Verified that blood type and crossmatch were completed if ordered by surgeon and that blood transfusions were available as needed.

    ____ ____ ____ _____

12. Instructed patient to void.

    ____ ____ ____ _____

13. Performed hand hygiene and applied clean gloves. Started IV line; referred to unit standards or surgeon's orders. Removed and disposed of gloves. Performed hand hygiene.

    ____ ____ ____ _____

14. Administered preoperative medications as ordered. Managed potential for postoperative nausea and vomiting.

    ____ ____ ____ _____

15. Option: Applied compression stockings.

    ____ ____ ____ _____

	S	U	NP	Comments

16. Option: Applied intermittent sequential compression devices (ISCDs) if ordered. Note: Compression stockings may or may not be used in combination with ISCDs. Verified order.

17. Applied clean gloves. Cleaned and prepared surgical site if ordered. Removed and disposed of gloves.

18. Option: Performed hand hygiene and applied sterile gloves. Inserted urinary catheter if ordered. Removed and disposed of gloves and performed hand hygiene.

19. Allowed patient to wear eyeglasses or hearing aid if possible before surgery so that patient could sign consents and read materials. Removed contact lenses, eyeglasses, hairpieces, and dentures just before surgery (saw checklist completed before surgery, noting that all items were removed before proceeding to OR).

20. Placed head cover over patient's head and hair.

21. Placed patient on bed rest with nurse call system within reach and forbid patient getting out of bed without help. Allowed family members to remain at bedside until patient was transferred to surgical area. Maintained quiet and relaxing environment.

22. Transferred patient via stretcher to OR. Raised side rails appropriately.

23. Disposed of all contaminated supplies in appropriate receptacle, removed and disposed of gloves, and performed hand hygiene.

EVALUATION

1. Had patient describe surgical procedure and its benefits and risks.

2. Had patient repeat preoperative instructions.

3. Monitored patient for signs and symptoms of anxiety and asked how patient and family were feeling.

4. Confirmed that IV was infusing at a keep-open or ordered rate.

5. Used Teach-Back. Revised instruction if patient or family caregiver were not able to teach back correctly.

DOCUMENTATION

1. Documented preoperative physical preparation on preoperative checklist.

2. Documented that informed consent was completed.

		S	U	NP	Comments

3. Documented disposition of patient valuables/belongings.

    —   —   —   ————————————

4. Documented evaluation of patient and family caregiver learning.

    —   —   —   ————————————

HAND-OFF REPORTING

1. Reported lack of signed and witnessed consent form or failure of patient to maintain NPO status and action taken.

    —   —   —   ————————————

2. Reported to nursing staff receiving patient in OR that preoperative physical preparation was successfully completed, any deviations from appropriate preparation, and that completed informed consent was available in the patient's record.

    —   —   —   ————————————

PERFORMANCE CHECKLIST SKILL 36.4 **PROVIDING IMMEDIATE ANESTHESIA RECOVERY IN THE POSTANESTHESIA CARE UNIT**

	S	U	NP	Comments
ASSESSMENT				
1. Identified patient using at least two identifiers.	___	___	___	_____
2. Received hand-off report from circulating nurse and anesthesia provider.	___	___	___	_____
3. On patient's arrival in PACU, reviewed surgeon's orders.	___	___	___	_____
4. Considered type of surgical procedure, restrictions to movement, and type of anesthesia used.	___	___	___	_____
5. Performed hand hygiene. Applied clean gloves. Performed thorough patient assessment. Assessed patient's surgical site and drains, skin integrity, safety, and anxiety level.	___	___	___	_____
6. Ensured that discharge criteria from phase I level of care was met, not a time limit. Criteria should have addressed assessment of airway patency, oxygenation, hemodynamic stability, thermoregulation, neurological stability, intake and output, tube patency, dressings, pain, and comfort management, and postanesthesia recovery score if used.	___	___	___	_____
PLANNING				
1. Determined expected outcomes following completion of procedure.	___	___	___	_____
2. Provided privacy and explained PACU activities to patient and family caregiver (when allowed into recovery).	___	___	___	_____
3. Removed and disposed of gloves. Performed hand hygiene and applied new pair of clean gloves. Organized and set up equipment for continued monitoring and care activities.	___	___	___	_____
IMPLEMENTATION				
1. While receiving hand-off report as patient entered PACU on stretcher/bed, immediately attached oxygen tubing to regulator, hung IV fluids, and checked IV flow rates. Connected any drainage tubes to gravity drainage or continuous or intermittent suction as ordered. Attached cardiac monitor. Ensured that indwelling catheter and bag were in drainage position and patent.	___	___	___	_____

	S	U	NP	Comments

2. Continued ongoing assessment of all vital signs every 5–15 min until patient stabilized, or more frequently if clinically indicated. Compared findings with patient's baseline. Provided warm blankets as needed for patient comfort. ___ ___ ___ _____

3. Maintained patent airway after general anesthesia: ___ ___ ___ _____

   a. Positioned patient on side with head facing down and neck slightly extended. Did not position patient with hands over chest. ___ ___ ___ _____

   b. Placed small, folded towel or small pillow under patient's head. If patient was restricted to supine position, elevated head of bed approximately 10–15 degrees, extended neck, and turned head to side. Had emesis basin available if patient became nauseated. ___ ___ ___ _____

   c. Encouraged patient to cough and deep breathe on awakening and every 15 minutes. ___ ___ ___ _____

   d. Suctioned artificial airway and oral cavity as secretions accumulated. ___ ___ ___ _____

   e. Once gag reflex returned, had patient spit out oral airway. Did not tape oral airway. ___ ___ ___ _____

   f. Avoided rapid position changes in patients who had spinal anesthesia. Maintained good body alignment. Maintained IV infusion. Encouraged fluid intake, if allowed. ___ ___ ___ _____

4. Called patient by name in normal tone of voice. If there was no response, attempted to arouse patient by touching or gently moving a body part. Explained that surgery was over, and that patient was in recovery area. ___ ___ ___ _____

5. Assessed circulatory perfusion by inspecting color of nail beds, mucous membranes, and skin. Palpated for skin temperature. Tested for capillary refill. ___ ___ ___ _____

6. Assessed closely for any behavioral or clinical changes reflecting potential cardiovascular and pulmonary complications of general anesthesia. Monitored laboratory findings. ___ ___ ___ _____

7. If patient had general anesthesia: As patient aroused, introduced self and oriented patient to surroundings. ___ ___ ___ _____

8. For spinal or epidural anesthesia, monitored sensory, circulatory, pulmonary, and neurological responses: ___ ___ ___ _____

   a. Monitored for hypotension, bradycardia, and nausea and vomiting. ___ ___ ___ _____

   b. Maintained adequate IV infusion. ___ ___ ___ _____

		S	U	NP	Comments

c. Kept patient supine or with head slightly elevated and maintained position. ___ ___ ___ _____

d. Assessed respiratory status, level of spinal sensation, and mobility in lower extremities. Drowsiness was apparent after IV sedation. Had patient close eyes and used alcohol wipe to test sensation along sensory dermatomes. Had patient identify if warm or cold. Reminded patient that loss of extremity sensation and movement was normal and would return in several hours. ___ ___ ___ _____

e. Observed patients in PACU until they regained movement in extremities. ___ ___ ___ _____

9. Monitored source of intake and output: ___ ___ ___ _____

a. Observed dressing and drains for any evidence of bright red blood. Inspected surgical incision for swelling or discoloration. Noted condition of surgical dressing. Marked dressing with circle around drainage using black pen. Placed time of marking and checked area every 10–15 minutes, marking any changes and noting vital signs. ___ ___ ___ _____

b. Reinforced pressure dressing or changed simple dressing if ordered. Continued to monitor condition of incision, surrounding tissue, and amount and color of any drainage if incision was exposed or covered with transparent dressing. ___ ___ ___ _____

c. Informed surgeon of unexpected bloody drainage and reinforced dressing as indicated. Applied direct pressure. Also looked underneath patient for any pooling of bloody drainage. Monitored for decreased BP and increased pulse. ___ ___ ___ _____

d. Inspected condition and contents of any drainage tubes and collecting devices. Noted character and volume of drainage. ___ ___ ___ _____

e. Observed amount, color, and appearance of urine from indwelling Foley catheter (if present). ___ ___ ___ _____

f. If nasogastric (NG) tube was present, assessed drainage. If not draining, checked placement and irrigated, if necessary, with normal saline. ___ ___ ___ _____

g. Monitored and maintained IV fluid rates. Observed IV site for signs of infiltration. ___ ___ ___ _____

10. Promoted comfort: ___ ___ ___ _____

a. Provided mouth care by placing moistened washcloth to lips, swabbing oral mucosa with dampened swab or soft toothbrush, or applying petrolatum to lips. ___ ___ ___ _____

	S	U	NP	Comments

b. Provided warm blanket or active warming device to promote warmth and minimize shivering. ___ ___ ___ _____

c. Helped with position changes and provided supportive pillows. Encouraged leg exercises. ___ ___ ___ _____

11. Continued monitoring pain as patient awakened and until transferred to surgical unit or discharge, including quality, severity, and location. Did not assume that all postoperative pain was incisional pain. ___ ___ ___ _____

   a. Provided pain medication as ordered and when vital signs stabilized. ___ ___ ___ _____

12. Explained patient's condition to patient and informed patient of plans for transfer to nursing unit or discharge to alternate setting. ___ ___ ___ _____

13. Appropriately disposed of supplies and equipment used in PACU setting. Removed and disposed of gloves. Performed hand hygiene. ___ ___ ___ _____

14. When patient's condition stabilized, contacted anesthesiologist to approve transfer to nursing unit or release to home. ___ ___ ___ _____

15. Before patient was discharged to home from ambulatory surgery unit, provided verbal and written instructions. ___ ___ ___ _____

16. For patients transferring to the next point of care by stretcher, raised side rails and requested transport team. Appropriately disposed of supplies and equipment used in PACU setting. Performed hand hygiene. ___ ___ ___ _____

EVALUATION

1. Compared all vital sign assessment measurements with patient's baseline and expected normal levels. ___ ___ ___ _____

2. Inspected surgical wound and dressings for drainage. Assessed for wound drainage under patient. ___ ___ ___ _____

3. Measured I&O. Urine output should have been at least 30–50 mL/h. ___ ___ ___ _____

4. Auscultated bowel sounds and asked if patient had passed flatus. ___ ___ ___ _____

5. Measured patient's perception of pain after implementing pain-relief measures. ___ ___ ___ _____

6. Completed system-specific physical assessments as appropriate according to patient's unique type of surgery. ___ ___ ___ _____

7. Used Teach-Back. Revised instruction if patient or family caregiver were not able to teach back correctly. ___ ___ ___ _____

	S	U	NP	Comments

DOCUMENTATION

1. Documented patient's arrival time at PACU; included vital signs, I&O, and other physical parameters; level of consciousness (LOC); and pain location and severity. Also included condition of dressings and tubes, character of drainage, condition of IV infusion, and all nursing measures.   ___ ___ ___ _____

2. Documented evaluation of patient and family care-giver learning.   ___ ___ ___ _____

HAND-OFF REPORTING

1. Reported any abnormal assessment findings and signs of complications to surgeon.   ___ ___ ___ _____

Student _____ Date _____

Instructor _____ Date _____

PERFORMANCE CHECKLIST SKILL 36.5 **PROVIDING EARLY POSTOPERATIVE (PHASE II) AND CONVALESCENT PHASE (PHASE III) RECOVERY**

	S	U	NP	Comments
ASSESSMENT				
1. Obtained phone report from postanesthesia care unit (PACU) nurse summarizing patient's current status.	___	___	___	_____
2. Performed hand hygiene and arranged equipment at bedside.	___	___	___	_____
3. Identified patient using at least two identifiers.	___	___	___	_____
4. If patient was transported by stretcher, prepared for transfer with bed in high position (level with stretcher), with sheet folded to side and room for stretcher to be placed beside bed easily. Transferred patient to bed using safe patient handling.	___	___	___	_____
5. Collected more detailed hand-off report from nurse accompanying patient.	___	___	___	_____
6. Collected an initial set of vital signs.	___	___	___	_____
7. Assessed character and location of patient's surgical pain; rated severity on scale of 0 to 10.	___	___	___	_____
8. Reviewed electronic health record (EHR) for information pertaining to type of surgery; postoperative complications; medications administered in PACU; preoperative medical risks; baseline vital signs, PACU vital signs, and other assessment findings; and patient's usual medications given/not given before surgery. Compared and validated with information from hand-off report	___	___	___	_____
9. Reviewed postoperative medical orders.	___	___	___	_____
10. Assessed patients risk for postoperative urinary retention (POUR), including patient factors, procedural factors, and anesthetic factors.	___	___	___	_____
11. Assessed patients risk for postoperative nausea and vomiting (PONV), including patient risk factors, anesthetic factors, and surgical factors.	___	___	___	_____
12. Referred to nurses' notes or, if necessary, reassessed a patient's/family caregiver's health literacy.	___	___	___	_____
13. Asked patient or referred to nurses' notes regarding a patient's knowledge, prior experience with surgery, and feelings about procedure.	___	___	___	_____

632

	S	U	NP	Comments

PLANNING

1. Determined expected outcomes following completion of procedure. ___ ___ ___ _____

2. Provided privacy and explained all postoperative care measures to patient. Provided postoperative teaching during all care measures. If applicable, taught patient how to report complications or side effects from surgery. ___ ___ ___ _____

3. Attached any existing oxygen tubing, hung IV fluids, verified IV flow-rate settings on infusion pump, and checked drainage tubes. ___ ___ ___ _____

IMPLEMENTATION

1. Performed hand hygiene. Applied clean gloves for any necessary procedures. ___ ___ ___ _____

2. Early recovery initial postoperative care:

   a. Maintained airway. If patient remained sleepy or lethargic, kept head extended and supported in side-lying position. ___ ___ ___ _____

   b. Assessed level of consciousness (LOC) and continued measuring vital signs per frequency of agency policy or health care provider order. Compared findings with vital signs taken in PACU and patient's baseline. ___ ___ ___ _____

   c. Encouraged coughing, deep breathing, and use of incentive spirometry and positive expiratory pressure (PEP) device to prevent atelectasis. ___ ___ ___ _____

   d. Assessed for return of bowel sounds. ___ ___ ___ _____

      (1) Managed postoperative nausea and vomiting PONV: opioid-sparing pain management, use of postoperative antiemetics, and nonpharmacologic techniques. ___ ___ ___ _____

      (2) If NG tube was present, checked placement and irrigated. Connected to proper drainage device. Connected all other drainage tubes to appropriate suction or collection device. Secured to prevent tension on tubing. ___ ___ ___ _____

   e. Inspected patient's surgical dressing for appearance, presence, and character of drainage. Unless contraindicated by surgeon, outlined drainage along edges with pen and reassessed in 1 hour for change. If no dressing was present, inspected condition of wound. ___ ___ ___ _____

	S	U	NP	Comments

f. Palpated abdomen for bladder distention or used bladder ultrasound when available. If Foley catheter was present, checked placement. Ensured that it was draining freely and properly secured. ___ ___ ___ _____

   (1) Managed postoperative urinary retention POUR: Used bladder ultrasound for high-risk patients who had not voided within 4 hours; if greater than 600 mL of urine was present, considered a single-time catheterization. ___ ___ ___ _____

   (2) If no urinary drainage system was present, explained that voiding within 8 hours after surgery was expected. Male patients may have voided successfully if allowed to stand. ___ ___ ___ _____

g. Measured all sources of fluid intake and output (I&O). ___ ___ ___ _____

h. Described purpose of equipment and frequent observations to patient and family caregivers. ___ ___ ___ _____

i. Provided pain management. Positioned patient for comfort, maintaining correct body alignment. Avoided tension on surgical wound site. Assessed last time analgesic was given. ___ ___ ___ _____

   (1) Patient-controlled analgesia (PCA) may have been used for pain control. Medicated patient as ordered either around the clock or PRN as ordered during first 24–48 hours. Gave PRN analgesic as soon as possible when patient reported increase in pain. Explained pain-management measures to patient. Knew the symptoms of opioid use and withdrawal. ___ ___ ___ _____

j. Placed that nurse call system in an accessible location within patient's reach. ___ ___ ___ _____

k. Raised side rails (as appropriate) and lowered bed to lowest position, locking into position. ___ ___ ___ _____

l. Disposed of all contaminated supplies in appropriate receptacle, removed and disposed of gloves, and performed hand hygiene. ___ ___ ___ _____

3. Continued postoperative care: ___ ___ ___ _____

a. Continued to assess vital signs at least every 4 hours or as ordered. ___ ___ ___ _____

b. Closely monitored progress of wound healing and changed dressings as needed or ordered. ___ ___ ___ _____

c. Monitored and maintained wound drainage devices such as Jackson-Pratt, Hemovac, or Penrose drains. ___ ___ ___ _____

d. Provided oral care at least every 2 hours as needed. If permitted, offered ice chips. ___ ___ ___ _____

	S	U	NP	Comments

e. Encouraged patient to turn, cough, and deep breathe, and used incentive spirometer and PEP device at least every 2 hours.

f. Applied or monitored function of sequential compression devices or elastic stockings on lower extremities. May have been applied preoperatively. Explained to patient that compression device would inflate and deflate intermittently.

g. Promoted early ambulation and activity per agency protocol. Assessed vital signs before and after activity to assess tolerance. Set goals for patient to increase ambulation progressively.

h. Progressed from clear liquids to regular diet as tolerated if nausea and vomiting did not occur.

i. Included patient and family caregiver in decision making; answered questions as they arose.

j. Provided opportunity for patients who must adjust to change in body appearance or function to verbalize feelings.

4. Convalescent phase:

a. Assessed patient's home environment for safety, cleanliness, and availability of community resources and help for patient. (NOTE: This may be done by a case manager and not a staff nurse). Used the information to revise any teaching as needed.

b. Provided instruction on care activities that patient or family caregiver would perform at home.

c. Kept patient and family caregiver informed of progress made toward recovery. Explained time expected for discharge from health care agency. Provided answers to individual patient questions or concerns.

d. Following any procedure, removed and disposed of gloves; performed hand hygiene.

e. Prepared patient for discharge home. Ensured that patient and family caregiver had all necessary printed instructions. Provided a hand-off report if patient was being discharged to an agency such as a long-term care facility.

EVALUATION

1. Auscultated breath sounds bilaterally.

2. Monitored trends in vital signs.

3. Evaluated I&O records. Assessed time of patient's first postoperative urination.

	S	U	NP	Comments

4. Auscultated bowel sounds and evaluated for nausea.

5. Asked patient to describe character of pain and rated acuity on a scale of 0–10 after moderate activity.

6. Inspected incision.

7. Monitored progress of patient ambulation.

8. Had patient or family caregiver describe incision care, dietary modifications or restrictions, activity restrictions, medication schedule, and plans for follow-up visit.

9. Used Teach-Back. Revised instruction if patient/family caregiver were not able to teach back correctly.

DOCUMENTATION

1. Documented patient's arrival at nursing unit; included vital signs, I&O, body system assessment findings, and all nursing measures initiated.

2. Continued to document assessment measures every 4 hours or more frequently as patient's condition warranted.

3. Documented evaluation of patient and family caregiver learning.

HAND-OFF REPORTING

1. Reported onset of any postoperative complications to surgeon or other health care provider immediately.

2. During hand-off report, communicated patient's assessment findings pertinent to surgery, patient response, and progress with postoperative instruction.

3. If transitioned to any other environment than home, reported preoperative course and postoperative summary, as well as current status, to receiving nurse.

Student _____ Date _____

Instructor _____ Date _____

PERFORMANCE CHECKLIST SKILL 37.1 **SURGICAL HAND ANTISEPSIS**

	S	U	NP	Comments

ASSESSMENT

1. Determined type and length of time for hand hygiene __ __ __ _____

2. Removed bracelets, rings, and watches. __ __ __ _____

3. Inspected fingernails, which must be short (2 mm), clean, and healthy. Checked with the agency policy to see if fingernail polish was permitted. Did not wear artificial nails or extenders. __ __ __ _____

4. Inspected condition of cuticles, hands, and forearms for presence of abrasions, cuts, or open lesions. __ __ __ _____

PLANNING

1. Determined expected outcomes following completion of procedure. __ __ __ _____

IMPLEMENTATION

1. Donned surgical shoe covers, cap or hood, face mask, and protective eyewear. __ __ __ _____

2. Performed prescrub wash at beginning of work shift: __ __ __ _____

   a. Turned water on using foot or knee control and adjusted to comfortable temperature. __ __ __ _____

   b. Wet hands thoroughly with water. Followed manufacturer directions for application of soap. __ __ __ _____

   c. Rubbed hands, covering all surfaces with lather, including backs of hands, fingertips, inner webs, and palms, washing for at least 15 seconds. __ __ __ _____

   d. Rinsed hands well. Dried hands thoroughly with disposable towel and discarded towel. __ __ __ _____

3. Surgical hand scrub (with sponge):

   a. Turned on water using foot or knee control. Cleaned under nails of both hands with disposable nail pick or cleaner. Rinsed hands and forearms under running water, keeping hands and forearms elevated and elbows down. __ __ __ _____

   b. Dispensed antimicrobial scrub agent according to manufacturer instructions. Applied agent to wet hands and forearms with soft, nonabrasive sponge. __ __ __ _____

		S	U	NP	Comments

c. Scrubbed for the length of time recommended by the manufacturer. Visualized each finger, hand, and arm as having four sides. Paid particular attention to cleansing fingernails. Washed all four sides of fingers effectively, keeping hand elevated, elbow down. Repeated for other hand, fingers, and arm. ___ ___ ___ _____

d. Avoided splashing surgical attire. Discarded sponges in appropriate container. ___ ___ ___ _____

e. Rinsed hands and arms, running water from fingertips to elbows in one continuous motion, holding hands higher than elbows. ___ ___ ___ _____

f. Turned off water using foot or knee controls and back into OR holding hands higher than elbows and away from surgical attire. ___ ___ ___ _____

g. Approached sterile setup and grasped sterile towel, taking care not to drip water on sterile field. ___ ___ ___ _____

h. Keeping hands and arms above waist and outstretched, carefully grasped one end of sterile towel to dry one hand thoroughly, moving from fingers to elbow in rotating motion. ___ ___ ___ _____

i. Used opposite end of towel to dry other hand. ___ ___ ___ _____

j. Dropped towel into linen hamper or into circulating nurse's hand, making certain that hands did not fall below waist level. ___ ___ ___ _____

4. Performed spongeless surgical hand scrub with alcohol-based hand-rub product: ___ ___ ___ _____

a. After prescrub wash (Step 2), turned on water using foot or knee control. Cleaned under nails of both hands with disposable nail pick or cleaner and rinsed hands and forearms under running water. Dried hands thoroughly with paper towel. Turned off water. ___ ___ ___ _____

b. Dispensed manufacturer-recommended amount of antimicrobial agent hand preparation. Applied agent to hands and forearms according to manufacturer instructions for application, recommended volume, and specified time. ___ ___ ___ _____

c. Repeated antimicrobial product application if indicated in manufacturer instructions. ___ ___ ___ _____

d. Rubbed thoroughly until completely dry. Proceeded to OR to don gloves. ___ ___ ___ _____

EVALUATION

1. Monitored patient after surgery for signs of surgical site infection (usually occurs 2–3 days after surgery). ___ ___ ___ _____

	S	U	NP	Comments

DOCUMENTATION

1. Documentation is not required for surgical hand asepsis. ___ ___ ___ _____

2. Documented area and description of surgical site after surgery to provide baseline for monitoring wound. ___ ___ ___ _____

HAND-OFF REPORTING

1. Reported area and description of surgical site after surgery. ___ ___ ___ _____

Student _____ Date _____

Instructor _____ Date _____

PERFORMANCE CHECKLIST SKILL 37.2   **DONNING A STERILE GOWN AND CLOSED GLOVING**

	S	U	NP	Comments

ASSESSMENT

1. Selected proper size and type of sterile gloves. Selected latex-free gloves if patient or surgical personnel latex sensitive was known.

2. Selected proper size and type of sterile surgical gown.

PLANNING

1. Determined expected outcomes following completion of procedure.

IMPLEMENTATION

1. Donned sterile gown:

   a. Opened sterile gown and glove package on clean, dry, flat surface. Scrub nurse (before scrubbing hands) or circulating nurse could assist, preferably on small table separate from sterile field containing sterile instruments and supplies.

   b. Performed surgical hand antisepsis. Dried hands thoroughly.

   c. Picked up gown (folded inside out) from sterile package, grasping inside surface at collar.

   d. Lifted folded gown directly upward and stepped back, away from table.

   e. Located neckband; with both hands grasped inside front of gown just below neckband.

   f. Keeping gown at arm's length away from body, allowed it to unfold with inside of gown toward body. Did not touch outside of gown or allow it to touch floor.

   g. With hands at shoulder level, slipped both arms into armholes simultaneously. Did not allow hands to move through cuff opening. Had circulating nurse pull gown over shoulders by reaching inside arm seams. Pulled gown on, leaving sleeves covering hands.

   h. Had circulating nurse tie gown at neck and waist. If gown was wraparound style, did not touch sterile front flap until scrub nurse/technician was gloved.

640

	S	U	NP	Comments

2. Applied gloves using closed-glove method:

   a. With hands covered by gown cuffs and sleeves, opened inner sterile glove package.

   b. Grasped folded cuff of glove for dominant hand with nondominant hand.

   c. Extended covered dominant hand and forearm forward with palm up and placed palm of glove against palm of dominant hand. Gloved fingers pointed toward elbow.

   d. While holding glove cuff through gown with dominant hand on which it was placed, grasped back of glove cuff with nondominant hand and turned glove cuff over end of dominant hand and gown cuff.

   e. Grasped top of glove and underlying gown sleeve with covered nondominant hand. Carefully extended fingers into glove, being sure that cuff of glove covered cuff of gown.

   f. Gloved nondominant hand in same manner with gloved, dominant hand. Kept hand inside sleeve. Ensured that fingers were fully extended into both gloves.

3. Donned wraparound gown:

   a. Grasped sterile front flap/paper tab with gloved hands and untied.

   b. Passed sterile paper tab to member of sterile surgical team or to nonsterile team member. Kept gown tie in right hand. Circulating nurse stood still as scrub nurse/technician turned.

   c. Allowing margin of safety, turned to left one-half turn, covering back with extended gown flap. Retrieved sterile tie only from team member and secured both ties in place.

EVALUATION

1. Monitored patient after surgery for signs of surgical site infection (usually occurs 2–3 days after surgery).

DOCUMENTATION

1. Documentation is not required for sterile gowning and gloving.

2. Documented area and description of surgical site after surgery to provide baseline for monitoring wound.

HAND-OFF REPORTING

1. Recorded area and description of surgical site after surgery.

PERFORMANCE CHECKLIST PROCEDURAL GUIDELINE 38.1 **PERFORMING A WOUND ASSESSMENT**

	S	U	NP	Comments

PROCEDURAL STEPS

1. Identified patient using at least two identifiers according to agency policy.

2. Examined the electronic health record (EHR) for findings from the last wound assessment to use as a comparison for this wound assessment. Reviewed the record to determine the etiology of the wound.

3. Reviewed EHR to determine patient's age and history of dehydration, malnutrition, exposure to radiation therapy, underlying chronic conditions, and edema of the skin, which increase patient's risk for medical adhesive–related skin injury (MARSI).

4. Determined agency-approved wound assessment tool and reviewed the frequency of assessment. Examined the last wound assessment to use as comparison for this assessment.

5. Assessed patient's/family caregiver's health literacy.

6. Assessed patient's knowledge, prior experience with wound assessment, and feelings about the procedure.

7. Assessed character of patient's pain and rated acuity on a pain scale of 0 to 10. Offered pain medication 30 minutes before assessment as needed.

8. Performed hand hygiene. Closed room door or bed curtains and positioned patient.

   a. Positioned comfortably to permit observation of wound in well-lit room.

   b. Exposed only the area of the wound.

9. Explained procedure of wound assessment to patient.

10. Formed a cuff on waterproof biohazard bag and placed near bed.

11. Applied clean gloves and removed soiled dressings; removed gauze one layer at a time.

	S	U	NP	Comments

12. Examined dressings for quality of drainage (color, consistency), presence or absence of odor, and quantity of drainage (noted if dressings were saturated, slightly moist, or had no drainage). Discarded dressings in waterproof biohazard bag. Removed and discarded gloves. ____ ____ ____ _____

13. Performed hand hygiene and applied clean gloves. ____ ____ ____ _____

14. Inspected wound and determined type of wound healing. ____ ____ ____ _____

15. Used agency-approved assessment tool and assessed the following: ____ ____ ____ _____

   a. Wound healing by primary intention (surgical wound): ____ ____ ____ _____

     (1) Assessed anatomical location of wound on body. ____ ____ ____ _____

     (2) Noted if incisional wound margins were approximated or closed together. ____ ____ ____ _____

     (3) Observed for presence of drainage. ____ ____ ____ _____

     (4) Looked for evidence of infection. ____ ____ ____ _____

     (5) Lightly palpated along incision to feel a healing ridge. ____ ____ ____ _____

   b. Wound healing by secondary intention: ____ ____ ____ _____

     (1) Assessed anatomical location of wound. ____ ____ ____ _____

     (2) Assessed wound dimensions: Measured size of wound (including length, width, and depth) using a centimeter measuring guide. Measured length by placing the disposable measuring guide over wound at the point of greatest length (or head to foot). Measured width from side to side. Measured depth by inserting cotton-tipped applicator in area of greatest depth and placing a mark on applicator at skin level; used measuring guide to determine depth. Discarded measuring guide and cotton-tipped applicator in a biohazard bag. ____ ____ ____ _____

     (3) Assessed for undermining: Used cotton-tipped applicator to gently probe wound edges. If undermining was present, measured depth and noted location using the face of a clock as a guide. Documented the number of centimeters that area extended from wound edge underneath intact skin. ____ ____ ____ _____

	S	U	NP	Comments

(4) Assessed extent of tissue loss: If wound was a pressure injury, determined the deepest viable tissue layer in wound bed and determined stage. Did not determine stage if necrotic tissue did not allow visualization of base of wound. If it was a pressure injury, used the staging system of the National Pressure Injury Advisory Panel.

(5) Observed tissue type, including percentage of granulation, slough, and necrotic tissue.

(6) Noted presence of exudate: amount, color, consistency and odor. Indicated amount of exudate by using part of dressing saturated (completely or partially saturated or in terms of quantity).

(7) Determined if wound edges were rounded toward wound bed. Described presence of epithelialization at wound edges (if present).

16. Inspected the periwound skin, including color, texture, and temperature, and described skin integrity.

17. Applied dressings per order. Placed time, date, and initials on new dressing.

18. Reassessed patient's pain and level of comfort, including pain at wound site, using a scale of 0 to 10 after dressing was applied.

19. Discarded biohazard bag and soiled supplies per agency policy. Removed and disposed of gloves. Performed hand hygiene.

20. Helped patient to a comfortable position.

21. Placed nurse call system in an accessible location within patient's reach.

22. Raised side rails (as appropriate) and lower bed to lowest position, locking into position.

23. Used Teach-Back. Revised instruction if patient/family caregiver was not able to teach back correctly.

24. Documented wound assessment findings and compared assessment with previous wound assessments to monitor wound healing.

25. Provided hand-off report to health care provider regarding any serious complication such as new bleeding or signs of dehiscence.

PERFORMANCE CHECKLIST SKILL 38.1   **PERFORMING A WOUND IRRIGATION**

	S	U	NP	Comments

ASSESSMENT

1. Identified patient using at least two identifiers according to agency policy.

2. Reviewed patient's electronic health record (EHR), including health care provider's order and nurses' notes. Noted previous status of wound and type of solution to be used.

3. Reviewed EHR for most current signs and symptoms related to patient's open wound.

   a. Extent of impairment of skin integrity, including size of wound

   b. Determined patient's age and history of dehydration, malnutrition, exposure to radiation therapy, underlying chronic conditions, and edema of the skin

   c. Number of drains present

   d. Drainage, including amount, color, consistency, and any odor noted

   e. Wound tissue color

   f. Culture reports

4. Assessed patient's/family caregiver's health literacy.

5. Assessed character of patient's pain and rated acuity on a pain scale of 0 to 10.

6. Assessed patient for history of allergies to antiseptics, solutions, medications, tapes, latex, or dressing material. If allergy identified, applied allergy wrist band.

7. Assessed if patient was taking an anticoagulant or had coagulopathy.

8. Assessed patient's and family caregiver's understanding of need for irrigation and signs of wound infection.

9. Assessed patient's knowledge, prior experience with wound irrigation, and feelings about procedure.

	S	U	NP	Comments

PLANNING

1. Determined expected outcomes following completion of procedure.

2. Performed hand hygiene. Administered analgesic at least 30 minutes before starting wound irrigation procedure.

3. Provided privacy and explained procedure to patient and family caregiver, instructed not to touch wound or sterile supplies.

4. Organized and set up any equipment needed and positioned patient to properly perform procedure.

   a. Positioned comfortably to promote gravitational flow of irrigating solution over wound and into collection receptacle.

   b. Ensured that the irrigant solution was at room temperature, and positioned the patient so wound was vertical to the collection basin.

   c. Placed padding or extra towel on bed under area where irrigation would take place.

IMPLEMENTATION

1. Performed hand hygiene.

2. Formed cuff on waterproof biohazard bag and placed near bed.

3. Applied PPE: gown, mask, and goggles as indicated; applied clean gloves and removed old dressing. Disposed of dressing in proper biohazard receptacle. Removed and discarded gloves. Performed hand hygiene.

4. Applied clean or sterile gloves. Cleaned periwound with either normal saline or cleansing agent recommended by health care provider or wound care consultant. Removed and disposed of gloves. Performed hand hygiene.

5. Applied clean or sterile gloves (checked agency policy). Exposed area near wound only, performed wound assessment, and examined recent documented assessment of patient's open wound.

6. Irrigated wound:

   a. Filled a 35-mL syringe with irrigation solution.

   b. Attached a 19-gauge angiocatheter.

   c. Held syringe tip 2.5 cm (1 inch) above upper end of wound and over area being cleaned.

646

	S	U	NP	Comments

d. Using continuous pressure, flushed the wound; repeated until solution draining into basin was clear. ___ ___ ___ _____

7. Irrigated deep wound with very small opening: ___ ___ ___ _____

   a. Attached soft catheter to filled irrigation syringe. ___ ___ ___ _____

   b. Gently inserted tip of catheter into opening about 1.3 cm (0.5 inch). ___ ___ ___ _____

   c. Using slow, continuous pressure, flushed wound. ___ ___ ___ _____

   d. While keeping catheter in place, pinched it off just below syringe. ___ ___ ___ _____

   e. Removed and refilled syringe. Reconnected it to catheter and repeated irrigation until solution draining into basin was clear. ___ ___ ___ _____

8. Cleaned wound with handheld shower: ___ ___ ___ _____

   a. With patient seated comfortably in shower chair or standing, if condition allowed, adjusted spray to gentle flow; made sure the water was warm. ___ ___ ___ _____

   b. Showered for 5 to 10 minutes with shower head 30 cm (12 inches) from wound. ___ ___ ___ _____

9. When indicated, obtained wound cultures only after cleaning with nonbacteriostatic saline. ___ ___ ___ _____

10. Dried wound edges with gauze; dried patient after shower. ___ ___ ___ _____

11. Removed and disposed of gloves. Performed hand hygiene. Applied clean or sterile gloves, per agency policy. Applied appropriate dressing and labeled with time, date, and initials. ___ ___ ___ _____

12. Removed and disposed of mask, goggles, and gown. ___ ___ ___ _____

13. Disposed of equipment and soiled supplies. Performed hand hygiene. ___ ___ ___ _____

14. Helped patient to a comfortable position. ___ ___ ___ _____

15. Raised side rails (as appropriate) and lowered bed to lowest position, locking into position. ___ ___ ___ _____

16. Placed nurse call system in an accessible location within patient's reach. ___ ___ ___ _____

EVALUATION

1. Had patient describe pain and rate level of comfort on scale of 0 to 10. ___ ___ ___ _____

2. Monitored type of tissue in wound bed. ___ ___ ___ _____

	S	U	NP	Comments

3. Inspected dressing periodically, per agency policy. ___ ___ ___ _____

4. Inspected periwound skin integrity. ___ ___ ___ _____

5. Observed for presence of retained irrigant. ___ ___ ___ _____

6. Used Teach-Back. Revised instruction if patient or family caregiver was not able to teach back correctly. ___ ___ ___ _____

DOCUMENTATION

1. Documented wound assessment before and after irrigation; appearance of wound before and after irrigation; amount, color, and odor of drainage on dressing removed; amount and type of solution used; irrigation device used; patient's tolerance of the procedure; and type of dressing applied after irrigation. ___ ___ ___ _____

2. Documented patient's and family caregiver's understanding through Teach-Back for reasons for wound irrigations. ___ ___ ___ _____

HAND-OFF REPORTING

1. Immediately reported to the health care provider any evidence of fresh bleeding, sharp increase in pain, retention of irrigant, or signs of shock. ___ ___ ___ _____

648

PERFORMANCE CHECKLIST SKILL 38.2 **REMOVING SUTURES AND STAPLES**

	S	U	NP	Comments

ASSESSMENT

1. Identified the patient using two identifiers according to agency policy.

2. Reviewed patient's electronic health record (EHR), including health care provider's order and nurses' notes for the following information:

   a. Reviewed specific directions related to suture or staple removal.

   b. Determined history of conditions that might pose risk for impaired wound healing: advanced age, cardiovascular disease, dehydration, diabetes, edema, immunosuppression, radiation, obesity, smoking, poor nutrition, and infection.

3. Assessed patient's/family caregiver's health literacy.

4. Assessed patient for history of allergies. If allergy was identified, applied an allergy wrist band.

5. Assessed character of patient's pain and rated acuity on a pain scale of 0 to 10.

6. Deferred direct assessment of wound and periwound skin to implementation, just before suture removal.

7. Assessed patient's knowledge, prior experience with suture removal, and feelings about the procedure.

PLANNING

1. Determined expected outcomes following completion of procedure.

2. Provided privacy, and explained to patient how staples or sutures would be removed and that removal was usually not a painful procedure, but patient might feel pulling or tugging of skin.

3. Administered prescribed analgesic, if needed, at least 30 minutes before procedure.

4. Organized and set up any equipment needed to perform procedure.

IMPLEMENTATION

	S	U	NP	Comments

1. Performed hand hygiene and positioned patient comfortably while exposing suture line. Ensured that direct lighting was on the suture line. ___ ___ ___ _____

2. Placed cuffed waterproof disposal bag within easy reach. ___ ___ ___ _____

3. Opened sterile packages of equipment needed for suture/staple removal: ___ ___ ___ _____

   a. Opened sterile suture removal kit or staple extractor kit. ___ ___ ___ _____

   b. Opened sterile antiseptic swabs and placed on inside surface of kit. ___ ___ ___ _____

   c. Obtained gloves (sterile gloves if policy indicated). ___ ___ ___ _____

4. Performed hand hygiene. Applied clean gloves. Removed any gauze dressing covering wound. Disposed of soiled dressing in proper receptacle. Inspected incision for healing ridge and skin integrity of suture line for uniform closure of wound edges, normal color, and absence of drainage and inflammation. Palpated around suture line gently, looked for expression of drainage, and noted any tenderness. Removed and disposed of gloves. Performed hand hygiene. ___ ___ ___ _____

5. Applied clean or sterile gloves as required by agency policy. ___ ___ ___ _____

6. Cleaned sutures or staples and healed incision with antiseptic swabs. Started at sides next to incision and then wiped across suture line using new antiseptic swab for each swipe. ___ ___ ___ _____

7. Removed staples: ___ ___ ___ _____

   a. Placed lower tips of staple extractor under first staple. As the nurse closed the handles, upper tip of extractor should have depressed center of staple, causing both ends of staple to be bent upward and simultaneously exit their insertion sites in dermal layer. ___ ___ ___ _____

   b. Carefully controlled staple extractor. ___ ___ ___ _____

   c. As soon as both ends of the staple were visible, lifted up and moved it away from skin surface and continued until staple was over refuse bag. Disposed of contaminated staples in a sharps container, if agency policy. ___ ___ ___ _____

   d. Released handles of staple extractor, allowing staple to drop into refuse bag. ___ ___ ___ _____

650

	S	U	NP	Comments

e. Repeated Steps 7a through 7d until all staples were removed.

8. Removed interrupted sutures:

a. Placed gauze few inches from suture line. Held scissors in dominant hand and forceps (clamp) in nondominant hand.

b. Grasped knot of suture with forceps and gently pulled up knot while slipping tip of scissors under knot of suture near skin.

c. Snipped suture as close to skin as possible at end distal to knot.

d. Grasped knotted end with forceps and, in one continuous smooth action, pulled suture through from the other side. Placed removed suture on gauze.

e. Repeated Steps 8a through 8d until every other suture was removed.

f. Observed healing level. Based on observations of wound response to suture removal and health care provider's original order, determined whether remaining sutures would be removed at that time. If so, repeated Steps 8a to 8d until all sutures removed.

g. If any doubt, stopped and notified health care provider.

9. Removed continuous and blanket stitch sutures:

a. Placed sterile gauze a few inches from suture line. Grasped scissors in dominant hand and forceps in nondominant hand.

b. Snipped first suture close to skin surface at end distal to knot.

c. Snipped second suture on same side.

d. Grasped knotted end and gently pulled with continuous smooth action, removing suture from beneath skin. Placed suture on gauze.

e. Repeated Steps 9a to 9d in consecutive order until entire line was removed.

10. Inspected incision to make sure that all sutures had been removed and identified any trouble areas. Gently wiped suture line with antiseptic swab to remove debris and clean incision.

	S	U	NP	Comments

11. To maintain contact between wound edges, applied Steri-Strips if any separation greater than two stitches or two staples in width was apparent. ___ ___ ___ _____

   a. Cut Steri-Strips to allow them to extend 4 to 5 cm (1 ½ to 2 inches) on each side of the incision. ___ ___ ___ _____

   b. Removed from backing and applied across incision. ___ ___ ___ _____

   c. Instructed patient to take showers rather than soak in bathtub, according to health care provider's preference. ___ ___ ___ _____

12. Removed and discarded gloves. Performed hand hygiene and applied new pair of gloves. Applied light dressing or exposed to air if no clothing would come in contact with suture line. Instructed patient about applying own dressing if needed at home. ___ ___ ___ _____

13. Disposed of sharps (disposable staple extractor and/or scissors) in designated sharps disposal bin. ___ ___ ___ _____

14. Removed and disposed of supplies; removed and disposed of gloves. ___ ___ ___ _____

15. Helped patient to comfortable position. ___ ___ ___ _____

16. Raised side rails (as appropriate) and lowered bed to lowest position, locking into position. ___ ___ ___ _____

17. Placed nurse call system in an accessible location within patient's reach. ___ ___ ___ _____

18. Perform hand hygiene. ___ ___ ___ _____

EVALUATION

1. Examined site where sutures or staples were removed; inspected condition of soft tissues, including skin. Looked for any pieces of removed suture left behind. ___ ___ ___ _____

2. Determined if patient had pain along incision and rated severity using pain rating scale. ___ ___ ___ _____

3. Used Teach-Back. Revised instruction if patient or family caregiver was not able to teach back correctly. ___ ___ ___ _____

DOCUMENTATION

1. Documented the time the sutures or staples were removed and the number of sutures or staples removed; documented the cleaning of the suture line, appearance of the wound, level of healing of the wound, and type of dressing applied; documented patient's response to suture or staple removal. ___ ___ ___ _____

	S	U	NP	Comments
2. Documented patient's and family caregiver's level of understanding following instruction.	___	___	___	_____

HAND-OFF REPORTING

1. Immediately reported to the health care provider if suture line separation, dehiscence, evisceration, bleeding, or purulent drainage occurred.　　　　___　___　___　_____

2. During hand-off, reported during hand-off the removal of staples/sutures, integrity of the incision, use of a dressing (if indicated), and patient's response to removal of staples/sutures.　　　　___　___　___　_____

PERFORMANCE CHECKLIST SKILL 38.3 **MANAGING WOUND DRAINAGE EVACUATION**

	S	U	NP	Comments

ASSESSMENT

1. Identified patient using at least two identifiers, according to agency policy.

2. Reviewed patient's electronic health record (EHR), including health care provider's order and nurses' notes. Noted presence, location, and purpose of closed wound drain and drainage system as patient returned from surgery.

3. Reviewed EHR to determine patient's age and history of dehydration, malnutrition, exposure to radiation therapy, underlying chronic conditions, edema of the skin, and presence of erythema, blistering, or excoriation of skin under or adjacent to adhesive's securing dressing.

4. Assessed patient's/family caregiver's health literacy.

5. Performed hand hygiene. Applied clean gloves. Assessed drainage present on patient's dressing. Identified number of wound drain tubes and what each one was draining. Labeled each drain tube with a number or label.

6. Inspected drainage system to determine presence of one straight tube or Y-tube arrangement with two tube insertion sites.

7. Inspected active drainage system to ensure proper functioning, including insertion site, drainage moving through tubing in direction of reservoir, patency of drainage tubing, airtight connection sites, and presence of any leaks or kinks in system. Removed and disposed of gloves. Performed hand hygiene.

8. Determined if drain tube needed self-suction, wall suction, or no suction by checking the health care provider's orders.

9. Identified type of drainage containers that patient had.

10. Assessed patient's knowledge, experience with drainage system, and feelings about procedure.

	S	U	NP	Comments

PLANNING

1. Determined expected outcomes following completion of procedure.

2. Provided privacy and explained procedure to patient.

3. Organized and set up any equipment needed to perform procedure.

IMPLEMENTATION

1. Performed hand hygiene and applied clean gloves.

2. Placed open specimen container or measuring graduate container on bed between nurse and patient.

3. Emptied Hemovac or ConstaVac:

   a. Maintained asepsis while opening plug on port indicated for emptying drainage reservoir.

     (1) Tilted suction container in direction of plug.

     (2) Slowly squeezed two flat surfaces together, tilting toward measuring container.

   b. Drained all contents into measuring container.

   c. Held open antiseptic swab in dominant hand. Placed suction device on flat surface with open outlet facing upward; continued pressing downward until bottom and top were in contact.

   d. Held device flat with one hand and using antiseptic swab, quickly cleaned opening, plugged with other hand, and immediately replaced plug; secured suction device on patient's bed.

   e. Checked device for reestablishment of vacuum, patency of drainage tubing, and absence of stress on tubing.

4. Emptied Hemovac with wall suction:

   a. Turned off suction.

   b. Disconnected suction tubing from Hemovac port.

   c. Emptied Hemovac as described in Step 3.

   d. Used an antiseptic swab to clean port opening and the end of suction tubing. Reconnected tubing to port.

	S	U	NP	Comments

e. Set suction level as prescribed or on low if health care provider did not specify suction level.

___ ___ ___ _____

5. Emptied JP suction drain:

___ ___ ___ _____

   a. Opened port on top of bulb-shaped reservoir. Opened device away from self to prevent sprays to face.

___ ___ ___ _____

   b. Tilted bulb in direction of port and drained toward opening. Emptied drainage from device into measuring container. Cleaned end of emptying port and plugged with antiseptic wipe.

___ ___ ___ _____

   c. Compressed bulb over drainage container. While compressing bulb, replaced plug immediately.

___ ___ ___ _____

6. Placed and secured drainage system below site with safety pin on patient's gown. Ensured that there was slack in tubing from reservoir to wound.

___ ___ ___ _____

7. Noted characteristics of drainage in measuring container: measured volume and discarded by flushing in commode.

___ ___ ___ _____

8. Discarded soiled supplies and removed and disposed of gloves. Performed hand hygiene.

___ ___ ___ _____

9. Applied clean gloves. Proceeded with dressing change around drain site and inspection of drain insertion site and periwound skin. If used, taped split-drain sponge dressings around drain tubes and taped in place.

___ ___ ___ _____

10. Removed and discarded contaminated material and supplies, removed and disposed of gloves, and performed hand hygiene.

___ ___ ___ _____

11. Helped patient to comfortable position.

___ ___ ___ _____

12. Raised side rails (as appropriate) and lowered bed to lowest position, locking into position.

___ ___ ___ _____

13. Placed nurse call system in an accessible location within patient's reach.

___ ___ ___ _____

EVALUATION

1. Observed for drainage in suction device.

___ ___ ___ _____

2. Inspected wound for drainage or collection of drainage fluid under skin.

___ ___ ___ _____

3. Measured drainage from drainage system, and documented on I&O form at least every 8 to 12 hours and as needed for large drainage volume (per agency policy).

___ ___ ___ _____

	S	U	NP	Comments

4. Inspected periwound skin for any signs of irritation from wound exudate or dressing adhesive material.

5. Used Teach-Back. Revised instruction if patient or family caregiver was not able to teach back correctly.

DOCUMENTATION

1. Documented emptying the drainage suction device; reestablishing vacuum in suction device; amount, color, odor of drainage; dressing change to drain site; and appearance of drain insertion site.

2. Documented amount of drainage.

3. Documented evaluation of patient and family caregiver learning.

HAND-OFF REPORTING

1. Immediately reported a sudden change in amount of drainage, either output or absence of drainage flow, to the health care provider. Also reported pungent odor of drainage or new evidence of purulence, severe pain, or dislodgement of the drainage tube to the health care provider.

PERFORMANCE CHECKLIST SKILL 38.4   **NEGATIVE-PRESSURE WOUND THERAPY**

	S	U	NP	Comments

ASSESSMENT

1. Identified patient using two identifiers, according to agency policy.

2. Reviewed patient's electronic health record (EHR), including health care provider's order and nurses' notes, for frequency of dressing change, amount of negative pressure, type of foam or gauze to use, pressure cycle (intermittent or continuous), and appearance of wound at last dressing change.

3. Reviewed EHR to determine patient's age and history of dehydration, malnutrition, exposure to radiation therapy, underlying chronic conditions, edema of the skin, and the presence of erythema, blistering, or excoriation of skin under or adjacent to adhesive's securing dressing.

4. Assessed patient's/family caregiver's health literacy.

5. Assessed character of patient's pain and rated acuity on a pain scale of 0 to 10.

6. Performed hand hygiene. Applied clean gloves and appropriate PPE. Assessed condition of skin around wound and status of NPWT dressing without disrupting NPWT. Removed and disposed of gloves. Performed hand hygiene.

7. Assessed patient's knowledge, prior experience with NPWT, and feelings about procedure.

PLANNING

1. Determined expected outcomes following completion of procedure.

2. Provided privacy and positioned the patient so that only the area currently being examined was exposed; used sheet to cover rest of the body.

3. Administered prescribed analgesic as needed 30 minutes before dressing change.

4. Organized and set up supplies at patient's bedside.

5. Explained procedure to patient and family caregiver, instructing patient not to touch wound or sterile supplies.

	S	U	NP	Comments

IMPLEMENTATION

1. Cuffed top of disposable waterproof biohazard bag and placed within reach of work area. _____ _____ _____ _____

2. Performed hand hygiene and applied clean gloves and PPE, if not previously applied. If risk for spray existed, applied protective gown, goggles, and mask. _____ _____ _____ _____

3. Followed manufacturer directions for removal and replacement (units will vary). (Following are steps for Wound Vac by KCI). Turned off NPWT unit by pushing therapy on/off button. _____ _____ _____ _____

   a. Closed clamp on dressing tubing. _____ _____ _____ _____

   b. Closed clamp on pump tubing. _____ _____ _____ _____

   c. Disconnected the tubes; allowed any fluid in pump tubing to drain into collection device. _____ _____ _____ _____

4. Removed transparent film by gently stretching and slowly pulling away from skin. _____ _____ _____ _____

5. Removed old foam one layer at a time and discarded in bag. Ensured all pieces of foam were removed. Observed drainage on dressing. Used caution to avoid tension on any drains that were present near the wound or surrounding area. Removed and disposed of gloves. _____ _____ _____ _____

6. Performed hand hygiene and conducted a wound healing assessment. Observed surface area and tissue type, color, odor, and drainage within wound. Measured length, width, and depth of wound as ordered. _____ _____ _____ _____

7. Removed and discarded gloves in biohazard bag. Avoided having patient see old dressing because sight of wound drainage might be upsetting. _____ _____ _____ _____

8. Cleaned wound per order/recommendations of WOCN or wound care specialist. _____ _____ _____ _____

   a. Performed hand hygiene. Applied sterile or clean gloves, depending on agency policy and wound status. _____ _____ _____ _____

   b. If ordered, irrigated wound with normal saline or other solution ordered by health care provider. Gently blotted periwound with gauze to dry thoroughly. _____ _____ _____ _____

9. Applied skin protectant, barrier film, solid skin barrier sheet, or hydrocolloid dressing to periwound skin. _____ _____ _____ _____

	S	U	NP	Comments

10. Filled any uneven skin surfaces with skin-barrier product. ___ ___ ___ _____

11. Removed and disposed of gloves. Performed hand hygiene. ___ ___ ___ _____

12. Depending on type of wound, applied sterile or new clean gloves, per agency policy. ___ ___ ___ _____

13. Applied NPWT dressing. ___ ___ ___ _____

   a. Prepared NPWT filler dressing. Consulted with wound-care expert for appropriate type. ___ ___ ___ _____

     (1) Measured clean wound and selected appropriate-size dressing. ___ ___ ___ _____

     (2) Using sterile scissors, cut filler dressing foam to wound size, making sure to fit exact size and shape of wound, including tunnels and undermined areas. ___ ___ ___ _____

   b. Placed filler dressing in wound following manufacturer instructions. Ensured that filler dressing was in contact with entire wound base, margins, and tunneled and undermined areas. Counted number of filler dressings and documented in patient's chart. ___ ___ ___ _____

   c. Applied NPWT transparent dressing over foam wound dressing. ___ ___ ___ _____

     (1) Trimmed dressing to cover wound and dressing so it extended onto periwound skin approximately 2.5 to 3 cm (1–2 inches). ___ ___ ___ _____

     (2) Applied transparent dressing. ___ ___ ___ _____

       (a) Retained blue handling tab on portion of dressing used. Peeled back one side of layer one. Then placed adhesive side down over wound. ___ ___ ___ _____

       (b) Removed remaining side of layer one. ___ ___ ___ _____

       (c) Removed green striped stabilization layer two. Removed blue handling tabs. ___ ___ ___ _____

     (3) Applied connecting pad and tubing to dressing: ___ ___ ___ _____

       (a) Identified site over dressing for pad application. Pinched transparent dressing and cut at least a 2 cm round hole. ___ ___ ___ _____

       (b) Removed backing layers from pad. Placed connecting tube opening of pad directly over hole in dressing. ___ ___ ___ _____

	S	U	NP	Comments

(c) Applied gentle pressure to secure. Removed any remaining stabilization layer and discarded. ___ ___ ___ _____

(d) Connected pad tubing to canister tubing and opened all clamps. ___ ___ ___ _____

14. Turned on power to vac unit and set appropriate mode and pressure levels. ___ ___ ___ _____

15. Secured tubing several centimeters away from dressing, avoided pressure points. ___ ___ ___ _____

16. Removed and disposed of gloves. Performed hand hygiene. ___ ___ ___ _____

17. Inspected NPWT system. ___ ___ ___ _____

a. Verified that the system was on. Checked agency policy and procedure for specific information. ___ ___ ___ _____

b. Verified that all clamps were open and all tubing was patent. ___ ___ ___ _____

c. Examined system to be sure that seal was intact and therapy was working. ___ ___ ___ _____

d. If a leak was present, used strips of transparent film to patch areas around edges of wound. ___ ___ ___ _____

18. Wrote initials, date, and time on new dressing. ___ ___ ___ _____

19. Disposed of sharps (scissors) in designated sharps disposal bin, removed gloves if not already removed, and performed hand hygiene. ___ ___ ___ _____

20. Helped patient to comfortable position. ___ ___ ___ _____

21. Raised side rails (as appropriate) and lowered bed to lowest position, locking into position. ___ ___ ___ _____

22. Placed nurse call system in an accessible location within patient's reach. ___ ___ ___ _____

EVALUATION

1. Inspected condition of wound, wound bed, and periwound area on an ongoing basis; noted drainage and odor. ___ ___ ___ _____

2. Asked patient to describe character of pain and rate severity pain using scale of 0 to 10. ___ ___ ___ _____

3. Verified airtight dressing seal and correct negative-pressure setting. ___ ___ ___ _____

4. Measured wound drainage output in canister on regular basis. ___ ___ ___ _____

5. Used Teach-Back. Revised instruction if patient or family caregiver was not able to teach back correctly. ___ ___ ___ _____

	S	U	NP	Comments

DOCUMENTATION

1. Documented appearance of wound, characteristics of drainage, placement of NPWT (time and type of dressing, pressure mode and setting), and patient response to dressing change. ___ ___ ___ _____

2. Documented whether the patient or caregiver was participating in changing the NPWT dressing. ___ ___ ___ _____

3. Documented evaluation of patient and family caregiver learning. ___ ___ ___ _____

HAND-OFF REPORTING

1. Reported brisk, bright-red bleeding; evidence of poor wound healing; evisceration or dehiscence; and possible wound infection to health care provider immediately. ___ ___ ___ _____

PERFORMANCE CHECKLIST SKILL 39.1 **RISK ASSESSMENT, SKIN ASSESSMENT, AND PREVENTION STRATEGIES**

	S	U	NP	Comments

ASSESSMENT

1. Identified patient using at least two identifiers, according to agency policy.

2. Reviewed electronic health record (EHR) to determine patient's age and history of dehydration, malnutrition, exposure to radiation therapy, underlying chronic conditions, erythema, and edema of the skin.

3. Reviewed patient's EHR, including health provider's orders and nurses' notes, to assess patient's risk for pressure injury formation.

4. Selected agency-approved risk assessment tool. Performed risk assessment when patient entered health care setting and repeated on regularly scheduled basis or when there was significant change in patient's condition.

5. Obtained risk score and evaluated its meaning based on patient's unique condition and risk factors.

6. Assessed patient's/family caregiver's health literacy.

7. Provided privacy and explained procedure.

8. Performed hand hygiene. Assessed condition of patient's skin over regions of pressure. Applied clean gloves as needed with open and/or draining wounds.

   a. Inspected for skin discoloration and tissue consistency (firm or boggy feel) and/or palpated for abnormal sensations.

   b. Palpated discolored area on skin and under and around medical devices, released fingertip, and looked for blanching.

   c. Inspected for pallor and mottling.

   d. Inspected for absence of superficial skin layers.

   e. Inspected for changes in skin temperature, edema, and tissue consistency, especially in individuals with darkly pigmented skin.

   f. Inspected for wound drainage.

9. Assessed skin and tissue around and beneath medical devices at least twice daily for areas of potential pressure injury resulting from medical devices.

   a. Nares: NG tube, oxygen cannula

b. Ears: oxygen cannula, pillow

c. Tongue and lips: oral airway, ET tube

d. Forehead: pulse oximetry device

e. Drainage or other tubing

f. Indwelling urethral catheter

g. Orthopedic and positioning devices such as casts, neck collars, splints

h. Compression stockings

i. Immobilization device and restraints

10. Removed and disposed of gloves and performed hand hygiene.

11. Observed patient for preferred positions when in bed or chair.

12. Observed ability of patient to initiate and help with position changes.

13. Assessed knowledge and prior experience of patient with pressure injury prevention techniques, and feelings about procedure.

PLANNING

1. Determined expected outcomes following completion of procedure.

2. Closed room door or pulled the curtain around the bed and positioned the patient so that only the area being examined would be exposed.

3. Prepared and organized equipment. Ensured that the correct risk-assessment tool was at bedside.

4. Explained procedure(s) and purpose to patient and family caregiver.

5. Arranged for extra personnel to help as necessary. Organized supplies at bedside.

IMPLEMENTATION

1. Implemented Pressure Injury Prevention Guidelines according to agency policy.

2. Performed hand hygiene and applied clean gloves.

3. Raised bed to appropriate working height. Raised side rail on opposite edge of bed and lowered side rail on working side.

4. Following initial assessment, continued to inspect skin at least once a day.

a. Observed patient's skin; paid particular attention to bony prominences and areas around and under medical devices and tubes. If a reddened area was found, gently pressed area with gloved finger to check for blanching. If area did not blanch, suspected tissue injury and rechecked in 30 minutes to 1 hour.

664

	S	U	NP	Comments

b. If patient had darkly pigmented skin, looked for color changes that differed from patient's normal skin color. ___ ___ ___ _____

5. Each shift, checked all treatment and assistive devices for potential pressure points. ___ ___ ___ _____

   a. Verified that device was correctly sized, positioned, and secured. ___ ___ ___ _____

   b. Considered shielding underlying at-risk skin with protective dressing. ___ ___ ___ _____

6. Removed and disposed of gloves; performed hand hygiene. ___ ___ ___ _____

7. Reviewed patient's pressure injury risk assessment score. ___ ___ ___ _____

8. If immobility, inactivity, and/or poor sensory perception were risk factors for patient, considered one of the following interventions. ___ ___ ___ _____

   a. Repositioned patient based on frequent assessment findings of individual's skin condition and risk factors to identify early signs of pressure damage. If skin changes occurred, reevaluated the positioning plan. ___ ___ ___ _____

   b. When patient was in side-lying position in bed, used 30-degree lateral position. Avoided 90-degree lateral position. ___ ___ ___ _____

   c. Placed patient (when lying in bed) on pressure-redistribution surface. ___ ___ ___ _____

   d. Placed patient (when in chair) on pressure-redistribution device and shifted points under pressure at least every hour. ___ ___ ___ _____

9. If friction and shear were identified as risk factors, considered the following interventions: ___ ___ ___ _____

   a. Used safe patient-handling guidelines to reposition patient. ___ ___ ___ _____

   b. Ensured that heels were free from bed surface by using a pillow under calves to elevate heels or used a heel-suspension device; knees should have been in 5- to 10-degree flexion. ___ ___ ___ _____

   c. Maintained head of the bed (HOB) at 30 degrees or lower or at the lowest degree of elevation consistent with patient's condition (did not lower HOB if patient was at risk for aspiration). ___ ___ ___ _____

10. If patient received low score on moisture subscale, considered one of the following interventions: ___ ___ ___ _____

   a. Applied clean gloves. Cleaned and dried the skin as soon as possible after each incontinence episode. Applied moisture barrier ointment to perineum and surrounding skin after each incontinence episode. ___ ___ ___ _____

	S	U	NP	Comments

b. If skin was denuded, used protective barrier after each incontinence episode.
_____ _____ _____ _____

c. If moisture source was from wound drainage, considered frequent dressing changes, skin protection with protective barriers, or collection devices.
_____ _____ _____ _____

11. If friction and shear were risk factors and patient was chairbound:

a. Tilted patient's chair seat to prevent sliding forward, and supported arms, legs, and feet to maintain proper posture.
_____ _____ _____ _____

b. Limited amount of time patient spent in a chair without pressure relief.
_____ _____ _____ _____

c. For patients who could reposition themselves while sitting, encouraged pressure relief every 15 minutes using chair push-ups, forward lean, or side to side.
_____ _____ _____ _____

12. Educated patient and family caregiver regarding specific pressure injury risk factors and prevention.
_____ _____ _____ _____

13. Removed and disposed of gloves and performed hand hygiene.
_____ _____ _____ _____

14. Helped patient to a comfortable position.
_____ _____ _____ _____

15. Raised side rails (as appropriate) and lowered bed to lowest position, locking into position.
_____ _____ _____ _____

16. Placed nurse call system in an accessible location within patient's reach.
_____ _____ _____ _____

17. Performed hand hygiene.

EVALUATION

1. Observed patient's skin for areas at risk for tissue damage, noting change in color, appearance, or texture.
_____ _____ _____ _____

2. Observed tolerance of patient for position change by measuring level of comfort on pain scale.
_____ _____ _____ _____

3. Compared subsequent risk assessment scores and skin assessments.
_____ _____ _____ _____

4. Used Teach-Back technique. Revised instruction if patient or family caregiver was not able to teach back correctly.
_____ _____ _____ _____

DOCUMENTATION

1. Documented any skin changes, patient's risk score, and skin assessment. Described positions, turning intervals, pressure-redistribution devices, and other prevention measures. Noted patient's response to the interventions.
_____ _____ _____ _____

2. Documented evaluation of patient's and family caregiver's understanding of the need for frequent skin and pressure injury assessment education.
_____ _____ _____ _____

HAND-OFF REPORTING

1. Reported need for additional consultations for the high-risk patient to health care provider.
_____ _____ _____ _____

666

Student _____ Date _____

Instructor _____ Date _____

PERFORMANCE CHECKLIST SKILL 39.2 **TREATMENT OF PRESSURE INJURIES**

	S	U	NP	Comments

ASSESSMENT

1. Identified patient using at least two identifiers, according to agency policy.

2. Reviewed patient's electronic health record (EHR), including health care provider's orders and nurses' notes. Noted previous dressing change for wound assessment, types of topical medications, types of analgesia if needed, and wound care supplies.

3. Reviewed EHR to determine patient's age and history of dehydration, malnutrition, exposure to radiation therapy, underlying chronic conditions, and edema of the skin.

4. Assessed patient's/family caregiver's health literacy.

5. Assessed patient's knowledge, prior experience with treatment of pressure injuries, and feelings about procedure.

6. Assessed character of patient's pain and rated acuity on a pain scale of 0 to 10. If patient was in pain, determined if PRN pain medication had been ordered and administered.

7. Asked patient and checked EHR for history of allergies. Checked allergy bracelet. Determined if patient had allergies to topical agents.

8. Provided privacy and explained procedure.

9. Positioned patient to allow dressing removal and positioned plastic bag for dressing disposal.

10. Performed hand hygiene and applied clean gloves. Removed and discarded old dressing.

11. Assessed patient's wounds using wound parameters and continued ongoing wound assessment per agency policy. Note: This may have been done during wound care procedure.

   a. *Wound location:* Described body site where wound was located.

   b. *Stage of wound:* Described extent of tissue destruction.

	S	U	NP	Comments

c. *Wound size:* Length, width, and depth of wound were measured per agency protocol. Used disposable measuring guide for length and width. Used cotton-tipped applicator to assess depth. ___ ___ ___ _____

d. *Presence of undermining, sinus tracts, or tunnels:* Used sterile cotton-tipped applicator to measure depth, undermining, or sinus tracts. ___ ___ ___ _____

e. *Condition of wound bed:* Described type and percentage of tissue in wound bed. ___ ___ ___ _____

f. *Volume of exudate:* Described amount, characteristics, odor, and color. ___ ___ ___ _____

g. *Condition of periwound skin:* Examined skin for breaks, dryness, and presence of rash, swelling, redness, or warmth. Modified assessment based on patient's skin color. ___ ___ ___ _____

h. *Wound edges:* With a gloved finger, examined wound edges for condition of tissue. ___ ___ ___ _____

12. Assessed periwound skin; checked for maceration, redness, or denuded tissue. ___ ___ ___ _____

13. Removed gloves and discarded in appropriate receptacle. Performed hand hygiene. ___ ___ ___ _____

14. Assessed for factors affecting wound healing: poor perfusion, immunosuppression, or preexisting infection. ___ ___ ___ _____

15. Assessed patient's nutritional status. ___ ___ ___ _____

16. Assessed patient's knowledge, prior experience with prevention and treatment, and feelings about procedure. ___ ___ ___ _____

PLANNING

1. Determined expected outcomes following completion of procedure. ___ ___ ___ _____

2. Explained procedure to patient and family caregiver. ___ ___ ___ _____

3. Provided privacy. ___ ___ ___ _____

4. Organized and set up equipment and supplies: ___ ___ ___ _____

   a. Wash basin, warm water, equipment, and supplies ___ ___ ___ _____

   b. Normal saline (NS) or other wound-cleaning agent ___ ___ ___ _____

   c. Prescribed topical agent: ___ ___ ___ _____

   (1) Enzyme-debriding agents. (Followed specific manufacturer directions for frequency of application.) OR ___ ___ ___ _____

   (2) Topical antibiotics ___ ___ ___ _____

	S	U	NP	Comments

d. Selected appropriate dressing based on pressure injury characteristics, principles of wound management, and patient care setting. ___ ___ ___ _____

e. Obtained hypoallergenic tape or adhesive dressing sheet. ___ ___ ___ _____

IMPLEMENTATION

1. Performed hand hygiene. ___ ___ ___ _____

2. Opened sterile packages and topical solution containers. Kept dressings sterile. Wore goggles, mask, and moisture-proof cover gown if potential for contamination from spray existed when cleaning wound. ___ ___ ___ _____

3. Raised bed to appropriate working height. If side rails were in use, raised side rail on opposite side of bed and lowered side rail on working side. ___ ___ ___ _____

4. Placed waterproof pad under patient. ___ ___ ___ _____

5. Arranged patient's gown to expose injury and surrounding skin. Kept remaining body parts draped. ___ ___ ___ _____

6. Cleaned wound thoroughly with normal saline or prescribed wound-cleaning agent from least contaminated to most contaminated area. For deep injuries, cleaned with saline delivered with irrigating syringe as ordered. Removed gloves and discarded. ___ ___ ___ _____

7. Performed hand hygiene and applied clean or sterile gloves. (Referred to agency policy.) ___ ___ ___ _____

8. Applied topical agents to wound using cotton-tipped applicators or gauze as ordered: ___ ___ ___ _____

   a. Enzymes

      (1) Applied small amount of enzyme-debridement ointment directly to necrotic areas in pressure injury. Did not apply enzyme to surrounding skin. ___ ___ ___ _____

      (2) Placed moist gauze dressing directly over injury and taped in place. Followed specific manufacturer recommendation for type of dressing material to use to cover a pressure injury when using enzymes. Taped dressing in place. ___ ___ ___ _____

   b. Antibacterial ___ ___ ___ _____

9. Applied prescribed wound dressing: ___ ___ ___ _____

   a. Hydrogel:

      (1) Covered surface of injury with thick layer of amorphous hydrogel or cut sheet to fit wound base. ___ ___ ___ _____

      (2) Applied secondary dressing such as dry gauze; taped in place. ___ ___ ___ _____

	S	U	NP	Comments

(3) If using impregnated gauze, packed loosely into wound; covered with secondary gauze dressing and tape.

    b. Alginate, such as calcium alginate:

      (1) Lightly packed wound with alginate using sterile cotton-tipped applicator or gloved finger.

      (2) Applied secondary dressing and taped in place.

    c. Transparent film dressing, hydrocolloid, and foam dressings

10. Repositioned patient comfortably off the pressure injury.

11. Removed and disposed of gloves. Disposed of soiled supplies in appropriate receptacle. Performed hand hygiene.

12. Raised side rails (as appropriate) and lowered bed to lowest position, locking into postion.

13. Placed nurse call system in an accessible location within patient's reach.

14. Performed hand hygiene.

EVALUATION

1. Observed skin surrounding injury for inflammation, edema, and tenderness.

2. Inspected dressings and exposed injuries, observing for drainage, foul odor, and tissue necrosis. Monitored patient for signs and symptoms of infection: fever and elevated white blood cell (WBC) count.

3. Compared subsequent injury measurements, using one of the scales designed to measure wound healing such as PUSH Tool or BWAT.

4. Used Teach-Back technique. Revised instruction if patient or family caregiver was not able to teach back correctly.

DOCUMENTATION

1. Documented type of wound tissue present in injury, measurements of the injury, periwound skin condition, character of drainage or exudate, type of topical agent used, dressing applied, and patient's response.

2. Documented evaluation of patient's and family caregiver's understanding of frequent observation and measuring of wound.

HAND-OFF REPORTING

1. Reported any deterioration in injury appearance to nurse in charge or health care provider.

PERFORMANCE CHECKLIST SKILL 40.1 **APPLYING A DRESSING (DRY AND MOIST DRESSINGS)**

	S	U	NP	Comments

ASSESSMENT

1. Identified patient using at least two identifiers, according to agency policy.

2. Reviewed patient's electronic health record (EHR), including health care provider's orders and nurses' notes. Noted previous dressing change, including equipment used and patient response.

3. Reviewed EHR to determine patient's age and history of dehydration, malnutrition, exposure to radiation therapy, underlying chronic conditions, edema of the skin, and the presence of erythema, blistering, excoriation, or erosion of skin or a rash under or adjacent to adhesive's securing dressing.

4. Assessed patient's/family caregiver's health literacy.

5. Assessed patient for allergies, especially antiseptics, tape, or latex. Had patient describe allergic response and acquired specific orders for dressing change.

6. Asked patient to rate level of wound pain acuity on a pain scale of 0 to 10. Administered prescribed analgesic as needed 30 minutes before dressing change.

7. Reviewed EHR to identify patients at risk for poor wound-healing.

8. Performed hand hygiene and applied clean gloves. Assessed condition of skin around wound, existing dressing, and presence of drainage on outer gauze. Removed and disposed of gloves and performed hand hygiene.

9. Assessed patient's and family caregiver's knowledge, prior experience with dressing change, and feelings about procedure.

PLANNING

1. Determined expected outcomes following completion of procedure.

	S	U	NP	Comments

2. Provided privacy and explained procedure. Explained to patient any sensations that might be felt during dressing change.

     ____ ____ ____   _____

3. Performed hand hygiene. Organized and set up any equipment needed to perform procedure at bedside.

     ____ ____ ____   _____

4. Placed biohazard bag within reach of work area. Folded top of bag to make a cuff.

     ____ ____ ____   _____

5. Positioned patient comfortably and draped to expose only wound site. Instructed patient not to touch wound or sterile supplies.

     ____ ____ ____   _____

IMPLEMENTATION

1. Performed hand hygiene and applied clean gloves. Applied gown, goggles, and mask if risk for splashing existed.

     ____ ____ ____   _____

2. Gently removed tape, bandages, or ties. Using two hands, slowly removed adhesive at a low angle, parallel to the patient's skin, while supporting the skin at the tape-skin interface. If dressing was over hairy area, removed in direction of hair growth. Got patient permission to clip or shave area (checked agency policy). Removed any adhesive from skin.

     ____ ____ ____   _____

3. With gloved hand or forceps, removed dressing one layer at a time, observing appearance of drainage on dressing. Carefully removed outer secondary dressing first, and then removed inner primary dressing in contact with wound bed. If drains were present, slowly and carefully removed dressings and avoided tension on any drainage devices. Kept soiled dressing from patient's sight.

     ____ ____ ____   _____

   a. If bottom layer of a moist dressing adhered to wound, gently freed dressing while alerting patient of discomfort.

     ____ ____ ____   _____

   b. If dry dressing adhered to wound that was not to be debrided, moistened with normal saline first, waited 1 to 2 minutes, and then removed.

     ____ ____ ____   _____

4. Inspected wound and periwound for appearance, color, size (length, width, and depth), drainage, edema, presence and condition of drains, approximation, granulation tissue, or odor. Used measuring guide or ruler to measure size of wound. Inspected periwound area for signs of MARSI and MASD and gently palpated wound edges for bogginess or patient report of increased pain.

     ____ ____ ____   _____

672

	S	U	NP	Comments

5. Folded dressings with drainage contained inside and removed gloves inside out. With small dressings, removed gloves inside out over dressing. Disposed of gloves and soiled dressing according to agency policy. Covered wound lightly with sterile gauze pad and performed hand hygiene. _____ _____ _____ _____

6. Described appearance of wound and any indicators of wound healing to patient. _____ _____ _____ _____

7. Created sterile field with sterile dressing tray or individually wrapped sterile supplies on over-bed table. Poured any prescribed solution into sterile basin. _____ _____ _____ _____

8. Cleaned wound. _____ _____ _____ _____

   a. Performed hand hygiene and applied clean gloves. Used gauze or cotton ball moistened in saline or antiseptic swab (per health care provider order) for each cleaning stroke, or sprayed wound surface with wound cleaner. _____ _____ _____ _____

   b. Cleaned from least to most contaminated area. _____ _____ _____ _____

   c. Cleaned around any drain (if present) using circular strokes, starting near drain and moving outward and away from insertion site. _____ _____ _____ _____

   d. Used sterile dry gauze to blot wound bed in same manner. _____ _____ _____ _____

9. Applied antiseptic ointment (if ordered) with sterile cotton-tipped applicator or gauze along wound edges. Disposed of gloves. Performed hand hygiene. _____ _____ _____ _____

10. Applied dressing, per agency policy: _____ _____ _____ _____

   a. Dry sterile dressing:

   (1) Applied clean gloves, per agency policy. _____ _____ _____ _____

   (2) Applied loose woven gauze as contact layer. _____ _____ _____ _____

   (3) If drain was present, applied precut, split 4 × 4-inch gauze around drain. _____ _____ _____ _____

   (4) Applied additional layers of gauze as needed. _____ _____ _____ _____

   (5) Applied thicker woven pad for the outermost dressing if needed. _____ _____ _____ _____

   b. Moist dressing:

   (1) Applied sterile gloves, per agency policy. _____ _____ _____ _____

   (2) Placed fine-mesh or loose 4 × 4-inch gauze in container of prescribed sterile solution. Wrung out excess solution thoroughly. _____ _____ _____ _____

(3) Fluffed the damp fine-mesh or open-weave gauze and applied as single layer directly onto wound surface. If wound was deep, gently packed gauze into wound with sterile gloved hand or forceps until all wound surfaces were in contact with damp gauze, including dead spaces from sinus tracts, tunnels, and undermining. Ensured that gauze did not touch periwound skin.

___ ___ ___ _____

(4) Applied dry moisture retentive sterile dressing over moist gauze.

___ ___ ___ _____

(5) Covered with ABD pad, Surgipad, or gauze.

___ ___ ___ _____

11. Secured dressing:

___ ___ ___ _____

a. Tape: Applied nonallergenic tape over gauze and 2.5 to 5 cm (1 to 2 inches) beyond dressing.

___ ___ ___ _____

b. Montgomery ties:

(1) Ensured that skin was clean. Application of skin barrier recommended.

___ ___ ___ _____

(2) Exposed adhesive surface of tape ends.

___ ___ ___ _____

(3) Placed ties on opposite sides of dressing over skin barrier.

___ ___ ___ _____

(4) Secured dressing by lacing ties across dressing snugly enough to hold it secure but without placing pressure on skin.

___ ___ ___ _____

c. For protective window:

(1) Cut hydrocolloid pad into four strips used to form a "window" around the wound.

___ ___ ___ _____

(2) Used skin barrier to wipe areas of skin where strips would be applied.

___ ___ ___ _____

(3) Applied hydrocolloid dressing strips to frame a "window" around the wound using four strips, one on each side, one on the top, and one on the bottom of the dressing material.

___ ___ ___ _____

(4) Applied dressing and secured tape ends to stomahesive or hydrocolloid strips.

___ ___ ___ _____

d. For dressing on an extremity, secured with rolled gauze or elastic net.

___ ___ ___ _____

	S	U	NP	Comments

12. Disposed of all dressing supplies. Removed cover gown and goggles, removed gloves inside out, and disposed of all items according to agency policy. Performed hand hygiene. ___ ___ ___ _____

13. Labeled tape over dressing with initials and date dressing was changed. ___ ___ ___ _____

14. Helped patient to comfortable position. ___ ___ ___ _____

15. Raised side rails (as appropriate) and lowered bed to lowest position, locking into position. ___ ___ ___ _____

16. Placed nurse call system in an accessible location within patient's reach. ___ ___ ___ _____

EVALUATION

1. Compared observations of the wound and periwound area with previous assessment and observed appearance of wound for healing: measured size of wound; and observed amount, color, and type of drainage and periwound erythema, rash, excoriation, or swelling; and observed forigns associated with MARSI and MASD. ___ ___ ___ _____

2. Asked patient to describe character of wound pain and rate acuity on a pain scale of 0 to 10. ___ ___ ___ _____

3. Inspected condition of dressing at least every shift. ___ ___ ___ _____

4. Used Teach-Back technique. Revised instruction if patient or family caregiver was not able to teach back correctly. ___ ___ ___ _____

DOCUMENTATION

1. Documented appearance and size of wound, characteristics of drainage, presence of necrotic tissue, type of dressing applied, periwound skin integrity, patient's response to dressing change, and level of comfort. ___ ___ ___ _____

2. Documented patient's and family caregiver's understanding through Teach-Back. ___ ___ ___ _____

HAND-OFF REPORTING

1. Reported any unexpected appearance of wound drainage, accidental removal of drain, or bright red bleeding. ___ ___ ___ _____

2. Reported any changes in periwound skin or signs of MARSI or MASD. ___ ___ ___ _____

3. Reported any change in wound integrity. ___ ___ ___ _____

Student _____ Date _____

Instructor _____ Date _____

PERFORMANCE CHECKLIST SKILL 40.2 **APPLYING A PRESSURE BANDAGE**

	S	U	NP	Comments

ASSESSMENT

1. If situation permitted, identified patient using at least two identifiers, according to agency policy.

2. Performed hand hygiene and applied clean gloves. Anticipated patients at risk for unexpected bleeding, including traumatic injury, arterial puncture, donor graft site, postoperative incision, wounds after surgical debridement, and surgical patient with history of bleeding disorder.

3. Looked for visible presence of blood or blood pulsating from arterial site.

4. If situation permitted, assessed patient for allergies to antiseptics, tape, or latex. If patient was nonresponsive and no history was available, used nonlatex or nonallergenic supplies.

5. Quickly assessed patient's anxiety level.

6. If possible, reviewed electronic health record (EHR) for patient's baseline vital signs before onset of hemorrhage.

7. After the initial crisis and if the situation permitted, assessed patient's/family caregiver's health literacy.

PLANNING

1. Determined expected outcomes following completion of procedure.

2. Provided privacy and, if possible, explained procedure and what was occurring to patient.

3. Performed hand hygiene. Obtained specialized equipment, such as chest tube tray and hemocclusive dressing material.

4. If not already present, arranged for extra personnel to help as needed.

IMPLEMENTATION

Phase I: Immediate Action—First Nurse

1. Performed hand hygiene and applied clean gloves. Identified external bleeding site. Turned patients to observe underneath those who had large abdomens.

676

	S	U	NP	Comments

2. Used both hands and pressed as hard as possible to apply immediate manual pressure to bleeding site.

3. Remained with the patient and sought help. Had another person notify patient's health care provider as appropriate.

Phase II: Applying Pressure Bandage—Second Nurse

4. If the situation permitted, performed hand hygiene and applied clean gloves. Quickly identified source of bleeding.

5. Elevated affected body part if possible.

6. First nurse continued to apply direct pressure as second nurse unwrapped elastic rolled bandage and placed within easy reach. Second nurse quickly cut three to five lengths of adhesive tape and placed them within reach; did not clean wound.

7. In simultaneous coordinated actions:

   a. Rapidly covered bleeding area with multiple thicknesses of gauze compresses. The first nurse slipped fingers out as other nurse exerted adequate pressure to continue controlling bleeding.

   b. Placed adhesive strips 7 to 10 cm (3 to 4 inches) beyond width of gauze dressing with even pressure on both sides of fingers as close as possible to central bleeding source. Secured tape on distal end, pulled tape across dressing, and kept firm pressure as proximate end of tape was secured.

   c. Removed fingers temporarily and quickly covered center of area with third strip of tape.

   d. Continued reinforcing area with tape as each successive strip was overlapped on alternating sides of center strip. Kept applying pressure.

   e. If pressure bandage was on extremity, applied gauze directly over bleeding site. Then, applied elastic rolled bandage over gauze: Applied two circular turns tautly on both sides of fingers that were pressing gauze. Compressed over bleeding site. Simultaneously removed finger pressure and applied rolled bandage over center. Continued with figure-eight turns, moving from distal to proximal moving toward the patient's heart. Secured end with two circular turns and strip of adhesive.

	S	U	NP	Comments

8. Once bandage was applied, disposed of any contaminated supplies; removed and disposed of gloves. Performed hand hygiene. ___ ___ ___ _____

9. If the situation permitted, helped patient to a comfortable position. ___ ___ ___ _____

10. Raised side rails (as appropriate) and lowered bed to lowest position, locking into position. ___ ___ ___ _____

11. Placed nurse call system in an accessible location within patient's reach. ___ ___ ___ _____

EVALUATION

1. Observed dressing for control of bleeding. ___ ___ ___ _____

2. Evaluated adequacy of circulation (distal pulse, skin temperature, and color). ___ ___ ___ _____

3. Estimated volume of blood loss. ___ ___ ___ _____

4. Monitored vital signs. ___ ___ ___ _____

DOCUMENTATION

1. Documented location of bleeding, assessment findings, application and type of pressure dressing, and patient response. ___ ___ ___ _____

HAND-OFF REPORTING

1. Reported immediately to health care provider present status of patient's bleeding control, time bleeding was discovered, estimated blood loss, nursing interventions (including effectiveness of applied pressure bandage), apical and distal pulses, blood pressure, mental status, signs of restlessness, and need for health care provider to administer to patient without delay. ___ ___ ___ _____

Student _____ Date _____

Instructor _____ Date _____

PERFORMANCE CHECKLIST SKILL 40.3 **APPLYING A TRANSPARENT DRESSING**

	S	U	NP	Comments

ASSESSMENT

1. Identified patient using at least two identifiers, according to agency policy.

2. Reviewed patient's electronic health record (EHR), including health care provider's order for frequency and type of dressing change.

3. Reviewed previous nurses' notes in EHR or chart, noting location, wound assessment, size of wound, and patient response to dressing changes.

4. Reviewed EHR to determine patient's age and history of dehydration, malnutrition, exposure to radiation therapy, underlying chronic conditions, edema of the skin, and the presence of erythema, blistering, excoriation, or erosion of skin or a rash under or adjacent to adhesive's securing dressing.

5. Reviewed EHR for patient's medical history indicating risks for impaired wound healing

6. Assessed patient's/family caregiver's health literacy.

7. Assessed patient for allergies, especially antiseptics, tape, or latex. Had patient describe allergic response.

8. Asked patient to describe character of any wound pain and to rate severity using pain scale of 0 to 10. Administered prescribed analgesic as needed 30 minutes before dressing change.

9. Assessed patient's knowledge, prior experience with transparent dressing, and feelings about procedure.

PLANNING

1. Determined expected outcomes following completion of procedure.

2. Provided privacy and explained procedure.

3. Performed hand hygiene. Organized and set up any equipment needed to perform procedure at bedside.

4. Placed biohazard bag within reach of work area.

679

	S	U	NP	Comments

5. Positioned patient comfortably and draped to expose only wound site. Instructed patient not to touch wound or sterile supplies.   ____ ____ ____ _____

IMPLEMENTATION

1. Performed hand hygiene and applied clean gloves. Applied PPE as needed if there was a risk for splashing.   ____ ____ ____ _____

2. Removed old dressing by stretching film in direction parallel to wound rather than pulling.   ____ ____ ____ _____

3. Disposed of soiled dressing in waterproof bag, removed gloves by pulling them inside out, disposed of them in waterproof bag, and performed hand hygiene.   ____ ____ ____ _____

4. Prepared dressing supplies. Used sterile supplies for new wounds, per agency policy.   ____ ____ ____ _____

5. Poured saline or prescribed solution over 4 × 4-inch sterile gauze pads.   ____ ____ ____ _____

6. Applied clean or sterile gloves, per agency policy.   ____ ____ ____ _____

7. Cleaned wound and periwound area gently with 4 × 4-inch sterile gauze pads moistened in sterile saline or spray with wound cleaner. Cleaned in direction from least to most contaminated area.   ____ ____ ____ _____

8. Patted skin around wound in same direction as Step 7; dry thoroughly with dry 4 × 4-inch sterile gauze pads.   ____ ____ ____ _____

9. Inspected wound for tissue type, color, odor, and drainage; measured size if indicated.   ____ ____ ____ _____

10. Removed and disposed of gloves and performed hand hygiene.   ____ ____ ____ _____

11. Applied clean gloves and applied transparent dressing according to manufacturer's directions. Did not stretch film during application and avoided wrinkles.   ____ ____ ____ _____

    a. Removed paper backing, taking care not to allow adhesive areas to touch one another.   ____ ____ ____ _____

    b. Placed film smoothly over wound without stretching.   ____ ____ ____ _____

    c. Used fingers to smooth and adhere dressing.   ____ ____ ____ _____

12. Discarded soiled dressing materials properly. Removed gloves by pulling them inside out and discarded in prepared bag. Performed hand hygiene.   ____ ____ ____ _____

13. Labeled dressing with date, initials, and time of dressing change on outer label of dressing.   ____ ____ ____ _____

14. Helped patient to comfortable position.   ____ ____ ____ _____

	S	U	NP	Comments

15. Raised side rails (as appropriate) and lowered bed to lowest position, locking into position. ⎯ ⎯ ⎯ ⎯⎯⎯⎯⎯⎯⎯

16. Placed nurse call system in an accessible location within patient's reach. ⎯ ⎯ ⎯ ⎯⎯⎯⎯⎯⎯⎯

EVALUATION

1. Inspected appearance of wound and characteristics and amount of drainage. Measured wound size. ⎯ ⎯ ⎯ ⎯⎯⎯⎯⎯⎯⎯

2. Inspected condition of periwound areas. ⎯ ⎯ ⎯ ⎯⎯⎯⎯⎯⎯⎯

3. Asked patient to describe character of pain and rate severity of wound pain using scale of 0 to 10. ⎯ ⎯ ⎯ ⎯⎯⎯⎯⎯⎯⎯

4. Used Teach-Back technique. Revised instruction if patient or family caregiver was not able to teach back correctly. ⎯ ⎯ ⎯ ⎯⎯⎯⎯⎯⎯⎯

DOCUMENTATION

1. Documented appearance of wound, presence and characteristics of drainage, type of dressing applied, patient's response to dressing change, and level of comfort. ⎯ ⎯ ⎯ ⎯⎯⎯⎯⎯⎯⎯

2. Documented patient's and family caregiver's understanding through Teach-Back for effective application of dressing. ⎯ ⎯ ⎯ ⎯⎯⎯⎯⎯⎯⎯

HAND-OFF REPORTING

1. Reported any signs of infection, changes in skin integrity, or signs of pressure injury to the health care provider. ⎯ ⎯ ⎯ ⎯⎯⎯⎯⎯⎯⎯

Student _____ Date _____

Instructor _____ Date _____

PERFORMANCE CHECKLIST SKILL 40.4 **APPLYING A HYDROCOLLOID, HYDROGEL, FOAM, OR ALGINATE DRESSING**

	S	U	NP	Comments

ASSESSMENT

1. Identified patient using at least two identifiers, according to agency policy.

2. Reviewed patient's electronic health record (EHR), including health care provider's orders and nurses' notes for frequency and type of dressing change.

3. Reviewed EHR to determine patient's age and history of dehydration, malnutrition, exposure to radiation therapy, underlying chronic conditions, edema of the skin, and the presence of erythema, blistering, excoriation, or erosion of skin or a rash under or adjacent to adhesive's securing dressing.

4. Reviewed patient's EHR, including health care provider's orders and nurses' notes, for frequency and type of dressing change. Noted possible need to use customized shape or size of dressing to fit difficult body parts.

5. Assessed patient's/family caregiver's health literacy.

6. Assessed for presence of allergies, especially antiseptics, tape, or latex. Had patient describe allergic response.

7. Asked patient to describe character of wound pain and to then rate severity of pain using scale of 0 to 10. Administered prescribed analgesic as needed 30 minutes before dressing change.

8. Performed hand hygiene and applied clean gloves. Inspected location, size, and condition of wound. Removed and disposed of gloves and performed hand hygiene.

9. Assessed patient's knowledge and prior experience with dressings, and feelings about procedure.

PLANNING

1. Determined expected outcomes following completion of procedure.

	S	U	NP	Comments

2. Provided privacy and explained procedure. ___ ___ ___ _____

3. Performed hand hygiene. Organized and set up any equipment needed to perform procedure at bedside. ___ ___ ___ _____

4. Placed biohazard bag within reach of work area. Folded top of bag to make a cuff. ___ ___ ___ _____

5. Positioned patient comfortably and draped to expose only wound site. Instructed patient not to touch wound or sterile supplies. ___ ___ ___ _____

IMPLEMENTATION

1. Performed hand hygiene and applied clean gloves. Applied appropriate PPE as needed if there was a risk for splashing. ___ ___ ___ _____

2. Draped patient and exposed wound site. Instructed patient not to touch wound or sterile supplies. ___ ___ ___ _____

3. Using nondominant hand, gently removed tape, bandages, or ties of existing dressing. Pulled tape parallel to skin and toward dressing. If dressing was over hairy areas, removed tape in direction of hair growth and got patient's permission to clip or shave area before applying new dressing (checked agency policy). Removed any adhesive from skin. ___ ___ ___ _____

4. With gloved hand or forceps, removed old dressing one layer at a time. Noted amount and character of drainage. Used caution to avoid tension on any drains. ___ ___ ___ _____

5. Folded dressings with drainage contained inside and removed gloves inside out. With small dressings, removed gloves inside out to enclose dressing. Disposed of gloves and soiled dressing according to agency policy. Covered wound lightly with a sterile 4 × 4-inch gauze pad. Performed hand hygiene. ___ ___ ___ _____

6. Prepared sterile field with sterile dressing kit or individually wrapped sterile supplies on over-bed table. Poured prescribed solution into sterile bowl. ___ ___ ___ _____

7. Removed gauze cover over wound. ___ ___ ___ _____

8. Cleaned wound: ___ ___ ___ _____

   a. Applied clean gloves. Sterile gloves optional, per agency policy. Used 4 × 4-inch gauze cotton ball moistened in saline or an antiseptic swab (per health care provider order) for each cleaning stroke. Option: Sprayed wound surface with wound cleaner. ___ ___ ___ _____

	S	U	NP	Comments

b. Cleaned in direction from least contaminated to most contaminated.

c. Cleaned around any drain using circular stroke starting near drain and moving outward away from insertion site.

9. Used sterile dry gauze to blot dry wound bed and on skin around wound using same direction as Steps 8b and c.

10. Inspected appearance and condition of wound. Measured wound size and depth.

11. Removed and disposed of gloves and performed hand hygiene. Applied clean gloves. Sterile gloves optional, per agency policy.

12. Applied dressing (per manufacturer directions).

a. Hydrocolloid dressings:

(1) Selected proper size wafer, allowing dressing to extend onto intact periwound skin at least 2.5 cm (1 inch).

(2) Applied skin barrier wipe to surrounding skin that would come in contact with any adhesive or gel.

(3) For deep wound, applied hydrocolloid granules, impregnated gauze, or paste before the wafer.

(4) Removed paper backing from adhesive side and placed over wound. Did not stretch and avoided wrinkles or tenting. Held dressing in place for 30 to 60 seconds after application.

(5) If cut from larger piece, taped edges with nonallergenic tape to avoid rolling or adherence to clothing.

b. Hydrogel dressings:

(1) Applied skin barrier wipe to surrounding skin that would come in contact with any adhesive or gel.

(2) Applied gel or gel-impregnated gauze directly into wound, spreading evenly over wound bed. Filled wound cavity with gel about one-third to one-half full or packed gauze loosely, including any undermined or tunneled areas. Covered with moisture-retentive dressing or hydrocolloid wafer.

684

	S	U	NP	Comments

(3) Cut hydrogel sheet containing glycerin so that it extended 2.5 cm (1 inch) out onto intact periwound skin. Covered with secondary moisture-retentive dressing if needed.   ___ ___ ___ _____

(4) Secured dressing with nonallergenic tape if secondary dressing was not self-adhering.   ___ ___ ___ _____

  c. Foam dressings:

(1) Displayed understanding of removal and application characteristics of specific brand of foam dressing.   ___ ___ ___ _____

(2) Applied skin barrier wipe to surrounding skin that would come in contact with thin foam dressing adhesive.   ___ ___ ___ _____

(3) Cut foam sheet to extend 2.5 cm (1 inch) out onto intact periwound skin. (Verified which side of foam dressing should be placed toward wound bed and which side should be facing away from it; checked product instructions.)   ___ ___ ___ _____

(4) Cut foam to fit around drain or tube.   ___ ___ ___ _____

(5) Covered with secondary dressing, such as loose gauze, as needed.   ___ ___ ___ _____

  d. Alginate dressings:

(1) Cut sheet or rope to fit size of wound or loosely packed into wound space, filling one-half to two-thirds full.   ___ ___ ___ _____

(2) Applied secondary dressing, such as transparent film, foam, or hydrocolloid.   ___ ___ ___ _____

13. Labeled dressing with initials and date dressing changed.   ___ ___ ___ _____

14. Discarded soiled dressing materials properly. Removed gloves by pulling them inside out and then discarding into prepared bag. Performed hand hygiene.   ___ ___ ___ _____

15. Helped patient return to a comfortable position.   ___ ___ ___ _____

16. Raised side rails (as appropriate) and lowered bed to lowest position, locking into position.   ___ ___ ___ _____

17. Placed nurse call system was in an accessible location within patient's reach.   ___ ___ ___ _____

	S	U	NP	Comments

EVALUATION

1. Compared observations of the wound and periwound area with previous assessment and observed appearance of wound for healing. Measured size of wound; observed amount, color, and type of drainage; and observed presence of periwound erythema or swelling; and observed for signs associated with MARSI or MASD. Palpated around wound for tenderness.

2. Evaluated patient's level of comfort by having patient describe character of pain and rate severity on scale of 0 to 10.

3. Inspected condition of dressing at least every shift or as ordered.

4. Used Teach-Back technique. Revised instruction if patient or family caregiver was not able to teach back correctly.

DOCUMENTATION

1. Documented size and appearance of wound, characteristics of drainage, presence of necrotic tissue, type of dressings applied, patient's response to dressing change, and level of comfort.

2. Documented evaluation of patient learning.

HAND-OFF REPORTING

1. Reported location and condition of wound, type of dressings used, and any change in wound management.

2. Reported signs of infection, necrosis, or deteriorating wound status to health care provider immediately.

3. Reported any unexpected appearance of wound drainage, bright red bleeding, evidence of wound dehiscence or evisceration, and any change in exudate, odor, pain, or localized edema to health care provider.

686

Student _____ Date _____

Instructor _____ Date _____

PERFORMANCE CHECKLIST PROCEDURAL GUIDELINE 40.1   **APPLYING ROLLED GAUZE AND ELASTIC BANDAGES**

	S	U	NP	Comments

PROCEDURAL STEPS

1. Identified patient using at least two identifiers, according to agency policy.

2. Reviewed patient's electronic health record (EHR) for specific orders related to application of rolled gauze or elastic bandage. Noted area to be covered, type of bandage required, frequency of change, and previous response to treatment.

3. Assessed patient's/family caregiver's health literacy.

4. Assessed patient's level of comfort by asking patient to describe character of pain and rate severity on a pain scale of 0 to 10. Administered prescribed analgesic 30 minutes before dressing change as needed.

5. Performed hand hygiene. Assessed adequacy of circulation by palpating temperature of skin and pulses, presence of edema, and sensation (distal to area to be bandaged). Observed skin color and movement of body part to be wrapped.

6. Applied clean gloves. Inspected skin of area to be bandaged. Noted alterations in integrity such as presence of abrasion, blistering, discoloration, or chafing. Paid close attention to areas over bony prominences or under medical adhesive.

7. Inspected the condition of any wound for appearance, size, and presence and character of drainage, and ensured that it was covered with a proper dressing. If not, reapplied dressing (checked agency policy for type of gloves to use). Removed and disposed of gloves and performed hand hygiene.

8. Assessed for size of bandage:

    a. Rolled gauze or basic elastic bandage to secure a dressing: Assessed size of area to be covered. Each successive rolled gauze/elastic should have overlapped previous layer. Used smaller widths for upper extremities and larger widths for lower extremities.

	S	U	NP	Comments

b. Elastic bandage to provide simple compression: Assessed circumference of lower extremity before or shortly after patient got out of bed in the morning or after patient had been in bed for at least 15 minutes. Selected width that would cover and overlap without bulkiness.

9. Assessed patient's/family caregiver's knowledge, prior experience with bandaging, and feelings about procedure.

10. Performed hand hygiene. Gathered and organized supplies at bedside.

11. Provided privacy and explained procedure. Positioned patient comfortably in an anatomically correct supine position in bed.

12. Performed hand hygiene and applied clean gloves.

13. Applied gauze or elastic bandage to secure dressings:

a. Elevated dependent extremity for 15 minutes before applying elastic bandage to promote venous return.

b. Verified that primary dressing over wound was securely in place.

c. Began elastic bandage application at the distal body part. Held elastic bandage in dominant hand and used other hand to lightly hold beginning layer.

d. Applied even tension during application and began with two circular turns to anchor bandage. Continued to maintain even tension and transferred roll to dominant hand as nurse wrapped bandage.

e. Applied bandage from distal point toward proximal boundary, using appropriate turns to cover various body parts.

(1) Rolled gauze, overlapping each layer by one-half to two-thirds the width of the bandage.

(2) Used figure-eight dressing to cover joint. To apply overlap turns, alternated ascending and descending over bandaged part, each turn crossing the previous one to form a figure-eight pattern.

(3) Unrolled and slightly stretched bandage.

(4) Overlapped turns by one-half to two-thirds the width of bandage roll.

688

	S	U	NP	Comments

(5) Secured bandage with clip before applying additional rolls.

(6) Ended bandage with two circular turns; secured end of gauze or elastic bandage to outside layer of bandage, not skin, with tape or clips.

14. Applied elastic bandage over stump:

    a. Elevated stump with pillow or supported it with the help of another person.

    b. Secured bandage by wrapping it twice around proximal end of stump or person's waist (depending on size of stump).

    c. Made half-turn with bandage perpendicular to its edge.

    d. Brought body of bandage over distal end of stump.

    e. Continued to fold bandage over stump, wrapping from distal to proximal points.

    f. Secured with metal clips, self-gripping fastener if provided, or tape.

15. Removed and disposed of gloves if worn and performed hand hygiene.

16. Helped patient to comfortable position.

17. Raised side rails (as appropriate) and lowered bed to lowest position, locking into position.

18. Placed nurse call system in an accessible location within patient's reach.

19. Assessed degree of tightness of bandage, wrinkles, looseness, and presence of drainage.

20. Assessed distal extremity circulation when bandage application was complete, at least twice during next 8 hours, and then at least every shift.

    a. Observed skin color for pallor or cyanosis.

    b. Palpated skin for warmth.

    c. Palpated distal pulses and compared bilaterally.

    d. Asked patient to describe character of any pain and to rate severity on a pain scale of 0 to 10. Asked patient to note if any numbness, tingling, or other discomfort was present to evaluate for neurological and vascular changes.

21. Observed mobility of extremity as patient turned or repositioned.

	S	U	NP	Comments

22. Used Teach-Back technique. Revised instruction if patient or family caregiver was not able to teach back correctly.

    ___   ___   ___   _____

23. Documented patient's level of comfort, circulation status, type of bandage applied, presence of swelling, and range of motion at baseline and after bandage application on flow sheet in EHR.

    ___   ___   ___   _____

24. Reported any changes in neurological or circulatory status to health care provider.

    ___   ___   ___   _____

25. Hand-off reporting:

   a. Immediately reported any changes in circulatory status to health care provider and to nurse in charge.

   b. Reported any changes in wound or skin integrity to nurse in charge.

Student _____ Date _____

Instructor _____ Date _____

PERFORMANCE CHECKLIST PROCEDURAL GUIDELINE 40.2 **APPLYING AN ABDOMINAL BINDER**

	S	U	NP	Comments

PROCEDURAL STEPS

1. Identified patient using at least two identifiers, according to agency policy.

2. Reviewed electronic health record (EHR) for order for binder, per agency policy.

3. Reviewed EHR and nurses' notes to identify data regarding size of patient, and appropriate binder to use to ensure proper fit (saw manufacturer's guidelines).

4. Assessed patient's/family caregiver's health literacy.

5. Observed patient who needed support of thorax or abdomen; observed ability to breathe deeply, cough effectively, and turn or move independently.

6. Performed hand hygiene and applied clean gloves. Inspected skin for actual or potential alterations in integrity. Observed for irritation, abrasion, and skin surfaces that come in contact with the binder.

7. Inspected any surgical dressing for intactness, presence of drainage, and coverage of incision. Changed any soiled dressing before applying binder (using clean gloves). Disposed of soiled dressings in appropriate container, removed and disposed of gloves, and performed hand hygiene.

8. Determined patient's level of comfort by assessing character of pain and measuring acuity on a pain scale of 0 to 10.

9. Assessed patient's knowledge of purpose of binder, previous experience, and feelings about procedure.

10. Provided privacy and explained procedure to patient. Prepared supplies at bedside.

11. Performed hand hygiene and applied clean gloves.

	S	U	NP	Comments

12. Applied abdominal binder:

   a. Positioned patient in supine position with head slightly elevated and knees slightly flexed.

   b. Helped patient roll on side away from nurse toward raised side rail while firmly supporting abdominal incision and dressing with hands. Fan-folded far side of binder toward midline of binder.

   c. Placed binder flat on bed, right side up. Fan-folded far side of binder toward midline of binder.

   d. Placed fan-folded ends of binder under patient.

   e. Instructed or assisted patient to roll over folded binder. For overweight patients, has a second nurse or AP assist.

   f. Unfolded and stretched ends out smoothly on far side of bed. Then, stretched out ends on near side of bed.

   g. Instructed patient to roll back into supine position.

   h. Adjusted binder so that supine patient was centered over binder, using symphysis pubis and costal margins as lower and upper landmarks.

   i. If patient was very thin, padded iliac prominences with gauze bandage.

   j. Closed binder. Pulled one end of binder over center of patient's abdomen. While maintaining tension on that end of binder, pulled opposite end of binder over center and secured with Velcro closure tabs or metal fasteners. This provided continuous wound support and comfort.

13. Assessed patient's comfort level and adjusted binder as needed. Asked patient to describe character of pain and rate severity on a pain scale of 0 to 10.

14. Removed and disposed of gloves and performed hand hygiene.

15. Helped patient to a comfortable position. Raised rails (as appropriate), and lowered bed to lowest position, locking into position.

16. Placed nurse call system in an accessible location within patient's reach.

	S	U	NP	Comments

17. Removed binder and surgical dressing to assess skin and wound characteristics at least every 8 hours.

    —— —— —— ————————————

18. Evaluated patient's ability to ventilate properly, including deep breathing and coughing, every 4 hours to determine presence of impaired ventilation and potential pulmonary complications.

    —— —— —— ————————————

19. Used Teach-Back. Revised instruction if patient/family caregiver was not able to teach back correctly.

20. Documented baseline and post binder condition of skin and wound, integrity of underlying dressing, and patient's comfort level in the EHR.

    —— —— —— ————————————

21. Hand-off reporting: Reported any complications to nurse in charge.

22. Report reduced ventilation to health care provider immediately.

    —— —— —— ————————————

Student _____ Date _____

Instructor _____ Date _____

PERFORMANCE CHECKLIST SKILL 41.1 **HOME ENVIRONMENT ASSESSMENT AND SAFETY**

	S	U	NP	Comments

ASSESSMENT

1. Identified client using at least two identifiers according to agency policy.

2. Assessed client's and family caregiver's health literacy level and knowledge of safety risks.

3. Reviewed risk factors that predispose clients to accidents within the home (shared these with client and family caregiver during assessment).

4. Instructed client who had a near fall or actual fall to maintain a fall diary.

5. Determined if client had fear of falling using the Falls Efficacy Scale (FES-1) or the Activities-specific Balance Confidence (ABC) scale.

6. Shared with client and family caregiver any risk factors identified in initial assessment and how they affect mobility in the home.

7. Partnered with client and family caregivers to conduct home safety assessment.

   a. Assessed front and back entrances.

   b. Assessed kitchen.

   c. Assessed bathroom.

   d. Assessed bedroom.

   e. Assessed living room/family room.

   f. Assessed areas around the house.

   g. Assessed general fire safety.

   h. Assessed general electrical safety.

   i. Assessed carbon monoxide prevention.

8. Assessed client's financial resources; determined monthly income used for ongoing expenses.

9. Assessed client's and family caregiver's willingness to make changes. Determined how important functional independence was for client.

10. Assessed the client's goals or preferences for how suggested home modifications would be implemented. Assessed family caregiver's perceptions as well.

694

	S	U	NP	Comments

PLANNING

1. Determined expected outcomes following completion of procedure.   ___ ___ ___ _____

2. Prioritized with client and family caregiver environmental barriers that posed the greatest risk.   ___ ___ ___ _____

3. Recommended calling in reliable contractor if major home repairs were necessary and acceptable to client and family.   ___ ___ ___ _____

IMPLEMENTATION

1. General home safety: ___ ___ ___ _____

   a. Provided direct light source in areas where client reads, cooks, uses tools, or conducts hobby work.   ___ ___ ___ _____

   b. Considered satin and non-glossy finishes for walls, cabinets, and countertops in kitchen. Had sheer curtains or adjustable shades in other living areas.   ___ ___ ___ _____

   c. Applied colored tape or paint to color code controls of stove, oven, dryer, toaster, and other appliances.   ___ ___ ___ _____

   d. Considered installing rotating tray or pull-out drawers with glide mechanisms in kitchen cabinets. Installed C-ring handles in lower cabinets.   ___ ___ ___ _____

   e. Installed automatic door openers, level doorknob handles, and hook-and-chain locks.   ___ ___ ___ _____

2. Fall prevention steps:

   a. Painted edges of concrete stairs bright yellow, orange, or white.   ___ ___ ___ _____

   b. Installed treads with uniform depth of 22.5 cm (9 inches) and 22.5-cm (9-inch) risers (vertical face of steps).   ___ ___ ___ _____

   c. Rearranged furniture to open up space through hallways and major rooms.   ___ ___ ___ _____

   d. Reduced clutter within living areas.   ___ ___ ___ _____

   e. Secured all carpeting, mats, and tile; placed nonskid backing under small rugs and doormats. Removed throw rugs/mats in nonessential (dry) areas.   ___ ___ ___ _____

   f. Padded floor and used specialized tile that absorbs impact of falls.   ___ ___ ___ _____

   g. Used low-rise beds, futon beds, or mattress on floor if not contraindicated.   ___ ___ ___ _____

	S	U	NP	Comments

h. Had enough electrical outlets installed to be able to plug light or electronic device into nearby outlet. Secured electrical cords against baseboards.   ___ ___ ___ _____

i. Installed nonskid strips on surface of bathtub and/or shower stall. Ensured that floor was clean and dry.   ___ ___ ___ _____

j. Had grab bar installed in studs at tub, toilet, and/or shower. Had client select vertical or horizontal placement if choice was available. Ensured that bar was different color than wall and easy to see.   ___ ___ ___ _____

k. Had handrails installed along side of any stairway. Ensured that stairways were well lit, with switches at top and bottom of steps.   ___ ___ ___ _____

l. Installed appropriate broad-beam lighting for outside walkways.   ___ ___ ___ _____

m. Kept lighted phone easily accessible, next to client's bed.   ___ ___ ___ _____

n. Installed motion-sensor exterior lighting for walkways/driveway.   ___ ___ ___ _____

o. Offered option for client to use padding or types of clothing that would cushion bony prominences.   ___ ___ ___ _____

3. Prevention of food borne illness:

a. Taught client and family caregiver cleaning practices to prevent the spread of infection.   ___ ___ ___ _____

b. Instructed client not to share eating and drinking utensils.   ___ ___ ___ _____

c. Instructed client to clean appliances and surfaces daily.   ___ ___ ___ _____

d. Instructed client in safe food preparation and storage. Referred to guidelines in https://www.cdc.gov/foodsafety/.   ___ ___ ___ _____

4. Fire safety:

a. Had smoke detectors installed near each bedroom, in kitchen, and in home basement. Ensured that detector was on each floor of home.   ___ ___ ___ _____

b. Had client select fire extinguisher that was easy to handle and manipulate. Asked client to read instructions and demonstrate its proper use.   ___ ___ ___ _____

c. Had area around furnace cleared of any flammable items.   ___ ___ ___ _____

	S	U	NP	Comments

d. Instructed client to be sure that portable space heater had a thermostat, overheat protection, and auto shutoff and that equipment housing and electrical cords were intact. ____ ____ ____ _____

e. Had client make appointments for maintenance of furnace and chimney cleaning in appropriate season. ____ ____ ____ _____

f. Had client check light-bulb wattage in all fixtures. ____ ____ ____ _____

g. Had client establish routine during cooking that kept client in kitchen. Ensured that cooking range was clean and that items such as potholders and towels were away from burners. ____ ____ ____ _____

h. If client was a smoker, reviewed need to keep ashtrays clean and emptied. ____ ____ ____ _____

i. Strongly discouraged smoking in bed, smoking in chair when there was possibility of falling asleep, smoking near oxygen source, and smoking after taking medication that diminished alertness. Instructed client/family caregiver to put cigarette or cigar out all the way at first sign of feeling drowsy ____ ____ ____ _____

j. Warned clients to not charge e-cigarettes with phone or tablet charger; not to charge an e-cigarette overnight; to store loose batteries in a case. ____ ____ ____ _____

k. Recommended that client install power strips or surge protectors for plugging in multiple appliances/devices. ____ ____ ____ _____

5. Burn safety:

a. If children or elderly lived in the home, set hot water heater thermostat at 48.8° C (120°F). If immunocompromised persons lived in the home, set hot water heater thermostat at 60° C (140°F). ____ ____ ____ _____

b. Instructed client to always turn cold water on first. ____ ____ ____ _____

c. Installed touch pads on lamps. ____ ____ ____ _____

d. Used color codes of red for hot and blue for cold on water faucets. (If client had difficulty distinguishing those colors, chose two that were easily distinguished.) ____ ____ ____ _____

6. Carbon monoxide safety:

a. Had condition of furnace venting checked annually just before turning on furnace. ____ ____ ____ _____

b. Cautioned clients against using gas stove or barbecue grill for heating inside home. ____ ____ ____ _____

	S	U	NP	Comments

c. Had battery-operated carbon monoxide detector installed in home; checked or replaced battery when changing clocks in fall and spring. ___ ___ ___ _____

7. Firearm safety:

a. Taught client about dangers associated with keeping guns in home. ___ ___ ___ _____

b. If guns were in home, taught client how to safely store a firearm, to install trigger locks, and to store guns unloaded in locked cabinet. Taught client to store ammunition in secured area separate from guns. Stored keys in place inaccessible to children. ___ ___ ___ _____

EVALUATION

1. Had client and family caregiver(s) identify safety risks revealed in home safety assessment. ___ ___ ___ _____

2. During follow-up visit or call, asked client to discuss plans for making any modifications and observed changes client had implemented. ___ ___ ___ _____

3. During follow-up visits or calls, asked if client had experienced any falls or other injuries within home. ___ ___ ___ _____

4. During subsequent home visits, reassessed for progression of dementia if applicable. ___ ___ ___ _____

5. Used Teach-Back technique. Revised instruction if client or family caregiver were not able to teach back correctly. ___ ___ ___ _____

DOCUMENTATION

1. Retained copy of home safety assessment in client's home care record. ___ ___ ___ _____

2. Documented any instruction provided, client's and family caregiver's response, and changes made within environment. ___ ___ ___ _____

Student _____ Date _____

Instructor _____ Date _____

PERFORMANCE CHECKLIST SKILL 41.2 **ADAPTING THE HOME SETTING FOR CLIENTS WITH COGNITIVE DEFICITS**

	S	U	NP	Comments

ASSESSMENT

1. Identified client using at least two identifiers. ___ ___ ___ _____

2. Assessed client over several short periods of time and was ready to adapt assessment if client had sensory disabilities. If client did not speak English, had a professional interpreter assist. ___ ___ ___ _____

3. Assessed client's/family caregiver's health literacy and knowledge of adapting the home environment. ___ ___ ___ _____

4. Determined if client had family caregiver who helped with self-care or home-management responsibilities. ___ ___ ___ _____

5. Ensured that meeting room was well lit with minimal outside noises or interruptions. Listened carefully and spoke clearly and in normal tone of voice. ___ ___ ___ _____

6. Asked client to describe own level of health and describe how it affected ability to perform ADLs and IADLs. Asked family caregiver (if available) to confirm description. Screened for risky behaviors. ___ ___ ___ _____

7. Asked how client was handling home-management responsibilities. ___ ___ ___ _____

8. Assessed client's medication history and adherence to taking medications. Reviewed number and type of medications prescribed compared with those being taken, client's understanding of purpose as prescribed or as chosen for over-the-counter (OTC) medications, time of day taken, and dosages. Conducted pill count over course of a week (had family caregiver help as needed). Assessed where client stored medications. Gave special attention to pain medications, anticonvulsants, antihypertensives (especially beta-adrenergic blockers), diuretics, digoxin, aspirin, and anticoagulants. ___ ___ ___ _____

9. During discussion, observed client's dress, non-verbal expressions, appearance, and cleanliness. ___ ___ ___ _____

10. Observed immediate home environment. ___ ___ ___ _____

	S	U	NP	Comments

11. If a cognitive or mental status change was suspected:

   a. Completed Mini-Mental State Examination (MMSE) or the Mini-Cog for dementia.

   b. Completed Geriatric Depression Scale Short Form (GDS-SF) for depression.

   c. When client demonstrated signs of dementia, conducted a Home Safety Inventory (HSI).

12. If risk for wandering was suspected or evidence of wandering was present, observed for following behaviors (and/or asked family caregivers to provide information as well):

- Repeated shadowing or seeking whereabouts of family caregiver
- Wanting "to go home" even when at home.
- Inability to locate familiar places (bathroom, kitchen) or getting lost in familiar settings
- Going into unauthorized or private places
- Searching for "missing" people or places
- Walking with no apparent destination or purpose
- Haphazard or continuous moving, restless walking, or pacing
- Walking that cannot easily be redirected

13. Assessed whether the client was right- or left-handed.

14. Assessed which current environmental strategies family caregivers were using to deal with wandering and their effectiveness.

15. Assessed family caregiver for signs and symptoms of stress.

- Withdrawal from friends and family
- Loss of interest in activities previously enjoyed
- Feeling irritable, hopeless, and helpless
- Changes in appetite, weight, or both
- Changes in sleep patterns
- Getting sick more often
- Feelings of wanting to hurt self or the person for whom the individual is caring
- Emotional and physical exhaustion
- Irritability

700

	S	U	NP	Comments

PLANNING

1. Determined expected outcomes following completion of procedure.

2. If client had difficulty with self-care or fine-motor skills, referred family caregiver to OT, homemaker services, or respite care provider as appropriate.

3. Considered client's level of cognitive impairment when making changes in the living environment.

4. Determined best time of day for approaches that result in desired response.

IMPLEMENTATION

1. If client had difficulty remembering when to perform tasks, helped to create lists or post reminder notes in conspicuous location.

2. If client had difficulty remembering when to take medicines, involved family caregiver in finding best solutions: reinforcement with a reminder list or note, provided medication container organized by days of week, or recommended wristwatch with alarm or schedule of text messages to signal medication administration times.

3. When client had difficulty completing tasks such as writing checks for bills or bringing groceries into home from store, reduced steps to complete tasks. Consolidated steps or simplified tasks.

4. If client had difficulty bathing, dressing, writing, or feeding, offered assistive devices.

5. Helped client and family caregiver determine routine schedule for ADLs, such as eating, bathing, daily exercise, home cleaning, and napping. Had large calendar posted in conspicuous area to write in appointments or special planned events.

6. Instructed family caregiver to focus on client's abilities rather than disabilities. Used abilities in modifying approaches to perform daily activities.

7. Considered different activities the person could do to stay active. Matched the activities to what the person could do.

8. Had family caregiver help set up activities so client could complete tasks.

701

	S	U	NP	Comments

9. Discussed with client, family caregiver, pharmacist, and health care provider options for making medication self-administration safer including scheduling multiple medications: ___ ___ ___ _____

   a. Made sure client could read and understand the name of the medicine, as well as the directions on the container and on the color-coded warning stickers on the bottle. If a label was hard to read, asked pharmacist to use larger type. ___ ___ ___ _____

   b. Had medications that were likely to cause confusion prescribed to be given at bedtime. ___ ___ ___ _____

   c. Spaced antihypertensives and antiarrhythmics at different times to minimize side effects. ___ ___ ___ _____

   d. When possible, reduced number of pain medications used. ___ ___ ___ _____

   e. Had diuretics taken early in day and not at night. ___ ___ ___ _____

   f. Discussed with health care provider the possibility of taking medications at same time. ___ ___ ___ _____

   g. Discussed use of medication organizer and dispenser. ___ ___ ___ _____

10. Taught family caregiver how to use simple and direct communication: ___ ___ ___ _____

   a. Sat or stood in front of client in full view. ___ ___ ___ _____

   b. Faced client with hearing impairment while speaking; did not cover mouth and did not speak in a loud tone. ___ ___ ___ _____

   c. Used calm and relaxed approach. Respected personal space. ___ ___ ___ _____

   d. Used eye contact and touch. ___ ___ ___ _____

   e. Spoke slowly, in simple words and short sentences. ___ ___ ___ _____

   f. Reminded the person who nurse was if client didn't remember. Encouraged two-way conversation for as long as possible. ___ ___ ___ _____

   g. Used nonverbal gestures that complemented verbal messages. ___ ___ ___ _____

11. Placed clocks, calendars, and personal mementos throughout rooms within home. Enhanced environment with addition of tactile boards or three-dimensional art. ___ ___ ___ _____

12. Had family caregiver routinely orient client to who family caregiver was and which activities were going to be completed. ___ ___ ___ _____

13. Ensured that client had regular naps or rest periods during day. ___ ___ ___ _____

	S	U	NP	Comments

14. Had family caregiver encourage and support frequent visits by family and friends. Taught family caregiver how to use humor and reminiscences about favorite stories to promote social interaction. ___ ___ ___ _____

15. Provided safe place for person to wander. ___ ___ ___ _____

16. Recommended that family of wandering client install door locks or electronic guards. ___ ___ ___ _____

17. Created calm, safe setting that was appropriate for client's abilities. ___ ___ ___ _____

18. Regularly monitored client for personal comfort. ___ ___ ___ _____

19. Considered having client wear Global Positioning System (GPS) device to help manage location. Installed motion detector near exit site, with portable alarm that could accompany family caregiver. ___ ___ ___ _____

20. Collaborated with family caregiver to consider need for full-time care. ___ ___ ___ _____

EVALUATION

1. During follow-up visits, asked client to review home-management activities completed the morning of that day and previous day. ___ ___ ___ _____

2. Reviewed with client and family caregiver revised schedule for medication administration. ___ ___ ___ _____

3. Checked pill count that client/family caregiver maintained for a week. ___ ___ ___ _____

4. Asked family caregiver to describe ways that would increase client's success in completing home-management and self-care activities. ___ ___ ___ _____

5. Had family caregiver show schedules of daily routines and review specific approaches used. Observed environment for presence of reality orientation cues. ___ ___ ___ _____

6. Had family caregivers describe options for minimizing wandering. ___ ___ ___ _____

7. Had family caregivers report number of occurrences of wandering. ___ ___ ___ _____

8. Used Teach-Back technique. Revised instruction if family caregiver was not able to teach back correctly. ___ ___ ___ _____

DOCUMENTATION

1. Documented all assessment findings, including client's functional, cognitive, and mental status; availability of family caregiver; recommended interventions; and client's and family caregiver's response. ___ ___ ___ _____

REPORTING

1. Reported to health care provider any change in client's behavior that reflects a decline in cognitive or mental status. ___ ___ ___ _____

PERFORMANCE CHECKLIST SKILL 41.3   **MEDICATION AND MEDICAL DEVICE SAFETY**

	S	U	NP	Comments

ASSESSMENT

1. Identified client using at least two identifiers.

2. Assessed client's/family caregiver's health literacy and knowledge of medication and medication devices.

3. Assessed client's sensory, musculoskeletal, and neurological function, specifically hand strength, ability to read doses on syringe, ability to prepare medicine in a syringe, and ability to open medication container.

4. Determined if client had family caregiver who helped with self-care or home-management responsibilities. If family caregiver provided routine help, asked family caregiver if there were any concerns about being able to care for client.

5. Assessed client's medication regimen and length of time that client had been receiving each medication. Asked client to describe doses taken daily for each medication. Queried family caregiver if necessary.

6. Asked client to show where medications were stored in home. Looked at each container.

7. Assessed temperature of storage area.

8. Assessed client's daily schedule for medication administration. Asked client to describe schedule and whether there were any problems in following that schedule. Used family caregiver as resource, if appropriate.

9. If client self-administered injections, asked to see where client stored supplies and what was used to dispose of used syringes and needles.

10. If client used glucose-monitoring device, asked to see where monitor, lancets, and glucose strips were stored. Also asked about how client disposed of lancets.

PLANNING

1. Determined expected outcomes following completion of procedure.

	S	U	NP	Comments

IMPLEMENTATION

1. Taught client and family caregiver the following principles of safe medication use:

   a. Never take medicine prescribed for another person.

   b. Do not take any medicine more than 1 year old or after expiration date on container.

   c. Always keep medicines in original container.

   d. Always finish prescribed medication; do not save for future illness.

   e. Do not take medicine that has changed color, texture, or smell, even if it has not expired.

   f. Wash hands before and after administering/taking medication.

2. Recommended approaches for preparation of medications:

   a. For clients with weakened grasp or pain in hands and fingers, had local pharmacist place medications in screw-top container.

   b. For clients with visual alterations, had pharmacy type larger labels on all medication containers.

   c. For clients who were legally blind, had Braille labels placed on medication containers.

   d. For clients taking multiple medications, asked if they wished to try to introduce a color-coding system. Used same color for medications that client needed to take at same time. Marked tops of bottle caps with colored marking pen.

   e. Provided specially designed syringes with large numerals or syringe magnifier for clients with visual alterations.

   f. For clients who had difficulty manipulating syringes, offered spring-loaded needle insertion aid.

   g. Taught family caregivers how to properly draw up prescribed volume of medication into syringe. When necessary, had family caregiver prepare extra prefilled syringes for client's use when caregiver was absent.

	S	U	NP	Comments

3. Recommended approaches for safe medication and supply storage:

a. Store medications in safe, dry place, preferably in dresser drawer or a kitchen cabinet away from the stove, sink, and any hot appliances. *Option:* Store medicine in a storage box, on a shelf, or in a closet. ___ ___ ___ _____

b. Keep liquid medications and parenteral drugs, especially insulin, in cool place. ___ ___ ___ _____

c. Keep medical supplies, such as syringes, dressing supplies, and glucose meter, in airtight container and store in cool place such as bedroom closet. ___ ___ ___ _____

d. Instructed client and family caregiver to use new needle with each medication administration. ___ ___ ___ _____

4. Reviewed with client and family caregiver proper techniques for disposal of unused parts of medications or outdated medications properly using these guidelines: ___ ___ ___ _____

a. The best way to dispose of most types of old, unused, unwanted, or expired medicines (both prescription and over the counter) is to drop off the medicine at a medication take-back site, location, or program immediately. ___ ___ ___ _____

b. Do not flush unused medications. Certain medications should be flushed if medication take-back site is not available because of their abuse potential. Read the instructions on the medication and talk to a pharmacist or go to the FDA (2020) website for a list of medications that can be flushed. ___ ___ ___ _____

c. Many medicines, except those on the FDA flush list can be thrown into household trash. Follow these steps: ___ ___ ___ _____

(1) Remove the medications from their original containers and mix them with something undesirable, such as used coffee grounds, dirt, or cat litter. ___ ___ ___ _____

(2) Put the mixture in something you can close. ___ ___ ___ _____

(3) Throw the container in the garbage. ___ ___ ___ _____

(4) Scratch out or remove the label containing all personal information on the empty medicine packaging. Throw the packaging away. ___ ___ ___ _____

706

	S	U	NP	Comments

d. Check for approved state and local collection programs, or with area hazardous waste facilities. ___ ___ ___ _____

5. Reviewed with client and family caregiver proper techniques for disposal of sharps and disposable medical supplies: ___ ___ ___ _____

   a. Obtain sharps container from medical supply store or IV equipment supplier. (If finances are limited, have client use small-neck plastic bottle such as soda bottle.) Dispose of all needles and lancets in container. ___ ___ ___ _____

   b. Caution against filling sharps container to point where needles protrude out of opening. Discard when three-fourths full, securing top with duct tape or adhesive tape. ___ ___ ___ _____

   c. Store sharps container in area inaccessible to children. ___ ___ ___ _____

   d. Dispose of soiled dressings and use glucose testing reagent strips and IV tubing in separate, sealed, plastic garbage bag. Place in second plastic bag (double bagged) and discard appropriately as trash. ___ ___ ___ _____

   e. Consult local public health department or community authorities regarding proper way to dispose of waste. ___ ___ ___ _____

EVALUATION

1. Had client and/or family caregiver describe steps to take to ensure that medications were safe to use. ___ ___ ___ _____

2. Observed client and/or caregiver prepare and administer medication dose. ___ ___ ___ _____

3. Observed home setting for location of medications and supplies. ___ ___ ___ _____

4. Had client describe how sharps or medical equipment were discarded. ___ ___ ___ _____

5. Performed pill counts (pills remaining in containers) at successive intervals such as twice a week for 2 weeks. ___ ___ ___ _____

6. Used Teach-Back technique. Revised instruction if patient or family caregiver were not able to teach back correctly. ___ ___ ___ _____

DOCUMENTATION

1. Documented assessment findings, instructions, and recommendations to client and family caregiver and results of return demonstrations. ___ ___ ___ _____

REPORTING

1. Reported to health care provider any unsafe situation found within the home. ___ ___ ___ _____

Student _____ Date _____

Instructor _____ Date _____

PERFORMANCE CHECKLIST SKILL 42.1   **TEACHING CLIENTS TO MEASURE BODY TEMPERATURE**

	S	U	NP	Comments

ASSESSMENT

1. Identified client using at least two identifiers.

2. Assessed client's electronic health record (EHR) including health care provider's orders and nurses' notes. Noted previous teaching sessions (if any) about body temperature measurement and client's/ family caregiver's response to teaching.

3. Assessed client's/family caregiver's health literacy.

4. Assessed client's/family caregiver's ability to manipulate and read thermometer. Had client put on eyeglasses if necessary.

5. Assessed client's/family caregiver's knowledge of normal temperature range for client, symptoms of fever and hypothermia, and client's risk for body temperature alterations.

6. Assessed client's/family caregiver's ability to determine appropriate type of thermometer to be used in varying situations.

7. Assessed client's/family caregiver's learning readiness and ability to concentrate; considered presence of pain, nausea, or fatigue and client's interest in instruction.

8. Assessed client's/family caregiver's goals or preferences for how skill was to be performed or what was expected.

9. Assessed knowledge and experience of client's/ family caregiver's skill to be performed and feelings about procedure.

PLANNING

1. Determined expected outcomes following completion of procedure.

2. Selected setting in home where client was most likely to measure temperature and was a good location for teaching session:

   a. Selected room that was well lit with comfortable seating.

	S	U	NP	Comments

b. Provided privacy and prepared and organized equipment

c. Ensured that client was close and could see nurse clearly.

d. Controlled sources of noise and distractions (asked if children could be taken to another room; pets taken outside; audio noises turned off).

3. Discussed with client/family caregiver normal temperature ranges for client and demonstrated how to measure body temperature.

IMPLEMENTATION

1. Demonstrated steps of thermometer preparation, insertion, and reading. Provided rationale for steps to client/family caregiver.

a. Instructed client to take oral temperature 20–30 minutes after smoking or ingesting hot or cold liquids or foods and to wait at least an hour after hot bath or vigorous exercise. Explained indications for selecting temperature site other than oral.

b. Performed hand hygiene (applied gloves if needed). Instructed family caregiver to wear clean, disposable gloves if in contact with body fluids.

c. Taught client/family caregiver proper way to position client for temperature measurement.

d. Demonstrated temperature measurement technique and had client/family caregiver perform each step with guidance. Did not rush the client.

e. Explained any special precautions in using thermometers: oral thermometer must be placed in sublingual pocket; rectal thermometers must be lubricated with water-soluble lubricant; use rectal thermometer only for measuring rectal temperatures; never force rectal thermometer into rectum.

f. Discussed typical time frame needed for each type of temperature to register (based on thermometer type) and how to take reading.

g. Taught proper method for removing, cleaning, and storing thermometer (when applicable) and selected suitable storage location.

h. Removed and disposed of gloves in appropriate receptacle and performed hand hygiene.

2. Discussed common symptoms of fever: warm, dry, flushed skin; feeling warm; chills; piloerection; malaise; and restlessness.

S   U   NP   Comments

3. Discussed common signs and symptoms of hypothermia: cool skin, uncontrolled shivering, loss of memory, and signs of poor judgment. Explained that people with inadequate home heating, older adults, or those unaware of potential dangers of cold conditions are at risk.

___ ___ ___ _____

4. Discussed importance of notifying health care provider when temperature elevations occur. Collaborated with health care provider on the range of acceptable temperature readings for the specific client and when notification should be done. Reviewed common therapies for temperature reduction that are safe to perform at home, including using antipyretics; exposing skin to air; reducing room temperature; increasing air circulation; applying cool, moist compresses to skin; and drinking fluids.

___ ___ ___ _____

5. Provided set of written guidelines for client's/family caregiver's reference at appropriate level of health literacy.

___ ___ ___ _____

6. Gave client/family caregiver paper or digital logbook to time and recorded temperature if frequent monitoring was required. Instructed client to use written record to report temperatures to health care provider.

___ ___ ___ _____

7. Helped client assume comfortable, safe position.

___ ___ ___ _____

8. Removed gloves if worn and disposed in appropriate receptacle. Performed hand hygiene.

___ ___ ___ _____

EVALUATION

1. Had client/family caregiver independently demonstrate technique for temperature measurement, including body placement and ability to read thermometer three separate times.

___ ___ ___ _____

2. Asked client/family caregiver to identify normal temperature range and influence of smoking and hot and cold liquids or foods on oral readings; discussed safety implications for temperature measurement.

___ ___ ___ _____

3. Had client/family caregiver describe common signs and symptoms of fever and hypothermia and methods for control.

___ ___ ___ _____

4. Watched client/family caregiver clean and store equipment.

___ ___ ___ _____

5. Watched client record temperature values and times in log. Reviewed client's log periodically to ensure that temperatures are being recorded correctly.

___ ___ ___ _____

6. Used Teach-Back. Revised instruction if client/family caregiver was not able to teach back correctly.

___ ___ ___ _____

710

	S	U	NP	Comments

DOCUMENTATION

1. Documented client's temperature and information taught and client's and family caregiver's return demonstration. ____ ____ ____ _____

HAND-OFF REPORTING

1. Reported location of session, who participated, type of thermometer used, content discussed, client's and/or family caregiver's response to procedures, and evaluation of client learning. ____ ____ ____ _____

2. Reported to health care provider any high and low temperatures. ____ ____ ____ _____

Student _____ Date _____

Instructor _____ Date _____

PERFORMANCE CHECKLIST SKILL 42.2   **TEACHING BLOOD PRESSURE AND PULSE MEASUREMENT**

	S	U	NP	Comments

ASSESSMENT

1. Identified client using at least two identifiers.

2. Assessed client's electronic health record (EHR) including health care provider's orders and nurses' notes. Noted previous teaching sessions (if any) about BP and pulse measurement and client/family caregiver's response to teaching.

3. Assessed client's/family caregiver's health literacy.

4. Assessed client's/family caregiver's psychomotor function: visual (see dial and clock) and auditory (hear Korotkoff sounds) acuity, ability to manipulate BP monitoring equipment, and ability to feel pulse.

5. Assessed client's/family caregiver's knowledge of normal BP and pulse range for client and the symptoms of high or low readings. (Consulted with health care provider regarding normal range desired.)

6. Assessed client's/family caregiver's knowledge of what BP and pulse measure, specific medical issues that affect them, and why awareness of variations is important to client's health.

7. Assessed client's/family caregiver's learning readiness and ability to concentrate; considered presence of pain, nausea, or fatigue and client's interest in instruction.

8. Assessed home environment for favorable place to measure BP and pulse. Assessed the quality of home BP equipment.

9. Assessed client's/family caregiver's knowledge and experience in measuring blood pressure and pulse.

10. Assessed client's/family caregiver's goals or preferences for how skill was to be performed or what was expected.

PLANNING

1. Determined expected outcomes following completion of procedure.

712

	S	U	NP	Comments

2. Selected setting in home where client was most likely to measure temperature and was a good location for teaching sessions:

   a. Selected room that was well lit with comfortable setting.

   b. Provided privacy and prepared and organized equipment.

   c. Ensured that client was close and could see nurse clearly.

   d. Controlled sources of noise and distraction (asked if children could be taken to another room; pets taken outside; audio noises turned off).

3. Encouraged client/family caregiver to perform measurements on routine schedule for long-term monitoring plan.

4. Encouraged client to avoid exercise, caffeine, and smoking for 30 minutes before assessment to avoid inaccuracy. Recommended the client sit quietly without any distractions such as reading for 5 minutes before taking the measurement.

5. Prepared for client/family caregiver to perform measurement in comfortable position, with arm supported at heart level and feet flat on floor and in warm and quiet environment.

IMPLEMENTATION

1. BP measurement:

   a. Performed hand hygiene.

   b. Explained importance of having client sit quietly for 5 minutes with back supported and feet on floor before measurement. If client could not sit in this position, selected position that client could maintain. Separated repeat blood pressure readings by at least 1 minute.

   c. Discussed with client/family caregiver best sites for assessing BP. If client could not sit in this position, selected position that client could maintain. Explained to avoid applying cuff to arm with intravenous (IV) catheter with or without fluids infusing; arteriovenous shunt; breast or axillary surgery; and trauma, inflammation, or disease.

   d. Demonstrated steps for measuring BP.

      (1) Use of sphygmomanometer and stethoscope:

         (a) Taught palpating artery, positioning cuff, wrapping cuff, placing stethoscope, inflating and releasing cuff, and listening for Korotkoff sounds.

	S	U	NP	Comments

(b) Described sounds of measurement and relationship to observation of gauge during BP reading. Cautioned client/family caregiver about level and length of time appropriate for cuff inflation. ___ ___ ___ _____

(c) Taught client/family caregiver to routinely clean diaphragm and earpieces of stethoscope with rubbing alcohol or damp cloth between uses. ___ ___ ___ _____

(2) Use of electronic BP monitor:

(a) Taught correct placement of cuff and use of electronic equipment for proper cuff inflation (followed manufacturer's directions). ___ ___ ___ _____

2. Pulse measurement:

a. Discussed with client/family caregiver best sites for assessing pulse: radial and carotid. ___ ___ ___ _____

b. Reinforced need for the family caregiver's fingers to be warm enough to accurately assess the pulse. ___ ___ ___ _____

c. Demonstrated steps for palpating pulse: position of artery on wrist or neck, how to locate artery, using fingertips for palpation, compressing artery, palpating pulse before counting, counting pulse, and calculating pulse rate. ___ ___ ___ _____

(1) Instructed in use of gentle pressure; reinforced not to press hard over pulse site. ___ ___ ___ _____

(2) Instructed in use of watch or clock with second hand to count pulse. ___ ___ ___ _____

(3) Instructed to count for full 60 seconds, starting with second hand at 12-o'clock position. ___ ___ ___ _____

3. Educated client/family caregiver about normal desired BP and pulse ranges, purposes for monitoring, and when to take measurements. ___ ___ ___ _____

4. Described symptoms that indicate need to perform BP and/or pulse measurement. ___ ___ ___ _____

5. Had client/family caregiver attempt each step of skill on nurse or family member. ___ ___ ___ _____

6. Observed client/family caregiver demonstrate techniques to measure BP and pulse. When measuring BP, did not allow multiple repetitive BP attempts on any one limb. ___ ___ ___ _____

7. Taught client/family caregiver to monitor BP and pulse even if they remained in normal range. ___ ___ ___ _____

714

	S	U	NP	Comments

8. Provided client/family caregiver with printed instructions with written or pictorial guide or an electronic format for demonstration of procedure if possible.

9. Gave client/family caregiver log to record BP and pulse and time they were taken. In addition, client documented whether or not medications that affect BP or pulse were taken. Instructed client to bring written record to follow-up appointments to report readings to health care provider.

10. Instructed client/family caregiver in proper care of equipment.

11. Helped client assume comfortable and safe position.

12. Performed hand hygiene.

EVALUATION

1. Observed client/family caregiver demonstrate technique for BP and/or pulse measurement on at least three different occasions and verified that client added information to logbook correctly.

2. Asked client/family caregiver if readings were within desired range and when to report abnormal readings to health care provider.

3. Asked client/family caregiver to describe reason for BP and pulse monitoring and any related medications or treatment.

4. Had client/family caregiver demonstrate proper care of equipment.

5. Used Teach-Back. Revised instruction if client/family caregiver was not able to teach back correctly.

DOCUMENTATION

1. Documented BP and pulse and teaching, client and family caregiver responses, and demonstration.

HAND-OFF REPORTING

1. Reported location of teaching session for BP and pulse, who participated, equipment used, content discussed, and client's and/or family caregiver's response to procedure and evaluation of client learning.

2. Reported abnormal readings of BP and/or pulse to health care provider.

Student _____ Date _____

Instructor _____ Date _____

PERFORMANCE CHECKLIST SKILL 42.3 **TEACHING INTERMITTENT SELF-CATHETERIZATION**

	S	U	NP	Comments

ASSESSMENT

1. Identified client using at least two identifiers.

2. Assessed client's electronic health record (EHR) including health care provider's orders and nurses' notes. Noted if any previous teaching session on CISC was performed and client's/family caregiver's response to teaching.

3. Assessed client's/family caregiver's health literacy.

4. Asked client and checked EHR for history of allergies.

5. Performed hand hygiene. Assessed client's/family caregiver's knowledge about CISC and observed performance of CISC if client had performed previously. If family caregiver would perform CISC, had individual also perform hand hygiene and put on clean gloves.

6. Assessed client's/family caregiver's ability to manipulate and handle the catheter and reach the perineum.

7. Assessed client's/family caregiver's goals or preferences for how skill was to be performed or what was expected.

PLANNING

1. Determined expected outcomes following completion of procedure.

2. Helped client/family caregiver select catheter that was easiest to use, caused least amount of trauma, and was most comfortable.

3. Selected setting in home that client/family caregiver would most likely use when performing CISC and was a good place for teaching session.

4. Explained procedure to client/family caregiver.

5. Provided privacy. Organized and set up equipment needed to perform procedure.

716

	S	U	NP	Comments

IMPLEMENTATION

1. Had client/family caregiver perform appropriate hand hygiene using soap and water. If family caregiver was performing skill, instructed how to apply pair of disposable clean gloves. ___ ___ ___ _____

2. Performed hand hygiene. Helped client get into comfortable position. Positioned client in place that had adequate lighting. ___ ___ ___ _____

3. Taught client/family caregiver how to clean urethral meatus: ___ ___ ___ _____

   a. *For women:* Had client spread labia with one hand. Used other hand to clean urethral opening with a washcloth containing warm soapy water, and then used a clean moist washcloth to rinse. Had female clean in direction from urethral meatus toward rectum. If menses were present, had client/family caregiver cleanse the perineum using a different washcloth. Cleaned and dried before beginning inserting catheter. ___ ___ ___ _____

   b. *For men:* If client was not circumcised, taught him to retract foreskin to expose urethral meatus. Taught client to hold penis perpendicular to body with one hand, use other hand to clean urethral opening with a washcloth containing warm soapy water, and then use a clean moist washcloth to rinse. Had male clean in circular motion from meatus outward. ___ ___ ___ _____

4. Taught female client/family caregiver how to insert catheter: ___ ___ ___ _____

   a. Catheter selection depends on client preference; had client select catheter. ___ ___ ___ _____

   b. Using mirror, helped client locate meatus. Explained that it was just below clitoris and just above vaginal opening. ___ ___ ___ _____

   c. If an uncoated catheter was selected, had client lubricate tip of catheter with water-soluble jelly by rotating tip to spread lubricant around bottom 2.5–5 cm (1–2 inches) of catheter. ___ ___ ___ _____

   d. Placed outflow end of catheter into urine collection container or let hang over toilet bowl. Slowly and gently inserted tip of catheter 5–10 cm (2–4 inches) into meatus until urine began to flow. ___ ___ ___ _____

5. Taught male client/family caregiver how to insert catheter: ___ ___ ___ _____

   a. Catheter selection depends on client preference and other factors such as ability to learn the skill. ___ ___ ___ _____

	S	U	NP	Comments

b. Lubricated tip of uncoated catheter with water-soluble jelly by rotating tip to spread lubricant around bottom 13–18 cm (5–7 inches) of catheter.   _____ _____ _____ _____

c. Placed outflow end of catheter into urine collection container or let hang over toilet bowl. Slowly and gently inserted tip of catheter 15–20 cm (6–8 inches) into meatus until urine began to flow. For uncircumcised male, retracted foreskin before inserting catheter. Told client that catheter often needs to be inserted all the way for urine to begin to flow. Pulled foreskin back to normal position when catherization was complete.   _____ _____ _____ _____

6. Instructed client/family caregiver to hold catheter in place while urine flowed into container or toilet.   _____ _____ _____ _____

7. When urine stopped, slowly removed the catheter. Pinched the catheter end closed.   _____ _____ _____ _____

8. Discarded single-use catheters after self-catheterization was complete.   _____ _____ _____ _____

9. Helped client to assume comfortable position.   _____ _____ _____ _____

10. Removed and disposed of gloves. Performed hand hygiene.   _____ _____ _____ _____

11. Gave client log to record amount of urine if needed.   _____ _____ _____ _____

EVALUATION

1. Observed while client/family caregiver independently demonstrated technique for CISC.   _____ _____ _____ _____

2. Asked client to identify plan for timing of CISC and steps to take when problems arise.   _____ _____ _____ _____

3. Reviewed client's logbook and watched client enter information about urine output if indicated.   _____ _____ _____ _____

4. Used Teach-Back. Revised instruction if client/family caregiver was not able to teach back correctly.   _____ _____ _____ _____

DOCUMENTATION

1. Documented teaching, client and family caregiver responses, and demonstration.   _____ _____ _____ _____

2. Documented urine output in home care record and home documentation system.   _____ _____ _____ _____

HAND-OFF REPORTING

1. Reported signs and symptoms of UTIs and difficulty performing CISC to health care provider.   _____ _____ _____ _____

Student _____ Date _____

Instructor _____ Date _____

PERFORMANCE CHECKLIST SKILL 42.4   **USING HOME OXYGEN EQUIPMENT**

	S	U	NP	Comments
ASSESSMENT				
1. Identified clilent using at least two identifiers.	—	—	—	_____
2. Assessed client's electronic health record (EHR) including health care provider's orders and nurses' notes. Noted previous teaching sessions about home oxygen therapy and client's/family caregiver's response to teaching.	—	—	—	_____
3. Determined appropriate backup systems for compressor in event of power failure. Had spare oxygen tank available for emergency use.	—	—	—	_____
4. Assessed client's/family caregiver's health literacy.	—	—	—	_____
5. Completed a risk assessment that included assessment of client and household member(s) smoking status and other household risks of fire, trips, and falls.	—	—	—	_____
6. Assessed client's/family caregiver's knowledge and experience with home oxygen.	—	—	—	_____
7. Assessed client's/family caregiver's learning readiness and ability to concentrate; considered presence of pain, nausea, or fatigue and client's interest in instruction.	—	—	—	_____
8. Assessed client's/family caregiver's goals or preferences for how skill was to be performed or what was expected.	—	—	—	_____
PLANNING				
1. Determined expected outcomes following completion of procedure.	—	—	—	_____
2. Selected setting in home where client was most likely to use oxygen equipment and that was conducive to a teaching session:	—	—	—	_____
a. Selected a room that was well lit with comfortable seating.	—	—	—	_____
b. Ensured that client was close and could see nurse clearly.	—	—	—	_____
c. Controlled sources of noise and distractions.	—	—	—	_____
d. Provide privacy and prepare and organize equipment.	—	—	—	_____

719

		S	U	NP	Comments

IMPLEMENTATION

1. Taught client/family caregiver how to perform hand hygiene before handling oxygen equipment. ___ ___ ___ _____

2. Placed oxygen-delivery system in clutter-free environment that was well ventilated; away from walls, drapes, curtains, bedding, and combustible materials; and at least 2.4 meters (8 feet) from heat sources. ___ ___ ___ _____

3. Demonstrated steps for preparation and maintenance of oxygen therapy: ___ ___ ___ _____

   a. Compressed oxygen system:

      (1) Turned cylinder valve counterclockwise two to three turns with wrench. ___ ___ ___ _____

      (2) Checked cylinders by reading amount on pressure gauge. ___ ___ ___ _____

      (3) Stored wrench with oxygen tank or in another safe place near the tank. ___ ___ ___ _____

   b. Oxygen concentrator system:

      (1) Plugged concentrator into appropriate outlet. ___ ___ ___ _____

      (2) Turned on power switch. Alarm would sound for a few seconds. ___ ___ ___ _____

   c. Liquid oxygen system:

      (1) Checked liquid system by depressing button at lower right corner and reading dial on stationary oxygen reservoir or ambulatory tank. ___ ___ ___ _____

      (2) Collaborated with DME provider to provide instruction in refilling ambulatory tank when it becomes empty. ___ ___ ___ _____

      (3) To refill liquid oxygen tank:

         (a) Wiped both filling connectors with clean, dry, lint-free cloth. ___ ___ ___ _____

         (b) Turned off flow selector of ambulatory unit. ___ ___ ___ _____

         (c) Attached ambulatory unit to stationary reservoir by inserting female adapter from ambulatory tank into male adapter of stationary reservoir. ___ ___ ___ _____

         (d) Opened fill valve on ambulatory tank and applied firm pressure to top of stationary reservoir. Stayed with unit while it was filling. A loud hissing noise should have been heard. Tank should have filled in about 2 minutes. ___ ___ ___ _____

720

	S	U	NP	Comments

(e) Disconnected ambulatory unit from stationary reservoir when hissing noise changed and vapor cloud began to form from stationary unit. ___ ___ ___ _____

(f) Wiped both filling connectors with clean, dry, lint-free cloth. ___ ___ ___ _____

4. Connected oxygen-delivery device to oxygen-delivery system. ___ ___ ___ _____

5. Adjusted oxygen flow rate (L/min) to ordered rate. ___ ___ ___ _____

6. Had client/family caregiver apply oxygen-delivery device correctly. Ensured that client had two sets of oxygen-delivery devices and tubing. ___ ___ ___ _____

7. Instructed client and family caregiver not to change oxygen flow rate. ___ ___ ___ _____

8. Had client/family caregiver perform each step with guidance. Provided written material at appropriate health literacy level for reinforcement and review. ___ ___ ___ _____

9. Instructed client/family caregiver to notify health care provider if signs or symptoms of hypoxia occur. ___ ___ ___ _____

10. Discussed emergency plans for power loss, natural disaster, and acute respiratory distress. Had client/family caregiver call 9-1-1 and notify health care provider and home care agency. ___ ___ ___ _____

11. Instructed client and family caregiver in safe home oxygen practices, including placing "No Smoking/Oxygen in Use" signs at each entrance to home, not allowing smoking in house, keeping oxygen tanks 2.4 meters (8 feet) away from open flames, potential trip hazards of tubing and cylinders, and storing oxygen tanks upright. ___ ___ ___ _____

12. Helped client assume safe and comfortable position. ___ ___ ___ _____

13. Placed a bell or other type of sound-making device in a location within client's reach. ___ ___ ___ _____

14. Removed and disposed of any extraneous supplies. Performed hand hygiene. ___ ___ ___ _____

EVALUATION

1. Monitored rate at which oxygen was being delivered during each home visit. ___ ___ ___ _____

2. Asked client/family caregiver about ease of use or problems associated with home oxygen. ___ ___ ___ _____

	S	U	NP	Comments

3. Asked client/family caregiver to state safety guidelines, emergency precautions, and emergency plan.

    ____ ____ ____ _____

4. Used Teach-Back. Revised instruction if client/family caregiver was not able to teach back correctly.

    ____ ____ ____ _____

DOCUMENTATION

1. Documented teaching plan, information provided to client, and client's and family caregiver's ability to discuss information.

    ____ ____ ____ _____

2. Documented oxygen-delivery system, related supplies, and prescribed oxygen flow rate.

    ____ ____ ____ _____

HAND-OFF REPORTING

1. Reported reason for oxygen, type of equipment, contact information for supplier, safety measures in the home, client's or family caregiver's response to teaching, and evaluation of client or family caregiver leaning.

    ____ ____ ____ _____

2. Reported respiratory complications/concerns to health care providers involved in client's care.

    ____ ____ ____ _____

Student _____   Date _____

Instructor _____   Date _____

PERFORMANCE CHECKLIST SKILL 42.5   **TEACHING HOME TRACHEOSTOMY CARE AND SUCTIONING**

	S	U	NP	Comments
ASSESSMENT				
1. Identified client using at least two identifiers.	——	——	——	_____
2. Assessed client's electronic health record (EHR) including health care provider's orders and nurses' notes. Noted previous teaching sessions about tracheostomy care and suctioning and client's/family caregiver's response to teaching.	——	——	——	_____
3. Assessed client's/family caregiver's health literacy.	——	——	——	_____
4. Assessed client's/family caregiver's vision and fine motor function for ability to perform tracheostomy care and suctioning properly. Also assessed client's level of consciousness and ability to problem solve. Asked client/family caregiver to explain what to do for the following:	——	——	——	_____
a. Tracheostomy care: observed for excess intratracheal secretions, and soiled or damp tracheostomy dressing/ties.	——	——	——	_____
b. Suctioning: assessed client's perceived need for suctioning, presence of gurgling, wheezes on inspiration or expiration, restlessness, ineffective coughing, tachypnea, cyanosis, acutely decreased level of consciousness, tachycardia or bradycardia, acutely shallow respirations, or acute dyspnea.	——	——	——	_____
5. Assessed client's/family caregiver's ability to assess pulse rate and respirations.	——	——	——	_____
6. Assessed client's learning readiness and ability to concentrate; considered presence of pain, nausea, or fatigue and client's interest in instruction.	——	——	——	_____
7. Performed hand hygiene.	——	——	——	_____
8. Assessed client's/family caregiver's goals or preferences for how skill was to be performed or what client expected.	——	——	——	_____

	S	U	NP	Comments

PLANNING

1. Determined expected outcomes following completion of procedure. ___ ___ ___ _____

2. Selected setting in home in which client/family caregiver was most likely to perform tracheostomy tube care and that was conducive to teaching. ___ ___ ___ _____

   a. Selected room that was well lit with comfortable seating. ___ ___ ___ _____

   b. Ensured that client was close and could see nurse clearly. ___ ___ ___ _____

   c. Controlled sources of noise and distractions. ___ ___ ___ _____

   d. Provide privacy and prepare and organize equipment. ___ ___ ___ _____

3. Performed hand hygiene and applied clean gloves. ___ ___ ___ _____

4. Demonstrated to client and family caregiver how to organize and set up any equipment needed to perform procedure. ___ ___ ___ _____

5. Discussed and demonstrated with client/family caregiver proper position for procedure (high-Fowler position in front of mirror). ___ ___ ___ _____

IMPLEMENTATION

1. Suctioning:

   a. Verified health care provider's orders for suctioning. Ensured that client and family caregiver understood suctioning order. ___ ___ ___ _____

   b. Taught client/family caregiver techniques for hand hygiene and application of clean gloves. ___ ___ ___ _____

   c. Explained and demonstrated step-by-step preparation and completion of tracheostomy tube suctioning using either open or closed suctioning. ___ ___ ___ _____

   d. After client/family caregiver suctioned tracheostomy, taught how to suction nasal and oral pharynx and perform mouth care. Encouraged client/family caregiver to brush teeth with small soft toothbrush 2 times a day and use mouth moisturizer to moisturize lips every 2–4 hours. ___ ___ ___ _____

   e. At conclusion of procedure, had client take two to three deep breaths; reassessed status of breathing. ___ ___ ___ _____

   f. Demonstrated how to disconnect suction catheter and coil and discard catheter in appropriate receptacle. If catheter was to be cleaned and disinfected, set aside. Had client/family caregiver remove soiled gloves and dispose of in appropriate container; performed hand hygiene. ___ ___ ___ _____

724

	S	U	NP	Comments

2. Tracheostomy care:

a. Had client sit at table with mirror. Instructed client/family caregiver how to perform hand hygiene and apply clean gloves with nurse. Taught techniques for cleaning stoma and tracheostomy tube and changing tracheostomy ties and dressing. *Exception:* Cleaned inner cannula with approved cleaning solution such as hydrogen peroxide and small brush.

b. Had client/family caregiver remove and dispose of gloves. Performed hand hygiene.

c. Instructed client/family caregiver to apply clean gloves. Demonstrated technique for cleaning reusable supplies in warm soapy water. Rinsed thoroughly and dried between two layers of clean paper towels. Stored supplies in loosely closed clear plastic bag; labeled bag.

d. Had client/family caregiver remove and dispose of gloves. Performed hand hygiene.

3. Disinfecting supplies:

a. Explained procedure for disinfecting reusable supplies. To disinfect supplies, used one of following methods after performing hand hygiene and donning gloves:

(1) *Method 1:* Soaked reusable supplies that touched membranes in prepared solution of 3% hydrogen peroxide for 30 minutes.

(2) *Method 2:* Soaked reusable supplies that touched membranes in prepared solution of 70% isopropyl for 5 minutes. Rinsed usable supplies in saline or sterile saltwater.

(3) *Method 3:* Soaked reusable supplies that touched membranes in 1:50 prepared dilution of 5.25%–6.15% sodium hypochlorite (household bleach) for 5 minutes. Rinsed reusable supplies in saline or sterile saltwater.

4. Had client/family caregiver perform each step with guidance from nurse.

5. Helped client assume comfortable position.

6. Taught client/family caregiver signs and symptoms of the following:

a. Stoma infection

b. Respiratory tract infection

c. Transesophageal fistula

	S	U	NP	Comments

7. Placed a bell or other type of sound-making device in an accessible location within client's reach.   ___ ___ ___ _____

8. Removed and disposed of gloves. Performed hand hygiene.   ___ ___ ___ _____

EVALUATION

1. Observed as client/family caregiver demonstrated technique for tracheostomy tube care and suctioning.   ___ ___ ___ _____

2. Asked client/family caregiver to describe signs and symptoms indicating need for tracheostomy care and suctioning and the factors that influence tracheostomy airway functioning.   ___ ___ ___ _____

3. Had client and family caregiver explain the problems that need to be reported to their health care provider.   ___ ___ ___ _____

4. Asked client/family caregiver to describe how to clean and disinfect reusable supplies.   ___ ___ ___ _____

5. Used Teach-Back. Revised instruction if client/family caregiver was not able to teach back correctly.   ___ ___ ___ _____

DOCUMENTATION

1. Documented client instruction and client's and family caregiver's ability to demonstrate tracheostomy care, suctioning skills, and disinfecting skills.   ___ ___ ___ _____

2. Developed a system of documenting for client or family caregiver to describe appearance of trach and secretions, patient tolerance, and tracheostomy care provided.   ___ ___ ___ _____

HAND-OFF REPORTING

1. Reported location of tracheostomy teaching session, who participated, content discussed, client's and/or family caregiver's response to procedure, and evaluation of client learning.   ___ ___ ___ _____

2. Reported any unexpected outcomes or concerns, such as a hardened or reddened stoma, to health care providers involved in client's care.   ___ ___ ___ _____

PERFORMANCE CHECKLIST SKILL 42.6   **TEACHING MEDICATION SELF-ADMINISTRATION**

	S	U	NP	Comments

ASSESSMENT

1. Identified client using at least two identifiers.

2. Assessed client's electronic health record (EHR) including health care provider's orders and nurses' notes. Noted previous teaching sessions about medication self-administration and client's/family caregiver's response to teaching.

3. Assessed client's/family caregiver's health literacy.

4. Asked client and checked EHR for history of allergies. If client had allergies, checked with pharmacist if any of the prescribed medications could cause an allergic reaction.

5. Assessed client's/family caregiver's learning readiness and ability to concentrate (considered presence of pain, nausea, or fatigue and client interest in instruction) and learning style preference.

6. Assessed client's/family caregiver's belief in need for medication therapy. Considered prior experiences, ethnic values, religious beliefs, personal experiences with medications, and family caregivers' values about medications.

7. Assessed client's prescribed and over-the-counter (OTC) medications, including use of herbal supplements.

8. Ensured that family caregiver knew client's drug allergies and type of allergic response.

9. Consulted with health care provider to review medications that client was receiving and simplified regimen if possible.

10. Assessed client's/family caregiver's goals or preferences for how skill was to be performed or what client expected.

PLANNING

1. Determined expected outcomes following completion of procedure.

2. Selected setting in home in which client/family caregiver was likely to prepare and administer medications:

	S	U	NP	Comments

a. Selected room that was well lit and offered comfortable seating.

b. Ensured that client was close and could see nurse clearly.

c. Controlled sources of noise and distractions.

3. Prepared teaching materials:

   a. Planned approach that matched client's/family caregiver's learning preference (visual, auditory, reading/writing, kinesthetic):

     (1) Written materials were printed in large bold letters (set in 14-point or larger type)

     (2) DVD or Internet instructional programs

     (3) Illustrations of medication safety guidelines

     (4) Handling equipment and supplies

4. Considered mobile health (mHealth) applications delivered through smart phones or tablet devices.

5. Ensured that client was wearing glasses or hearing aids if needed during teaching session.

6. Arranged teaching time to allow participation of client with family caregivers.

IMPLEMENTATION

1. Instructed client/family caregiver about importance of performing hand hygiene before medication self-administration.

2. Presented information clearly and concisely:

   a. Faced learner in well-lit room.

   b. Used short sentences and spoke in slow, low-pitched voice.

   c. Provided descriptions in understandable terms.

   d. *Option:* Provided tables for explaining actions, side effects, or schedules; offered bar charts to show when medications reach peak effects.

3. Frequently paused during instruction so that client/family caregiver could ask questions and express understanding of content.

4. Instructed client/family caregiver on following content: purpose of regularly scheduled and prn (as needed) medications and their desired effects, how medication works and why it helps, dosage schedules and rationale, common side effects, what to do to relieve side effects, what to do if dose was missed, when to call health care provider with problems, whom to call with problems, medication safety guidelines, and implications when medications are not taken.

	S	U	NP	Comments

5. Instructed client/family caregiver in appropriate route of medication delivery. ____ ____ ____ _____

6. Provided frequent, short teaching sessions. Planned to have several teaching sessions, especially if client needed to take multiple medications. ____ ____ ____ _____

7. Provided teaching about OTC medications and herbal supplements. ____ ____ ____ _____

8. Provided client with written schedules or individualized instruction sheets for review. Offered special charts, diagrams, learning aids, written information, weekly pill organizers, and Internet/Intranet resources. ____ ____ ____ _____

9. Offered help as client practiced preparing medication. ____ ____ ____ _____

10. Had pharmacy provide clear, large-print labels for medication bottles and medication teaching handouts if appropriate. ____ ____ ____ _____

11. Had pharmacy provide containers that client could open independently if manual dexterity was limited. ____ ____ ____ _____

12. Facilitated arrangements for pharmacy to receive written prescriptions in timely fashion if required for dispensing. Arranged for pharmacy to deliver medications to home if client was unable to arrange for transportation to pharmacy. ____ ____ ____ _____

13. Discussed with client/family caregiver how to dispose of discontinued or expired medications. ____ ____ ____ _____

14. Helped client assume comfortable position. ____ ____ ____ _____

EVALUATION

1. Asked client/family caregiver to explain information about each drug: purpose; actions; routes; timing of medications and maximum frequency of use of either prescribed or OTC medications; side effects and interactions; and foods, herbals, or OTC medications to avoid. ____ ____ ____ _____

2. Asked client/family caregiver to describe when to call health care provider or refer to printed information for resources. ____ ____ ____ _____

3. Had client/family caregiver prepare and administer doses for all prescribed medications. ____ ____ ____ _____

4. Used Teach-Back. Revised instruction if client/family caregiver was not able to teach back correctly. ____ ____ ____ _____

DOCUMENTATION

1. Documented instruction provided and learning outcomes achieved by client and family caregiver. ____ ____ ____ _____

	S	U	NP	Comments

2. Developed a system of recording (client diary) for client or family caregiver to use to document adherence to dosage schedules and self-monitoring of any problems. ____ ____ ____ _____

3. Left a phone number and instructions about how to reach home care nurse if needed. ____ ____ ____ _____

HAND-OFF REPORTING

1. Reported location of session, who participated, content discussed, client's and/or family caregiver's response to procedure, and evaluation of client learning. ____ ____ ____ _____

Student _____ Date _____

Instructor _____ Date _____

PERFORMANCE CHECKLIST SKILL 42.7   **MANAGING FEEDING TUBES IN THE HOME**

	S	U	NP	Comments
ASSESSMENT				
1. Identified client using at least two identifiers.	___	___	___	_____
2. Assessed client's electronic health record (EHR) including health care provider's orders and nurses' notes. Noted previous teaching sessions about enteral feedings and client's/family caregiver's response to teaching.	___	___	___	_____
3. Assessed client's/family caregiver's health literacy.	___	___	___	_____
4. Assessed client's and family caregiver's physical (visual, fine motor) function. Also assessed emotional, financial, and community resources.	___	___	___	_____
5. Assessed environmental conditions of home (sanitation, storage of equipment, work area, supplies, and power source).	___	___	___	_____
6. Assessed client's/family caregiver's understanding of purpose of enteral feedings and positive expected outcomes.	___	___	___	_____
7. Assessed client's/family caregiver's understanding of storage and management of equipment and supplies as well as where and how to obtain supplies.	___	___	___	_____
8. Assessed client's learning readiness and ability to concentrate (considered presence of pain, nausea, or fatigue and client interest in instruction); and learning style preference.	___	___	___	_____
9. Performed hand hygiene.	___	___	___	_____
10. Observed client/family caregiver administer an enteral feeding (when previously ordered).	___	___	___	_____
11. Assessed client's/family caregiver's knowledge and experience in managing a feeding tube.	___	___	___	_____
12. Assessed client's/family caregiver's goals or preferences for how skill was to be performed or what was expected.	___	___	___	_____
PLANNING				
1. Determined expected outcomes following completion of procedure.	___	___	___	_____
2. Select setting in home in which client/family caregiver is likely to prepare and administer enteral feedings:	___	___	___	_____

	S	U	NP	Comments

a. Selected room that was well lit with comfortable seating.

b. Ensured that client was close and could see nurse clearly.

c. Controlled sources of noise and distractions.

3. Provided privacy and prepared and organized equipment and supplies.

IMPLEMENTATION

1. Performed hand hygiene. Instructed family caregiver to wear clean, disposable gloves.

2. Helped client/family caregiver determine feeding schedule that would maintain nutritional requirements, fit within client's or family's schedule, and fit health care provider's order.

3. Had client/family caregiver apply clean gloves with nurse. If a client had a nasoenteral tube, demonstrated how to identify placement of feeding tube: aspirating gastric fluid, checking pH of gastric fluid, and acceptable pH range.

4. Observed as client/family caregiver demonstrated how to check correct placement of nasally placed tube.

5. When client had a gastrostomy tube, watched client/family caregiver check for gastric residual volume by aspirating gastric contents.

6. Discussed use of medical asepsis in setting up and changing administration sets, mixing formulas (did not add formula to hanging bag), refrigerating unused formula, limiting amount of formula "hung" at one time to amount that could be infused in 4- to 6-hour period (less time in warmer weather), and maintaining and caring for bag.

7. Instructed client/family caregiver that client needed to sit up in chair or have head of bed elevated at least 30 degrees, preferably 45 degrees, while receiving feedings or medications or when tube was flushed.

8. Observed client/family caregiver mixing, administering, and storing formulas. Discussed flushing of tube after administration of feedings or medications.

9. Watched client/family caregiver change administration sets and clean bags. Had them dispose of supplies, remove and dispose of gloves, and perform hand hygiene.

732

	S	U	NP	Comments

10. Observed client/family caregiver administering medications and flushing tube.

11. Discussed and observed use of infusion pump if client was receiving continuous feeding.

12. Discussed measures to stabilize feeding tube in clients with abdominal tubes and to clean and protect skin insertion site.

13. Provided contact information for ordering equipment and supplies or whom to call in case of equipment failure.

14. Placed a bell or other type of sound-making device in an accessible location within client's reach.

15. Discussed emergency plan and actions to take for signs and symptoms of aspiration such as elevating head of bed, oral suctioning, and calling health care provider.

16. Discussed whom to contact and when for signs of diarrhea, constipation, or weight loss.

17. Removed and disposed of gloves. Performed hand hygiene.

EVALUATION

1. Asked client/family caregiver to state purpose of home enteral nutrition therapy, feeding schedule, and signs and symptoms of complications.

2. Observed client/family caregiver performing medical asepsis techniques, checking tube placement, aspirating residuals, administering medications and feedings, and using and cleaning equipment.

3. Asked client/family caregiver to state measures used to prevent complications.

4. Asked client/family caregiver how to care for open formula cans.

5. Used Teach-Back. Revised instruction if client/family caregiver was not able to teach back correctly.

DOCUMENTATION

1. Documented instructions given to client and family caregiver and their response.

2. Documented specifics of enteral feeding plan, including type and size of tube in home, formula, and amounts to be administered in specific time frames.

3. Had client or family caregivers record I&O, daily weights, amount of gastric fluid aspirated before each feeding (or every 4 hours if receiving continuous feeding), date and time of feedings, amount and type of formula, any additives, and date and time that administration sets were changed.

___   ___   ___   _____

HAND-OFF REPORTING

1. Reported reason for enteral feeding, type of tube and equipment, contact information for supplier, client's or family caregiver's response to teaching, and evaluation of client or family caregiver leaning.

___   ___   ___   _____

2. Reported complications and concerns to health care providers involved in client's care.

___   ___   ___   _____

734

Student _____ Date _____

Instructor _____ Date _____

PERFORMANCE CHECKLIST SKILL 42.8 **MANAGING PARENTERAL NUTRITION IN THE HOME**

	S	U	NP	Comments
ASSESSMENT				
1. Identified client using at least two identifiers.	___	___	___	_____
2. Assessed client's electronic health record (EHR) including health care provider's orders and nurses' notes. Noted any previous teaching sessions for parental nutrition and client's/family caregiver's response to teaching.	___	___	___	_____
3. Assessed client's/family caregiver's health literacy.	___	___	___	_____
4. Assessed client's fluid and electrolyte levels, serum albumin, total protein, transferrin, prealbumin, triglycerides, and glucose levels. Assessed body composition and consulted with registered dietitian nutritionist.	___	___	___	_____
5. Performed hand hygiene. Instructed family caregiver to apply clean gloves.	___	___	___	_____
6. Assessed client's venous access device for edema, drainage, tenderness, and signs of inflammation. Measured circumference of upper arm if client had peripherally inserted central catheter (PICC); marked place on arm where measurement was taken.	___	___	___	_____
7. Removed and disposed of gloves and performed hand hygiene.	___	___	___	_____
8. Verified health care provider's order for PN, including amino acids, dextrose, fat emulsions, vitamins, minerals, trace elements, electrolytes, and flow rate.	___	___	___	_____
9. Assessed client's learning readiness, anxiety and ability to concentrate (considered presence of pain, nausea, or fatigue and client interest in instruction), and learning style preference.	___	___	___	_____
10. Assessed client's/family caregiver's previous knowledge and experience in managing PN in home. Had client/family caregiver perform return demonstration if able to perform skill.	___	___	___	_____
11. Assessed client's/family caregiver's goals or preferences for how skill was to be performed or what was expected.	___	___	___	_____

735

	S	U	NP	Comments

PLANNING

1. Determined expected outcomes following completion of procedure.

2. Selected setting in home where client was most likely to administer PN and that was conducive to a teaching session.

   a. Selected room that was well lit with comfortable seating.

   b. Organized supplies.

   c. Ensured that client was close and could see nurse clearly.

   d. Controlled sources of noise and distractions.

   e. Explained procedure to client.

IMPLEMENTATION

1. Provided name and phone number of people or resources available 24 hours a day, 7 days a week in case problems arise.

2. Explained type/name of infusion, volume and infusion rate, expected outcomes, and components of PN. Explained that PN needs to be stored in refrigerator.

3. Had client/family caregiver perform each of the following steps with guidance from nurse. Did not rush client.

4. Instructed client/family caregiver to inspect the IV solution bag label, ensured that client's name was on label, ensured that solution had not expired, and checked bag for leaks.

5. Suggested taking PN solution out of refrigerator for 30–60 minutes before scheduled infusion time.

6. Explained need to inspect fluid in bag for color and precipitates.

7. Had client/family caregiver perform hand hygiene and apply clean gloves with the nurse. Demonstrated how to attach IV tubing to bag, how to attach filter to IV tubing (optional), how to prime IV tubing, and how to load IV tubing into electronic infusion pump.

8. Wiped CVC port with alcohol and showed how to flush CVC and connect IV tubing to port. Used needleless system whenever possible.

9. Explained how to determine appropriate rate of infusion and program infusion pump. Cautioned client and family caregiver against changing rate to "catch up."

736

	S	U	NP	Comments

10. Had client and family caregiver remove and dispose of gloves; performed hand hygiene.

11. When infusion was completed, explained and demonstrated how to disconnect IV tubing and flush CVC. Ensured that client/family caregiver performed hand hygiene before and after disconnecting line.

12. Described appropriate use and storage of infusion pump and supplies. Explained appropriate tubing replacement schedules.

13. Helped to develop plan for appropriate disposal of supplies, including needles, syringes, and unused medications or solutions, using principles of Standard Precautions.

14. Demonstrated appropriate care of CVC site; discussed how to change dressings, frequency of dressing changes, and signs of infection.

15. Taught client and/or family caregiver about signs and symptoms that indicate potential complications from PN therapy and when to call for help.

16. Demonstrated how to use a glucose monitor for testing and monitoring blood glucose. Explained frequency of testing, normal glucose values, and what to do if values fall outside of expected range.

17. Helped client to a comfortable position.

18. Placed a bell or other type of sound-making device in an accessible location within client's reach.

19. Removed and disposed of gloves. Performed hand hygiene.

20. Provided client with logbook to document administration of PN, weights, intake and output (I&O), and blood glucose levels.

21. Helped client develop plan to reorder supplies, PN fluid, and prescribed additives; for emergencies; and for home safety.

EVALUATION

1. Had client/family caregiver independently demonstrate initiation, infusion, and discontinuation of PN infusion and CVC site care.

2. Watched client/family caregiver clean and store PN, equipment, and supplies.

3. Asked client/family caregiver to identify expected outcomes of nutritional therapy.

	S	U	NP	Comments

4. Had client/family caregiver independently demonstrate blood glucose monitoring and documentation. ___ ___ ___ _____

5. Watched client/family caregiver document information in log. Reviewed client's/family caregiver's log periodically to ensure that information was being documented correctly. ___ ___ ___ _____

6. Used Teach-Back. Revised instruction if client/family caregiver was not able to teach back correctly. ___ ___ ___ _____

DOCUMENTATION

1. Documented information taught, client's and family caregiver's response, and outcomes of PN therapy in home care log. ___ ___ ___ _____

2. Documented appearance of CVC site, infusions, glucose monitoring results, client's weight in home care log. ___ ___ ___ _____

HAND-OFF REPORTING

1. Reported location of PN teaching session, who participated, content discussed, client's and/or family caregiver's response to PN procedure, and evaluation of client learning. ___ ___ ___ _____

2. Reported any signs and symptoms of complications from PN or CVC to healthcare providers involved in client's care. ___ ___ ___ _____